GLENCOE

Health

A Guide to Wellness

FOURTH EDITION

Mary Bronson Merki, Ph.D.

Don Merki, Ph.D.

Contributing Authors
Eddye Eubanks, Ph.D.
Gale Cornelia Flynn
Charlotte Sorrel

GLENCOE
Macmillan/McGraw-Hill

New York, New York   Columbus, Ohio   Mission Hills, California   Peoria, Illinois

CONTRIBUTING WRITERS

CONFLICT RESOLUTION

Jean M. Brainard, Ph.D.
Consulting Medical Anthropologist
Fredericktown, Ohio

CULTURALLY SPEAKING

Karen Muir, Ph.D.
Instructor
Columbus State Community College
Columbus, Ohio

HELP WANTED

Rich Smith, M.S.
Director of Guidance
Westerville North High School
Westerville, Ohio

PERFORMANCE ASSESSMENT

K. Michael Hibbard, Ph.D.
Assistant Superintendent
Pomperaug Regional School District 15
Middlebury, Connecticut

Susan E. Kurtain
Thinking Skills Teacher
Bleyl Junior High School
Houston, Texas

Send all inquiries to:
Glencoe/McGraw-Hill
936 Eastwind Drive
Westerville, Ohio 43081

ISBN: 0-02-652600-X (Student Text)
ISBN: 0-02-652602-6 (Teacher's Wraparound Edition)
Printed in the United States of America

5 6 7 8 9 10 VH/LP 00 99 98 97 96 95 94

X 21704

MENTAL HEALTH

Rodney Page
Health Teacher
McNeil High School
Austin, Texas

Roger F. Puza
Health Educator
Central High School
LaCrosse, Wisconsin

FAMILY AND SOCIAL HEALTH

Gayle S. Jenkins
Health Education Program Specialist
Wake County Public School System
Raleigh, North Carolina

George E. Serednesky, Ph.D.
Psychologist
Child and Adult Guidance Center
Columbus, Ohio

THE LIFE CYCLE

Charles Balling
Superintendent of Leisure Services
Elmhurst Park District
Elmhurst, Illinois

Michael E. Childers, Ph.D.
Health and Physical Education Teacher
Clifton Middle School
Houston, Texas

BODY SYSTEMS

Bernadette L. Norris
Health and Physical Education Teacher
Lake View High School
Chicago, Illinois

PERSONAL HEALTH and PHYSICAL FITNESS

Doug Monaghen
Coordinator of Health Education
Alief Independent School District
Alief, Texas

Tinker D. Murray, Ph.D.
Associate Professor
Department of Health, Physical Education,
and Recreation
Southwest Texas State University
San Marcos, Texas

Don Rainey
Department Head, Physical Education and Health
Edward Marcus High School
Flower Mound, Texas

Rudiger K. Zimmerman
Health and Physical Education Department Chair
Gar-Field High School
Woodbridge, Virginia

NUTRITION

Roberta Duyff
Nutrition Education Consultant
Duyff Associates
St. Louis, Missouri

EDUCATIONAL CONSULTANTS

MEDICINES and DRUGS

John R. Lauritsen, Ph.D.
Community Relations Representative
Parkside Lodge of Columbus
Columbus, Ohio

Michael D. McNeer, M.D.
Associate Medical Director
Parkside Lodge of Columbus
Columbus, Ohio

Sandy Moreland
Drug Education, Health and
Physical Education Teacher
Arsenal Technical High School
Indianapolis, Indiana

Richard C. Rapp
Project Director
Substance Abuse Intervention Programs
Wright State University School of Medicine
Dayton, Ohio

Dolores Salazar
Health Educator
Homer Hanna High School
Brownsville, Texas

DISEASES and DISORDERS

Nita Auer
Health Educator
North Side High School
Fort Wayne, Indiana

Susan A. Tilgner
Epidemiologist
Columbus Health Department
Columbus, Ohio

COMMUNITY and
ENVIRONMENTAL HEALTH

Charles Balling
Superintendent of Leisure Services
Elmhurst Park District
Elmhurst, Illinois

CONSUMER HEALTH

Robert D. Barrett
Administrative Resident
Prison Health Services
Xavier University
New Castle, Delaware

SAFETY and EMERGENCY CARE

Denise J.K. Abbott
Teacher, Registered Nurse
Timpriew High School
Provo, Utah

Lynn Gustafson Haley
Health Teacher
Mackenzie Junior High
Lubbock, Texas

Debra McMillan
Health and Physical Education Teacher
Douglas Byrd Junior High School
Fayetteville, North Carolina

MULTICULTURAL EDUCATION

Addie E. Pettaway
Education Consultant
Madison, Wisconsin

C O N T E N T S

UNIT 3: FAMILY AND SOCIAL HEALTH

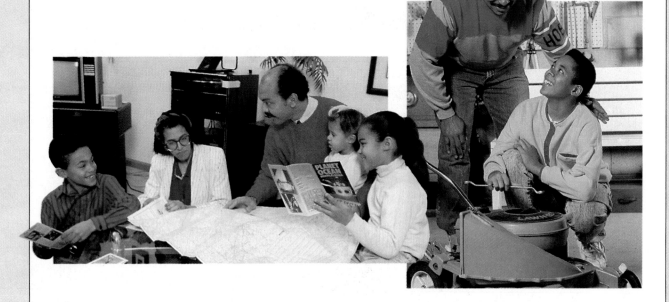

C O N T E N T S

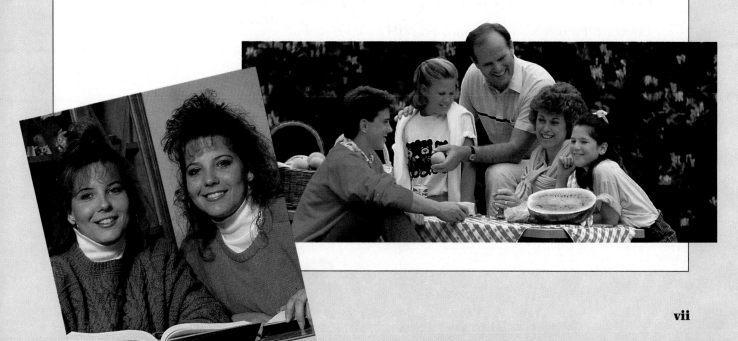

C O N T E N T S

C O N T E N T S

C O N T E N T S

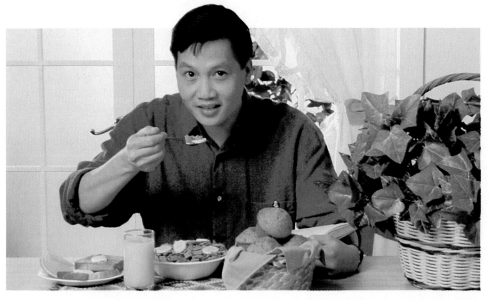

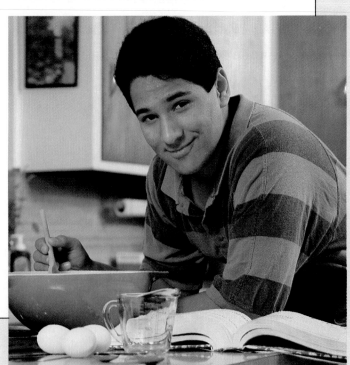

C O N T E N T S

CONTENTS

C O N T E N T S

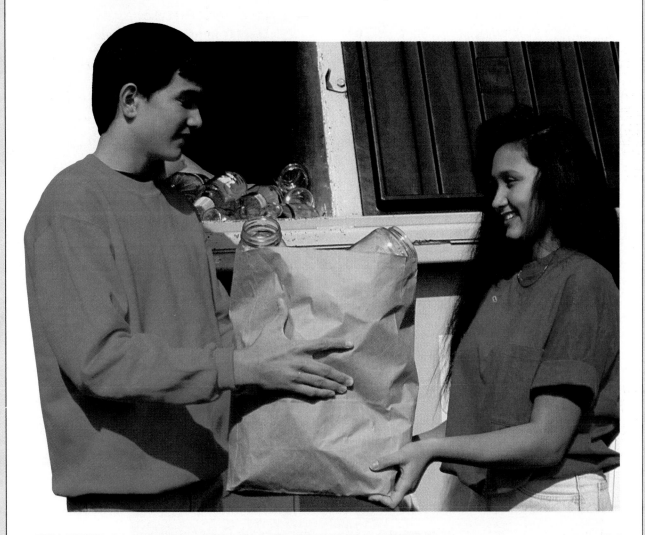

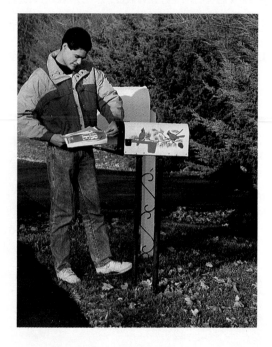

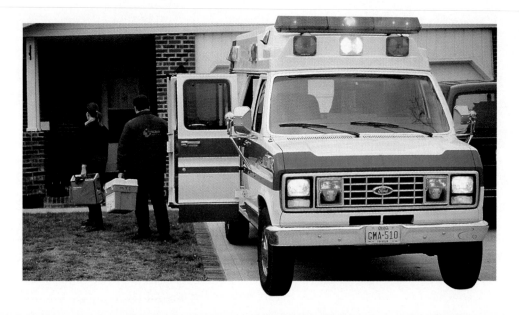

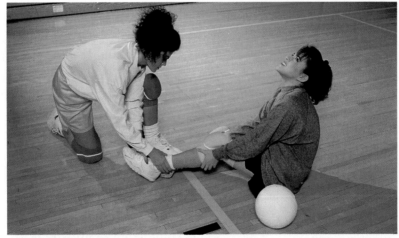

CONFLICT RESOLUTION

Overcoming The Odds

Self-Inventory

HEALTH UPDATE

S P E C I A L   F E A T U R E S

Culturally Speaking

HELP WANTED

FINDING HELP

YOUR HEALTH

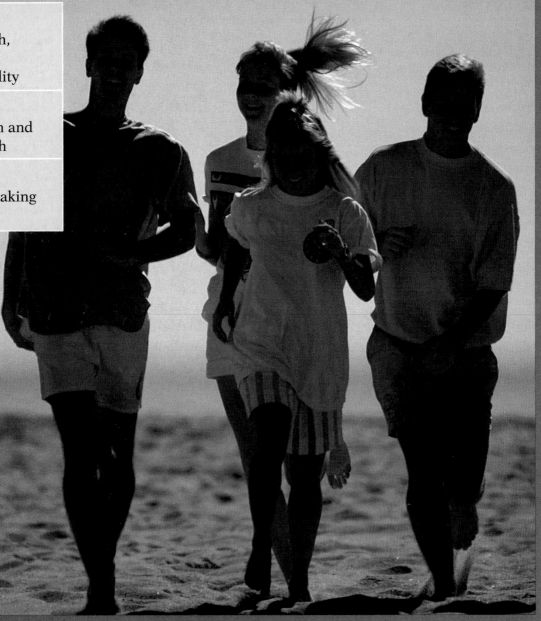

YOUR HEALTH, YOUR RESPONSIBILITY

How do you feel this minute? Are you awake and alert? Do you have energy? Are you ready to face the day's challenges and stresses? Is your outlook generally upbeat? Are you happy to be alive?

What about yesterday? Did you eat well, exercise hard, get a good night's sleep? Did you spend time with people who make you feel good about yourself? Did you have a specific, positive goal that you worked at or achieved? Did you also find some time to relax, smile, and laugh?

Your answers to all of these questions may be a tip-off about your general level of health. Of course, you may be having an "off day." Everyone does sometimes. However, the health decisions you made yesterday or this morning may have more to do with how you feel this very minute than you suspect.

Taking Responsibility for Your Health

Imagine that the story of your health were made into a video. The video would portray your health from the day you were born until today. This video would show how well you felt and functioned at each stage of your life and how the health decisions you made along the way or that others made for you have affected your overall well-being.

Now imagine that you can keep adding to the video day after day, showing how the decisions you make today will affect your health tomorrow or how the decisions you make this year may affect the rest of your life. Do you like the way the story of your health is progressing?

The fact is that the remainder of the video—the story of your personal health for the rest of your life—is, for the most part, in your hands. True, there may be some factors influencing your health that are out of your control; but most of the choices and decisions affecting your health are yours to make. You, nobody else, are this video's director. So sit down in the director's chair, and get ready to take responsibility for your health—and your life.

The Many Definitions of Health

There are many ways to talk about health. The word *health* comes from an Old English word meaning "to make sound, whole, or well." Not surprisingly, it derives, or comes, from the same root as the word *heal*.

In the past the word *health* was defined as the absence of disease. Many people still think that if they are not sick, they are healthy. Others think that if they are physically fit or if they look good on the outside, they are healthy. Still others think they are healthy because they have never broken a bone, had stitches, or spent the night in the hospital. These definitions, however, are limited and inaccurate.

LESSON 1 FOCUS

TERMS TO USE
- Health
- Health education
- Wellness
- Holistic
- Life-style factors
- Quality of life
- Prevention

CONCEPTS TO LEARN
- Your health is your responsibility.
- Health education provides information to apply in all areas of your life.
- Your health is influenced by your life-style.

ATTITUDES AND BEHAVIORS TO EVALUATE
- Self-Inventory, page 22.
- Building Decision-Making Skills, page 23.

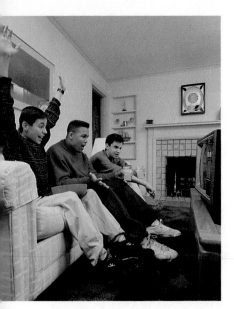

The three elements of your health—physical health, mental health, and social health—are related to each other and contribute to your total health. The more they are in balance, the better your health will be.

These days the definition of health has returned to the broader idea of wholeness. In its fullest sense, **health** is the state of total physical, mental, and social well-being, not just freedom from sickness or ailments. Someone who is totally healthy has a healthy body and mind as well as a positive attitude about life. Someone who is totally healthy has many relationships that enrich his or her life.

Your personal level of health affects everything about you. It affects how you look, how you feel, even how you act. It affects your attitudes and performance in school, work, and recreation. It affects how you feel about yourself and how successful you are in your relationships. It may even determine some of your goals and your ability to accomplish them.

Even though heredity and environment play a part in your one-of-a-kind health story, what you do to keep yourself healthy or to make yourself healthier is probably the greatest factor in your overall well-being.

The Importance of Health Education

Since health is so critical to the quality of your life, learning how to get and stay healthy should be a priority. That is why health education is so important. **Health education** is the providing of health information in such a way that it influences people to change attitudes so that they take positive action about their health. Its goal is to help people live long, zestful, and productive lives.

Health education is about gaining the tools to achieve and maintain total well-being. It is not just about teaching health facts. Its goal is to get students—and that includes you—to put these facts to use in all areas of their lives.

The Three Elements of Your Health

Notice that people ask, "How are you?" not "Do you have any diseases?" or "Are all your systems functioning properly?" That is because how you are doing involves much more than the absence of physical disease or the proper functioning of your body's many processes. It also includes how you are doing mentally and socially. To obtain a complete picture of your health, you must take into consideration all of these elements.

K E E P I N G   F I T

Improving Your Social Health

Are you often lonely? Do you sometimes feel like there's nowhere that you fit in? Be creative and improve your social health at the same time.

For example, consider Handicap Introductions, a New Jersey-based social dating service that matches people with disabilities from all over the world.

What creative techniques might you try?

- Join a club with people who have a similar interest or talent. Or start one.
- Get a part-time job where you expand your contacts to new people.
- Have a party where everyone brings someone no one else knows.

Physical Health

Physical health means that all parts and systems of the body work well together. It means that your body has the ability to withstand the stresses of normal daily life. It means having strength and energy to pursue physical, mental, emotional, and social challenges and changes.

To gain or maintain physical health, you need to have proper nutrition, adequate exercise, and enough rest and sleep. You also need to develop healthy skills, practice cleanliness in order to prevent disease, and get medical and dental checkups and care when needed.

Mental Health

Mental health includes how you like, accept, and feel about yourself; how well you relate to others; and how you meet the demands of daily life. A person with good mental health is in touch with his or her emotions and expresses them in acceptable, healthful ways. Such an individual can usually deal with the problems and frustrations of life without being overwhelmed by them.

Mental health also calls for a person to use his or her mind to develop thinking skills. People with good mental health enjoy learning and know that striving for information and understanding can be an exciting, lifelong process.

Social Health

Social health involves the way you get along with others. It includes your ability to make and keep friends and to work and play in cooperative ways, seeking and lending support when necessary. It involves communicating well and sharing your feelings with others.

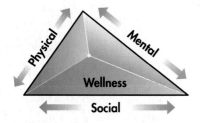

When you neglect one area of your health, the other areas are affected. If you do not exercise regularly, for example, you will not be as alert in class, or able to enjoy certain activities with your friends.

Your Health Triangle

Have you ever been very tired or hungry? How did that feeling affect the way you acted toward others? Did it affect your work? If it went on too long, did it affect your physical well-being? A direct relationship exists among physical, mental, and social health. To be truly healthy, you must work hard in each of these areas.

An equilateral triangle illustrates these connections and the need for a balanced approach to health. To achieve and maintain a high level of health, you must develop all three sides—physical, mental, and social. Conversely, your health triangle can become lopsided and unbalanced if you do not work to develop any one of the sides, or if you spend too much time in one area.

The Health Continuum

Wellness means an overall state of well-being, or total health. It comes from a way of living each day that includes making decisions and choosing behaviors that are based on sound health knowledge and healthful attitudes. It implies a threefold commitment to physical health, mental health, and social health. This approach to health is called a holistic approach. **Holistic** means "whole," and the holistic approach considers physical, mental, and social influences on the whole person and his or her health.

A continuum is a chart, spectrum, or sliding scale showing the progress of an activity, movement, or cycle. The Health Continuum below shows the wide range of wellness and illness within which people may live and through which they may move back and forth over time.

As you study the Health Continuum, keep in mind that it is always changing. You experience different levels of total health, from day to day and from year to year. In any of the areas that affect health, there can be sudden change. Conversely, a person may slide from one side of the continuum to the other so gradually that he or she is not even fully aware of the change.

The sad fact is that too many people settle for functioning below their health midpoint—the place where they are not exactly sick but neither are they fully happy or functioning at their best. They make health choices that keep them from enjoying and living their lives to the fullest.

This continuum has opposite states of health and wellness at the ends with varying degrees in between. The choices you make will influence your level of wellnesss. Accept the responsibiltiy of maintaining a high level of wellness for yourself.

Health Continuum

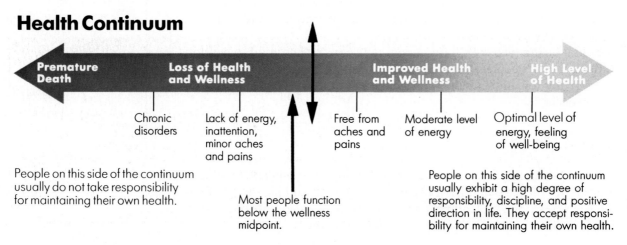

| Premature Death | Loss of Health and Wellness | | Improved Health and Wellness | High Level of Health |

| Chronic disorders | Lack of energy, inattention, minor aches and pains | Free from aches and pains | Moderate level of energy | Optimal level of energy, feeling of well-being |

People on this side of the continuum usually do not take responsibility for maintaining their own health.

Most people function below the wellness midpoint.

People on this side of the continuum usually exhibit a high degree of responsibility, discipline, and positive direction in life. They accept responsibility for maintaining their own health.

Promoting Your Health

Recent discoveries in medicine have helped wipe out many of the diseases that killed people 100, 50, even 30 years ago. Yet the way we live today poses new threats to our health and our lives. Millions of people get sick, become disabled, or die each year because of the decisions they make and the way they live. Their decision-making skills and personal behavior are directly related to their deaths. Many of these deaths could be prevented if people practiced a few simple health habits.

Life-Style Factors

After years of studying many groups of people, experts have identified seven habits that make a difference in people's overall health, happiness, and longevity—or how long they live. People who regularly practice these seven important habits tend to be healthier and live longer. These habits are called life-style factors. **Life-style factors** are repeated behaviors related to the way a person lives, which help determine his or her level of health. The following are important life-style factors:

- Get between 7 and 8 hours of sleep per night.
- Eat three meals a day at regular times.
- Refrain from smoking.
- Eat breakfast daily.
- Participate in aerobic exercise at least 20 to 30 minutes 3 to 4 times a week.
- Do not use alcohol.
- Maintain your recommended weight.

How many of these basic health habits do you practice regularly? If you do not practice them regularly, what are the reasons? What changes in habits can you make? Keep in mind that not following these guidelines can prove hazardous to your health and take years off your life.

Life Expectancy: Quantity of Life

Life expectancy is the average number of years a group of people is expected to live. It is dependent on many factors, including gender, heredity, environment, culture, access to medical care and, most importantly, basic health habits.

KEEPING FIT

An Attitude of Gratitude

Sometimes it's difficult to concentrate on what we have to be grateful for, particularly when things seem to be falling apart. However, with practice, you can learn to create an attitude of gratitude—reminding yourself to be grateful for what you have. Try one or more of these attitude boosters, and elevate your mood and overall health in the process.

- Learn to separate your wants from your needs.
- Identify what you can and can't change. Concentrate on the former. Let go of the latter.
- Be grateful just to be alive. This is the only life you've got!
- Use your humor. Laugh.

Life expectancy in the United States is almost twice as long as it was at the beginning of the twentieth century. In 1900 the average expected life span was 49 years, while in 1989 it was 75. Life expectancy has increased 9 years for women and 8 for men just since 1950.

At the turn of the century, the leading causes of death were pneumonia, flu, and tuberculosis—all communicable diseases spread from person to person. In contrast, the four leading causes of death today are not communicable. They are due to life-style factors. The leading causes of death in the United States today are heart disease, cancer, stroke, and accidents. The leading causes of death for 15- to 24-year-olds are injuries, murders, suicide, and cancer.

Life expectancy varies from country to country. For example, a person born in the United States in 1989 has an overall life expectancy of 75 years, while a person born in Ethiopia has a life expectancy of only 41 years. This is because of differences in availability and access to health care services, health education, immunizations, and medications, as well as to differences in nutrition, sanitation, and standards of living.

Life Enjoyment: Quality of Life

Just living a long time is not enough. Quality of life is as important as quantity of life. **Quality of life** means the level of health and satisfaction that a person has in being alive. Being able to function physically, mentally, and socially at a high level adds to the enjoyment and productivity of a person's life regardless of age. Practicing sound decision-making skills and health habits now can contribute to a good quality of life not only today but also in the future.

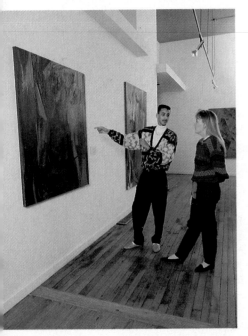

The quality of your life will be enhanced as you explore new ideas and learn from others.

Your Attitudes, Your Health

Practicing good health habits involves much more than just knowing what to do. Your attitudes also affect how well you take care of yourself. For example, in order to practice good health habits, you must believe that there is some benefit for you, and believe that by not practicing good health habits, problems will develop.

You also need to become aware of your overall attitude, or outlook, on life since this can play a major role in both your quality of life and your health.

Studies have shown that optimists, people who tend to see the positives in situations, are less likely to suffer illnesses and die young than are pessimists, those who look for and see the negative in situations. Other studies have concluded that it is not what happens to a person but the person's attitude about what happens that determines how well that person will cope and how happy he or she will be with his or her quality of life.

Even if you live in a very difficult situation, it can be helpful to try to find something positive about your situation and try to build on that. By gradually improving your outlook on life, you can get to a point where you can really believe that you can make a difference in your health and your life.

Toward a Healthy 2000

In 1991 Dr. Louis Sullivan, Secretary of the U.S. Department of Health and Human Services, made public 300 new health goals for the United States. These were aimed at making America healthier and stronger as the year 2000 approaches. Among the many health goals he recommended were reducing infant mortality rates, reducing the cancer rate, limiting the number of AIDS cases, and getting people to be more responsible for their own health by doing the following:

- giving up smoking
- becoming physically active daily
- limiting dietary fat intake
- learning to deal with stress in positive ways
- never drinking and driving
- always wearing seat belts
- seeking current and reliable health information
- getting early prenatal care when pregnant
- immunizing children against communicable diseases
- teaching how to make safe decisions about health-risk behaviors such as smoking, drinking, using drugs, or having sex

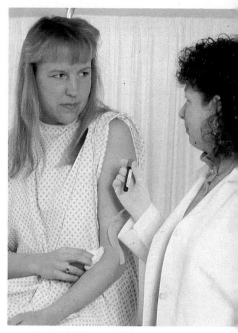

Having regular checkups is a good preventive habit. You can learn about your health status and ask questions about maintaining or improving your health.

According to Dr. Sullivan, Americans tend to use the health care system to patch themselves up rather than to prevent the very health problems that later need patching. Instead, **prevention,** or practicing healthy habits to keep a person well and free from disease and other ailments, should be the focus of everyone's personal health goals.

You, like many others, may think only in terms of today. You may not relate your present actions to how they will affect you in the future. Keep in mind, however, that the habits you practice now are setting the stage for how healthy or unhealthy you will be in your adult life.

LESSON 1 REVIEW

Reviewing Facts and Vocabulary

1. In a paragraph define the terms *health*, *health education*, and *wellness*, and explain how these terms are related to one another.
2. What are the three elements of health?
3. What is the Health Continuum?

Thinking Critically

4. **Analysis.** Analyze some of the reasons that even health-informed teens do not always practice basic health habits.
5. **Synthesis.** From all the factors you have studied in Lesson 1, identify the most important influences on your health and life expectancy.

6. **Analysis.** What are some behaviors that might lead to the top three causes of death for teens? Do you or any of your friends engage in these behaviors? How might these top three categories of death be prevented? Which, if any, of these prevention techniques might you need to apply to your own life?

Applying Health Knowledge

7. Draw your own health triangle. Are its three sides equal? If not, how are they lopsided? What steps can you take to make them more equal?

SELF-ESTEEM AND YOUR HEALTH

LESSON 2 FOCUS

TERMS TO USE
- Self-esteem
- Goal

CONCEPTS TO LEARN
- Your self-esteem is related to your health.
- Certain skills can improve self-esteem.
- Setting and achieving goals is important to your self-esteem.

ATTITUDES AND BEHAVIORS TO EVALUATE
- Self-Inventory, page 22.
- Building Decision-Making Skills, page 23.

Think of five adjectives that describe you. How many of them are positive descriptions? How many are based on how others see you? How many are based on how you see yourself? Now close your eyes. Imagine looking in the mirror. What do you see? How do you feel about what you see? Now imagine that there was a mirror that would let you see your mind, your creative abilities, and various qualities of your personality. What would you see? How would you feel about what was reflected back at you?

Self-Esteem

Self-esteem is the confidence and worth that you feel about yourself. Your self-esteem influences everything you do, think, feel, and are. It is, in fact, one of the most important factors in your overall sense of well-being. How well you feel physically, mentally, and socially can affect your self-esteem. In turn, your level of self-esteem can directly affect your physical, mental, and social health.

Some of the messages about who you are and how likable you are come from outside yourself. They are called external messages. Others come from inside yourself. They are called internal messages.

Did you ever get a compliment that you were unable to accept? Negative internal messages can get in the way of and erase even the most positive of external messages. That is why working on those internal messages you give yourself is so important.

Many people base their self-esteem on external factors—on how they look, what they have, how they perform, how others see them, or with whom they are friends. In reality, however, self-esteem comes from knowing, accepting, and liking not what you have, whom you know, or what you do, but who you are.

Some Signs of High Self-Esteem

Your level of self-esteem varies from day to day—even from hour to hour. However, your basic level of self-esteem probably falls most often within one portion of a high-to-low self-esteem continuum.

If you have a high level of self-esteem, you can accept yourself, including any weaknesses, illnesses, or handicaps you may have. You can admit mistakes and take responsibility for your actions. You may have self-doubt sometimes—everyone does—but most days you basically like yourself. Besides that, you know you can always make changes when you realize there are things about yourself that you do not like.

If you have high self-esteem, you probably feel competent in some areas and are willing to learn and try new things in other areas. You are willing to take chances and even to fail sometimes. You see mistakes as part of the learning process. You use your abilities and talents and take

Overcoming The Odds

Virginia Vasquez is 17. She works hard at her studies, has a part-time job in a snack bar, and is even taking flying lessons. Now she is making plans to go to college.

This is a good time in Virginia's life, but it has not always been that way. In fact, she has overcome great obstacles to get where she is today.

For much of Virginia's life, her mother, Maria Leyva, was a migrant farm worker, moving from place to place throughout the Southwest to find work harvesting onions. Virginia says, "The longest we lived in one place was in an apartment for three years. My sister and I didn't have fun in the summers back then. We had to wake up at 4 o'clock in the morning and go with my mom to her work in the fields. We had to go because we didn't have a baby-sitter, and we'd sleep in the back of the truck. It was cold. I first went to work in the fields myself picking onions when I was about 12 or 13.

"I now have a room of my own," she continues, "and it's big." The room Virginia refers to is her own bedroom at a center for homeless people in California. She lives there with her mother, stepfather, and younger half-brothers and sis-

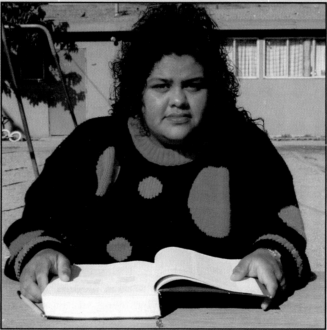

ter. Her mother now works in the thrift store at the shelter and her stepdad works selling furnishings. Her sister, Lupe, who also lived at the center, attends college but comes "home" to visit. The family is living at the shelter while they wait for affordable housing. They have been on a government waiting list for over two years.

"We came to the center about three years ago," she says. "Things have gotten a lot better since then. We eat better, we're more comfortable, and there's even a basketball team here. I played basketball until I hurt my knees. We have a doctor who comes here every week from the county. My knee ligaments are messed up, and I have to wear two braces. The doctors are now helping me with this.

"There are also people who care here at the center like Dr. Judy." Dr. Judy, who has a Ph.D. in psychology, works at the center, counsels Virginia, and provides her with encouragement and advice. He even asks to see her report card on a regular basis, and she sometimes works in his office.

Virginia also has other role models. "I also use my sister Lupe (who is a junior at Stanford University) as an example, too. Dr. Judy tells me if my sister can do it, I can do it, too. He always advises me not to give up.

"As for my plans," she says, "well, I'm going to graduate from high school. Then I want to study psychology."

And how does Virginia feel about herself? "I feel pretty good about myself," she says.

1. How do we do people a disservice when we assume they can't achieve goals just because they are from a particular race, socioeconomic level, age, or for any other reason?
2. What effects might such attitudes have on their self-esteem? On our self-esteem?

part in activities whether or not you are good at them. You believe that you are worthwhile as a human being and that you do not have to over-achieve to prove your worth. You have healthful habits and do not engage in self-destructive behaviors.

People with high self-esteem usually have healthful relationships. They seek out people who respect them. In turn, they respect others. They show respect for people of all races, religions, cultural back-grounds, and ages. They reach out to help people and to know them.

Some Signs of Low Self-Esteem

People with low self-esteem tend to let others influence them in nega-tive ways. They may engage in people-pleasing and approval-seeking behaviors. They may get their identity from external rather than internal sources, and they may trust others' reactions more than their own. In short, they may worry too much about what others think of them. In addition, their self-esteem goes up and down like a thermometer, often depending on how others react toward them.

To seem cooler, tougher, or more confident than they feel on the inside, they may engage in unhealthy behaviors to try to gain recogni-tion or to escape their insecurities. They may engage in activities that jeopardize their or others' health. For example, teens with low self-esteem are more likely to have sex early, get pregnant, drop out of school, engage in violent behavior, commit crimes and acts of prejudice, even commit suicide. They may use food, alcohol, tobacco, other drugs, and engage in unhealthful behaviors as ways of temporarily relieving the constant pain of not liking and accepting who they are.

Rather than using their time and energy to enjoy their lives, people with low self-esteem spend time and energy defending themselves, avoiding new challenges, trying to pump up their fragile egos, or putting down others in attempts to feel better.

People with low self-esteem often have few satisfying relationships. They may boast too much, bully too much, or even threaten others they see as weaker than themselves. They may go to great, even very danger-ous, lengths to prove how smart, rich, tough, attractive, right, or talented they are. However, these attempts usually backfire when their behavior turns off or frightens away other people.

People with low self-esteem may get caught in a vicious cycle. They may think that they cannot succeed, so they do not try. In not trying, they may feel even worse about themselves. Living with low self-esteem can be a terribly painful way of life, but it does not have to stay that way.

K E E P I N G F I T

Goals

Most teens would probably agree that what they want is to be loved, to be healthy, and to get a job they really enjoy.

Take time to ask yourself, "What do *I* really want more than any-thing else?" Then set goals that will help you work toward getting what you want.

Try these suggestions:
- List short- and long-range goals.
- Break major goals into smaller ones.
- Stay flexible. If one method of

achieving your goal doesn't pan out, try others. Be creative in your approaches.
- Start small. Set one small goal today that you wish to achieve by tomorrow.

Skills for Improving Your Self-Esteem

There are many positive steps that you can take to begin to improve your self-esteem. Doing so will not only increase your self-esteem, it may also improve your relationships and your overall level of health. Here are some simple ways that you can begin to make these changes:

- Assist others when appropriate.
- Find something that you can enjoy doing and that gives you a feeling of success. Make time to do that activity regularly.
- Stop making life a contest. Recognize that there will always be people both more and less able than you are in all areas of life.
- Aim for improvement, not perfection.
- Build a network of supportive relationships.
- Surround yourself with people who respect, approve, and accept you as an individual.
- Accept mistakes and errors as learning tools rather than as signs of your failure.
- Reject any negative feedback from others that is intended to put you down.
- Practice visualizing situations in which you are successful.
- Whenever you look at your weaknesses, spend equal time considering your strengths.
- Give yourself credit for all accomplishments or improvements, even the smallest ones.
- Practice basic health habits, giving attention to your physical, mental, and social health.
- Stay in school.
- Improve your mind—read a book, write a story.
- Use your creative talents on a regular basis.
- Get some training in an area of interest.
- Make lists of your qualities, skills, and talents. Read them often.
- Avoid engaging in self-destructive behaviors to escape your shyness or lack of social success. Doing so will just make matters worse.
- Do something nice for someone else. Do something nice for yourself.
- Set some realistic, achievable goals, and work at them.

CONFLICT RESOLUTION

Isabel is a freshman at the same school where her older sister Rosa is a junior. Both are good students, but they have very different personalities. Rosa is full of life and outgoing, while Isabel is quiet and reserved. Recent comments about how different Isabel is from Rosa have left Isabel feeling inadequate. Isabel has always envied her older sister's outgoing nature and busy social life. She's tried to be more outgoing in class, but doing so only makes her feel uncomfortable.

How do you think Isabel can improve her self-esteem and resolve the conflict she feels?

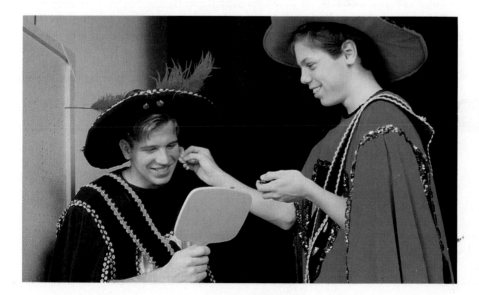

Try new activities. Volunteer to help in order to learn new skills and to discover new areas of interest.

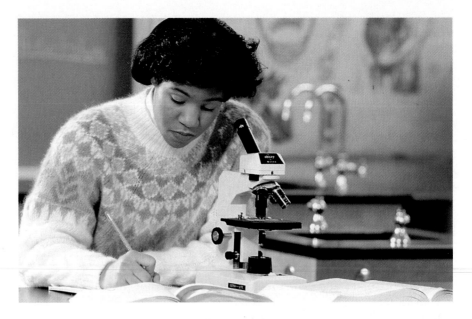

Choose a schedule of classes that will help you qualify for a future goal. You want to be ready to prepare for the career that interests you.

The Importance of Goals

Do you view your life as a series of events that simply happen to you? Do you see it as a work of art that you are constantly shaping and creating? How you view your life can have major effects on your health and your self-esteem.

Having and setting goals is one way to help shape your life in positive directions and enhance your self-esteem. A **goal** is something you aim for that takes planning and work. People who identify and work at achieving goals feel more satisfaction with themselves and with their lives.

If you do not have many personal goals, think about why not. Are you afraid of failure? Of success? Of standing out apart from your friends? Are you afraid of being made fun of? Are your standards of perfection so high that you would rather not even try?

If you do not have positive goals, the first question you must ask yourself is why? The second question is, How can I remove the roadblocks that stand in the way of my having positive goals?

Goal-setting is a skill. It involves a process that gives you direction, a framework within which to work, and a timetable for completing that work. Practicing the following steps will help you improve your goal-setting skills and, in turn, your self-esteem:

K E E P I N G   F I T

Take a Stroll Down Memory Lane

The memories you hold of yourself in the past can affect your present feelings of self-esteem.

For a few minutes, close your eyes, and remember times when you felt loved, cared for, or valued by others. Think, too, of times when you did something nice for somebody else, helping them feel loved, cared for, or valued. Experience the feelings that come with each of these esteem-building positive memories.

Open your eyes. Think of someone you know now who gives you positive feedback. Then think of someone in your life now to whom you can give some positive feedback. Reaching out to others is one good way to boost your own self-esteem.

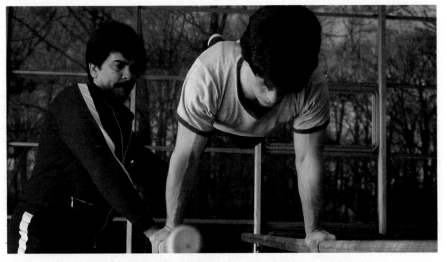

Practice is involved in reaching some goals. A coach can help you set realistic short-term goals in order to be ready to meet your long-term goal.

1. Select one goal to work toward.
2. List what you will do to reach this goal.
3. Identify others who can help you and support your efforts.
4. Give yourself an identified period of time to reach your goal.
5. Build in several checkpoints to evaluate how you are doing.
6. Give yourself a reward once you have achieved your goal.

When setting a goal, keep these additional guidelines in mind:

- Make certain your goal will not harm your health or anyone else's.
- Be sure that your goal shows respect both for you and for everyone else affected by it.
- Ask yourself, Whose goal is this? Make sure the goal is what you want and what is good for you rather than what you think someone else wants for you.
- Set a goal because it will help you grow, not because you want to outdo someone else or win someone else's attention.
- Avoid setting unachievable, unreasonable goals.
- Break down long-term goals into achievable short-term goals.
- If you fail to reach your goal, use what you learn from the failure to set a new goal.

LESSON 2 REVIEW

Reviewing Facts and Vocabulary

1. Use the term *self-esteem* in a paragraph.
2. Identify some of the steps a person can take to improve his or her self-esteem.
3. Identify at least three important steps to follow in goal attainment.

Thinking Critically

4. **Analysis.** Write one sentence that describes your general level of self-esteem. Then analyze what factors might be at least in part responsible for the way you view yourself.
5. **Synthesis.** Write a song, poem, story, or skit in which there are two characters—one with high self-esteem, one with low self-esteem. Have them interact.

Applying Health Knowledge

6. Write a one-page paper about how your level of self-esteem has affected one important relationship in your life.

DECISION MAKING AND HEALTH

LESSON 3 FOCUS

TERMS TO USE
- Decision
- Risk
- Precaution
- Consequence

CONCEPTS TO LEARN
- Health and well-being are affected by one's decisions.
- Decisions involve some degree of risk.
- Practicing decision making can help prepare you for real-life situations.

ATTITUDES AND BEHAVIORS TO EVALUATE
- Self-Inventory, page 22.
- Building Decision-Making Skills, page 23.

D o you ever feel as if you have no power? Does it seem that one minute people expect a lot of you but the next minute they treat you like a child? Most teens feel that way at least some of the time. The truth is, you have more power than you ever suspected. You have personal power. Each time you make a major decision, you are exerting enormous power—power over how healthy, happy, and productive you may be for the rest of your life. That is why learning decision-making skills is so important. Some of the decisions you make may not only make or break your day; they could make or break your whole life.

Big Decisions, Little Decisions

What is a decision? A **decision** is the act of making a choice or coming to a solution. You make hundreds of decisions every day. Many of these are not very important in the overall scheme of things. Should you have ice cream or frozen yogurt? Which shoes should you wear? Should you go to the movies or to the mall? Other decisions, however, are very important because they may affect

- your health and well-being,
- someone else's health or well-being,
- your future,
- someone else's future.

Imagine that you find three beautifully wrapped boxes at your front door along with a note that states, "Whichever box you choose will determine how your life proceeds." At first they all seem identical. Then you notice that on each box is a card. One says, "Decisions that will keep you healthy." One says, "Decisions that will make you unhealthy." One says, "Decisions that will kill you." Which box would you choose?

The answer seems clear-cut, right? Yet when you make actual decisions in your everyday life, do you stop to think which one of these outcomes you might be choosing?

Some of the big decisions that teens face include:

- Should I drink?
- Should I try drugs?
- Should I have sex?
- Should I be a passenger in the car of a driver who has been drinking?
- Should I stay in school?
- Should I get married?
- Should I further my education?
- Should I get some help with a particular problem?
- Should I smoke?
- Should I tell someone I am being abused?
- Should I get a job?

Making decisions about major life issues like these must be done carefully and deliberately. These are the kinds of decisions for which you must stop and really think about which of the three boxes you are choosing.

Sometimes there are conflicts in your life between what might appear to be a good choice at the moment and what ultimately may be best for you. These conflicts are very real, so it helps to know and use an effective decision-making model to ease you through such conflicts safely with your health and self-esteem intact.

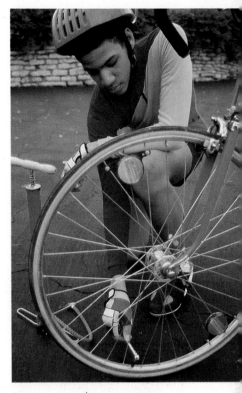

In any sport, there are many precautions you can take to reduce the chances of getting hurt. Can you identify the risks that are lessened by each piece of equipment shown?

Reasonable and Unreasonable Risks

Many activities involve risk. A **risk** is a behavior with an element of danger that may cause injury or harm. If you take a risk, you expose yourself to these possible dangers.

Some risks are unavoidable. You take a risk in getting hurt when you cross the street or ride a bike. Reasonable risks are those in which the likelihood of damaging your or someone else's safety or health is low. Trying out for the school play may be scary but can bring you great enjoyment and heightened self-esteem.

Unreasonable risks are ones in which the likelihood that someone may get hurt now or in the future is high. Many unreasonable risks are taken by people trying to make up for low self-esteem. Remember, however, that there are healthy ways to boost self-esteem without putting life and limb at risk.

You can cut down on the risks in a situation when you plan ahead and take precautions. A **precaution** is a planned, preventive action taken before an event to increase the chances of a safe outcome. Learning to ski, for example, though risky, is less risky if you receive proper instruction and use safe equipment. Some activities have dangers involved, but you have to do them anyway. For example, riding in a car is risky business, but taking a precaution like wearing a seat belt can decrease the chances you will get hurt, even if things go wrong.

Most accidents involve high-risk behaviors and making high-risk decisions. Before making any big decision, it is important to consider what the risks involved will be. Then ask yourself these questions:

■ Are they necessary risks?
■ Are they reasonable risks?

K E E P I N G   F I T

Get Up and Go

Resisting exercise? Consider the following benefits that can be yours if you simply get up and go. Exercise
■ strengthens your cardiovascular system,
■ helps you control weight,

■ burns off unnecessary fat,
■ improves your appearance,
■ improves your sleep,
■ improves your breathing,
■ reduces stress,
■ improves your mood and outlook,

■ decreases your appetite,
■ gives you more energy and decreases fatigue,
■ uses time productively,
■ reduces boredom,
■ provides social opportunities,
■ boosts your self-esteem!

- If they are reasonable and you plan to take them, what precautions can you take to increase your chances of a safe outcome?
- If they are to show off or to get recognition, what more healthful alternative actions can you take to increase your self-esteem?

The Decision-Making Model

The decision-making model is effective to use when you are faced with a situation that requires a major decision. It is designed to help you make decisions that will protect your rights, health, and self-esteem while also respecting the rights, health, and self-esteem of others.

Think of approaching a busy intersection in the road as the driver of a car. You would not continue at a high rate of speed. You would slow down and look for approaching cars, then proceed with caution. Failing to use caution puts your health and life at risk.

Now think of approaching a big life decision in the same way. How well you come through to the other side of the decision will depend in great part on how prepared you are when you enter the decision-making process, how carefully you look and proceed, and which road you finally choose to take. All of these factors can have major effects on your health and life. There are five basic steps that you need to take when faced with making a major decision.

1. State the situation that requires a decision.
2. List the possible choices.
3. Consider the consequences and your values—personal, family, religious, spiritual, moral, and legal.
4. Make a decision based on everything you know, and act on it.
5. Evaluate your decision.

State the Situation

It is important that you clearly identify the problem or situation. It is sometimes helpful to ask questions such as these:

- Why is there a decision to make?
- Why am I in this situation?
- Who is involved?
- How much time do I have to decide?

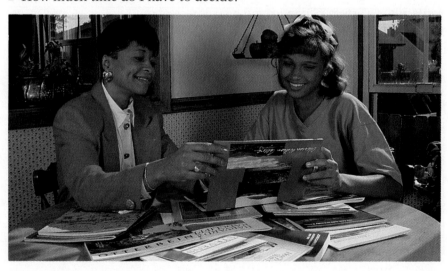

Use the decision-making model when faced with a major decision.

List the Possible Choices

Ask yourself, What are all the possible choices that I could make? Write them down if this will help. Remember to include "not act at all" if such an option is appropriate.

Consider the Consequences

A **consequence** is the result of an action. You need to consider both positive and negative results of each choice as well as the possible short-term and long-term consequences. You need to think about how risky each of the alternatives may be. At this point in the decision-making process, you need to consider the many possible costs to you or others of making a particular decision. Some of the obvious costs of a decision might be time or money. Among the other questions you might ask yourself are these:

- Is it safe? Is it a reasonable risk?
- Am I comfortable with this possible outcome?
- How will it affect my health triangle?
- How will it affect my self-esteem?
- How will it affect others?
- How will my family feel about this decision?
- Is my decision something I will feel proud of?
- Is it legal?
- How might this decision affect my life goals?
- How might this decision affect other decisions I have made?

You may also decide that you need more time to gather some up-to-date health data, consider others' opinions, analyze alternatives, and weigh the possible consequences. You may also decide at this point that you want to consult various resource people, such as a doctor, teacher, parent, or counselor. Bouncing decision-making thoughts off someone knowledgeable and understanding can be a terrific help in guiding you in healthful directions.

Make a Decision and Act

Use everything you know at this point to make a decision. Remember, you are not perfect. There are no guarantees about results. However, as you move ahead, you can feel good that you have prepared so carefully.

DID YOU KNOW?

- Want to swim the English Channel, or at least its equivalent of 21 miles? Avoid the waves and the cold and try swimming 1,848 laps of a pool instead. Want to climb Mt. Everest? To do so would be the equivalent of climbing 49,762 stairs.
- The number one dessert ordered in restaurants these days is not chocolate ice cream or frosted cake. It's fresh fruit!

K E E P I N G   F I T

Twelve Attitudes that Can Hurt Your Health

Could your attitude be getting in the way of your total health? Are you stuck in any of these attitudes too much of the time?

- That could never happen to me.
- I'm too young.
- I don't know anyone who ever got in trouble doing that.
- What I do won't matter.
- I'll show him (or her)!
- I'll get around to a checkup when I'm older.
- I'll start tomorrow.
- But everybody's doing it.
- We're all going to die someday anyway.
- I've never been sick.
- Nobody else cares about me, so why should I?
- I'm in control. I can stop any time I want.

If you get some last-minute information that changes the situation, you may want to go back to the first step and start the process over again.

Once you have made the decision, you need to take action. Timing can be important. You may need to set a deadline for yourself. Be sure you are ready to take action. If you have strong doubts, do not proceed.

Evaluate

After you have made the decision and taken the necessary action, reflect on what happened. Ask yourself these questions:

- What was the outcome?
- Was it what I expected?
- How did it affect each element of my health triangle?
- How did it affect my self-esteem?
- What was the effect of my decision on others?
- Would I make the same decision again? Why or why not?
- What can I take from this experience that I can apply in healthful ways to my next major decision-making experience?

One Big Decision: A Walk-Through

Consider the following situation and how one teen uses the model for decision making to make an important life decision:

Steve is 15. He will not get his driver's license for another 6 months. His friend Ben, who is 16, has driven him to a party.

When it is time to go home, Steve realizes that Ben has had a lot to drink. He is nervous about riding with him. He cannot offer to drive because he does not have a license. He cannot walk home because it is too far. There is no one else he knows well enough to ask for a ride home.

If Steve were to use the decision-making model, his thinking might go something like this:

1. **State the Situation.** I have to get home from this party, but I do not want to ride with a driver who has been drinking. What should I do?
2. **List the Choices.**
   a. I can ride home with Ben.
   b. I can ask someone here I do not know for a ride.
   c. I can borrow money and take a taxi or bus home.
   d. I can ask to spend the night and call Dad when he gets home.
3. **Consider the Consequences of Each Choice.** Steve might reason that if he rides home with Ben, there could be two possible positive consequences: Ben would not be mad at him, and they might get home without incident. Then Steve considers the many negative consequences of this possible choice: Ben could be arrested for drunk driving or cause a crash. Now Steve would think of the pros and cons for the other possible choices he has listed, thinking about the risks involved and the short-term and long-term effects of each.
4. **Make a Decision and Act.** Steve does not know if Ben is legally drunk, but he knows he is not in full control, so he decides that riding home with Ben is not an acceptable choice. He also discounts

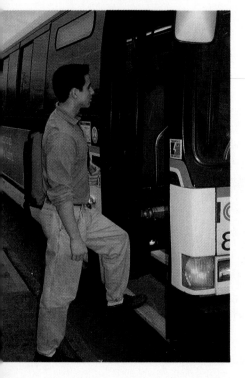

After considering the consequences of his choices, Steve chose a safe ride home.

riding with someone he does not know, since other people have been drinking. He calls his dad, who says he has to work a double shift, and after consulting with him, Steve decides to borrow the money from the host of the party and take the long bus ride home. Though it is hard for him to do, Steve tells Ben why he is not riding home with him and borrows the money from the host. He asks Ben to come with him on the bus, but Ben declines. Then Steve heads for the bus stop.

5. **Evaluate.** The next day Steve reflects on the situation. He thinks he made the right decision. He realizes that next time he should bring a few dollars with him in case that situation arises again. He also knows that from now on he will try to ride to parties with drivers who do not drink. He knows, too, that the next time he is faced with a friend who is drinking and who wants to drive, he will try to get the car keys away from the person.

The Benefits of Practice

Obviously, in situations like these, you may not feel comfortable sitting down and writing out all the options or walking through the decision-making model step-by-step with a friend. That is why practicing this model and walking yourself through the many kinds of situations and problems you are likely to face should be done ahead of time as a precaution. Doing so can make you prepared for those times when real-life risky situations occur, the same way practicing fire drills can prepare you for real fires.

Caring for your health is primarily your responsibility. The benefits gained from choosing healthy habits and making healthy decisions will be mostly yours to enjoy. Who would deliberately pass up opportunities for improved physical, mental, and social health; for higher self-esteem; or for a better quality of life? So go for it! Start today. Aim for total health!

LESSON 3 REVIEW

Reviewing Facts and Vocabulary

1. Define and use the terms *decision, risk, precaution,* and *consequence* in a paragraph, describing how they relate to one another.
2. What are the five steps in the decision-making model?
3. Why are the questions about consequences so important when using the decision-making model?

Thinking Critically

4. **Analysis.** Analyze some of the reasons a teen might take an unreasonable risk.

5. **Synthesis.** Write an interior monologue (the thoughts of one person written from the "I" point of view) in which a teen uses the decision-making model to decide whether or not to smoke a cigarette.

Applying Health Knowledge

6. Think about an important decision you have made. Analyze how you made the decision. Now rethink it, using the decision-making model.

Self-Inventory

What Is Your Level of Wellness?

HOW DO YOU RATE?

Number a sheet of paper from 1 through 36. Read each item below and write *true* for each one that accurately describes you or your behavior. Total the number of *true* responses. Then proceed to the next section.

Physical Health

1. I get at least 8 hours of sleep each night.
2. I brush my teeth and use dental floss after each meal.
3. I do not use tobacco, and I try to avoid passive smoke.
4. I keep within 5 pounds of my ideal weight or within the normal weight range for people of my age, height, frame, and sex.
5. I use a seat belt and refuse to ride in cars with drivers who have been using alcohol or other drugs.
6. I do at least 20 minutes of aerobic exercise at least 3 times a week.
7. I eat a healthy breakfast every day.
8. I do not use alcohol or illegal drugs or misuse standard medicines.
9. I relax 10 minutes each day.
10. I eat a balanced diet.
11. I use sunscreen when necessary.
12. I get dental and medical checkups once each year.

Mental Health

13. I generally like and accept who I am.
14. I ask for help when I need it.
15. I can express my emotions in healthy ways.
16. I can enjoy being alone.
17. I can name 3 good qualities about myself.
18. I feel okay about crying.
19. I can accept constructive criticism.
20. I can be satisfied when I have done my best.
21. I express my thoughts and feelings to others.
22. I have at least 1 hobby that I enjoy.
23. I deal with stresses as they happen and don't let them build up.
24. Sometimes I feel afraid, angry, sad, or jealous, but I am not overwhelmed by these emotions.

Social Health

25. I am generally satisfied with my relationships with others.
26. I meet people easily and am usually comfortable entering into conversations.
27. I can be myself when I'm with people I know well.
28. I can still participate in an activity even though I don't get my way.
29. I have at least 1 or 2 close friends.
30. I do not abuse others or allow them to abuse me.
31. When working in a group, I can accept other people's ideas and suggestions.
32. I can say *no* to my friends and peers, especially when they ask me to do things that might damage my or someone else's health, safety, or self-esteem.
33. I can accept the differences in people.
34. If I have a problem with someone, I try to work it out.
35. I avoid gossiping about people.
36. I make important life decisions carefully.

HOW DID YOU SCORE?

Give yourself 1 point for each *true* response. A score of 10–12 in any of the 3 areas indicates a *very good* level of health in that area; 7–9 is *good;* 4–6 is *fair;* below 4 is *poor.* Then score your total health. 30–36 is *very good;* 21–29 is *good;* 12–20 is *fair;* below 12 is *poor.*

WHAT ARE YOUR GOALS?

Look over your scores and choose an area in which you scored low. Choose one item on which you need to work and use the goal-setting process below to begin making a change.

1. The behavior I would like to change or improve is ____.
2. If this behavior were completely changed, the benefits I would receive are ____.
3. The steps involved in making this change are ____.
4. The people I will ask for support and assistance are ____.
5. My reward for achieving this goal will be ____.

Building Decision-Making Skills

Stacy is a freshman whose brother is a junior basketball star. Dewayne, a friend and teammate of her brother, has begun to notice that Stacy has "grown up," and Stacy considers his attention very flattering since Dewayne is very good-looking and popular. Unfortunately his attention has progressed from casual comments to suggestive remarks.

Today he stopped by the apartment while Stacy's brother and parents were gone and acted in ways that made her very uncomfortable. Luckily her brother returned before Dewayne forced himself on Stacy any further. What should Stacy do? Some choices include the following:

A. Tell her brother, knowing he might harm Dewayne.

B. Tell her brother everything is OK at the time, but later confide in him and ask him to talk with Dewayne but not to harm him.

C. Don't tell anyone else, but tell Dewayne she doesn't want trouble and she doesn't want him touching her.

D. Tell Dewayne she likes him, but not his behavior.

WHAT DO YOU THINK?

1. **Choices.** What other options does Stacy have?

2. **Consequences.** How will everyone involved react to each of these options? How will her actions affect her relationship with Dewayne, other kids in school, her parents, and others?

3. **Consequences.** How would the different parts of Stacy's health triangle be affected by each possible action?

4. **Consequences.** What might happen if Stacy doesn't tell anyone?

5. **Decision.** What do you think Stacy should do?

6. **Decision.** Would the decision be different if the person were not her brother's friend?

7. **Evaluation.** Do you believe that there are certain ages when self-esteem and social maturity are strong enough that people are able to handle such situations? If you do, how can you prevent being in such situations before then? How have you handled such situations?

8. **Evaluation.** In similar situations what has been the best way for you to let the other person know how you differentiate between appropriate and inappropriate activity?

9. **Evaluation.** What have you found to be the best way to let others know your limits?

Carla is a senior in high school who is working part-time. Her grades are slightly below average. She plays on the basketball team and is on student council. After working at Yogurt Palace for six months, Carla has been asked to manage the evening shift. With this promotion comes a 20 percent raise—and the satisfaction of knowing she'll be the youngest manager the store has ever had. She will have to increase her work hours from 16 to 24 hours a week. Should she accept this promotion?

WHAT DO YOU THINK?

10. **Choices.** What are Carla's choices?

11. **Consequences.** What are the advantages of each choice?

12. **Consequences.** What are the disadvantages of each choice?

13. **Consequences.** How might Carla's goals affect this decision?

14. **Consequences.** How might Carla's parents be affected by this decision?

15. **Consequences.** How might Carla's health triangle be affected by this decision?

16. **Consequences.** How might her friends be affected by this decision?

17. **Consequences.** What risks are involved in this decision?

18. **Decision.** What do you think Carla should do? Explain your answer.

Using Health Terms

On a separate sheet of paper, write the term that best matches the definitions given below.

LESSON 1

1. The average number of years a group of people is expected to live.
2. The level of health and satisfaction that a person has in being alive.
3. Practicing healthful habits to keep one well and free from disease.

LESSON 2

4. The confidence and worth that you feel about yourself.
5. Something to aim for that takes planning and work.

LESSON 3

6. The result of an action.

Building Academic Skills

LESSON 1

7. **Writing.** Write an outline for a personal health video of your life. Divide your life into segments. Describe your health during each period, and tell what you or other family members did to promote your health. For each period, include information about your diet, exercise, diseases and injuries, relationships, and other activities that contributed to your overall health.

LESSON 2

8. **Writing.** Rewrite the following sentences using appropriate spelling, capitalization, and punctuation:
    Mike has decided to improve his Self-Esteem by trying out for the wressling team asking Sandy to the dance on friday and Studying three extra hours a week.

LESSON 3

9. **Reading.** In the following sentence, what is the meaning of *fork?* We came to a fork in the road.

Recalling the Facts

LESSON 1

10. Who is the most important person affecting your health?
11. What factors affect physical health?
12. Name two characteristics of a mentally healthy person.
13. What is meant by the health triangle?
14. List four life-style factors that promote good health.
15. List three factors on which a person's life expectancy is based.
16. What are the four leading causes of death in the United States today?
17. What causes differences in life expectancy from one country to another?
18. Why is health education important?

LESSON 2

19. List three factors that can affect your self-esteem.
20. Explain the difference between external and internal messages related to self-esteem.
21. What are two characteristics of people with high self-esteem?
22. What are two characteristics of people with low self-esteem?
23. List three ways in which you can improve your goal-setting skills.

LESSON 3

24. What are the factors that make a decision important?
25. Name two activities that involve risk. Describe the risks involved and tell how they can be reduced.
26. What is the purpose of the decision-making model?
27. List five factors you should consider in assessing the consequences of a decision.
28. During the decision-making process, what people might you consult for help?
29. After you have made a decision, what is the next step?
30. List five things you might consider in evaluating a decision you have made.

Thinking Critically

LESSON 1

31. Analysis. Consider the seven life-style factors. Decide whether each one applies to you always, sometimes, or never. What conclusions can you draw from this experience?

32. Analysis. Anita is the starting forward on the girls' basketball team. She also runs cross-country. She eats three nutritious meals a day and gets eight hours of sleep every night. On school days, Anita spends three hours studying in the evening. Anita has never attended a high school social function. Draw a health triangle for Anita. Which side is the shortest? What can Anita do to balance her health triangle?

LESSON 2

33. Evaluation. Evaluate your self-esteem. In what areas do you feel competent? In what areas are you willing to try new things?

34. Analysis. Make a list of your best physical, mental, and social accomplishments. Then list some of your failures. Decide what contributed to your successes and what caused your failures. Describe how you could have turned your failures into successes.

LESSON 3

35. Synthesis. What precautions could a person take to reduce the risks involved of being in a car accident?

Making the Connection

LESSON 1

36. Social Studies. From the bubonic plague in Europe in the 1300s to epidemics carried to Central America by Spanish explorers in the 1500s, public health problems have always influenced history. Research how health problems of the past compare with today's public health issues including AIDS, environmental pollution, and population growth. Report how current health problems might affect the future.

Applying Health Knowledge

LESSON 1

37. Would you describe yourself as an optimist or a pessimist? Does this description change from time to time? Explain your answer.

LESSON 2

38. Choose an area in which you would like to improve your self-esteem. Make a poster listing five things you could do to build self-esteem in this area. Hang the poster in your room, and read it every morning when you get up. Do two of the items on the list every day.

LESSON 3

39. For each question below, write *important* if the decision you make could affect your health or the rest of your life. Write *unimportant* if it could not. Write a sentence justifying your answer to each question.
- Should I go to college?
- Should I buy the brown or the black shoes?
- Should I ask Sandy to go to the dance?
- Should I quit school and get a job when I turn sixteen?
- Should I transfer to a vocational high school?
- Should I smoke cigarettes?

Beyond the Classroom

LESSON 1

40. Community Involvement. Survey five people of different ages. Ask them what good health means to them. Compare your findings with other members of your class.

LESSON 3

41. Parental Involvement. Ask a parent or other adult at home to tell you about an important decision he or she had to make as a teen. Find out how the decision was made and if he or she believes it was the right choice.

CHAPTER

2

MENTAL HEALTH

LESSON 1
What Is Mental Health?

LESSON 2
Understanding Your Needs, Understanding Personality

LESSON 3
Understanding Emotions

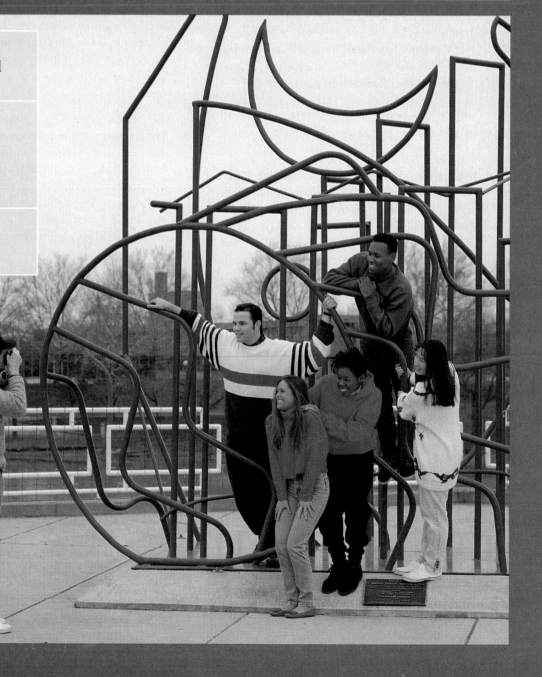

WHAT IS MENTAL HEALTH?

Like a collage made up of many different materials and shapes, the definition of mental health has many parts and can take many different forms. **Mental health** means generally accepting and liking oneself and adapting to and coping with the emotions, challenges, and changes that are part of every human being's life.

Mental health, like physical health, cannot be taken for granted. Working to achieve and maintain a high level of mental health should be a specific goal in each person's plan for achieving total health.

Everyone has varying levels of mental health at different times. Mental health does not mean feeling happy all the time. It does not mean always being in control. It does not mean never falling apart or never feeling angry, afraid, or insecure. In fact, being able to feel and deal with a variety of emotions and situations are key components of a person's "mental health collage." Being down, identifying why, doing something about it, and bouncing back can give a person a true sense of accomplishment and worth—and strengthen his or her mental health in the process.

LESSON 1 FOCUS

TERMS TO USE
- Mental health
- Feedback

CONCEPTS TO LEARN
- Mental health means much more than not being mentally ill.
- There are varying levels of mental health.
- Self-esteem is directly related to your general level of wellness.

ATTITUDES AND BEHAVIORS TO EVALUATE
- Self-Inventory, page 44.
- Building Decision-Making Skills, page 45.

A GREAT NATURAL FEELING

Did you know you can improve your feelings of well-being with strenuous exercise? When you engage in high intensity exercise, your body, specifically your brain, produces hormonelike substances called endorphins. These are released into your blood during intense exercise. Endorphins target your nervous system and can affect your sleep, eating behavior, body temperature, memory, ability to learn, and can reduce your response to pain. Besides feeling good, another benefit of exercise is that you will discover that success at exercise gives you good feelings about yourself.

Your Mental Health

It is difficult to identify specific standards for evaluating a person's mental health. However, some general characteristics of good mental health do exist. By looking at these characteristics, you can get an idea of what it means to be mentally healthy. You can also begin to determine your personal level of mental health. Keep in mind, however, that no one has every one of the characteristics described below all of the time. Still, knowing what the basic components of mental health are can help you define and work toward your own mental health goals.

A person with good mental health is described as one who

- feels good about herself or himself,
- feels comfortable with other people,
- is able to meet the demands of life.

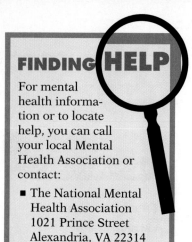

Feeling Good about Yourself

When you feel good about yourself, you have self-respect. You take care of yourself. For the most part, you accept who you are and do not overestimate or underestimate your abilities. You recognize your value as a human being and do not consider yourself more or less important than other people. You try to make decisions that will add to your physical and emotional well-being. When you feel good about yourself, you are not overwhelmed by emotions for long periods of time, and when you do feel strong emotions, you find ways to express them that do not hurt you or others. You take pleasure in everyday things. You enjoy your own company. You are not too hard on yourself when you make a mistake, and you do not try to do things perfectly. Sometimes, you can even laugh at yourself.

Feeling Comfortable with Other People

Feeling comfortable with other people means allowing others to get close to you and allowing yourself to get close to them. It means feeling free to be who you really are. It does not mean that you are never shy or never feel uncomfortable or angry with others. It does suggest that you generally like and trust people and respect the differences in their appearance, race, religion, interests, and abilities. When you are comfortable with others, you make friends and find these friendships satisfying. You nurture friendships that are important to you and maintain at least some of them over time. You recognize when a relationship is hurting you and work to change or end relationships that are damaging to your physical or mental health. You consider the needs and rights of others but not at the expense of your own safety or self-respect.

Meeting the Demands of Life

Meeting life's demands means facing problems when they arise. It means being able to deal with the minor crises of daily life, and when the big problems come along, being able to reach out and ask for help. Meeting life's demands means not staying paralyzed when problems are big, but working to try to solve them instead. It means making positive changes when you can and letting go when you cannot. It means developing decision-making and coping skills and putting them to use. You become willing to learn from mistakes and disappointments. You plan

KEEPING FIT

Knowing When To Get Help

How do you tell the difference between normal ups and downs of daily life and more serious mental problems?

Consider getting help when

■ you feel unhappy, sad, or numb for weeks at a time;

■ your efforts to solve a major problem continue to fail;

■ most of your energy goes into keeping it together instead of into enjoying daily life;

■ you feel yourself withdrawing from others;

■ you feel so insecure that you are sure people are watching you;

■ you are living with or affected by someone else's illegal drug use, mental illness, or abusive behavior.

Overcoming The Odds

Daryl is 15, and things in his family and in his neighborhood have been tough for a long time. As he puts it, "I was always the guy who stood out. I was real skinny and real tall. Friends used to call me names like Stick and Jav, for javelin, when I was younger. It hurt. Then I turned it around and became the best basketball player in the neighborhood. I showed them all. I put all my height and time and hope into it, you know, but I never figured my knees would give out. All of a sudden the one thing that made me feel like I was somebody was taken away. There I was again, with no hope and no way out.

"Things at home weren't any better. Since my mom split, I was doing a lot of the care for my two brothers and sister. We had money troubles. My dad had to work all the time. Sometimes I thought I would go out of my mind. I felt like there was this giant scream building up inside me and nowhere to go with it—not even to the basketball court.

"One night my dad slapped me around. He said I wasn't doing my part. I know now he was just totally stressed out, too, but it really hurt. I figured, what good am I? I can't do anything right. So I just took off.

"I went downtown and roamed around for a few days. I was lonely, scared, and confused. I had only a few bucks. I was hungry. All I knew was that I wanted to get as far away from home as possible.

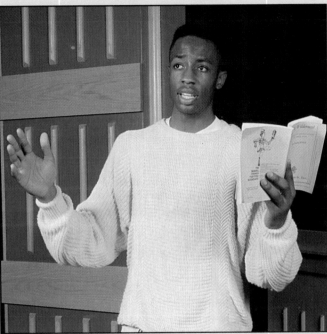

But if things at home were bad, things on the street were even worse. I'll spare you the details.

"The third night out this man gave me a card. He had a stack of them. It was for a runaway hotline. He told me to call them so at least they could let my father know I was okay. He said they wouldn't rat on me either. Then he showed me that on the back of the card was the address of a temporary shelter. He gave me money for the bus and wished me well. I had my doubts about him and that the place was what he said it was, but it was legit. I stayed there for three weeks.

"I'm back home now and things still aren't great. But this Youth at Risk group the shelter hooked me up with is helping me to learn that everything wrong in my life isn't my fault, that I have value, that I matter. I don't feel alone or crazy any more. Leon, the group leader, keeps telling us to remind ourselves that we've done really well considering all we've had to deal with. He also keeps telling us to tell ourselves when the tough stuff happens, 'This, too, shall pass.'

"I can't play ball, but I'm taking acting classes now at the High School of Performing Arts, and they're telling me I've got what it takes. And you know what? I'm starting to believe them."

1. What factors do you think were influencing Daryl's self-esteem when he ran away? Are any of these factors negatively affecting your self-esteem? If they are, what steps can you take to get help?
2. What factors or people helped him begin to recognize his own worth? Explain.

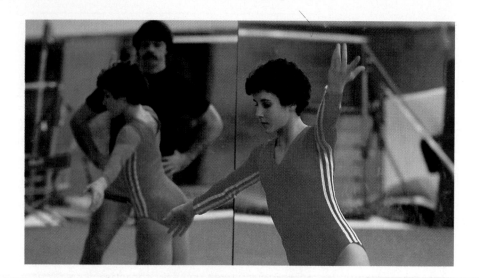

Positive feedback plays an important role in building self-esteem.

ahead for the future, welcoming new people, ideas, challenges, and experiences along the way. With good mental health, you work to put your talents and abilities to good use.

Self-Esteem and Your Mental Health

Self-esteem is directly related to your general level of wellness. How you feel mentally and physically, as well as how you take care of yourself—your health habits—are all affected by what you think of yourself. Having high self-esteem promotes good mental health.

The Role of Positive and Negative Feedback

How is self-esteem formed? Over the years you have received **feedback**—messages from others that tell you how they feel about you. You have received positive and negative feedback from many sources—from the adults who first took care of you, your brothers and sisters, extended family, neighbors, teachers, coaches, friends, and your peers.

From the moment you were born, you began to receive, process, and store these messages. Some messages were nonverbal ones. People hugged you, patted you, and smiled at you. Perhaps they frowned at you or ignored you. All of these actions made deep impressions on you. These first caretakers gave you verbal messages, too, like "Oh, what a

KEEPING FIT

Giving the Other Person a Break

One of the keys to good mental health is to realize that you have no real control over how others feel and act; you have control only over how you act.

The next time you feel someone has not lived up to your expecta-tions, try to remember that
■ everyone makes mistakes;
■ everyone has value, even if they do not behave as you would like;
■ most people who do and say awful things are themselves

hurting;
■ having compassion will help the other person feel better about his or her mistake;
■ people are not in this world to make you happy.

cute baby!" or "Bad boy!" With all of these verbal and nonverbal messages that you took in, you began to develop your self-esteem.

By the time you reached school age, other factors started to play a part in how you viewed yourself. Now, in addition to how your family responded to you, your feelings about yourself were influenced by how friends, teachers, and coaches reacted to you and by how well you could perform in the classroom and on the playing field. More importantly, you often set the stage for how others would respond to you by how you felt about yourself.

So what does self-esteem have to do with overall mental health? A person who has received mostly positive feedback probably has higher self-esteem and better mental health than a person who has received mostly negative feedback. On the other hand, someone who has received lots of negative messages may be more likely to have low self-esteem and more fragile mental health. This person may also misinterpret the feedback he or she gets from others, sometimes assuming messages are negative even when they are not. It is never too late to begin improving your self-esteem and, in turn, your mental health. Spending time with people who give you positive feedback and choosing healthy activities and environments can be an important step in working to achieve full mental health.

Culturally Speaking

Knowing Your Heritage

There are 27 colleges that are controlled by Native American tribes. All of these are on or near reservations and collectively serve about 12,000 students. Tribal colleges teach standard academic courses but also teach Native Americans about their cultures and traditions. Classes include Native American history, music, philosophy, and languages of one or more Native American peoples.

What cultures are emphasized in schools in your area? What art, music, or languages have you learned that reflect your heritage?

WHEN CARING IS THERE

Many teens who come from troubled families or face other difficult situations growing up do turn out to be mentally healthy, productive young adults. They seem to bounce back more easily than others. Perhaps the strongest factor in their growing up successfully was not some inborn ability to cope with stress but the continual presence of a caring adult figure in that young person's life. This might have been someone inside or outside the family, such as a grandparent, a coach, or a neighbor. Whoever it was, though, the message is clear: the caring made the difference.

LESSON 1 REVIEW

Reviewing Facts and Vocabulary

1. Describe the characteristics of mental health.
2. Define *mental health*. Discuss in a paragraph how self-esteem is related to mental health.

Thinking Critically

3. **Analysis.** Make two lists—one of the positive feedback and one of the negative feedback that you received as a child. Describe how this feedback affected your self-esteem.

4. **Synthesis.** Using material in the chapter and your own experience, write a 10-step plan for improving mental health.

Applying Health Knowledge

5. Think of a caring adult who has been important in your life and who has given you positive feedback. Write a letter to this person, thanking him or her for caring and listing ways the positive feedback made an impact on your life.

UNDERSTANDING YOUR NEEDS, UNDERSTANDING PERSONALITY

LESSON 2 FOCUS

TERMS TO USE

- Hierarchy of needs
- Aesthetic
- Self-actualization
- Personality
- Values

CONCEPTS TO LEARN

- All human beings have basic needs.
- Individuals set priorities in meeting their needs.
- Personality is influenced by a variety of factors.

ATTITUDES AND BEHAVIORS TO EVALUATE

- Self-Inventory, page 44.
- Building Decision-Making Skills, page 45.

All of us have basic needs. Getting these needs met is essential to a person's physical and mental health. Most human behavior reflects an attempt to get these needs met, and when they are not or cannot be met, the result is often physical illness, mental illness, or both.

A Hierarchy of Needs

Abraham Maslow, an American psychologist, presented human needs in the form of a pyramid. His idea is that we all have needs, but some are more basic than others. Consequently, there is a **hierarchy of needs**—that is, a ranked list of those things human beings must have to survive and thrive. The most basic needs come first. We must meet these before we even become aware of the other needs. For example, if the first level of physical needs is not satisfied, we have little awareness of our other needs. Our behavior is aimed entirely at satisfying our hunger or thirst. Once these needs are met, we move to the next level and begin to satisfy our needs for safety and security. It is not until these needs are met that we address our emotional needs, and so on.

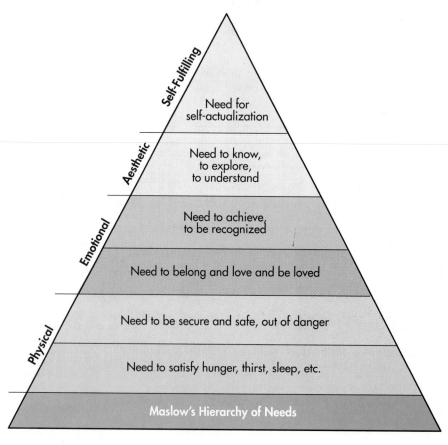

Self-Fulfilling
Need for self-actualization

Aesthetic
Need to know, to explore, to understand

Emotional
Need to achieve, to be recognized

Need to belong and love and be loved

Physical
Need to be secure and safe, out of danger

Need to satisfy hunger, thirst, sleep, etc.

Maslow's Hierarchy of Needs

Physical Needs

The most basic human needs (those on the bottom of the pyramid) are physical needs. These include the need to satisfy hunger, thirst, sleep, and so on. People who are denied food or water not only become physically weak, they become mentally weak as well. Food and water can preoccupy their thinking until these physical needs are met.

SLEEP AND MENTAL HEALTH

Our needs for sleep vary. At different ages and stages, we need different amounts of sleep. For example, a premature baby may sleep up to 20 hours a day. Adults need half the sleep they needed as young babies. Children spend more time than adults in the deepest stages of sleep—when the growth hormone is secreted. Children seem to tire out most quickly just before puberty. On average, teens need more sleep than they get.

So what happens when people do not get enough sleep? Effects of sleep deprivation include slowed reaction time, lack of concentration, increased sensitivity to pain, blurred vision, perceptual difficulties, and depression. Constant interruption of REM, or dream-state sleep, can result in disorientation and hallucinations. A good night's sleep, then, should be part of your mental health plan.

Emotional Needs

Meeting your emotional needs can have a great effect on your mental and physical health. The emotional needs—the need to love and be loved, the need to belong, and the need to feel worthwhile have an impact on your self-esteem. After we meet our physical needs, most of our behavior is an attempt to meet emotional needs.

The Need to Be Loved. Everyone needs to give love and to feel that he or she is loved in return. This is a basic need. Studies have shown that babies who are not picked up and talked to are stunted physically, emotionally, and mentally. They fail to thrive. Some even die.

The Need to Belong. Everyone has the need to belong. Human beings are social beings; that is, they need to be with and interact with people.

DID YOU KNOW?

- The amount of time parents devote to discussing emotions with their children may affect how sensitive these children will be to others' feelings when they become adults.
- Experts estimate that 90 percent of people feel shy in certain social situations, and 30 to 40 percent of the population is shy on a regular basis.

K E E P I N G   F I T

Stopping the Urge To Be Superhuman

Many people expect too much of themselves. Trying to be superhuman adds to your mental and physical stress and can lead to poor mental health.

To avoid these superhuman tendencies, try these suggestions:

- Don't try to be good at everything. It's okay not to win or not to be the best.
- Allow yourself to make mistakes.
- Take time to relax when busy times arise.

- Take a good hard look at why you stay so busy or so intent on being perfect. Remember, you deserve to be valued for who you are as much as for what you do.

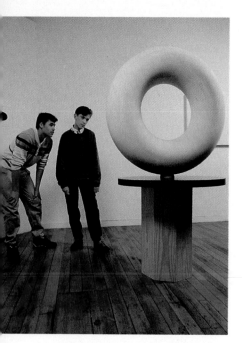

Admiring art, in any form, can bring rhythm, order, and beauty into our lives.

We need to feel like we belong to and are a valued member of a group. When we are mentally healthy, we meet these needs in positive ways that benefit ourselves and those to whom we are connected. When we are not mentally healthy, we may isolate ourselves from others or become overly attached to them.

The Need to Be Valued and Recognized. Another emotional need that all human beings have is feeling that they have personal value or worth. We have a need to achieve—to have ourselves and others recognize that we are competent at something and that we can make a positive contribution to the world. We must have something that we can do well, and we need recognition from others.

It is important to find healthy, positive ways to meet these needs for recognition. This is such a strong need that some people will seek negative attention just to be recognized.

Think of the child who is constantly being scolded for misbehaving. That child has probably learned that one sure way to get attention is to act up. How do you think this child might act as an adolescent or as an adult in order to meet the need to be recognized?

Aesthetic Needs

Maslow's hierarchy includes **aesthetic** needs. The word *aesthetic* means artistic; it means responding to or appreciating that which is beautiful. Aesthetic needs include our appreciation of beauty in its many forms. These needs also include the desire for order and balance in our lives. Our senses are constantly stimulated by the rhythms, forms, and colors around us, which can, in turn, affect our behavior and mental health.

Self-Fulfilling Needs

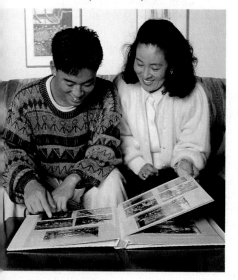

Inherited traits help determine one's personality.

Finally, it is Maslow's theory that we each have a need to reach or strive for our full potential as a person. This striving to be the best that one can be is called **self-actualization.**

You can certainly survive with only the basic physical and emotional needs met. For a rich and full quality of life, however, you need to have goals and ideals that motivate and inspire you. Defining and meeting your self-fulfilling needs is a lifelong process, not something you simply achieve in one day. Each of us is continually striving to satisfy this need, and when the need is neither acknowledged nor met, depression, boredom, and other mental disorders can set in.

According to Maslow, in order to feel fulfilled, people need not only to do what they are capable of doing, but also to do it as well as they can. By challenging ourselves, Maslow theorized, we find a greater sense of fulfillment in life.

Personality and Mental Health

Everyone has a personality. Your **personality** is that complex set of characteristics that makes you unique and distinguishes you from everyone else. It encompasses all of your traits, attitudes, feelings, behaviors, and habits. It includes your strengths, weaknesses, likes, and dislikes. It includes how you see yourself and the way you respond to your friends, your family, and the world. All of these factors go together to make up the person that you are and the person that others see.

Three main factors influence the development of your personality: heredity, environment, and personal behavior. To some extent, these factors work to influence your personality throughout your life.

Personality and Heredity

Heredity is the first influence on your personality. You inherit some basic traits from your parents and relatives. The most obvious traits are physical ones such as the color of your hair and eyes, the shape of your nose and ears, and your body type and size. You also inherit basic intellectual abilities. What you do with these abilities determines how well they develop. There is increasing evidence that heredity also plays an important role in your emotions and perhaps even some of your behaviors.

Personality and Environment

The second factor influencing the development of your personality is your environment. Your environment includes all of your surroundings—your family, where you grew up, where you live now, and all of your experiences.

People who come from unhealthful environments may suffer from poor mental health as a result of exposure to rejection, physical or verbal abuse, hostility, or other negative behaviors.

People who live in healthful environments have support from others. These relationships help them feel good about themselves. Feeling good about themselves enables them to reach out and support others.

Personality and Personal Behavior

The third factor affecting your personality is the one you have the most control over—your behavior. The way you choose to act within your environment and with your inherited abilities has a very important impact on who you are.

Many factors affect how you act. You have already read how your basic human needs affect your behavior. Another very important factor in how you act is your values. **Values** are those principles that you find important and that guide the decisions you make and how you live. You develop your values primarily from your family, but values are also shaped and developed by your personal beliefs, religion, school, friends, the media, and society.

How do values affect your behavior and, in turn, affect your mental health? Your actions are reflections of what is important to you. For example, if you value good health—that is, good physical and mental health is important to you—you will practice good health habits. You will actively work to take care of yourself and will choose behaviors that promote health. It is unlikely that you will take risks that threaten your health or the health of others.

LESSON 2 REVIEW

Reviewing Facts and Vocabulary

1. In one paragraph, define *personality* and describe three factors that influence the development of a person's personality.
2. Over which of the three factors that influence a person's personality does a person have the most control? Why?

Thinking Critically

3. **Analysis.** Compare the environment in which you grew up with that of a friend's. How has your environment affected your personality?

4. **Synthesis.** Give an example of a situation in which a person would have two different levels of needs present but would make a choice to meet the more basic need.

Applying Health Knowledge

5. List five ideals that you value most, such as honesty or loyalty. Pick one of these. For a week record how your behavior reinforces or supports this value or ideal.

UNDERSTANDING EMOTIONS

How do you feel right now? Are you in a good mood? Are you down or bored? Your feelings, or **emotions,** influence everything you do. They affect your thinking, your relationships with the people around you, your behavior, and even your success or failure at accomplishing a given task. Your emotions have an impact on your mental and physical health.

Having Mixed Emotions

Being a teen can be an especially emotional time. You want to be treated as an adult, but sometimes you still feel like a child. You get confusing signals both from inside and outside yourself. This pressure and turmoil can trigger all kinds of emotional responses. Sometimes these emotions may feel so strong that you want to act on them right away before you have had a chance to think them through.

You are experiencing what most young people do as they go through adolescence. This time of rapid growth and change is caused by body chemicals called **hormones.** Besides physical changes, hormones also cause emotional changes. It is important that you know that emotions are normal. Emotions themselves are neither healthy nor unhealthy. How you express your emotions, however, can be healthy or unhealthy.

Recognizing Your Emotions

Recognizing your emotions and handling them effectively are two of the most important skills a person can learn. Perhaps one of the most critical aspects of good mental health is learning to recognize and express feelings in a healthful manner. The key here is that this expression of emotions is learned.

LESSON 3 FOCUS

TERMS TO USE
- Emotions
- Hormones

CONCEPTS TO LEARN
- Your emotions influence everything you do.
- Chemicals called hormones cause growth and changes in the body.
- There are positive and negative ways to handle emotions.

ATTITUDES AND BEHAVIORS TO EVALUATE
- Self-Inventory, page 44.
- Building Decision-Making Skills, page 45.

THE RESPONSE

When you say that you are bored, what do you really mean?
- There's nothing to do that's fun.
- I'm feeling tired and can't get motivated.
- I'm lonesome.
- I'm not getting enough attention.
- No one asked me to go to the party.
- I have too much homework and don't know where to start.
- I'm depressed and don't really feel like doing anything.
- I'm totally stressed out.

If you focus on the real meaning behind your response, you will be in a better position to do something about it. What solution(s) would you give for each of the statements above?

Learning healthy ways to express emotions is a key to good mental health.

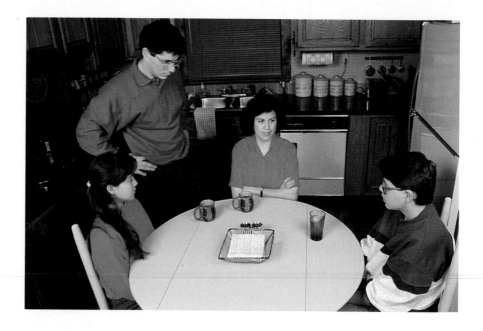

In growing up, you have probably learned various ways of expressing your emotions. We learn from watching others, from our environment, and from our own experiences. Suppose that as a young child you were repeatedly told that crying is a sign of weakness. Do you think that now you would be likely to express an emotion of sadness by crying? How have you learned to express joy and excitement?

Handling Emotions in Healthy Ways

Emotions are neither positive nor negative. The way that a particular emotion is expressed differs from person to person and from time to time. The way emotions are expressed can be either healthful or unhealthful, positive or negative.

Learning to recognize emotions and deal with them in healthful ways are two of the most important skills leading to good mental health. Both kinds of skills can be developed with practice. If you learned unhealthful ways to express your emotions growing up, it is never too late to learn new, healthful ways.

Certainly the ways you express your emotions may have to do with your personality. You may be easily brought to tears or quick to fly off the handle. Many of the ways you express your feelings have been

---

KEEPING FIT

Foods and Moods

Scientists have found that low-fat proteins tend to stimulate while carbohydrates tend to calm you down. Among the brain booster foods are low-fat milk, skinned chicken, and dried beans. Mood soother foods include bread, pasta, and cereals.

Need to stay awake to study? Don't load up on bagels. Need to get a good rest and calm down after a stressful day? Try a bowl of cereal or a piece of toast.

Do an experiment. Try to eat only low-fat proteins for a snack. Record your mood and mental alertness one, two, and three hours after you eat. The next day, repeat the experiment snacking only on carbohydrates. Compare your results.

learned from observing others. Perhaps in your family, people have family meetings and talk about their feelings openly. Maybe they express themselves indirectly with looks or smiles or with behaviors like crying or slamming doors. Perhaps they do not talk much at all, and you learned from their example that emotions were something not to be shared. Even so, you can still learn healthful ways to express feelings. It takes practice.

As you read about the emotions described in the following sections, think about how you generally handle each of them. Think, too, about how, when, where, and from whom you probably learned these ways of expression. Evaluate whether or not the ways you express emotions are mentally healthy and add to the quality of your life. If you discover that there are more healthful ways to deal with your emotions, begin changing the way you respond to them.

Fear

Everyone has fears. If you did not have some fears, you probably would not have survived this long. Fear can be a safeguard, a protection from danger.

As with all emotions, fear produces a physical reaction in your body. When you experience fear, your sympathetic nervous system (see Chapter 12) responds by preparing your body for necessary action. Hormones cause your heart to beat faster and increase the force of each contraction. This sends an increased supply of blood to your heart and muscles, while blood vessels in other parts of your body constrict. Your breathing rate increases. These responses are ways your body prepares to protect itself from danger. When the situation causing fear is gone, your body returns to its normal state. Some people like the response the body gets during times of fear. You may know someone who enjoys going to scary movies or doing daring acts.

Psychologists believe that most fears are learned, except for possibly the fear of loud noises and the fear of falling. What are some fears you learned as a child? Before you were old enough to reason and to recognize potential danger, someone probably instilled some fears in you to help protect you. For example, fear of playing with matches or playing in the street probably helped keep you safe when you were young. As you grew older, you may have developed fear about being hurt in a car accident. This fear may have helped you decide to wear a seat belt every time you ride in a car.

Other fears are not helpful and can even be destructive. Unrealistic fears, fears that immobilize us, and fears that damage potentially healthy relationships are not healthy. They can, in fact, greatly affect a person's total health.

Healthful Ways to Deal with Fear. In dealing with fear, it is important to identify what your fears are and find someone you trust to share your fears with. Perhaps together you can think of ways to help lessen your fear. This person may give you a perspective you may not have thought of or suggestions on ways to deal with your fear. This person may know about other resources you can contact for help. Working to increase your confidence may also help you overcome your fear and/or give you alternatives in dealing with it.

DID YOU KNOW?

- Both males and females cry. Perhaps because of different levels of the hormone prolactin, when males cry they are more likely just to get watery eyes; when females cry, tears fall down their cheeks.
- On average, females cry 5 times more often than males.
- The average cry lasts 6 minutes.
- Peak times for crying are between 7 and 9 P.M.
- Though public speaking is the number one fear among Americans, at least 100,000 people a day make speeches in the United States. If they were all waiting in line for a turn to speak, the line would stretch out over 28 miles.

A team of researchers asked 3,000 Americans, "What are you most afraid of?" They received the following replies:

1.	Speaking before a group	41%
2.	Heights	32%
3.	Insects and bugs	22%
4.	Financial problems	22%
5.	Deep water	22%
6.	Sickness	19%
7.	Death	19%
8.	Flying	19%
9.	Loneliness	14%
10.	Dogs	11%
11.	Driving/riding in a car	9%
12.	Darkness	8%
13.	Elevators	8%
14.	Escalators	5%

According to a poll of 160,000 teens, the 3 greatest fears of 13- to 18-year-olds were losing their parents (58 percent), dying (28 percent), and not getting a good job or not being thought of as successful (21 percent).

DID YOU KNOW?

The word *phobia* comes from the Greek word *phobos*, which means "terror" or "flight." In Greek mythology, Phobos was the god who could inspire terror or panic, causing mortals to flee.

Among the phobias from which people suffer are:

- bibliophobia (fear of books),
- brontophobia (fear of thunder),
- claustrophobia (fear of closed spaces),
- murophobia (fear of mice),
- pyrophobia (fear of fire),
- aerophobia (fear of flying),
- zoophobia (fear of animals).

Anger

Anger is often thought of as a negative emotion. Perhaps this is because anger is often expressed in negative or violent ways. Keep in mind, however, that anger is a normal emotion that everyone experiences from time to time. Learning how to express anger in healthful ways is a sign of good mental health and emotional maturity. This can be difficult to learn, but it can be accomplished with practice.

Think of some ways you have seen anger expressed. Perhaps you have seen a child throw a temper tantrum or seen someone kick a wall or take a swing at someone else. Some people let their anger build up, without saying or doing anything, until they explode and strike out at anyone who happens to be around.

Healthful Ways to Express Anger. How can you express your anger in a constructive way? As in the case of other emotions, you must first recognize your feelings and, if possible, identify the source of your feelings. Sometimes there is nothing you can do about what is causing the anger,

K E E P I N G   F I T

Some Tips to GROW By

GROW is a community mental health movement led by people in recovery from mental illness.

To handle an emotionally upsetting time, GROW suggests that you ask yourself these questions:

- What exactly am I troubled about?
- Is it certain, probable, or only possible that what I fear will, in fact, happen?
- How important is it?

- What shall I do about it?

The answers to these questions may help you see things more clearly and help you decide on the best course of action.

but you can find ways to cope with the anger so that it does not build up. Letting your anger out in safe and nondestructive ways can help you reduce the risk that you might act on impulse and be sorry later.

Here are some suggestions:

- Channel your energies into productive work or recreational activity. Hammer, paint, build, play the drums, draw, or sew.
- Get away by yourself, or have a good cry. Often underneath the anger you will find sadness or hurt.
- Do hard physical exercise. Run, race-walk, swim, or play basketball.
- Punch a pillow or a punching bag.
- Count to 10 very slowly. Take a deep breath as you do, then slowly exhale to the count of 10. Repeat this breathing exercise several times to help you relax.
- Pick up the phone. Call a good friend and talk it out.
- Close your eyes and listen to good music. Let it take your mind off the situation.
- Write down exactly how you are feeling and why. Express yourself freely. No one needs to see what you write.

Learn to channel your anger in safe ways. Acting irrationally could prove dangerous to your or someone else's health.

What do you gain from trying to express feelings like anger? First, you have identified the emotion and expressed it. It is over, so you do not carry the feeling around with you, wasting energy by seething over it. Chances are you will feel better. The knot in the stomach that is usually present in emotions like anger subsides, or goes away.

The most important gain is that you are more likely to carry on healthful relationships with people you are close to. How is this so? Getting angry with someone is normal and likely if you spend much time with that person. You clear the air if you express the emotion. If you bury or ignore it, you will carry it around with you. Then it can begin to affect how you feel about the other person, which can be unhealthful for you and the relationship.

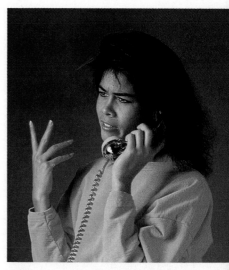

Talking with a friend is one way of channeling anger.

TALKING IT OVER

When you are angry with another person, follow these guidelines as you discuss the situation.
1. Tell what has happened and how you feel.
2. Start all your statements with the word *I*. Try not to use the word *you*. By using the word *I*, you are taking responsibility for how you feel rather than blaming someone else. When you use *I*, people have no need to be defensive and are more likely to talk out the problem with you because they do not feel attacked.
3. Tell the other person how your anger involves him or her.
4. Discuss what measures you think will reduce your anger and how the other person can help you. Offer to do your part.

Following these steps does not ensure that you will solve the problem. The other person may choose not to talk about the problem. You have no control over how the other person responds or reacts. However, you have expressed your feelings in a healthful, constructive manner, and you will feel better for doing it.

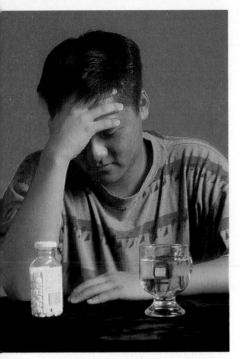

Strong emotions can produce tension. It is important for people to find healthy ways to express emotions. Taking a pill is not a healthy way to deal with emotions.

Understanding the Body-Mind Connection

Your physical and mental health are closely connected. Emotions can greatly affect your physical health. Strong emotions like anger cause physical changes to take place in your body. Your heart beats faster, you may perspire, your muscles tense, your stomach tightens. If you do not do something to deal with the emotions, the body does not relax. It stays in this state of tension. Over a period of time, fatigue can set in and physical illnesses may develop.

It is unhealthy to keep feelings inside, for you put an added strain on your body. In addition, you are not learning constructive ways to deal with emotions.

Consider these facts:

- People who hold emotions in and become highly stressed may experience an increased heart rate and rising blood pressure.
- Young people who have positive attitudes are likely to live longer than young people who have negative attitudes.
- Women with breast cancer who have positive attitudes are more likely to survive for longer periods of time than those who feel hopeless.
- Living with higher mental stress can lead to panic attacks and a lowered ability to handle pain.
- People who are frequently hostile have a higher rate of heart attacks.
- People under 30 tend to get sick more often from the daily hassles of life than do those in middle and later years. This may be because they feel emotions more deeply and do not yet have the perspective and the coping skills of older people. That is why learning these skills is so important to your overall health.

If negative patterns are developing, they may follow you throughout your adult life. The longer you practice them, the harder they are to change. Try some different ways of expressing your feelings. Learn new, healthful ways to deal with emotions. Try out some of the suggestions you have read about in this section.

DAILY EXPRESS

A new study suggests that writing and sharing your feelings in a journal can actually strengthen your body's immune responses—its ability to fight infections. In this study 25 adults kept a journal over a 5-day period, describing the most disturbing events that had happened in their lives and their emotional reactions to them. A control group of 25 people kept journals with insignificant details about their lives. When their immune systems were measured after 6 weeks and again after 6 months, the first group had an improved immune response, while the control group's immune response stayed the same.

Improving Your Mental Health

Throughout your life there will be periods when your emotions may seem to be stronger than usual. You may for a time feel overwhelmed, very frustrated, enraged, disappointed, or depressed. You also will have times when you feel really good about yourself. Regardless of how you feel, you know that there are steps you can take to feel better and keep improving your mental health.

Ways to Improve Your Mental Health

Emotions are like weather. You cannot accurately predict them. They are always there but are also always changing. They may come quickly from out of nowhere and pass just as quickly. Sometimes they bring sunshine, sometimes storms. In either case, you can choose healthful ways to deal with them by remembering these key points:

- Acknowledge that you are feeling an emotion strongly.
- Identify that emotion. Then identify the source of the emotion—what exactly you think triggered it.
- Express that emotion in a constructive way—one that will not damage you or anyone else.
- If possible, share your feelings with someone safe or neutral—someone not involved with the situation or person that has upset you.
- Remember that feelings are not facts. Do not feel guilty for feeling negative things. We all do. Do distinguish between the way you are feeling and the way you act about it. You may not have control over what you feel, but you do have control over how you act.
- Remember, too, that no matter how upsetting the emotion may be, it will pass—just like the weather.
- If a strong and disturbing emotion stays with you for too long and begins to affect your relationships or the quality of your life, get help. There are lots of people available to help you through a tough time. Remember that everyone needs help sometimes to deal with his or her emotions.

Many studies have concluded that it is not what happens to a person but rather that person's attitude toward what happens that makes a difference in his or her overall sense of happiness and mental health. So think positive. Be good to yourself. Be good to others. Take one thing at a time. Enjoy your life.

LESSON 3 REVIEW

Reviewing Facts and Vocabulary

1. What are some healthful ways to express anger?
2. How do emotions affect your overall level of health?

Thinking Critically

3. **Analysis.** What does the statement "emotions are neither positive nor negative" mean? Give examples to support the statement.

4. **Synthesis.** Write a dialogue in which a mind and a body talk to one another about the influence each has on the other's well-being.

Applying Health Knowledge

5. Keep track of positive and negative ways that you handle anger for one week. During the second week, stop yourself when using a negative approach and switch over to a positive one.

Self-Inventory

Rate Your Mental Health

HOW DO YOU RATE?

Number a sheet of paper from 1 to 10, 11 to 20, and 21 to 30. Leave a space between the three sections. Read each item below and write *yes* for each item that describes you all or most of the time. Total the number of *yes* responses in each part. Then proceed to the next section.

Part 1. Feeling Comfortable about Myself

1. I can express my thoughts and feelings.
2. I am not overcome by my emotions.
3. I can cope with both disappointment and success.
4. I recognize my own personal shortcomings.
5. I can laugh at myself.
6. I am generally optimistic and active.
7. I know my limits as well as my abilities.
8. I live by a set of values and know what is important.
9. I like and accept who I am.
10. I enjoy spending time alone.

Part 2. Feeling Comfortable with Others

11. I get along well with others.
12. I trust most people and want them to trust me.
13. I continue to participate when I do not get my way.
14. I do not try to dominate or control others.

15. I can accept differences in other people.
16. I feel I am part of a group.
17. I am interested in and enjoy being with others.
18. I have several satisfying personal relationships.
19. I do not feel consumed by fear, suspicion, or jealousy of others.
20. I am considerate of other people's needs and rights, but I respect my own needs and rights, too.

Part 3. Meeting the Demands of Life

21. I face my problems rather than avoid them.
22. I can ask for help when it is needed.
23. I do not make excuses for my actions.
24. I set realistic personal goals and have a plan for working toward them.
25. I can cope with change and see challenges and experiences as opportunities for growth.
26. I avoid trying to be perfect all the time.
27. I can relax and do nothing.
28. I know how to have fun and relax.
29. On important issues, I weigh the consequences before taking action.
30. I am generally happy to be alive.

HOW DID YOU SCORE?

Give yourself 1 point for each *yes* response. The highest possible score in each part is 10; the highest total score is 30. If you answered between 8 and 10 in any part, that suggests good mental health in that area. A score between 6 and 8 suggests acceptable mental health, though there is room for improvement. A score of 5 or less suggests that this is an area in which you need to set some specific goals for change and get some help. If your overall score is 25 to 30, that suggests good mental health; 20 to 25 suggests acceptable mental health; 16 to 20 suggests fair mental health. If your overall score is 15 or less, you should probably act now in seeking professional help.

WHAT ARE YOUR GOALS?

Write down one item from each of Parts 1, 2, and 3 in which you would like to improve. Under each of these three general goals, record three items for how you will go about improving that area of mental health. For example, under "I can express my thoughts and feelings" you might write: 1. Call one friend on the phone each day; 2. Read one book on communication skills. Include what resources you will use for making these changes and your timetable for achieving each goal. Record the progress you make with each of the three goals at the end of one, two, three, and four weeks.

Building Decision-Making Skills

A udrey is a senior at a suburban high school that sends a large percentage of its students to college. Much of the discussion in the school centers around the question, "Where are you going to college?" Audrey has given in to peer and parental pressure for three years and has taken college-prep courses. She has even passed up vocational opportunities that were appealing because of her percep- tion of this pressure. However, as she enters her senior year, she doesn't want to take more college-prep courses. Instead she has chosen an interesting work-study program in marketing. She hopes to attend the local community college to obtain a two-year associate's degree. What should Audrey do? Here are some possible choices:

A. Tell her parents she feels this is an adult decision she must be allowed to make in accordance with her own life goals, and that she is prepared to pay her own way if necessary.

B. Using her counselor's and teacher's help, work with her parents to help them understand that this is the best alternative for her.

C. Play the game, so that she can get their financial help and go ahead to college and have a good time, then quit at some point and go to community college or to work.

D. Give her parents' plan an honest try.

WHAT DO YOU THINK?

1. **Situation.** Who will be affected by this decision? In what ways?

2. **Situation.** Where can Audrey get information about the differences between her plan and her parents' plan?

3. **Choices.** What other choices does Audrey have?

4. **Consequences.** What are the advantages of each choice?

5. **Consequences.** What are the disadvantages of each choice?

6. **Consequences.** Should parents or the student have the final say in this matter?

7. **Consequences.** How might Audrey's self-esteem be affected?

8. **Decision.** What do you think Audrey should do?

9. **Evaluation.** Have you been in situations in which you've chosen to ignore someone with more experience because you just knew your decision was right for you? Explain. How did you feel afterward? Would you handle the same situation in the same way now?

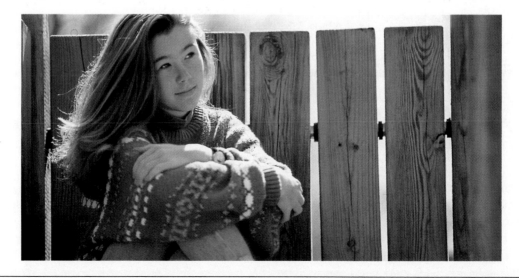

REVIEW

Using Health Terms

On a separate sheet of paper, write the term that best matches each definition given below.

LESSON 1
1. When you feel good about yourself.
2. Messages from others that tell you how they feel about you.

LESSON 2
3. The need to love and be loved, to belong, and to feel worthwhile.
4. Artistic; responding to and appreciating what is beautiful.
5. Striving to be the best one can be.
6. Traits or characteristics that are inherited through parents.
7. Everything that makes up a person's surroundings.
8. Principles that are important to a person and that guide his or her decision making.

LESSON 3
9. Feelings.
10. Body chemicals that cause emotional changes.
11. The relationship between your physical and mental health.

Building Academic Skills

LESSON 1
12. **Reading.** What is the main idea of the following paragraph?

    Meeting life's demands means facing problems and working to solve them. It means using decision-making skills and learning from mistakes and disappointments. It means setting goals for the future and using your talents.

LESSON 3
13. **Writing.** Rewrite the following passage to eliminate sentence fragments and run-on sentences.

    Emotions are like weather you can't predict them. Always changing.

Recalling the Facts

LESSON 1
14. Identify each characteristic listed below that is a sign of good mental health.
    - Feeling happy all the time.
    - Lacking self-respect.
    - Dealing successfully with a variety of emotions and situations.
    - Feeling comfortable with others.
    - Setting realistic goals.
    - Being in control all the time.
15. List five characteristics of people who have self-respect.
16. How is self-esteem formed?
17. Who are some of the people that contribute to a person's self-esteem?
18. Give an example of positive feedback.
19. Give an example of negative feedback.
20. How can a person improve his or her self-esteem?

LESSON 2
21. What is the theory underlying Maslow's hierarchy of needs?
22. What are the most basic human needs in Maslow's hierarchy?
23. What are some effects of not getting enough sleep?
24. What three main factors influence the development of your personality?
25. How can people meet their need for self-actualization?
26. What are some effects of not fulfilling the need for self-actualization?

LESSON 3
27. Give an example of expressing emotions indirectly.
28. If parents do not talk about their feelings, what conclusions are the children in the family likely to draw?
29. Describe the body's physical reaction to fear.
30. What are two advantages of expressing anger in healthful ways?
31. List five guidelines for dealing with strong emotions in healthful ways.

REVIEW

Thinking Critically

LESSON 1

32. Evaluation. Make a list of ten events that took place during your day. How did each one affect your self-esteem?

33. Synthesis. Decide whether each statement below is likely to raise or lower the self-esteem of the person who receives it.
- "Thanks for cleaning the garage without being asked."
- "I see you cleaned up the kitchen, but why didn't you take out the garbage?"
- "Another *F!* Do you think you'll ever be able to pass an English test?"

LESSON 2

34. Analysis. Label each section below as a positive or negative way to fulfill the need for recognition.
- Getting a good grade on a test.
- Using offensive language.
- Stealing a car.
- Cleaning your room.
- Destroying someone else's property.
- Doing volunteer work in a hospital.

35. Analysis. Label each activity below as a healthy or unhealthy way to express anger.
- Breaking dishes.
- Running around the block.
- Punching a pillow.
- Counting to ten slowly.
- Talking to a friend about the anger.

36. Evaluation. Are there appropriate and inappropriate times and places in which to express emotions? Explain.

Making the Connection

LESSON 3

37. Art. A photographer is often able to capture emotional moments on film. Using pictures from magazines, newspapers, and personal photos, make a book that shows the emotions of teens. Study each photograph carefully and write a caption to go with each one.

Applying Health Knowledge

LESSON 1

38. How are relationships with others important to mental health?

39. Give five examples of how people with good mental health meet life's demands.

40. Describe a problem you have encountered at some time in your life. Tell how you coped with it.

41. Describe a relationship you've had that harmed your mental health in some way.

LESSON 2

42. What are some things parents can do to fulfill an infant's need to be loved?

43. Interview five people. Ask them to tell you three things they do well. Write a report summarizing their responses.

LESSON 3

44. Discuss one of your fears with a friend or classmate who has the same fear and another one who does not. Find out how each of them deals with situations in which this fear might arise.

Beyond the Classroom

LESSON 1

45. Community Involvement. Find out what kinds of mental health organizations exist in your community. Arrange to interview an employee of one of these organizations. Find out what the organization does to help people with mental health problems and how this person specifically helps others deal with their problems.

LESSON 3

46. Parental Involvement. Share with your parents and other family members the guidelines for discussing anger. Have all family members share one thing that makes them angry. Try to get everyone to follow the guidelines, but do not force any individual to participate. Be accepting of differences, even if you disagree.

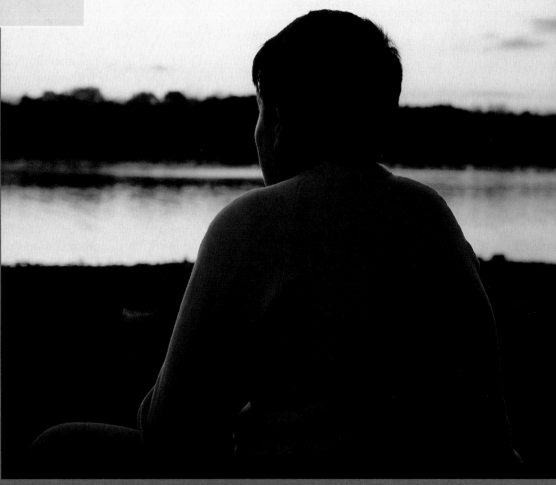

CHAPTER

3

MENTAL DISORDERS AND MENTAL HEALTH

LESSON 1
What Are Mental
Disorders?

LESSON 2
Knowing When
Someone Needs
Help

WHAT ARE MENTAL DISORDERS?

Perhaps no area of health is less understood than that of mental illness. **Mental illness** is a medical disease or disorder that affects the mind and prevents a person from leading a happy, healthful life. People who suffer from some form of mental illness are often identified by their inability to cope in healthful ways with life's changes, traumatic experiences, and losses.

Mental illness carries a stigma in American society. A stigma means a mark of shame. People who have been treated for mental illness say that their biggest problem is their inability to be accepted by other people. Mental health professionals are working to help people better understand mental illness and thus lessen some of the negative attitudes that exist toward it.

Types of Mental Disorders

The term *mental disorders* is used to describe many different types of mental and emotional problems. Mental disorders are classified into one of two general categories: organic or functional.

When a disorder is caused by a physical illness or an injury that affects the brain, it is called an organic disorder. Brain tumors, alcoholism, infections such as syphilis and meningitis, and stroke are all possible causes of organic disorders.

Functional disorders occur as a result of psychological causes in which no brain damage is involved. These disorders result from conditions such as stress, emotional conflict, fear, or poor coping skills. The main categories of functional disorders are anxiety disorders, somatoform disorders, affective disorders, and personality disorders.

Anxiety Disorders

Most people experience some form of anxiety from time to time, but their fears do not affect their daily lives. Not so with people who have anxiety disorders. **Anxiety disorders** are disorders in which real or imagined fears prevent a person from enjoying life. People with anxiety disorders often arrange their lives so as to avoid that which makes them anxious or fearful. Four types of anxiety disorders are phobias, obsessive-compulsive disorders, general anxiety disorders, and post-traumatic stress disorders.

Phobia.   When a person goes to extreme measures to avoid a fear and reacts in a way that limits normal functioning, it is called a **phobia.** A person with a phobia may be unable to carry out daily activities. Some mental health professionals believe that a phobia is related to some past experience that was upsetting to the individual. Although there is no longer a true threat or danger, the fear is still very real to the individual.

LESSON 1 FOCUS

TERMS TO USE
- Mental illness
- Anxiety disorders
- Phobia
- Hypochondria
- Manic-depressive disorder
- Schizophrenia

CONCEPTS TO LEARN
- Stigmas against the mentally ill take a variety of forms.
- Mental illness at any level poses special problems for the individual, the therapist, and society.
- Suicide affects the family, friends, and society.

ATTITUDES AND BEHAVIORS TO EVALUATE
- Self-Inventory, page 60.
- Building Decision-Making Skills, page 61.

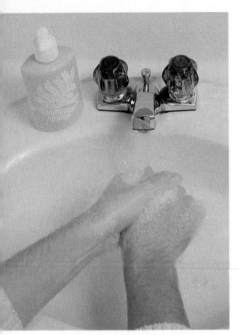

Washing hands every few minutes for no particular reason would be an example of obsessive-compulsive behavior.

Claustrophobia, the fear of closed spaces, and arachnophobia, fear of spiders, are two examples of phobias.

Obsessive-Compulsive Disorder. A person who has an unreasonable need to think and act in a certain way has an obsessive-compulsive disorder. Obsessions are persistent thoughts or ideas that keep people from thinking about other things. Compulsions are urgent, repeated behaviors. For example, an individual with this disorder may feel the need to wash his or her hands 20 or 30 times a day, or to avoid stepping on cracks in the sidewalk. When these activities interfere with other daily functions and cause the person to overlook other commitments, such as time with family and friends, they are considered a problem.

General Anxiety Disorder. A person with a general anxiety disorder feels anxious, fearful, and upset most of the time, but for no specific reason. This constant state of anxiety may lead to a panic disorder, a sudden attack of fear and terror often characterized by trembling, difficulty breathing, and a feeling of loss of control. A person with a panic disorder can be anywhere when the attack begins, although the attack is usually connected with certain situations.

Post-Traumatic Stress Disorder. Post-traumatic stress disorder is a condition in which a person who has experienced a traumatic event feels severe and long-lasting aftereffects. This disorder is common among veterans of military combat, rape survivors, and survivors of a natural disaster, such as a flood, or an unnatural disaster, such as a plane crash. Typical symptoms include dreams about the event, insomnia, feelings of guilt, or an extreme reaction to an image or sound that reminds the person of the event. Symptoms may appear six months or even years after the event.

Somatoform Disorders

A somatoform disorder describes a condition in which a person complains of disease symptoms, but no physical cause can be found.

Hypochondria, a preoccupation with the body and fear of presumed diseases, is an example of a somatoform disorder. A hypochondriac constantly feels aches and pains and worries about developing cancer, heart disease, or some other serious problem. Because hypochondriacs are convinced they are suffering from some imagined disease, they may refuse to believe doctors who tell them they are healthy.

Affective Disorders

Everyone has different moods. However, some mood swings are severe—from extreme happiness to extreme sadness—and last for a long period of time. When these mood swings interfere with everyday living, a person is said to be suffering from an affective disorder.

Clinical Depression. If feelings of sadness or hopelessness last for more than a few weeks and interfere with daily activities and interests, a person may be suffering from clinical depression. Clinical depression can occur over a single situation, or it can be about life in general. It can be a serious health problem that affects one's ability to concentrate, to sleep, to perform at school or work, or to handle everyday decisions and challenges.

Manic-Depressive Disorder. When a person's moods shift dramatically from one emotional extreme to another for no apparent reason, he or she may suffer from **manic-depressive disorder.** During manic periods, manic depressives may feel extremely happy or high. They may be overly talkative, often going rapidly from one topic of conversation to another. They may make lots of plans and take part in all sorts of activities. Manic depressives sometimes act impulsively or take unnecessary risks. Often this high period ends abruptly, and a period of depression sets in. Between episodes of extreme emotions, however, manic depressives may behave normally.

Although the exact causes of depression are unknown, depression tends to run in families. Any kind of emotional loss can cause depression. Unmet emotional needs and loneliness can also lead to feelings of depression. A healthy individual recognizes the feelings as a normal response to an event and looks for constructive ways to cope with feelings. It is when the person cannot cope with the feelings and is unable to get back into the swing of things that depression becomes a problem that could lead to thoughts of suicide.

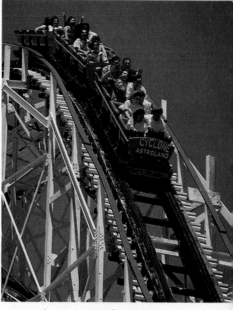

Manic-depressives often experience extreme shifts in their moods. These up and down feelings are often compared to a roller coaster ride. Can you explain the comparison?

Teenage Suicide. Suicide, the intended taking of one's own life, has become an increasing problem in the United States. Each year thousands of teenagers attempt suicide. In fact, suicide is now the second leading cause of death for people between the ages of 15 and 19. The rate of reported suicides among young people has nearly tripled in the last 30 years and continues to increase.

There are many possible causes of teen suicide. One explanation for suicide is that families are changing, and teenagers, like yourself, can have great difficulty coping with who they are, where they belong, and who cares about them. Teenagers also have many pressures to be responsible and to succeed. Failure in relationships, at school, or even at a job, can add to the depression. Pregnancy, alcohol and drug problems, having a sexually transmitted disease, or trouble with the law can be overwhelming to a teenager.

Sometimes feelings of failure or loss through death or divorce may be too much to bear. If you have experienced any of these situations and emotions, you know in a small way how bad a person can feel.

K E E P I N G   F I T

Dealing With the Blues

If you are feeling down, or blue, here are some steps that you can take to help the blues pass. In addition to getting lots of sleep, healthful food, and exercise, you can try the following:
■ Make contact with family and

friends. Go to the movies, get a jogging buddy, or talk on the phone.
■ Spend some time with someone whom you consider to be positive, productive, and in a good state of mind.

■ Try writing down all of your feelings in a journal. If you're afraid somebody may read your journal, rip up and throw away your writings each day.
■ Be around people who are active. Spend less time alone.

Teenagers who attempt suicide may be looking for some way to relieve the pain of a life that seems intolerable. Oftentimes suicide is accidental, a result of alcohol or drug abuse or misuse of firearms.

The vast majority of those who attempt suicide do not want to die. They are suffering and are making a plea for help. The lists below identify signs of potential suicides and suggest ways to help.

Warning signs of suicide can be verbal. Listen for

- direct statements, like "I want to die," "I don't want to live anymore," or "I wish I were dead";
- indirect statements, like "I want to go to sleep and never wake up," "They'll be sorry when I'm gone," "Soon this pain will be over," or "I can't take it anymore."

Warning signs of suicide can be reflected in a person's behavior. Look for

- depression, lack of energy;
- a change in sleeping patterns;
- an increase or decrease in appetite;
- withdrawal from usual social activities;
- loss of interest in hobbies, sports, job, or school;
- a good student's drop in grades or a poor student's new concern about grades;
- the giving away of possessions;
- increased risk-taking and other aggressive activity, such as driving a car recklessly;
- frequent accidents;
- personality changes—withdrawal, apathy, moodiness;
- previous suicide attempts (many of those who commit suicide have attempted suicide before).

Thoughts of suicide can also stem from certain situations. Look for warning signs if someone is

- experiencing a loss (death, divorce, breakup of a relationship);
- having difficulties with parents;
- encountering problems with school or employment;

CONFLICT RESOLUTION

Joyce is 15. She used to be a happy, popular student—that is, until her older brother Tim was diagnosed with schizophrenia two years ago. Now, her classmates often make remarks about how "crazy" Tim is and imply that Joyce might be "crazy" too. Joyce knows her mental health is fine and that, with good treatment, Tim may make a full recovery some day, but the cruel remarks have left her feeling bitter. Even though she loves her brother, she has started feeling resentful toward him. She thinks that if her classmates understood the illness better, especially the fact that, in Tim's case, it has a genetic cause, they would be less judgmental.

How can Joyce help her classmates understand Tim's condition?

HEARING SOMEONE'S CRY FOR HELP

Here are some suggestions for handling potential suicides:
- If a person threatens suicide, take him or her seriously.
- Ask whether the person has a specific plan and means to follow through with it.
- Be direct; talk openly and freely.
- Allow the person to express his or her feelings.
- Do not give advice. Express what you think, but do not be judgmental.
- Do not dare or challenge the person.
- Do not allow yourself to be sworn to secrecy.
- Be willing to listen. This affirms a person's feelings.
- Suggest to the person that he or she call a suicide center or crisis intervention center, or talk with a trusted teacher, counselor, doctor, member of the clergy, or other adult. If your friend refuses, talk to one of these people and your parents for advice on handling the situation.

- abusing drugs or alcohol;
- getting into trouble with the law;
- going through a time when there is no significant other person in his or her life (this is a critical factor, for a person who feels no one is interested in him or her has little reason to keep on trying);
- experiencing low self-esteem because of failure.

Personality Disorders

A variety of conditions are described as personality disorders. Unlike anxiety disorders, personality disorders have no apparent, distinct signs or symptoms. The individual continues to function, often effectively, in his or her environment. A person who has a personality disorder may respond inappropriately in certain situations or may interfere with others' interactions.

Antisocial Personality Disorder. One common personality disorder is termed the antisocial personality, characterized by a person's constant conflict with society. The antisocial individual may display behavior that is cruel, uncaring, irresponsible, and impulsive. Although he or she can distinguish right from wrong, the antisocial personality often does not care and therefore is usually in trouble with the law.

Passive-Aggressive Personality Disorder. People with passive-aggressive personality disorder are often uncooperative with others. They resent being told what to do, but they show their anger indirectly. For example, a passive-aggressive person who does not want to take part in a school activity may either forget to show up or may arrive late and leave early. He or she has not openly refused to participate, but the resentment is obvious by the failure to be reliable.

Schizophrenia. A mental disorder meaning *split mind*, **schizophrenia** disorder affects about 1 to 2 percent of the population and appears most frequently among people between the ages of 15 and 35. Schizophrenics are severely disturbed. They exhibit abnormal emotional responses or, in some cases, no emotional response at all. They may respond inappropriately in some situations. Some schizophrenics withdraw, often losing a sense of time and space. Others talk to themselves, act in an odd manner, or neglect to care for themselves. People with paranoid

K E E P I N G   F I T

Six Things to Remember When You're Down

1. Everyone has bad times and feels depressed now and then.
2. Remind yourself that you are not alone. There are many others who feel just as you do.
3. Be certain to take care of the basics when you're feeling down. Get enough sleep, eat regular and healthful meals, and get lots of exercise. Believe it or not, all of these efforts will improve your state of mind.
4. Avoid alcohol and other drugs, even caffeine. They will only add to the problem.
5. You, more than anyone else, control the way you feel.
6. It isn't what happens to you that counts as much as how you view what happens to you!

HEALTH UPDATE

LOOKING AT THE ISSUES

Who Has the Right to Prescribe?

Only psychiatrists—medical doctors who specialize in mental disorders—can prescribe medicines for people who suffer from mental disorders. Now there is a plan to allow psychologists—professionals trained in mental disorders, but not in medical school—to prescribe medicines.

Analyzing Different Viewpoints

ONE VIEW. Many psychiatrists state that only those with medical training understand the impact of medicines on the mind and body.

A SECOND VIEW. Some psychologists argue that most medicines prescribed for mental disorders are described and adequately explained in sources like the *Physician's Desk Reference*, a standard medical resource book.

A THIRD VIEW. Still others claim that there is such a shortage of professionals available to help the vast numbers of people with mental disorders that the expanded right to prescribe would only help the plight of the mentally ill.

Exploring Your Views

1. If you were being treated for a mental disorder would you also be comfortable getting your prescription from a pharmacist, physician's assistant, or nurse practitioner who had specific training regarding medicines? Why or why not?

schizophrenic disorder mistrust others and are often suspicious. They may believe that they are being followed and that others mean to harm them.

Much research is being carried out to better understand schizophrenia. Some doctors believe its causes stem from a physical disorder. Others think it is genetic in nature. The disorder may come and go throughout life. Professional help is always recommended.

LESSON 1 REVIEW

Reviewing Facts and Vocabulary

1. Define the term *mental illness*.
2. Define and give the cause of an organic disorder and a functional disorder.
3. Describe a person who suffers from a phobia.

Thinking Critically

4. **Evaluation.** Why do you think there is a stigma attached to mental illness?

5. **Synthesis.** What might happen if someone suffering from some type of mental disorder fails to get professional help?

Applying Health Knowledge

6. Prepare a presentation for a group of classmates that discusses methods of preventing teen suicide. Include posters that list the warning signs of suicide.

KNOWING WHEN SOMEONE NEEDS HELP

As you have read in this chapter, there are many different types of mental disorders. Within those types, the severity of the problems varies greatly. Unlike the symptoms of a cold or measles, specific symptoms of mental disorders are much more difficult to identify.

Signs of Mental Health Problems

Being aware of and recognizing early warning signs of mental disorders are the keys to getting help. Any of the following feelings or behaviors that persist over a period of days or weeks, and begin to interfere with other aspects of daily living, could be a sign that something is wrong:

- sadness over a specific event or for no reason
- hopelessness—the sense that one's life is out of control
- violent or erratic mood shifts
- inability to concentrate or to make decisions about daily life
- fear and anger at the world
- trouble getting along with others
- severe sleep disturbances—nightmares, insomnia
- compulsive self-destructive behavior—overeating, drinking, drug abuse
- frequent physical ailments, for which no medical cause can be found

Of course, no one symptom means a person has a mental disorder. However, any one of them may be an indication that stress in your life is building up and is something you need to look at closely, before more serious problems develop.

Health-Care Services for Mental Health

Often it is difficult to look in the mirror and do your own mental health checkup. Sometimes others are needed to help. Many times a friend may offer emotional first aid, that is, support and a listening ear, which may prevent more serious damage from taking place. However, this emotional first aid does not take the place of the aid that a mental-health professional can give.

The principal health-care providers for mental health are psychiatrists, psychiatric social workers, clinical psychologists, neurologists, and occupational therapists. These individuals may work in or outside a hospital setting.

Outside the hospital setting, help is available through marriage and family counselors, rehabilitation counselors, and pastoral counselors. In addition, there are various types of community services that deal specifically with rape, suicide, and family violence.

LESSON 2 FOCUS

TERMS TO USE
- Psychiatrist
- Therapy
- Neurologist
- Clinical psychologist

CONCEPTS TO LEARN
- Serious mental problems require the assistance of a mental health professional.
- Mental health professionals work to help individuals improve their perception of self and the outside world.

ATTITUDES AND BEHAVIORS TO EVALUATE
- Self-Inventory, page 60.
- Building Decision-Making Skills, page 61.

Psychiatrist

A **psychiatrist** deals with mental, emotional, and behavioral disorders of the mind. This person has completed four years of medical school and one year of internship and has passed a state licensing exam. Although this is all that is legally required, many psychiatrists have also spent several years as resident physicians in an institution that treats mental illness. Because psychiatrists are physicians, they can prescribe medicines.

The psychiatrist uses many **therapies,** or treatment techniques. Among them are the following:

- psychoanalysis—an analysis of a patient's past, particularly his or her early life, to determine the early roots of a mental problem
- psychotherapy—patient and psychiatrist discussions to understand the problem and find a solution
- medical therapy—the use of certain medications to reduce a mental disorder or to prepare for the above two treatments
- electroconvulsive therapy—electric shock given to a patient under anesthetic, usually on one side of the brain (a treatment that can sometimes help severely depressed patients)
- group therapy—meetings held with other people with similar problems, during which the participants pool their experiences and learn from one another, with the doctor as a guide

Neurologist

A **neurologist** is a physician who specializes in organic disorders of the brain and nervous system. This person has a degree in medicine, postgraduate training and experience in this field, certification as a specialist, and a state license permitting practice. Neurologists usually have received some training in psychiatry. Those who specialize in surgery are called neurosurgeons or neural surgeons. Consultation with and testing by a neurologist may be required for patients whose mental symptoms are suspected of being caused by an organic disease.

Clinical Psychologist

The **clinical psychologist** is a psychologist who diagnoses and treats emotional and behavioral disorders. The person may have any

---

K E E P I N G   F I T

When Does Depression Warrant Help?

According to the American Psychiatric Association, if you or someone you know has had four or more of the following symptoms for more than two weeks, help should be sought:
- change of appetite or weight
- change in sleeping patterns
- loss of interest in activities
- loss of energy or tiredness
- feelings of being worthless
- feelings of hopelessness
- feelings of inappropriate guilt
- problems with concentration, thinking, or decision making
- repeated thoughts of death
- overwhelming sadness
- disturbed thinking not based on reality
- physical symptoms such as stomachaches and headaches

Overcoming The Odds

Today, Dr. Warren A. Rhodes, a child psychologist, professor, and author, is a model of success. But it wasn't always that way. In fact, as a teen, he was a juvenile delinquent.

Rhodes started out in Baltimore, Maryland, where he lived with his parents and two siblings. He says, "Things were going well for me until the fifth grade when my mother's brother died. Two of his boys came to live with us. They fought with knives, skipped school, and eventually got in trouble with the law. One Christmas I got a lot of tips for selling papers. I hid the money in my sock to protect it from the people in my house who might steal it. While I was asleep, somebody cut the money out of my sock, and when I woke up, everybody was laughing about how they were slick enough to get my money. That's when I said if you can't beat 'em, join 'em."

"Joining them" took Rhodes onto a track that included failing sixth grade, failing eighth grade, and finally getting kicked out of school.

"I started shooting dope at 16." New at shooting, he almost killed himself accidentally by injecting air into his veins, but his brother stopped him. While still a teen, Rhodes was arrested three times.

Finally, a fight over a girl took Rhodes to his turning point. He says, "When someone broke up the fight, I told them I'd be back. I got my brother and 15 of his friends to go after those dudes. They were waiting for us. A shot

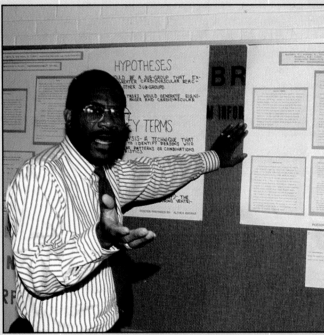

rang out. My brother was shot in the head near the temple. It grazed his head, but if his head had been turned differently, he could have died. That was the worst thing. I realized I had to change because, otherwise, I'd either be dead in a year or I'd kill somebody."

Rhodes signed up with the Job Corps where he stayed for eight months. "I got certificates for perfect attendance. Teachers saw something in me and kept encouraging me. Ultimately, I finished the pro-gram." He felt triumphant.

Rhodes then got a job and went to night school for three years to get his GED. He quit his job, determined that he'd go to college even if it took 20 years. "I didn't have great confidence. In fact, I thought I was dumb, but I would ask questions. To my surprise, I did very well."

He finally graduated from Morgan State College in Baltimore, got a fellowship to the University of Illinois that paid his way through graduate school, and went to the University of Mississippi Medical Center where he earned a postdoctoral degree in clinical child psychology.

These days, Rhodes is a professor at Delaware State College, where he focuses on kids who are in trouble with the juvenile justice system. He concludes, "We can never determine what's going to happen to a kid once he or she has become motivated." His advice to young people despite the tough odds they may have stacked against them: "Never give up. All things are possible."

1. At what point do you think Dr. Rhodes's self-esteem became positive?
2. How can turning one's pain into helping others increase a person's self-esteem?

Culture Shock

Culture shock occurs when people must function in a culture that is unfamiliar to them. Some people, like missionaries, business people, and anthropologists, move to other cultures to live. Even though they try to prepare, they find that ideas and behaviors are different. Everything seems "strange," such as the language, the food, and the way people act.

Culture shock may cause lack of appetite, inability to sleep, and stress. Fortunately, culture shock is usually a temporary problem. Humans are very flexible and, if they make the effort, can learn to understand and adapt to the new cultural rules. Humans can learn to function in many different cultural settings.

one of several college degrees: master of arts, master of science, doctor of philosophy in psychology, doctor of psychology, or doctor of education.

State law usually governs the title *psychologist*. Requirements include a doctoral degree, at least two years of supervised experience at a psychiatric hospital or clinic, and the passing of an examination.

The clinical psychologist can practice psychotherapy, group therapy, and individual counseling, in addition to testing for many kinds of specific mental disorders.

Educational Counselor

An educational counselor or school counselor is a person who generally works with young people, helping them in personal or educational matters. Counselors usually have a master's degree in counseling. They generally have special training in psychological testing, as well as in counseling students in a school or college setting. Some counselors address themselves to students' personal problems; others confine themselves to dealing with learning problems or assisting students in educational and vocational choices.

Pastoral Counselor

Informally, the clergy—ministers, priests, and rabbis—have been mental health practitioners for hundreds of years. A pastoral counselor helps people within the context of mental and social problems.

The American Association of Pastoral Counselors is a professional organization that has set standards for training and certification of individuals and institutions in the field of pastoral counseling. Today many members of the clergy receive formal education in counseling as part of their training. Those who are particularly interested in this aspect of their ministry usually take additional training.

Many members of the clergy provide counseling for couples and families.

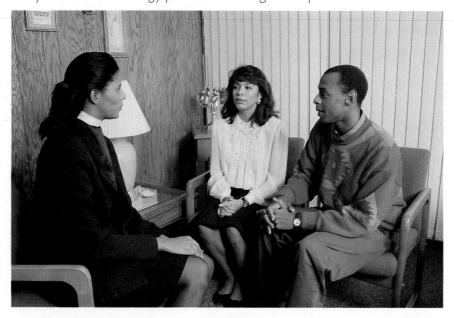

Social Worker

A social worker is a person who provides a link between the medical service center and the client and his or her family. The social worker has completed four years of college and two years of postgraduate study in a school of social work. A psychiatric or clinical social worker is one who has concentrated on psychiatric casework, doing fieldwork in a mental hospital, mental health clinic, or family service agency that provides guidance and treatment for clients with emotional problems.

A psychiatric social worker in a hospital maintains contact between patients and their families, serves as part of a treatment team (along with the psychiatrist, psychologist, nurses, and aides), helps the families understand and adjust to problems resulting from hospitalization, and supervises the rehabilitation of patients after they are released.

Occupational Therapist

The occupational therapist evaluates a person's abilities in light of his or her emotional or physical handicap. This person usually works in a psychiatric hospital or general hospital, conducting programs that involve work, recreation, and creative activities. An occupational therapist has completed a four-year college program with specialization in occupational therapy.

Behavioral Therapist

The behavioral therapist works with patients to help them change their habits. This technique is called behavioral therapy. This approach has become popular with people who want to give up smoking or drinking. The behavioral therapist also works with people who have phobias and other unreasonable fears. The behavioral therapist has completed a four-year college program, with further specialization in behavioral therapy.

LESSON 2 REVIEW

Reviewing Facts and Vocabulary

1. Select three mental health providers and create situations in which you would seek each for treatment or consultation.
2. Identify five signs of mental health problems.
3. Define the term *therapy*. List those therapies commonly used by a psychiatrist.

Thinking Critically

4. **Analysis.** Compare a psychiatrist with a neurologist.
5. **Synthesis.** Why might a psychologist refer a patient to a neurologist?

Applying Health Knowledge

6. After studying mental health disorders and different types of mental health professionals, create a Help Wanted ad that lists the personal qualities one would need to fill a position at a mental health clinic.
7. You have learned about support groups and how they can assist an individual. Develop an idea for a support group at your school. Identify the specific area of focus and why you think there is a need for this at your school.

Self-Inventory

Coping With Mental Disorders

HOW DO YOU RATE?

Number a sheet of paper from 1 through 20. Read each item below and respond by writing *agree* or *disagree* for each item. Then proceed to the next section.

1. Most people with mental disorders are not dangerous.
2. Most people with anxiety disorders should be hospitalized.
3. Most people who have been successfully treated for a mental disorder are usually able to hold down a job.
4. I would be embarrassed to tell my friends that someone in my family was suffering from a mental disorder.
5. Mental illness is sometimes incurable.
6. I feel that people with mental disorders are safer in clinics or institutions.
7. The media can help change people's negative views about mental disorders.
8. I have nothing in common with a person who has a mental disorder.
9. Mental illness is not the fault of the individual.
10. I would feel uncomfortable if a residence for people suffering from mental disorders was next door to my home.
11. I feel comfortable in the presence of someone with a mental disorder.
12. If I were an employer, I would not hire someone who had been treated for a mental disorder.
13. People with mental disorders have the same emotions as other people.
14. People who have recovered from a mental disorder are usually not interested in working.
15. People with mental disorders should not be discriminated against.
16. Anyone suffering from a mental disorder should not be out in public.
17. It is easy for me to see people with mental disorders as real people.
18. Those who have been treated for a mental disorder should live in a separate neighborhood.
19. Once a person suffers from a mental disorder, he or she can return to society and make many worthwhile contributions.
20. Mental illness is a problem only for those who have it.

HOW DID YOU SCORE?

Give yourself 1 point for each *agree* response to an odd-numbered item. Give yourself 1 point for each *disagree* response to an even-numbered item. Find your total to see how you scored. Then proceed to the next section.

18 to 20
Outstanding. You have a positive, healthful attitude about mental disorders.

12 to 17
Good. Although you have a good attitude about mental disorders, you could still make some improvements in your attitude toward mental illness.

Below 12
Needs Improvement. Your attitude toward those who have a mental disorder is an unhealthful one. It is time you know the facts about mental illness and consider a change in your attitude.

WHAT ARE YOUR GOALS?

If you received an *outstanding* or *good* score, complete the statements in Part A. If your score was rated *needs improvement,* complete Parts A and B.

Part A

1. I plan to learn more about mental disorders by ____.
2. My timetable for accomplishing this is ____.
3. I plan to share my information with others by ____.

Part B

4. The attitude or behavior toward those with a mental disorder that I would most like to change is ____.
5. The steps involved in making this change are ____.
6. The people or groups I will ask for support are ____.
7. My rewards for making this change will be ____.

Building Decision-Making Skills

Your good friend Victoria—a junior in high school and a popular classmate—committed suicide last night. The principal of your school is holding an emergency meeting with the teachers to determine how the school will handle this situation—with the students, with her friends, with her family, and with the community. What advice would you give the principal and the teachers?

WHAT DO YOU THINK?

1. **Choices.** What are several ways to help the students cope with this situation?

2. **Choices.** List several ways the school might help Victoria's friends cope with their loss.

3. **Choices.** Does the school have any responsibility toward Victoria's family?

4. **Choices.** Should the school get involved with the community in regard to this situation? If so, in what way?

5. **Consequences.** What are the advantages of each choice you listed in number 1?

6. **Consequences.** What are the disadvantages of each choice you listed in number 1?

7. **Consequences.** What will probably happen if the school takes no action?

8. **Decision.** What do you think the school should do to help Victoria's friends cope?

9. **Decision.** Do you think a different action is appropriate for the student body at large? Explain your answer.

10. **Evaluation.** Have you ever known someone who committed suicide? How did you feel? What helped you most as you coped with this loss?

Emily had a bad year last year. She had been depressed and experienced severe mood swings. Her friends were worried about her. Over the summer, Emily was treated by a psychiatrist. She is now on medication for a chemical imbalance. She is feeling much better, though she is embarrassed by her actions last year. It is now time to go back to school. Emily, her family, and her doctor are deciding what to tell other people about her condition.

WHAT DO YOU THINK?

11. **Situation.** What decisions need to be made by Emily?

12. **Situation.** Why do you think it is important for Emily to consider carefully exactly what she is going to say about her illness?

13. **Consequences.** How do you think her friends will react when they hear about this?

14. **Consequences.** How might her friends' reactions affect her recovery?

15. **Consequences.** How will her friends' reactions affect her self-esteem?

16. **Decision.** Who do you think should be told about this situation?

17. **Decision.** What should Emily tell each of the people you listed in number 16?

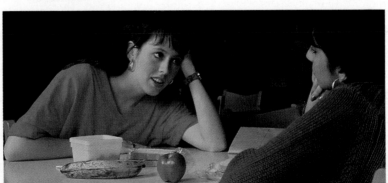

REVIEW

Using Health Terms

On a separate sheet of paper, write the term that best matches each definition given below.

LESSON 1

1. Disorders in which real or imagined fears prevent a person from enjoying life.
2. An extreme fear that causes a person to react in ways that limit normal functioning.
3. Persistent thoughts or ideas that keep people from thinking about other things.
4. An urgent need to repeat certain behaviors.
5. A condition in which a person who has lived through a traumatic event experiences severe and long-lasting aftereffects.
6. A preoccupation with the body and fear of imagined disease.
7. A type of mental disorder that is caused by a physical illness or injury that affects the brain.
8. A mental disorder characterized by feelings of sadness or hopelessness that lasts for more than a few weeks and interferes with daily activities and interests.

LESSON 2

9. A medical doctor who treats people with mental, emotional, and behavioral disorders of the mind.
10. A medical doctor who specializes in the treatment of organic disorders of the brain and nervous system.

Building Academic Skills

LESSON 1

11. **Reading.** Use the context clues in the following sentence to define *paranoid*.
    People with paranoid schizophrenic disorder mistrust others and are often suspicious.
12. **Math.** If schizophrenia affects 1 to 2 percent of the population, among a group of 1,000 people between the ages of 15 and 35, how many individuals are likely to be affected by schizophrenia?

Recalling the Facts

LESSON 1

13. What are the four main categories of functional disorders?
14. How do habits and compulsions differ?
15. What are three characteristics of a person with a general anxiety disorder?
16. Which of the following symptoms are characteristic of persons suffering from post-traumatic stress disorder?
    a. dreams about the event
    b. overeats
    c. can't sleep
    d. loses weight
    e. feels guilty
17. What is a somatoform disorder?
18. On which one of the following does an affective disorder have the most extreme effect: heart rate, sleeping patterns, moods, eating habits?
19. Write *good idea* or *not a good idea* for each suggestion below for handling potential suicides.
    a. Joke about it; don't take it seriously.
    b. Be willing to listen, but don't promise to keep it secret.
    c. Try to get the person to seek help.
    d. Don't dare or challenge the person.
    e. Give strong advice; tell the person what he or she is planning is wrong.
    f. Allow the person to express his or her feelings.
20. Name three types of personality disorders.

LESSON 2

21. Describe electroconvulsive therapy.
22. Which one of the following degrees is a clinical psychologist unlikely to have: master of science, doctor of psychology, doctor of medicine?
23. Which of the following mental health professionals can legally prescribe drugs: psychiatrist, neurologist, psychologist, social worker, educational counselor, pastoral counselor, occupational therapist, behavioral therapist?

REVIEW

Thinking Critically

LESSON 1

24. Evaluation. How do you think the stigma attached to mental illness could be eliminated?

25. Analysis. How are organic and functional disorders different?

26. Analysis. Compare three types of anxiety disorders and give an example of each.

27. Analysis. Compare the behavior of someone suffering from manic-depressive disorder with that of someone suffering from clinical depression.

28. Synthesis. Give an example of a passive-aggressive response on Joe's part to the following situation.

Joe is failing chemistry. So are four other students. Ms. Vronsky agrees to give them extra help every morning for an hour before school starts.

LESSON 2

29. Synthesis. After looking over the Self-Inventory on page 60, how would you describe the major challenges in coping with mental illness?

30. Synthesis. There are many types of mental health professionals. What common characteristics do they all share?

31. Evaluation. If you were to seek therapy from a psychiatrist, which of the therapies described in the text would you prefer? Which would you not want to consider?

32. Analysis. Compare and contrast the educational requirements and the responsibilities of an educational counselor, a pastoral counselor, and a social worker.

Making the Connection

LESSON 1

33. Language Arts. Read a synopsis of Shakespeare's *Romeo and Juliet* to explore the causes, futility, and tragedy of teenage suicide. Then write a less tragic ending.

Applying Health Knowledge

LESSON 1

34. Write *yes* for each statement below that might be a sign of an unhealthful mental attitude. Write *no* for each statement that indicates a healthful mental attitude.

  a. Jerry has asked me to the prom. This is the happiest day of my life.

  b. I don't think I did very well on the last biology quiz, but I'm going to study harder for the next one.

  c. I didn't get the job because I am female.

LESSON 2

35. If you want to be a psychiatrist, what is the minimum number of years of education and training you will need after you are graduated from high school?

36. A famous psychiatrist once said that the line between mental health and mental illness is a thin one that we cross over many times each day. How do you relate to that statement?

Beyond the Classroom

LESSON 1

37. Parental Involvement. Ask your parents if they know anyone who has suffered from any phobias during their lives. Ask them to tell you what they believe caused the phobia, how the individual conquered it or adjusted to it, and how it affected the individual's life.

38. Community Involvement. Investigate the resources in your community for suicide prevention. Find out what services are provided. Report your findings to the class.

39. Further Study. Read an article or watch a movie about the life of a person with multiple personalities. What caused this person's mental disorder? How did he or she cope with the disorder? What kind of professional help did he or she seek? Was it effective? What was the end result?

STRESS IN YOUR LIFE

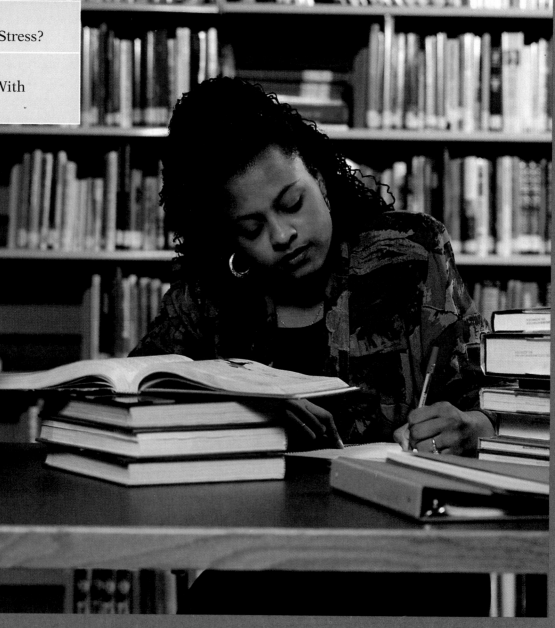

WHAT IS STRESS?

The word *stress* is used in many ways. To some people, it can mean an event that causes tension. It can mean a person's perception of an event or a response to a situation or demand on the body. Here, **stress** is defined as the body and mind's reactions to everyday demands. Stress requires the body to adjust so it can return to a normal state. The siren of an ambulance, the smell of fire, the hissing of a snake—all of these may cause the body to respond in a physical or psychological way. That response is different for each individual and may change for each situation.

Kinds of Stress

Stress is usually referred to in a negative sense. **Distress** is negative stress. Having too much stress, not knowing how to cope with stress, or experiencing a distressful situation causes distress. Having to play an away basketball game the night before a big test while a parent is ill at home can cause distress. Not all stress is bad. A certain amount of stress is necessary for life. As a matter of fact, experts say that moderate amounts of stress improve productivity. **Eustress** is positive stress. Eustress can help someone achieve his or her goals, such as studying for a test or working hard on a speech.

Factors Influencing Stress

Many reasons are given for the great variation in how well and how long people can hold up when feeling stress. Some people break down very quickly, while others endure for seemingly endless periods of time. What factors can you identify that might affect the way people respond to stressors? How might a person's life-style or attitude toward health affect his or her ability to endure stress?

The variation in the impact of a stressor on a person is related to the person's age, social status, income, state of health, diet, sleep habits, cultural background, and previous experience. Your response to a stressor also varies depending on how much control you think you have over a situation. If you feel you are helpless, the stress can be overwhelming.

What Is a Stressor?

Before looking at the problems related to stress, let us examine the relationship between stress and stressors. Imagine a bell sounding. Each time the bell sounds, you clench your fist. The sounding of the bell is known as a stressor. A **stressor** is any stimulus that produces a stress response. Stressors can be people, objects, places, or events. Think of some stressors you face during your day.

LESSON 1 FOCUS

TERMS TO USE
- Stress
- Distress
- Eustress
- Stressor
- Fatigue
- Chronic fatigue syndrome
- Psychosomatic (SY•KOH•SUH•MAT•IHK)

CONCEPTS TO LEARN
- A certain amount of stress is necessary for life.
- Stress can affect your mental, physical, and social health.

ATTITUDES AND BEHAVIORS TO EVALUATE
- Self-Inventory, page 78.
- Building Decision-Making Skills, page 79.

The clenching of your fist each time the bell rings is stress, or your response to that stressor. In this case, the response is voluntary; that is, you have conscious control over it. You can notice the tension in your fist as you clench it.

The stress response that takes place inside your body is involuntary. Sometimes we are completely unaware of the changes that occur. Other reactions, however, we can notice.

Have you ever been unable to sleep the night before a big event? Have you ever had knots in your stomach before a big game or a speech? Has your throat ever become dry when you were being confronted with a problem? All of these reactions were involuntary.

How the body responds to a stressor depends largely on how the individual perceives the stressor. What is stressful for one person may be a source of relaxation for another.

The Body's Response to Stressors

Two major body systems are active in the body's response to stressors: the nervous system and the endocrine system. You will study the nervous system and the endocrine system in Chapter 12, but here is some information on how these systems influence reactions to stressors.

The physical changes that are a part of stress begin in the hypothalamus, a nerve center in the brain, and a part of the endocrine system. When the hypothalamus is excited by a stressor, a complex series of changes takes place in the body. The result is a change in the functioning of almost every part of the body.

Nerve centers in the hypothalamus regulate some functions of the autonomic nervous system, the system that controls involuntary actions. Some of the nerves activate the pituitary gland. The pituitary gland secretes a hormone that stimulates the adrenal glands. The adrenal glands produce and secrete a hormone, called adrenaline, which prepares a person for a "fight or flight" response. Adrenaline is known as the "emergency" hormone.

Because of adrenaline, the heart speeds up its activity, providing more blood for the brain and muscles. Breathing becomes faster and deeper, providing more oxygen to the body. Saliva and mucus dry up, increas-

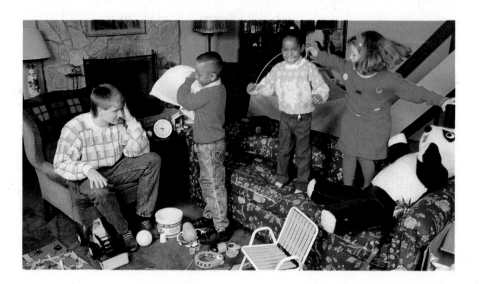

Stress increases when you feel out of control.

The Effects of Stress on the Body

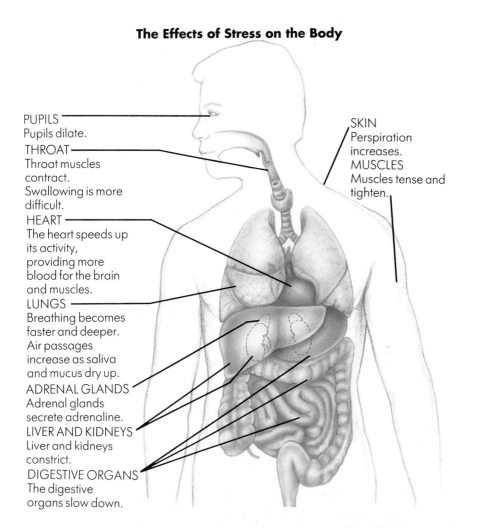

PUPILS
Pupils dilate.

THROAT
Throat muscles contract. Swallowing is more difficult.

HEART
The heart speeds up its activity, providing more blood for the brain and muscles.

LUNGS
Breathing becomes faster and deeper. Air passages increase as saliva and mucus dry up.

ADRENAL GLANDS
Adrenal glands secrete adrenaline.

LIVER AND KIDNEYS
Liver and kidneys constrict.

DIGESTIVE ORGANS
The digestive organs slow down.

SKIN
Perspiration increases.

MUSCLES
Muscles tense and tighten.

Many body organs respond to stressors.

ing the size of the air passages to the lungs. Throat muscles may contract, making swallowing difficult. Perspiration increases, helping to cool the body. Muscles tense and tighten to prepare the body for action. The pupils dilate. Other body functions, such as digestion, are suspended to conserve energy.

All of these changes take place when we are faced with something we perceive to be a stressor. Once the stressor has been dealt with, the body returns to normal. However, in cases where the stressor is prolonged or not dealt with, the body continues to work at the stimulated level. After a period of time, the body becomes exhausted. It becomes more susceptible to illness and accidents.

KEEPING FIT

Avoiding the Perfectionist Trap

Perfectionists have many characteristics in common. These include wanting their work to be better than everyone else's, being competitive even in noncompetitive situations, always looking for mistakes and ways to improve, not being really satisfied by the praise they've worked for once they get it, going to any lengths to avoid mistakes, and feeling overly ashamed by even minor mistakes. Perfectionists may also procrastinate, be indecisive, play it safe, or do one part of a task over and over until it is perfect.

If any of these characteristics describe you, perhaps it's time to work on accepting that you are just human. Everyone makes mistakes.

Overcoming The Odds

Marci is 17. A little over a year ago she tried to commit suicide. Since then, she has been in therapy and in a suicide survivor's group. These days she'd tell you she's grateful to be alive, but it hasn't been an easy journey. She says, "This is all really hard to talk about, but I guess I want to help anyone out there who may be facing the same kinds of stuff I faced. I guess you could say there have always been tensions in my family. I love them and all, but there was a lot of fighting along the way. Then my parents got divorced and my mom got remarried. When my dad remarried, it just felt like I didn't belong anywhere anymore. Even then, I didn't lose it in a big way until my cousin Paul. . . ."

Marci gets quiet. She is talking about Paul, her 18-year-old cousin, who committed suicide 2 years ago. "He was like a brother I never had. I knew he was in trouble, but I didn't know how badly. He was doing drugs. He painted and drew all kinds of weird pictures toward the end, and my aunt says he stayed in his room a lot, but I had no idea. One tip-off, looking back, is that he gave me our great-grandfather's stopwatch—this

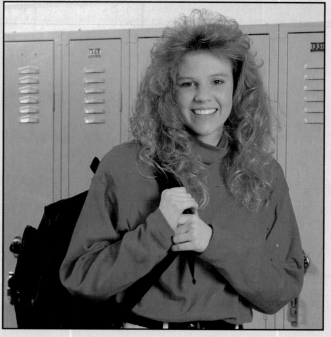

beautiful watch we always joked about his getting because he was the oldest cousin and hardly ever on time. I guess I should have known. Anyway, one weekend when his parents were out, he committed suicide in his garage. My uncle found him in his car.

"After that I just couldn't hold it together," Marci says. "I felt completely alone, like I was falling into this deep hole without a bottom. It felt like my parents didn't understand, that no one could understand, and there was no sense to anything any more. I saw what the pain was doing to Paul's family, but I got beyond caring. I was sleeping a lot, dropped out of stuff at school, and couldn't concentrate. All I can tell you is I felt incredibly bad, and then my boyfriend left me, and that did it. I took all these pills I'd been collecting. I don't even know if I cared if they found me or not, but they did, and now I'm grateful. I am incredibly grateful. I cry just thinking about it. I wish Paul had the same second chance."

For the last few months, Marci and her family have been getting professional help. "I guess we're getting a lot out in the open that needed to get out. I realize that those terrifying dark times do get better. I'm feeling better all the time. I don't feel so alone any more.

"I really want to say to any teen who's thinking about suicide, don't do it. Please. Things will get better. Trust me. They really will."

1. What factors led to Paul's suicide? To Marci's attempt? How did Paul's suicide affect her?
2. What signs of being in trouble did each display?
3. If you or someone you know has ever seriously thought about suicide, what lessons from Marci's story might you be able to apply? What message does her story give about getting help?

ADOLESCENT LIFE-CHANGE EVENT SCALE

The Social Readjustment Rating Scale

Life Events	Mean Value	Life Events	Mean Value
1. Getting married	101	23. Breaking up with boyfriend or girlfriend	53
2. Unwed pregnancy	92	24. Beginning to date	51
3. Death of parent	87	25. Suspension from school	50
4. Acquiring a visible deformity	81	26. Birth of a brother or sister	50
5. Divorce of parents	77	27. Increase in number of arguments with parents	47
6. Fathering an unwed pregnancy	77	28. Increase in number of arguments between parents	46
7. Becoming involved with drugs or alcohol	76	29. Loss of job by parent	46
8. Jail sentence of parent for one year or more	75	30. Outstanding personal achievement	46
9. Marital separation of parents	69	31. Change in parents' financial status	45
10. Death of a brother or sister	68	32. Being accepted at a college of your choice	43
11. Change in acceptance by peers	67	33. Beginning senior high school	42
12. Pregnancy of unwed sister	64	34. Serious illness requiring hospitalization of sibling	41
13. Discovery of being an adopted child	64	35. Change in father's or mother's occupation requiring increased absence from home	38
14. Marriage of parent to stepparent	63	36. Brother or sister leaving home	37
15. Death of a close friend	63	37. Death of a grandparent	36
16. Having a visible congenital deformity	62	38. Addition of third adult to family (i.e. grandparent)	34
17. Serious illness requiring hospitalization	58	39. Becoming a full fledged member of a church	31
18. Failure of a grade in school	56	40. Decrease in number of arguments between parents	27
19. Move to a new school district	56	41. Decrease in number of arguments with parents	26
20. Not making an extracurricular activity you wanted	55	42. Mother or father beginning to work	26
21. Serious illness requiring hospitalization of a parent	55		
22. Jail sentence of parent for 30 days or more	53		

Fatigue—It Is Not All Physical

Many illnesses and conditions have been linked to stress. One of the most common conditions is that of **fatigue**—a tired feeling that lowers your level of activity. Fatigue affects all levels of your health—physical, mental, and social. It interferes with work, school, relationships, and recreation. It affects your ability to successfully manage stress. It affects your general feeling of well-being.

Physical Fatigue

You have probably experienced one type of fatigue—physical fatigue, which is fatigue of the body in general. It occurs at the end of the day when the body signals a need for rest and sleep. It also occurs during exercise when the body produces waste products in the form of lactic acid from the muscles and carbon dioxide from all of the body's cells. A buildup of wastes in the muscles can produce soreness. When these wastes reach a certain level in the blood, the brain receives a message,

Scoring:

● If your total is below 150, you have a low stress level and your life has been stable in most areas.

● If your total is between 150 and 300, you have a moderate stress level and there has been a lot of change in your life.

● If your total is over 300, you have a high stress level and there have been major adjustments in your life.

and your activity level drops. Physical fatigue can build up to a point where the body cannot take any more effort.

The best solution for physical fatigue is rest. If getting regular periods of rest does not revive you, you might need to look for another cause of your fatigue.

Pathological Fatigue

A second kind of fatigue is pathological fatigue, which is fatigue brought on by the overworking of the body's defenses for fighting disease. When a disease does develop, your body becomes overworked trying to fight the disease and, at the same time, trying to keep you going. The result is fatigue.

The common cold, the flu, and anemia are all examples of illnesses brought on by pathological fatigue. Being overweight and having a poor diet are also causes of pathological fatigue. This type of fatigue is the body's way of warning you that it is not well and that you need to rest and care for yourself.

Psychological Fatigue

The third and most common type of fatigue is psychological fatigue, which is brought on by mental stress. Almost everyone experiences this type of fatigue. Depression, boredom, worry about schoolwork, home, dates, how you look, and being liked—all of these can cause fatigue. Trying to do too many activities and having conflicts also can cause it. Lack of exercise, which means that your body does not circulate oxygen fast enough, can also be a factor in psychological fatigue.

Unlike the answer to the other two types of fatigue, rest is not the answer to psychological fatigue; setting your priorities is. Choose activities such as exercise that promote your health. If fatigue continues, take a closer look at the source of it. Is there a problem you need to address? Perhaps you need to set a goal for changing a certain behavior. Perhaps you just need to talk to someone. Try to find out what is at the root of your fatigue. That is the first step toward eliminating it.

Remember, fatigue is your body's way of warning you that something is wrong. You risk further health problems by merely covering up the symptoms.

If you are not sure what kind of fatigue you are experiencing, examine what you were doing and how you were feeling before you got tired. Strong negative feelings can cause fatigue. So can worrying about something that is in your near future.

Chronic Fatigue Syndrome (CFS)

A new type of fatigue has been identified in the last few years. It is called **chronic fatigue syndrome (CFS).** The cause of this new disorder is unknown, and it is very difficult to diagnose.

The Centers for Disease Control and Prevention has identified these symptoms of the disease:

- persistent severe fatigue for at least six months
- mild fever and sore throat

- headaches and joint pains
- muscle weakness and pain
- sleep problems
- difficulty in thinking clearly
- fatigue after light exercise

There are many unanswered questions about CFS and how to treat it. Any long-term fatigue is a good reason for a medical checkup.

The Effects of Stress on Health

It is easy to look at stress in purely physical terms because the body's physical response to a stressor can be felt and seen. In recent years, however, the stress response has been associated with situations involving mental health. Situations causing anxiety, frustration, or tension trigger the stress response and can lead to the development of physical ailments. The term **psychosomatic,** involving both the mind and the body, is used to describe such illnesses.

A number of diseases, including cardiovascular disease, hypertension, asthma, ulcers, colitis, and migraine headaches, are thought to be related in some way to stress. In some cases stress seems to be a contributing factor in all of these diseases. However, it is hard to identify stress as the major factor because so many other factors can be involved.

One point is certain. There is increasing evidence that emotions cause physical reactions, which, over time, may be damaging to the body.

Stress has more than just a physical effect on the body. People feeling stress may not think as clearly as usual. Stress has been linked to accidents and injuries. People under stress may take more risks and may be less careful with their health. Stress also can affect your social health. When a person feels stress, he or she may not feel like being with others or may be impatient with them. If the effects of stress continue over time, relationships may suffer.

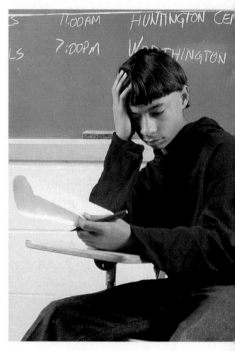

If this student had studied harder for this test, he probably wouldn't be feeling so stressed.

LESSON 1 REVIEW

Reviewing Facts and Vocabulary

1. Define *stress*. Why is stress necessary for life?
2. Give an example of an involuntary response to a stressor.
3. Define *stressor*. Give an example of a person, situation, and thought that could serve as a stressor.

Thinking Critically

4. **Analysis.** How might a person's response to a stressor affect his or her health?

5. **Analysis.** How might stress affect an individual's mental health? Social health?
6. **Analysis.** Compare eustress and distress, giving examples of each.
7. **Analysis.** Explain what makes the stress response such an individualized one.

Applying Health Knowledge

8. Give examples of at least five positive and negative stressors in your life. Discuss how they may or may not affect your health.

COPING WITH STRESS

LESSON 2 FOCUS

TERMS TO USE

- Time-management skills
- Defense mechanisms

CONCEPTS TO LEARN

- Practicing good health habits can help you cope with stress.
- Time is a major factor in stress management.
- Defense mechanisms are used to help deal with stressful situations in life.
- All of us manage stress, either successfully or unsuccessfully.

ATTITUDES AND BEHAVIORS TO EVALUATE

- Self-Inventory, page 78.
- Building Decision-Making Skills, page 79.

Although it is true that some stressors are good, even motivating, your body cannot distinguish between positive and negative sources of stress. The body's response is the same. You will need to identify the stressors in your life and learn to manage them. You can do this by following these guidelines:

- Identify your own sources of stress, and examine your methods of coping.
- Make conscious choices that help control the amount of stress you experience.
- Develop and use coping and relaxation techniques to diffuse the tension that builds up excess stress.
- Practice good health habits daily.

What is the relationship between health, fitness, and the ability to cope? Stress researchers believe that people who choose a healthful diet, get plenty of sleep, and exercise regularly are better able to cope with daily stress. When the unexpected does occur, a healthy body is better able to respond appropriately and efficiently.

Are you aware of your own needs, your anxieties, your motivations, and your goals? The better you know yourself, the better able you are to identify and manage stress-producing situations and your typical responses to stressors.

Personality Types

Several years ago two doctors developed a theory about personality types and their relationship to stress. You may have heard someone described as a type A or type B personality. Doctors Friedman and

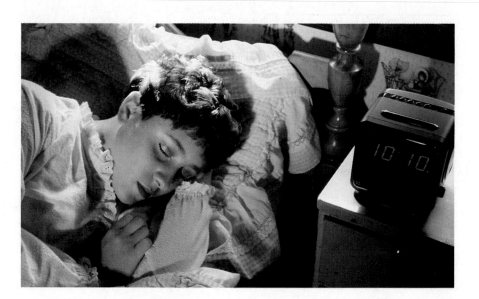

Good health habits help you cope with stress.

Rosenman have described these two personality types primarily on the basis of behavioral patterns.

Type A personalities seem to be more competitive, rushed, and time-oriented. Type B personalities appear to be more flexible and less rushed. While not wholly accurate, the theory is still a useful model.

Most people have characteristics of both type A and type B personalities. Think about your personality patterns. In different situations you may take on different characteristics. When you have a deadline for a paper, you may take on characteristics of a type A personality. When your homework is finished, and you are relaxing with friends, you may show a type B personality. Neither type A nor B determines intelligence, ambition, or success. Nor is one better than the other.

By being aware of your personality type, you can help eliminate some of your stress. Knowing how you respond to certain stress-producing situations can motivate you to plan ahead.

Time Management

In any discussion of stress, we must consider time. Time is a major factor in relieving stress. People who manage their time well are better able to control stress in their lives. They look at time as an ally and not as an opponent. How do you look at time? What are your **time-management skills**—your effective ways of arranging your time? Check yourself on the following behaviors:

- Are you always rushing?
- Do you bounce back and forth between unpleasant alternatives?
- Do you have trouble finding things?
- Do you find yourself tired from hours of nonproductive activity?
- Do you find you do not have enough time for rest or for personal relationships in your life?
- Do you regularly miss deadlines?
- Are you overwhelmed by demands and details?
- Do you find yourself doing several tasks at a time?
- Do you have trouble deciding what to do next?

If you answered yes to six or more of these questions, you may need to work on managing your time better.

Some people have difficulty managing their lives because they do not have good time-management skills. Part of this problem occurs because of a person's inability to say *no* to others. Sometimes you may be afraid to say *no* because it might offend someone. Perhaps you are afraid of what the other person will do if you say *no*. Saying *yes* to virtually anything that is proposed to you says that you have not established your priorities. It may also show that you do not think you are important. When you do not want to do something or have much to do, know when to say no. Make choices that help you do the tasks you must do to achieve your goals. This shows you can manage your life.

Defense Mechanisms

At times everyone uses **defense mechanisms,** which are strategies to deal with stressful situations. Defense mechanisms contribute to emotional health by providing relief from anxiety and helping someone cope

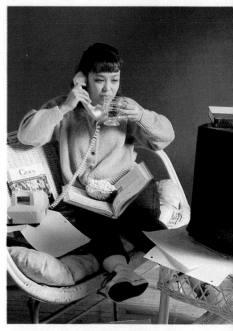

Trying to do many things at one time is not a good way of managing time—or reducing stress.

DID YOU KNOW?

- A yawn doesn't always mean you're tired; a sigh doesn't always mean you're in love. Sometimes these phenomena simply mean that your body is relieving itself of stress.
- Most workers in Europe get four to six weeks of vacation.
- In Australia, workers get four weeks of vacation and also receive a salary bonus during those weeks.
- In the U.S. the standard vacation time is two weeks per year.

with problems. However, too much dependence on them can lead to avoidance in facing the problems of day-to-day life.

The following are common defense mechanisms:

- **Denial.** Refusal to accept reality. Carol's pet dog has died. She had had the dog since she was a small child. Carol refuses to accept the dog's death. She refuses to talk about it and continues to act as if her dog is alive.

- **Escape, or fantasy.** Running away from a problem through day-dreams, books, and excessive sleep. Jim has failed to make the basketball team. He imagines that he is suffering from some hidden physical problem. When others find out about his problem, they will view his effort to make the basketball team as a success, rather than as a failure.

- **Rationalization.** An attempt to justify one's actions with an excuse rather than by admitting one's failure or mistake. Anne justifies flunking her math test because she was absent the day it was scheduled.

- **Projection.** An attempt to protect one's self-esteem by blaming unpleasant feelings or inappropriate actions on others. Getting poor grades and blaming it on the teacher's dislike for you is an example of evading personal responsibility.

- **Repression.** Blocking out thoughts about unpleasant things or experiences—forgetting on purpose. Repression is actually an unconscious method of escaping something unpleasant. You may have chores to do this weekend while your parents are away. You simply do not think about any of your responsibilities so that you can enjoy your weekend of fun with friends.

- **Identification.** Acting like or modeling one's behavior after a person one likes. Identification is a form of hero worship. However, it can take another form. People who have had a similar achievement or experience may identify with one another, sharing in something they all have in common.

- **Displacement.** Expressing feelings toward someone or something not associated with the source of the feelings. Suzanna is upset because she did not get picked for the team. When her sister greets her at home, Suzanna gives her a shove, says "Leave me alone," and slams the door to her room.

- **Regression.** Retreating to an earlier time that seems less threatening and requires less responsibility. Paul is having trouble adjusting to high school, with its challenges, greater number of students, and new atmosphere. He goes back and visits his former teachers and principal in junior high school, and entertains the idea that it would be nice to stay there.

- **Compensation.** An attempt to make up for something one did not have, or did not receive. Paul is not very good at basketball, but he is a first-rate swimmer.

- **Sublimation.** Transforming unacceptable behaviors into acceptable ones. Sublimation can involve redirecting specific behaviors. Jack is always fighting with people. He redirects this energy as a member of the wrestling team.

Managing Stress

You may not be able to control some stressors. However, you can control the effect you allow them to have on you. Five major ways to manage stress are planning, laughing, rechanneling your energy, learning to relax, and calling on your support system.

Planning

Planning is a major key to managing stress effectively. People who handle stress plan well, yet they know that even with the best plans, other things can happen to change those plans. By recognizing that changes can and often do occur, especially when other people are involved, people are better able to deal with changes, disappointments, frustrations, delays, or whatever might take place.

You further manage stress by being realistic about your plans and your expectations. Learn to anticipate the unexpected. Sometimes this simply means thinking ahead. Rather than concentrating on and living from moment to moment, think ahead to know what you might expect.

Of course, as in the case of each of these strategies, great variation exists. Some people spend so much time planning and anticipating what might happen that they do not enjoy the actual activity. This can be as stressful a situation as not planning at all. You have to decide what works for you.

Laughing

Another effective way to deal with stress is to laugh. There is the story of the little boy on his bicycle who went over a bump on the sidewalk and took a tumble. He got up, brushed himself off, and then burst out laughing.

Culturally Speaking

Working and Playing Worldwide

- According to a German publication called *Der Arbeitgeber*, or *The Employer*, the average employee in France works 33.8 hours per week, while the average worker in Great Britain works 34.1 hours per week; in Switzerland, 36 hours per week, in the U.S., 36.3 hours, and in Japan, 36.8 hours.

- In Japan, new attention is being paid to the importance of relaxation for better overall productivity and health. In fact, the National Recreation Association of Japan now offers training sessions for people to become leisure counselors, helping people to learn how and where to have fun and relax.

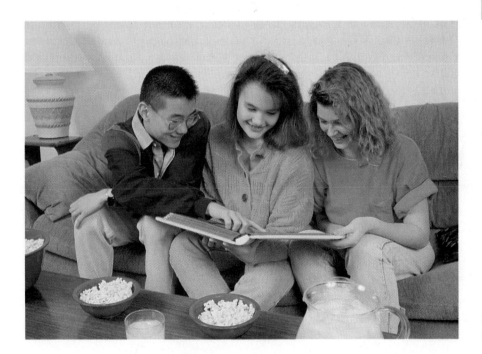

Laughing and relaxing help you relieve stress.

A man passing by, who saw no fun in the scraped knee and elbow, asked, "What's so funny? Why are you laughing?" The boy replied, "Mister, I'm laughing so I won't cry." Laughter can be a relief when things have gone wrong. By laughing, you accept the reality that you are human and realize that sometimes unfortunate things happen.

By laughing, you release the stress that builds up when things go wrong. This does not mean that you do not care about what happened. It simply means that you have chosen a healthful way to deal with the stress of that particular situation.

Rechanneling Your Energy

Transferring or rechanneling your energy is another way to manage stress. If you find that a situation is causing you to become tense, you might transfer your energy to some other activity—washing a car, taking a walk, cleaning your room, or just taking a break.

If you cannot physically get away from the situation, give your mind a break. Let it wander for a few minutes. Daydreaming can be an excellent stress reducer. Of course, be sure to know and use appropriate times to relax. Daydreaming when you are supposed to be taking notes or taking a test in class can be a source of added stress.

Learning to Relax

One effective way of relieving stress is physical exercise. It burns pent-up energy and clears the mind, allowing you to relax. Choose exercise you enjoy and do it in a peaceful environment. Choose a setting that prevents more stress from developing.

Calling on Your Support Group

A support group can help greatly in managing stress. What is a support group? *Support* means "to hold up." There are times when things get very difficult for you, and your energy and strength are worn down. On such occasions it is important for you to have a support system and to use it.

The supportive people in your life may include family, friends, a church leader, teachers, or employers. A strong support system might

KEEPING FIT

Avoid Getting "Testy" Over Tests

Studying for and taking tests can be very stressful. Consider these helpful hints:

- Use 2-hour blocks of time, then take a half-hour break, then return to work.
- Become aware of the messages you give yourself about your ability to take tests.
- Before taking the test, take the time to physically and mentally relax.
- First answer all the questions you are sure of. Then go back and answer the ones that are more difficult.
- Make an outline for any essay questions on a test.
- Remind yourself that tests are learning tools meant to help you improve.

HEALTH UPDATE

LOOKING AT TECHNOLOGY

Biofeedback

When you are stressed out, your body reacts. Your pulse races, your muscles tighten, and your hands sweat. One device—the biofeedback machine—monitors these bodily changes and shows them to the person hooked up to the machine. The machine may read brain waves, changes in the electricity and temperature of the skin, or muscle tension. It then "feeds back" information about the person's level of tension or relaxation by moving a temperature indicator, by emitting a certain tone, or by flashing lights. By showing a person what happens when he or she is stressed or relaxed, the person develops a greater awareness of what each state feels like and what physical signs indicate each one. With practice and by learning various relaxation techniques, the person can then learn to "tune in" to a more relaxed state. Once the person has learned to stop the beeping tone or slow down the flashing lights with his or her own relaxation response, the machine will no longer be needed.

include several of these people. This puts less pressure on any one person. It also reduces the problem of depending on only one person for some assistance and discovering that that person is not available at the time help is needed. Building a strong support system is perhaps one of the most important strategies for managing stress.

LESSON 2 REVIEW

Reviewing Facts and Vocabulary

1. Define the term *time-management skills*.
2. Which personality type—type A or type B—is more prone to stress? Explain.

Thinking Critically

3. **Synthesis.** How can setting priorities be an effective way of managing stress?
4. **Analysis.** Compare five defense mechanisms, giving an example of each.
5. **Evaluation.** Are there circumstances when being a type A personality is preferred over being a type B personality? Explain.

Applying Health Knowledge

6. Keep a journal of highly stressful situations at school, and record how you and others respond in those situations. Draw conclusions about the most effective ways to cope with stress.
7. On a sheet of paper list as many expressions as possible that include the word *time*. For example, "Time flies when you're having fun," "Time out," "Time is up." Choose one of these expressions and draw an illustration that shows a way you practice time management.

Self-Inventory

Stress—The Danger Signals

HOW DO YOU RATE?

Number a sheet of paper from 1 through 25. Read each item below and respond by writing *yes* or *no* for each item. Then proceed to the next section.

1. I am aware of when I am tense.
2. I try to be perfect at everything I do.
3. I like to work with others on projects.
4. I try to do everything right. If I cannot do something right, I do not do it at all.
5. I avoid eating on the run.
6. I have trouble expressing anger.
7. I offer help to others even when I get no personal gain from it.
8. I get angry with others easily.
9. I feel that my problems are no worse than anyone else's.
10. I am usually in a hurry.
11. I finish one thing before I start another.
12. I tend to do things the way I have always done them.
13. When I start making mistakes, I take a break from the task for a while.
14. It is hard for me to wait in lines.
15. It is easy for me to relax.
16. Things do not move fast enough for me.
17. When I have a problem, I like to share it with others.
18. I have trouble sleeping at night.
19. I use physical activity to help reduce my stress.
20. I can usually figure out what people are going to say before they say it.
21. I can laugh at myself when I make mistakes.
22. I find myself thinking about the next thing that I have to do while I am in the middle of something else.
23. I cry when I am hurt.
24. I keep my problems to myself.
25. I can enjoy what I am doing even before it is completely finished.

HOW DID YOU SCORE?

Give yourself 1 point for each *yes* response to an odd-numbered item. Give yourself 1 point for each *no* response to an even-numbered item. Find your total to see how you scored. Then proceed to the next section.

21 to 25
Excellent. You manage stress very well. Keep it up!

16 to 20
Very Good. You have a low-stress life-style.

11 to 15
Fair. You have low stress in some areas, but high stress in others. You need to make some changes in order to be a better stress manager.

Below 11
Needs Improvement. You do not handle stress well. This will have a negative impact on both your physical and mental health.

WHAT ARE YOUR GOALS?

If you received an *excellent* or *very good* score, complete the statements in Part A. If your score was *fair* or *needs improvement*, complete the statements in Parts A and B.

Part A

1. I plan to learn more about stress management by ____.
2. My timetable for accomplishing this is ____.
3. I plan to share my information with others by ____.

Part B

4. The behavior or attitude toward stress I would most like to change is ____.
5. The steps involved in making this change are ____.
6. My rewards for making this change will be ____.

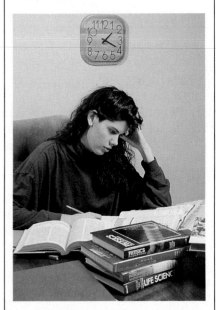

Building Decision-Making Skills

Marty is a 6′5″, 275-pound lineman whose speed makes him one of the top recruits in his state as he heads into his senior year. Currently he has a 2.5 GPA (out of a possible 4.0) in his school's college-preparatory core curriculum. His GPA is above the required 2.0 for an athletic scholarship. Marty's second set of ACT scores arrived in today's mail. He is very upset and depressed because his composite score of 15 is not high enough to qualify him for the athletic scholarship he's been offered. Although Marty's grades have always been above average, he has never done very well with standardized tests. He just doesn't seem to be able to handle the anxiety of those testing situations. What should Marty do?

WHAT DO YOU THINK?

1. **Situation.** Where might Marty get accurate information on which to base this decision?

2. **Situation.** What do you think causes Marty's anxiety: heredity, not being prepared, or some other factor?

3. **Choices.** What choices does Marty have?

4. **Consequences.** List the advantages of each choice.

5. **Consequences.** What are the disadvantages of each choice?

6. **Consequences.** What are the financial implications of this situation?

7. **Consequences.** How will each of these choices affect Marty's self-esteem?

8. **Decision.** What do you think Marty should do?

9. **Decision.** How should Marty respond to those who ask about his scores—friends, coaches, and the media?

Juanita and Allison have been good friends since elementary school. They live in the same neighborhood, hang out with the same group of friends, and even take the same courses in school. Last Saturday they spent the day at the local mall looking for the "perfect outfit" for their school's holiday dance. Juanita found her outfit early on. Allison, however, continued to try on many things only to find that with each outfit something just wasn't right. Either the color didn't work or her size wasn't available. Finally, in the last store, Allison found just what she was looking for. Juanita, too, thought it was perfect, and she left the fitting room to browse while Allison was getting dressed. When Allison came out of the dressing room she was carrying a package, but not the outfit. Juanita said, "Hey, where's your outfit?" Allison replied, "Oh, I decided not to spend the money."

The following weekend was the holiday dance and Juanita and Allison were double-dating. When Juanita picked up Allison she came out of her house wearing the new outfit. When Juanita asked her if she'd gone back to the store to get it Allison whispered, "Oh, I'm just borrowing it. That store will never know." What should Juanita do?

WHAT DO YOU THINK?

10. **Situation.** What decision does Juanita need to make?

11. **Choices.** What are Juanita's choices?

12. **Consequences.** What are the advantages and disadvantages of each choice?

13. **Consequences.** How might this decision affect Juanita and Allison's friendship?

14. **Consequences.** If Juanita does nothing, how may her self-esteem be affected?

15. **Consequences.** If Juanita confronts Allison and gets her to see her error, what action might Juanita expect Allison to take?

16. **Decision.** How do you think Juanita should handle this situation?

17. **Decision.** If Juanita decides to confront Allison, how and where should the confrontation take place?

Using Health Terms

On a separate sheet of paper, write the term that best matches each definition given below.

LESSON 1

1. The body's general reaction to everyday demands.
2. A nerve center in the brain that initiates physical changes associated with stress and is part of the endocrine system.
3. The "emergency" hormone.
4. A tired feeling that lowers a person's level of activity.
5. A type of fatigue that lasts for a long period of time and seems to have no identifiable cause.
6. A word used to describe physical ailments that seem to be triggered by the stress response.

LESSON 2

7. A personality type characterized by competitiveness and a desire to be active and busy.
8. A personality type characterized by a flexible and easygoing attitude toward life.
9. The things that are most important to an individual.
10. Strategies a person uses to deal with stressful situations.

Building Academic Skills

LESSON 1

11. **Math.** It is estimated that two-thirds of all office visits to family doctors are a result of stress-related symptoms. Using this figure, if a doctor sees 21 patients each day for 3 days, how many patients have stress-related symptoms?

LESSON 2

12. **Writing.** Write a paragraph explaining whether you think you are a type A or type B personality. Use details and examples to support your evaluation of your own personality type.

Recalling the Facts

LESSON 1

13. In what ways can stress be good?
14. List five factors that are related to the effect stressors have on a person's life.
15. How do voluntary stress responses differ from involuntary stress responses?
16. What two major body systems participate in the body's response to stressors?
17. What gland secretes a hormone that stimulates the adrenal gland to secrete adrenaline?
18. What is the best remedy for physical fatigue?
19. List three illnesses that can be brought on by pathological fatigue.
20. What are three causes of psychological fatigue?
21. List three ways to overcome psychological fatigue.
22. Name three conditions that can contribute to psychosomatic illnesses.

LESSON 2

23. How does the body distinguish between positive and negative stress?
24. List three strategies for managing stress and describe them.
25. What are three defense mechanisms people use to deal with stressful situations?
26. What theory regarding personality types was developed by Friedman and Rosenman? How does their theory relate to stress?
27. What does the phrase "Know when to say no" have to do with managing your time?
28. Explain how the management of time is related to a person's stress level.
29. What are some behaviors characteristic of a person who is using the defense mechanism of escape, or fantasy?
30. How might a person who is using the defense mechanism of projection behave if he or she gets a low grade on a test?
31. List five main ways to manage stress.
32. How can exercise help one manage stress?
33. What is a support system?

REVIEW

Thinking Critically

LESSON 1

34. **Synthesis.** Terri feels tired all the time. She has trouble sleeping at night. She cannot concentrate in school. She is having a lot of headaches, and her muscles and joints feel sore. Just walking up a flight of stairs exhausts her. She thinks she may have the flu. What might Terri's problem be, and what should she do?

LESSON 2

35. **Evaluation.** What are the limitations of trying to classify people according to personality types?

36. **Synthesis.** Which defense mechanism is each of the following people using?
    - Bob has an aggressive personality. He is always getting into fights with the other boys in the neighborhood. He decides to try out for the football team.
    - Rosita does not believe she can pass the algebra test on Monday. She spends the entire weekend reading novels instead of studying.
    - Harold missed several easy shots during the basketball game on Tuesday night. He tells his friends that the coach has not let him play enough in previous games.
    - Judy's best friend has begun taking ballet lessons. Although Judy has no interest in ballet, she has enrolled in a ballet class.
    - Matt tried out for the lead in the school play. Jeff got the part. When Matt got home, he slammed the door to his room.

Making the Connection

LESSON 1

37. **Music.** Many contemporary songs express themes of alienation, frustration, loneliness, interpersonal conflict, and other stressful emotions. Listen to two or three songs of various styles with these themes. Include rhythm and blues, country and western, and rap. Compare and contrast each artist's interpretation of these themes.

Applying Health Knowledge

LESSON 1

38. You have probably given some thought to the kind of job you would like to have when you finish school. Name three jobs you think would be highly stressful and explain why. Name three jobs you think would have low stress levels and explain why.

LESSON 2

39. Make a pie graph illustrating the percentages of time you spend on daily activities. Think about the following activities and include the ones that apply to your life: sleeping; attending classes; eating; engaging in extracurricular activities; exercising; watching television; reading; talking on the phone; going to and from school; studying; working at a job; doing household chores; and any other activities that take up more than an hour of your day.

40. Keep a diary of your activities for a week. Label each activity *A*, for high priority; *B*, for medium priority; or *C*, for low priority. Compare your priority labels with the pie graph you made in item 39. Is there a logical relationship between your priority labels and the amount of time you spend on each activity? What adjustments might you need to make?

Beyond the Classroom

LESSON 1

41. **Parental Involvement.** Ask your parents about the stressors they experience in their lives. Make a list of the things they find stressful about their jobs, how these stressors affect their relationships and their health, and how they cope.

LESSON 2

42. **Community Involvement.** Find out what kinds of support groups exist in your community to help people deal with stress. Make a list of these.

YOU AND YOUR FAMILY

LESSON 1
Looking at
Today's Families

LESSON 2
Looking at the
Health of the
Family

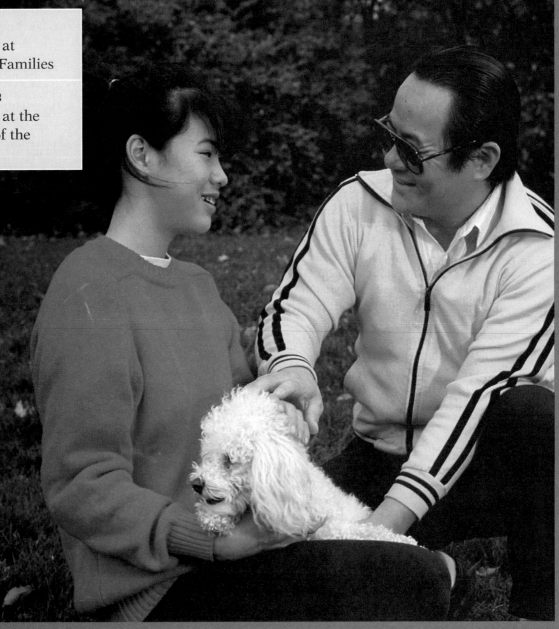

LOOKING AT TODAY'S FAMILIES

For many people the word *family* is often associated with warm feelings and pleasant scenes. Perhaps it reminds you of a holiday or vacation when all of the family, including aunts, uncles, cousins, and grandparents, got together for a celebration. Maybe the word brings to mind an older brother or sister who has moved away or a favorite aunt or uncle who comes for frequent visits. Although the word *family* means different things to different people, it often is defined as a group of people related by blood, marriage, or adoption. It is the group in which most people live their lives and in which people bring up children. The family is the basic unit of society.

LESSON 1 FOCUS

TERMS TO USE
- Mobile
- Blended family

CONCEPTS TO LEARN
- The family is the basic social unit of society.
- Many factors influence the health of the family.

ATTITUDES AND BEHAVIORS TO EVALUATE
- Self-Inventory, page 96.
- Building Decision-Making Skills, page 97.

The Family as a System

From the time you were born, your family exerted a strong influence on your life and personality. Families not only provide food, clothing, and shelter, but they also give family members a sense of security and a feeling of belonging. Families help children form their religious beliefs and values, and they pass on traditions and customs from one generation to the next.

Considering the family as a social system—knowing that what one person does affects every other person—can make you more aware of how your family works. A comparison can be made to the human body. For example, all parts of the body are interconnected to compose a whole being. Although separate elements can be identified, such as the heart or a specific muscle, no part exists in isolation. The body is in constant motion—taking in air, digesting food, healing itself—and it routinely deals with both the inner environment and the outside world. Just as your body functions because of the interrelationships of the different parts and the exchanges with the outside, so does your family.

As a system, the level of health—physical, mental, and social—of each family member affects the level of the total family's health. The reverse is also true. The health of the family system directly affects the health of its individual members. In addition, because the family is the basic social unit of society, society's health is directly related to the family's health. If we are to survive and maintain a healthy society, then everyone must work to promote healthy families.

Types of Families

There are many different types of families in today's world. Families vary in size, in relationships, and in the way in which they meet the needs of family members.

The Nuclear Family. The nuclear family unit is a common type of family. It consists of parents and one or more children sharing a household.

Love and care are two important characteristics of any healthy family structure.

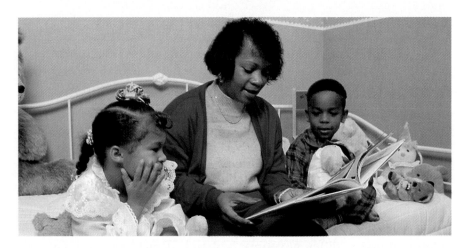

Culturally Speaking

Multigenerational Families

Many cultures live in multigenerational households. In China, a son traditionally brings his bride home to live in his parents' house. Each female will have her own kitchen area, but the house is shared. The Amish typically build a small living space onto the main house for when the parents wish to "retire" from farming. Several generations then live together on the farm. Some American fishing families on the east coast also maintain multigenerational family homes today.

Years ago, as employment in industry increased, many Americans left farm homesteads that housed several generations to live in nuclear families. Today, due to the increase in single-parent families and economic conditions, the multigenerational family is making a comeback.

The Single-Parent Family. Some families are single-parent families—that is, only one parent lives with the child or children. Most often the parent is the mother, especially in the case of a divorce, because she generally is awarded custody of the children. However, a growing number of fathers are now receiving custody of their children. Other types of single-parent families consist of a parent whose husband or wife has died or a single adult who has adopted one or more children.

The Extended Family. An extended family includes one or more relatives in addition to the nuclear family or single-parent family. Sometimes these relatives live in the same household as nuclear or single-parent families. This extended family may be composed of grandparents, aunts, uncles, and cousins who serve as an extra support system for the nuclear family.

Although newly married couples usually establish a separate home, family ties tend to remain intact with the extended family. However, as people become more and more **mobile,** or likely to move from place to place, there often is less direct involvement with the extended family. Transfers, job opportunities, and schooling can all mean moving away from the larger family unit. However, many people maintain contact in other ways—by letters, telephone calls, and visits. Mobile families also tend to establish other friends and relationships to maintain a support system that is important to a healthy family system.

The Blended Family. Many families, such as a blended family, reflect the effects of divorce and remarriage. A **blended family** is a type of nuclear family in which one or both people have been married before. Each may have a child or children from a previous marriage. *Stepparents, stepbrothers,* and *stepsisters* are terms frequently used to describe the various family members who are not related by birth.

The Adoptive Family. This type of family may be a nuclear, single-parent, or blended family. The children are not related by birth to the parents. Through a legal procedure, one or more children have become part of the family through adoption. The parent or parents are responsible for the children they have adopted as if they were their children by birth.

The Foster Family. A foster family can also be a nuclear, single-parent, or blended family. One or more of its children are not the birth children of the parent or parents. Through special arrangements with governmental agencies or foster parent and child organizations, the children are cared for by a particular family. Sometimes the children stay for extended periods of time. In some circumstances they are adopted later by the foster family.

Other Family Types.   Many groups do not consist of parents and children but are still considered families. An example is a married couple with no children. In other situations people who do not have families sometimes band together and take care of one another. These people function as a family because of the ways in which they meet one another's needs.

Functions of the Family

The family, as the basic social unit of society, serves two essential functions:

- It is the primary support system to which individuals turn in order to have their basic needs met.
- It is also the essential mechanism by which a child develops the capability to survive and to function independently in the world.

From the family come the first opportunities for physical well-being, learning, and loving. Some psychologists believe that a child's intelligence and personality are almost fully developed by age 4 or 5. The child's primary environment during those early years is in the family.

The Changing Family System

There have been major changes in family life-styles in the United States over the past 50 years. These changes directly affect the health of the family system. For example, in the mid-1900s, children may have spent a few hours a day interacting with various members of their immediate family. Today, many teenagers spend only minutes each day talking with their parents. Unfortunately, most of that time is often spent dealing with problems or family conflict. Families today also move more often due to parents' job changes. Thus, the extended family and neighborhood no longer have the significant role they used to have.

CONFLICT RESOLUTION

Hasso has a big problem—he feels totally responsible for his parents' recent breakup. Hasso and his dad were always fighting, and Hasso thinks that's why his father walked out six months ago. Hasso's mom refuses to discuss his dad—she just tries to act as if everything's normal. Yet Hasso is sure his mom blames him, and when she sometimes gets upset and cries about his dad, Hasso feels really guilty. At the same time, he can't help feeling relieved that his dad is out of the house and the fighting has stopped. Hasso's getting more confused about his conflicting feelings.

How has poor communication led to an unhappy situation for Hasso's family?

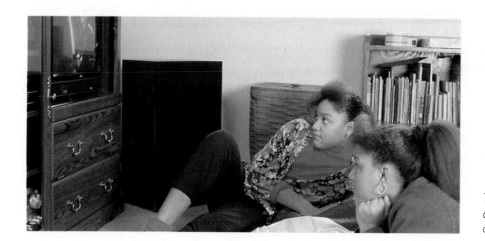

Through television, we are introduced to a variety of people and situations.

Some American children between ages 6 and 11 watch about 23 hours of television per week. Through television, young people are introduced to a variety of different role models, as well as many varied value systems. The role models and values may or may not support what the young person is being taught at home by the family.

Three significant changes are affecting the family system today:

- Family size tends to be smaller than in the past.
- More women are working outside the home.
- The number of single-parent heads of households is increasing.

Smaller Families

The decision of couples to have fewer or no children is often based on costs, health, the economy, jobs, or beliefs. Choosing to have fewer children is seen by some as a positive sign, because it may enable parents to better provide for the children they already have.

Working Wives and Mothers

The increase in the number of women entering the labor force stems largely from the fact that many of today's households need two incomes to support a family. The two-income family brings with it significant changes in traditional family roles. The impact on the health of the family system depends on how each family adjusts to these changes.

Another major reason for the growing numbers of working wives and mothers is the increasing divorce rate. Other women work outside the home because they want to use their talents and training—and there are more opportunities in the workplace now than in the past.

One of the greatest concerns that arises from the mother's working outside of the home is that of quality day care. Almost one-third of the women who are employed have preschool-aged children. Some studies have shown that when children receive quality care, the effects of day care are no different from those of care in the home.

Single-Parent Heads of Households

One of the greatest changes in the American family has been the increase in single-parent households. Over 11 million children—more than 1 out of every 4 under the age of 18—live in a single-parent home, either with a mother or a father.

The number of households headed by women is largely the result of an increasing divorce rate. The first divorce recorded in the United States was in the early 1600s, soon after Plymouth Colony was settled. By 1804, 1 marriage in 100 ended in divorce; and by the end of the 1920s it was 1 in 6. Today about half of all marriages end in divorce.

The term *single-parent family* is not an accurate description in some cases. Some youngsters in single-parent families are children of divorced parents; thus they still have two parents. Because their parents live in separate households, a more accurate term is *single-parent house-*

HEALTH UPDATE

LOOKING AT THE ISSUES

Should Adoptions Be Open or Closed?

Every year in the United States, about 100,000 children are adopted. Many of these adoptions are closed adoptions—adoptions in which records are sealed. This means that the names, addresses, and phone numbers of the birth parents remain unavailable to either the adoptive parents or the children.

Increasingly, however, there are open adoptions where information is made available to both sides in an adoption. Adoptive parents may meet birth parents or even be with the birth mother during the delivery.

Analyzing Different Viewpoints

ONE VIEW. Some people believe that records are sealed to protect the adoptive parents from unwanted contact by biological parents who have given up their children but may decide they want contact with them again.

A SECOND VIEW. Other people believe that laws that call for closed adoptions may also protect the biological parents from adoptive parents who want to find out more about the family background, or even, in some cases, try to return babies with problems to them.

A THIRD VIEW. Others maintain that people have a need for accurate medical information from their families of origin as well as an emotional need to know their roots.

A FOURTH VIEW. Some people believe that records should remain closed to protect the rights of the adoptive parents, the adoptees, and/or the biological parents and to avoid confusing the person who has been adopted. They fear that sharing families can prove unhealthy and confusing for all parties.

Exploring Your Views

1. Do you think adoptions should be open or closed? Do you think it should depend on the situation? Explain.
2. What might be gained from being able to contact one's birth parents? What might the risks be?
3. If you were an adoptive parent, would you support an adult adoptee's desire to find his or her natural parents? Explain.

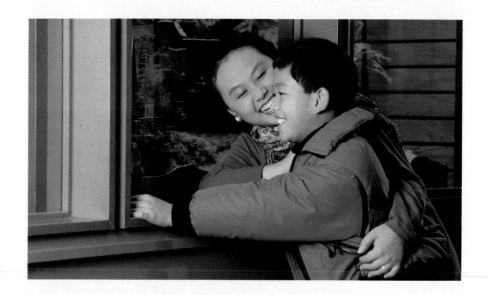

Single-parent families occur very frequently in our society.

hold. In spite of its inaccuracy, however, the term *single-parent family* has come to mean a family in which children live with one parent at a time.

In single-parent families everything may not be the same as when parents lived together, but the new arrangement can work. Single-parent families can be, and many times are, very healthy families. As in any family, it is necessary for all family members to work together to cope with changes and increased stress that may arise.

Each of these changes reflects the changing times in which we live. None of the changes are necessarily bad. And as individuals, we have little control over some of them. The important point is that they all influence the health of the family system. The healthy family copes with the changes while maintaining the family structure.

LESSON 1 REVIEW

Reviewing Facts and Vocabulary

1. Write a short paragraph describing nuclear, extended, and blended families.
2. Define the term *mobile*, and give an example of someone you know or have read about who is mobile.

Thinking Critically

3. **Evaluation.** Write a short skit or play, pointing out how trends toward smaller families, employed mothers, and increasing numbers of single-parent families have affected today's family unit.
4. **Analysis.** Read at least two magazines geared to teens. Write a short paper comparing how these magazines treat family issues. Discuss how the families and family issues reflected in these magazines compare with your family and its beliefs and values.

Applying Health Knowledge

5. Talk to an adult about his or her view of the ideal family. Write a brief report about the conversation.
6. Develop a list of questions to be used to interview an older individual, such as a family member, other relative, or adult friend, about the type of family in which he or she was reared. Ask this person to share his or her views about some of the changes affecting families today.

LOOKING AT THE HEALTH OF THE FAMILY

As mentioned in Lesson 1, the health of society depends on the health of families. It is important for us to be aware of the threats to the health of our families so that we can take steps to maintain a healthy family and thus, a strong society.

Troubled Families

A family system can break down for a variety of reasons. This breakdown may end in divorce, in which case the family system is restructured. In many cases the family system, though troubled, remains intact. If family members do not seek help for serious problems, however, the health of individual members can be threatened.

Recognizing Physical and Mental Abuse

The rising incidence of abused children, battered spouses, and runaways is evidence of troubled family systems. Family members may act out their hurts, miseries, and frustrations in numerous ways.

Spousal and Elder Abuse.   Persons with spouses who physically or mentally abuse them have become the subject of national attention. They are usually women who are married to men who are very authoritarian, who have low self-esteem, who do not handle stress well, or who become violent when drinking alcohol or using other drugs.

In the past many wives felt trapped in their situation. They usually had no means of employment and were dependent upon the husband's financial support. Their friends and neighbors often ignored the problem or did not want to get involved.

Elderly family members may also be the object of violence. A family member may take out his or her frustration on elderly parents or aunts or uncles who cannot defend themselves.

The problem of battered spouses and elders occurs in all levels of society. However, agencies and centers now exist in many communities to help provide support and, sometimes, a temporary place of refuge from the violence.

Child Abuse.   No one knows for sure how many children are abused in families. The statistics represent only reported cases, and it is likely that there are many more unreported cases. **Child abuse** can be physical harm, including sexual abuse, as well as emotional harm. The emotionally abused child is perhaps the most difficult to identify, because there may be no physical evidence of mistreatment.

Abuse of children can occur among any socioeconomic group, culture, or religious affiliation. Generally, the abusers are parents or close

LESSON 2 FOCUS

TERMS TO USE
- Child abuse
- Exploited
- Communication
- Compromise
- Crisis

CONCEPTS TO LEARN
- Because the family is the basic social unit of society, it is critical that we learn ways to improve and maintain the health of the family.
- Family violence continues to be a major problem in our society.

ATTITUDES AND BEHAVIORS TO EVALUATE
- Self-Inventory, page 96.
- Building Decision-Making Skills, page 97.

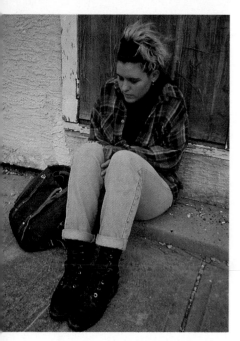

A teen who feels alone needs help either from family, friends, or a professional.

relatives, and the incidents happen repeatedly. In many cases abusive parents and other relatives were themselves abused children.

Abusive parents generally are isolated. They may have no one to turn to for relief from everyday frustrations. In many cases parents lack information about child development. They do not know what a child can reasonably be expected to do or how a child may act at certain ages. The tendency to abuse children is increased by such problems as unemployment, low self-esteem, poor stress-management skills, marital conflicts, and drug and alcohol use.

Over 4,000 children die each year in the United States from physical abuse. Many of these deaths occur in children under the age of 2 years. Aside from the risks of death or physical injury, the abused child tends to be depressed, fearful, and withdrawn. The abused child may also exhibit destructive behaviors.

A large number of child abuse cases involve sexual abuse. Typically, the sexually abused child is between 6 and 8 years of age and is victimized by someone in his or her own home—a father, stepfather, uncle, or some other trusted authority figure.

Reports of sexually abused boys and young girls are becoming more and more common. Sexual abuse can last for years and may never be reported. The child may be threatened with severe punishment, embarrassment, ridicule, or even death if he or she tells anyone.

It is important that the victim in this situation know that he or she is not at fault. The child has done nothing wrong—it is the abuser's behavior that is wrong. Victims should talk to some adult whom they trust, so that the adult can get help for them. If help does not come with the first try, it is important that victims seek assistance from other appropriate adults to get the help they need.

Young Runaways.   Some children and teens try to get out of an abusive home by running away. Unfortunately, because runaways usually have no money or job skills to help them survive, they often end up being **exploited,** or used for someone else's benefit. Runaway children are prime targets for people dealing in pornography and prostitution.

Running away is not the answer; help is available for the abused child or teenager. Before anyone can help an abused person, however, someone must report the abuse. All states now have laws requiring doctors and other health professionals to report suspected cases of child abuse. In many states, anyone who suspects or knows of an abuse situation is required to report it. Legally, children and teens can be removed from an abusive environment until it is corrected.

K E E P I N G   F I T

Keeping Family Fights Fair

Consider these strategies when arguing:
- Don't draw the names of relatives or friends who agree with you into the argument.
- Don't dredge up the past.
- Don't attack the person or his or her personality. Point to the behavior or situation that isn't working for you.
- Don't use labels or put-downs.
- Let the other person finish his or her sentences.
- Listen to the other person's point of view.
- Don't storm out, mid-argument.
- Don't yell or use the "silent treatment."
- Don't get into an argument with someone who's under the influence of alcohol or other drugs.

Family Counseling. Counseling is available for both the child and the parents. Many communities now have crisis intervention hot lines. Parents who realize that they are losing control can get immediate help.

Parents Anonymous is a national organization that helps parents overcome their tendencies toward violence. In meetings, parents make up a support system for one another. Parents learn how to help themselves and one another as they talk about their feelings and problems.

Just as important as the rehabilitation of abusive parents is the long-range prevention of abuse in society as a whole. Parents and prospective parents need opportunities for learning about family life, child development, and parent-child relationships.

Strengthening Your Family

When you hear about troubled families, families in crisis situations, violent families, and families on the edge of survival, you may conclude that only a few families are strong and able to function in a healthy manner. On the contrary, most families do work through their problems and resolve their conflicts—usually without outside help.

Healthy Family Systems

What characteristics go into making a family healthy and strong? What can family members do to change a hurting family into a healthy family? Loving, caring families do not just happen. There is no magic formula for building a healthy family, but there are some elements that healthy families seem to have in common. The following elements are characteristics of healthy families:

- Family members care about each other. They stick together even when times are tough.
- Family members communicate with each other. They listen and work to understand each other. **Communication,** or openness among family members, includes showing tenderness, warmth, and humor. It also means being able to express negative feelings. In general, members of a healthy family communicate with one another and approach life from a positive viewpoint.
- Family members support each other. Each member is recognized as a unique individual. Family members express their thoughts and feelings, and they listen to each other.

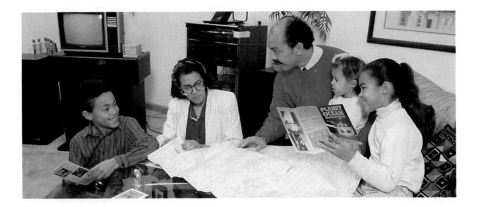

Open communication helps everyone in the family contribute to its well-being.

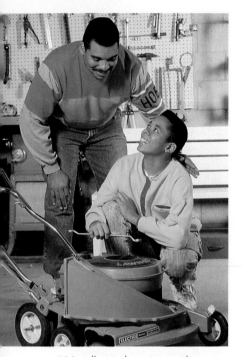

—We all need praise and encouragement to build up our self-esteem.

As you know, everyone has basic emotional needs. Individuals must meet these needs in order to feel good about themselves. The family can be the primary source of meeting these emotional needs. In supportive families, emotional needs are met in the following ways:

- Family members trust and respect each other. They do not gossip about family members; nor do they hide problems from one another —even serious ones such as addiction, abuse, and teen pregnancy. They are honest about their feelings toward all family members. They keep promises made to one another.
- Differences of opinion are allowed. Family members are able to disagree without attacking one another.
- Family members take time for one another and for the family as a whole. They share celebrations and traditions, and they find ways to have fun together.
- Everyone is included in important family decisions. Together, family members discuss issues that affect the entire family, such as finding a new place to live or deciding where to go on vacation.
- Everyone pitches in and shares responsibilities. Having each member do his or her share can go a long way.
- Family life has structure. People need structure—a certain rhythm in their lives and the realization of where they fit into society. Going to school, eating at certain times and at certain places, and playing on a team all give structure to your daily life. The family, too, needs structure. The members need to know their place in it and what their general functions are.
- Family members are willing to be flexible. Although there is structure in a healthy family, the leaders of the family, as well as the other members, need to be flexible and open to change when it is best for the family as a whole.

Doing Your Part

What can you do to help keep your family strong? What steps should you follow if your family is hurting? Here are some ways to show you care and to strengthen your family.

- Show appreciation for things done well. Saying "thank you" works at home, too.
- Encourage others, even your parents. Most people never get enough encouragement.
- Show concern when a family member has a problem. Offer to help or to get help.
- Stop criticizing. Be tactful and constructive. Avoid nagging.
- Show empathy by putting yourself in the other person's position. Try to see situations from his or her point of view.
- Listen to what other family members say. Listening is more than simply not talking. Avoid interrupting, daydreaming, jumping to conclusions, or just waiting for your turn to talk.
- Keep your promises. Do not make promises you cannot keep.
- Be dependable and on time. Your family must be able to depend on you. You owe family members your best.
- Be willing to compromise with family members. A **compromise** is a

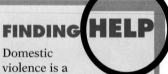

FINDING HELP

Domestic violence is a crime that can result in serious physical injury and even death. If you know that a battering incident is occurring, call the police immediately. Contacting the police does not always mean the abuser will be put in jail. It is simply the most effective way to protect the victim and the children from immediate harm.

way of solving a problem in which each person gives up something in order to find a solution that satisfies everyone. Being willing to give a little so that the other person will get something can result in a healthier relationship.

Getting Help

When people live together, conflicts are bound to occur. However, it is important to try to work out family problems as soon as they come up. If not resolved, minor concerns often become major problems.

Family problems range in size from small misunderstandings to major crises. A **crisis** is an extreme change in a person's life. There are many types of major crises. Five of the most common are financial problems, divorce, drug use, violence, and death. Help is available for coping with all of these crises.

Financial Problems. The causes of financial problems within the family vary greatly. Overdue bills, the loss of a job, serious illness, a natural disaster, or death could be the source of serious financial problems.

How your parents cope with financial loss directly affects you. You may notice a decrease in spending money if financial recovery takes a great deal of time. To resolve money problems, some single-parent families live together. Other families exchange help or share the expense of paying for services. Two or three parents might share a baby-sitter, for instance, and help each other with big jobs.

Some teens help with family money problems by learning how much such essentials as food and rent cost and doing their share to stay within the budget. They often try to get part-time jobs to pay for special clothes or entertainment. Most parents would view this type of assistance with pride and appreciation.

Divorce. To divorce is to end a marriage relationship, and it means a permanent separation. If your parents are divorcing, you might feel all alone, but you are not. In the United States, 12 million children under the age of 18 have divorced parents. Whether the mother or father leaves, it is important to remember that parents divorce each other—not their children. Although their feelings for each other have changed, their love for their children can stay the same. Parents who deliberately break the bond between parent and child may have deep, unsolved emotional problems of their own.

Most children of parents who are getting a divorce go through a difficult period of emotional adjustment. It is similar to the time of grief following the death of a loved one. They usually experience shock, disbelief, anger, sorrow, and finally, acceptance.

During the breakup of a marriage, children sometimes feel they are the cause of their parents' separation. However, divorce happens for many reasons, and children are seldom the cause.

Children of divorce must learn to cope with the lack of one parent's daily presence. This often leads to having less money and to a lower standard of living. Eventually, the children may find themselves faced with learning to accept a stepparent if one of their parents remarries.

If your parents are going through a divorce, share your feelings with them and try to understand their feelings. Find an older person with whom you can discuss your feelings.

Overcoming The Odds

She calls herself Leah. That's not her real name, but that doesn't matter. She's 19 years old and the victim of incest. She says, "I was sexually abused as a child from the time I was about 5 until I was about 13. The person who did it to me is my uncle. He is my mother's younger brother—younger by a lot—and for many years he lived with us. It started when he would babysit for my sister and me when my mom and dad had to work double shifts at their restaurant. He would come into my room. He would be real friendly and all, and then he would be . . . too friendly. I didn't really know what was going on, but I sensed, even as a young kid, that it wasn't right. He told me never to tell anyone or I would be in big trouble, and so I just kind of locked it all up inside.

"People say to me now, well, why didn't you tell anyone? I guess I was too afraid, and maybe I thought I somehow deserved it, like there was something wrong with me or this wouldn't be happening.

"Then, when my sister was about 23, she started to get some flashbacks of awful things happening to her when our uncle was around. So she joined some kind of group and started to talk about it all. The

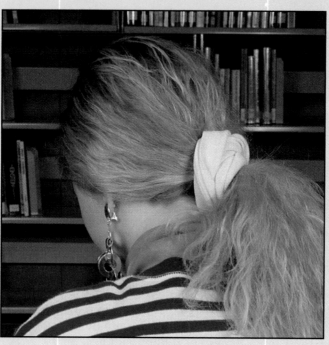

night she told my mom was an awful night. My mother said my sister must be crazy. My sister yelled and cried and stormed out. I stood in the kitchen just shaking. But after that, my sister and I started to really talk, and more and more about my uncle started to come back—for both of us.

"When I left home two years ago, I had lousy self-esteem. I felt like I couldn't trust anyone, like maybe I was crazy or making it up or it wasn't that bad after all. But with my sister's help and the help of an incest survivor's group I've joined, I'm coming to realize I didn't choose what happened to me as a child. It was done to me. Now I'm working on a letter to my uncle who lives on the other side of the country to

tell him how he hurt me, how he messed up my life, and that I hope he gets help before he does it to anyone else. I still have whole pockets of my childhood I can't remember," Leah says. "I still have some shame and a tendency to think that when things go wrong it's my fault. There's anger at my mom for not having realized what was going on. And I still have very bad days where I feel shaky about things. But I guess you'd have to say that knowing I'm not alone has helped. Knowing I'm not perverted or crazy helps, too. Just being able to say the word *molested* was a start. And my sister's support has been the greatest."

1. How did Leah's experience affect her self-esteem? Her ability to trust?
2. Why do you think the victims of incest often feel that it is somehow their fault or that they deserve it? How are these feelings unjustified? How do they get in the way of getting help?
3. If you or someone you know is the victim of incest or other sexual abuse, what safe steps can be taken to confront the situation?

Drug Use. Drug use within the family is almost always destructive. Parents—and others in the family—who are alcoholic or who use other drugs neglect their responsibilities, become very irritable, often lose their jobs, and may even abuse other family members.

When the health of the family is threatened by drug use, all of the members need help. By asking the right people for assistance, you can be the one who starts your family on its way back to a healthy life. The people most likely to help you are members of your extended family, a member of the clergy, a school counselor or trusted teacher, your school nurse, or a youth worker. Knowing how to get help is a way of caring for your family. These people can help you understand the problem and can help you get additional assistance.

Violence. Violent abuse is a real problem that happens in many families every year. Ignoring the problem never works; the code of silence does not help anyone. Family members in serious trouble may not be able to help themselves. Child welfare agencies, family doctors, school nurses, school counselors, religious leaders, or even the police are sources of help for a family experiencing violence.

Death. No family can escape death, and when there is a death in the family, there is grief. People go through grief in very different ways. Family members need to allow each other to mourn in their own ways.

Sometimes after a death it is difficult to determine what to do next. There are hundreds of details that a family must deal with when a member dies. Conflict among family members is common because of increased emotions during this time. Talking with each other—or with good friends or counselors—can be helpful in coping with this loss.

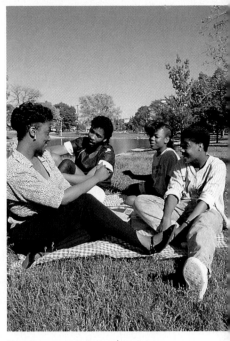

Enjoying recreational activities together is one way of keeping a family strong.

LESSON 2 REVIEW

Reviewing Facts and Vocabulary

1. Define the term *child abuse,* and summarize an article about a child abuse incident from a current newspaper or magazine.
2. Write a one- or two-minute public service announcement for families in trouble. Use the following terms in the announcement: *exploited, communication,* and *crisis.*

Thinking Critically

3. **Analysis.** Design a dance or pantomime contrasting the feelings of family members in troubled families with those in healthy family systems.
4. **Evaluation.** Do you think a child who complains of physical abuse should be returned to his or her family after a court hearing? Why or why not?

Applying Health Knowledge

5. Interview a school or family counselor, social worker, or other mental health professional about the occurrence of child, elder, and spousal abuse in the community. Make a list to share with the class of sources of available help.
6. Keep a log for one week of the number of hours you spend with each member of your family. Total these hours, illustrating them on a simple graph showing each 24-hour period. Write a brief summary of your feelings about the time spent with your family and how you might have improved the quality or the quantity of time spent with family members. Conclude by making a written plan for a special family activity for the following week.

Self-Inventory

You and Your Family

HOW DO YOU RATE?

Number a sheet of paper from 1 through 25. Read each item below, and rate yourself by writing *always*, *sometimes*, or *never* for each item. After you have rated yourself, ask a family member to use a separate sheet to rate you on each behavior. Total the number of *always*, *sometimes*, and *never* responses on each sheet. Then proceed to the next section.

1. Cares about others.
2. Communicates well.
3. Is trustworthy.
4. Respects differences of opinion.
5. Pitches in and helps when needed.
6. Shares responsibilities.
7. Is flexible when necessary.
8. Is appreciative.
9. Encourages others.
10. Shows concern for others.
11. Avoids criticizing others.
12. Tries to see others' point of view.
13. Listens well.
14. Avoids interrupting others.
15. Keeps promises.
16. Is dependable and punctual.
17. Is willing to compromise when necessary.
18. Cooperates with others.
19. Is cheerful.
20. Is enthusiastic.
21. Is hardworking.
22. Puts self in other's place.
23. Is loyal to other family members.
24. Is patient with others.
25. Works to solve conflicts in a positive way.

HOW DID YOU SCORE?

Give yourself 2 points for every *always* answer, 1 point for every *sometimes* answer, and 0 points for every *never* answer. Find your total from both sheets, and read below to see how you scored. Then proceed to the next section.

91 to 100
Excellent. You are making an exceptional contribution as a family member.

31 to 90
Good. You are a caring family member, but you could try harder.

Below 31
Poor. You need to improve your behavior toward family members. You are missing out on some terrific rewards that come from caring about others.

WHAT ARE YOUR GOALS?

If you received an *excellent* or *good* score, complete the statements in Part A. If your score was *poor*, complete the statements in Parts A and B.

Part A

1. I plan to learn more about healthy, caring behaviors by ____.
2. My timetable for accomplishing this is ____.
3. I plan to share my information with others by ____.

Part B

4. The behavior or attitude toward my family I would most like to change is ____.
5. The steps involved in making this change are ____.
6. My rewards for making this change will be ____.
7. My timetable for making this change is ____.
8. The people or groups I will ask for help are ____.

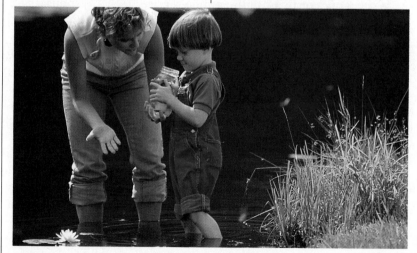

Building Decision-Making Skills

Shelley babysits for two cute little neighbor children. Lately she has become very concerned because she has seen some signs of possible child abuse. One child has a black eye, and the other has a sprained arm. When she asked about the injuries, the children seemed afraid, and their mother answered nervously that they had fallen down the stairs. The mother seems very unhappy, and the father seems very stressed out over business matters. What should Shelley do?

WHAT DO YOU THINK?

1. **Choices.** What choices does Shelley have?

2. **Consequences.** What potential danger exists and for whom?

3. **Consequences.** What are the probable consequences of each choice?

4. **Consequences.** How might Shelley's health triangle be affected by her decision?

5. **Consequences.** What might happen if Shelley tries to talk to the children about this?

6. **Consequences.** What will be the effect on everyone concerned if Shelley reports the problem but is wrong?

7. **Consequences.** What might happen if Shelley doesn't report the problem?

8. **Decision.** What would you advise Shelley to do?

Ava and her sister, Deb, have shared a room at home for several years. Just recently has it become a problem. Ava keeps her part of the room very neat. Deb, on the other hand, has started to leave things wherever they fall. Usually there's a pile of clothes on the floor, and it is not at all unusual for Deb to borrow clothes from Ava when they get ready for school. Ava wouldn't mind, if Deb returned them—clean. Instead, they too get left in a pile. Ava is getting really annoyed. What should she do?

WHAT DO YOU THINK?

9. **Situation.** Why does a decision need to be made?

10. **Choices.** List five possible ways Ava might handle the situation.

11. **Consequences.** What might be the outcome for each choice?

12. **Consequences.** How might Ava's health triangle be affected by this decision?

13. **Consequences.** How might Deb's health triangle be affected by this decision?

14. **Consequences.** How might this decision affect the girls' parents?

Rob is a senior in high school and is busy making plans for college next year. He hopes to attend the state university and live on campus. Until recently he has been cooperative and helpful around the house. Now, however, he has developed the habit of leaving wet towels on the floor of his room. His sister, Becki, just found two of them when she went into his room to get the sweatshirt he had borrowed from her. It was under the wet towels! How should Becki handle this situation?

WHAT DO YOU THINK?

15. **Choices.** What choices does Becki have?

16. **Consequences.** What are the consequences of each choice?

17. **Decision.** What should Becki do? Explain the reasons for your answer.

REVIEW

Using Health Terms

On a separate sheet of paper, write the term that best matches each definition given below.

LESSON 1

1. The basic unit of society; a group of people related by blood, marriage, or adoption.

LESSON 2

2. Talking about and expressing both positive and negative feelings.
3. A way of solving a problem in which each person gives up something in order to reach a solution that is satisfactory to everyone involved.
4. An extreme change in a person's life.

Building Academic Skills

LESSON 1

5. **Math.** If a family spends 10 to 12 minutes each day dealing with family conflict, how much total time is spent over a one-week period? Over a one-month period? In one year?
6. **Math.** Today by the time people reach the age of 18, they have spent an average of 18,000 hours watching television. Calculate the hours spent by a 36-year-old, a 42-year-old, and a 70-year-old.

LESSON 2

7. **Reading.** Use the context clues in the following sentence to define the word *compromise.*

    We were unable to agree on which restaurant to choose because no one was willing to compromise.

8. **Writing.** Write a composition of three to five paragraphs, beginning with the following words: "I can better contribute to and promote my family's health by. . . ." Before you begin writing, make an outline of the points you want to include. Use what you have learned in this chapter to generate ideas for your composition.

Recalling the Facts

LESSON 1

9. What do families provide besides food, clothing, and shelter?
10. Explain how the family is a system.
11. How does family health relate to the health of society as a whole?
12. List and describe two types of single-parent families.
13. What are the two essential functions of the family?
14. At what age do some psychologists believe that a child's intelligence and personality are almost fully developed?
15. What three significant changes are affecting the family system today?
16. Name three factors that may influence the decision of couples to have fewer children.
17. What are two reasons for the increase in the number of wives and mothers who work outside the home?
18. How can children be properly cared for if both parents work outside the home?

LESSON 2

19. How many children under the age of 2 die each year in the United States from physical abuse?
20. Why is it difficult for sexually abused children to seek help?
21. Describe several characteristics of a healthy family.
22. Describe the role of structure in family life.
23. List five things you can do to make your family healthy and strong.
24. What are the five most common types of crises in a person's life?
25. What emotions are children of divorced parents likely to feel? What adjustments might children of divorced parents have to make?
26. What are some ways children can cope with the divorce of their parents?
27. List three likely results of drug use in the family.

REVIEW

Thinking Critically

LESSON 1

28. **Analysis.** What is the difference between an extended family and a nuclear family?
29. **Evaluation.** How has television affected family life?
30. **Synthesis.** Keep a log of each family member's television viewing time for one week. Talk to family members about what programs they could give up in order to engage in family activities. Plan some family activities to take the place of watching television.

LESSON 2

31. **Evaluation.** Why do you think abused wives often stay in bad situations?
32. **Evaluation.** What do you think are three characteristics of a person who inflicts abuse on other family members?
33. **Synthesis.** What might you infer about a child in your neighborhood who tends to be depressed, fearful, and who sometimes exhibits destructive behaviors?
34. **Synthesis.** Summarize ways that healthy families can prevent abuse.
35. **Synthesis.** How could you help if your family experienced financial problems?

Making the Connection

LESSON 1

36. **Social Studies.** Television is a major part of many Americans' lives. How do you think television affects society? What impact is television having on your family? Is it a good or bad influence? Conduct a four-day study of your family's television viewing habits. Keep a log of what programs and the number of hours each member of your family watches television. What might your data suggest about the impact of television on your family? Make a list of healthful changes and alternatives to television viewing you can suggest to your family.

Applying Health Knowledge

LESSON 1

37. Label each type of family described below.
    a. Marisa and Miguel Esposito live in an apartment with their two children, Juan and Maria.
    b. Tom and Margaret Kenny have four children. Tom's sister, Anna, and her three children live with them.
    c. Alice Johnson is divorced. Her daughter, Sylvia, lives with her.
    d. Mary and Sam Gaines were not able to have children of their own. They adopted four Vietnamese children.

LESSON 2

38. Joyce and Judy are sisters who fight all the time. You are their best friend. What advice can you give them for getting along better?
39. Your cousin Angela's parents have recently separated. While they are trying to work out their problems, Angela is coming to live with your family. What can you do to help Angela get through this crisis in her life?

Beyond the Classroom

LESSON 1

40. **Parental Involvement.** Talk to your grandparents or two people you know who are over age 50. Ask them what they did in place of watching television when they were children. Evaluate their responses in relation to a healthy family life. Write a paragraph based on one of these people's early family life compared to your own. How does it compare?

LESSON 2

41. **Community Involvement.** The loss of a job and the death of a loved one are similar in many ways. Talk to at least two people who have experienced one or both of these crises. Find out what feelings they had after each event, how they dealt with the loss, whether they sought help and from whom.

YOUR RELATIONSHIPS WITH OTHERS

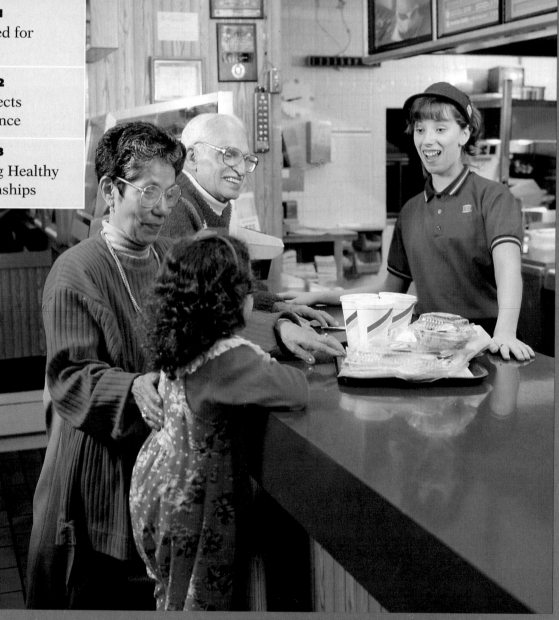

THE NEED FOR OTHERS

According to psychologist Abraham Maslow, everyone needs to be loved and to belong. Each of us also needs to feel safe, secure, valued, and recognized. By forming relationships, we are able to meet many of these basic human needs. A **relationship** is a bond or connection between people. Good relationships can affect a person's mental, social, and even physical health. You develop and learn from relationships throughout your life.

Who Matters to You?

Think of standing in one of those photo booths where you and a friend pull a curtain, drop four quarters into a slot, and get back four connected photos of the two of you. You are smiling or laughing, your faces side by side. Now imagine that you could have these four shots showing you with four different people with whom you have a significant connection—say, from your family; from your extended family, such as a grandparent or cousin; from your neighborhood; and from your school. Who would be with you in the four photos?

You have many relationships in your life, and all of them affect you. You are part of a network of people that includes your family, extended family, neighbors, friends, other peers, as well as people from social or religious organizations, sports teams, your town or city, your nation, and the world.

If you were suddenly plunked down on a desert island and removed from all of these relationships, you might like the peace and quiet for a short time, but chances are you would soon begin to get very lonely. Having relationships with others can, in fact, not only ward off loneliness; it can also have a direct effect on a person's total health.

Your Many Roles

You take on many roles in your relationships with others. A **role** is a part that you play, especially in a relationship. You may be a sister or brother, a daughter or son; a granddaughter or grandson; a member of the orchestra; a member of the volleyball team; a Scout; a student; an employee; a member of a synagogue, church, or mosque; and even someone's boyfriend or girlfriend—all at the same time.

Sometimes the roles you play are clear-cut. You know that when you mow the neighbor's lawn or wash his or her car, you are an employee and need to act as one. Sometimes, though, roles either switch suddenly or change gradually, depending on needs and situations. For example, some days you may be the caretaker for your disabled grandfather, but at other times he is a teacher and you are the student. Perhaps your lab partner becomes the person you are dating. Such changes in roles can be confusing. Sometimes you may not have a clue as to what your role is in a relationship. This can make it difficult for you to know how to act.

LESSON 1 FOCUS

TERMS TO USE
- Relationship
- Role
- Friendship
- Platonic relationship
- Peer pressure
- Manipulation
- Prejudice
- Stereotype

CONCEPTS TO LEARN
- Relationships affect your physical, mental, and social health.
- You play many roles in your relationships with others.
- Peer pressure is the control and influence people your age may have over you.
- Manipulation is one way people exert peer pressure.
- Prejudice is not based on experience, but rather on stereotypes.

ATTITUDES AND BEHAVIORS TO EVALUATE
- Self-Inventory, page 114
- Building Decision-Making Skills, page 115.

Choosing Relationships

As a small child, you had a limited circle of relationships. Now, that you are older, you have a larger circle from which to choose your relationships. You may realize for the first time that there are people of all ages, races, religions, and backgrounds from which you can choose relationships. You can choose people who support and encourage your best qualities. You can change or back out of relationships that have a negative influence on your health, your safety, your self-esteem, or your values. No relationship can be healthy unless both parties feel valued and want the relationship.

Friendship

A **friendship** is a significant relationship between two people, based on caring, consideration, and trust. A friend is someone whose companionship you enjoy and who can be a source of help when you have a problem. A friend also may be someone with whom you share confidences, interests, hobbies, or other friends. Having friends can help you define, understand, and reinforce your values. There are many kinds of friendships. Friendships vary in importance and in how challenging and complicated they are. Maintaining friendships can be hard work, but they are usually worth the effort.

Close Friendships. Having one or more close friends is important to your total health. Sitting with a group at ball games or in the cafeteria can make you feel socially connected. These casual relationships, however, do not fill some of the deeper needs humans have. A close friend is more likely to share what he or she is really feeling and thinking and, in turn, make you feel comfortable doing the same. You may trust a close friend with your secrets or go to this person when you are hurting, confused, or in trouble. He or she might give you honest criticism and make you apologize or be accountable for your mistakes. Because you may care deeply, a real friend is also more likely to make you angry or hurt. Losing or having to share a close friend with someone else can be painful. It is important to remind yourself that no one owns anyone else—that people must be free to choose with whom they want to be and when. Friends try to work through conflicts. This helps friendships stay healthy and grow.

KEEPING FIT

Your Friends, Your Self-Esteem

The friends you have or want to have can have a major impact on your self-esteem. Think of someone you consider to be a good friend. Then ask yourself the following questions:

- What qualities does the person have that you admire? What qualities bother you?
- How do you think this person feels about him- or herself?
- How does this person affect your health triangle?
- What positive peer pressure does the person put on you? What negative peer pressure?
- What positive effects does this person have on your self-esteem? What negative effects?
- What changes would make this relationship healthier?

Platonic Relationships.   Not all close friendships are made up of same-sex pairs. Sometimes a male and a female can become real buddies in what is a platonic relationship. A **platonic relationship** is one in which there is affection, but not romance. Such a relationship can be a wonderful way to grow to understand and feel comfortable with the opposite sex without feeling any of the pressures of dating. It can also help you begin to know that people of the opposite sex are human beings just like you, with the same kinds of fears, needs, and feelings.

Dating Relationships

Dating is part of the process of learning interpersonal skills. Dating provides an opportunity for you to get to know yourself better—to recognize your strengths and weaknesses. It also gives you an opportunity to interact with and feel comfortable with the opposite sex. By meeting and spending time with a variety of people, you learn what types of people you like and get along with best. In your dating experiences, you can practice your decision-making and communication skills and, in so doing, broaden your own development.

Dating often leads to an ongoing relationship with one person. There are some advantages to this type of relationship. However, teenagers who date only one person may be closing themselves off from meeting other people too early in their social development. Although this type of relationship may be convenient and ensures that you have a date, it may not be helpful in developing a healthy relationship.

It is important to remember that adolescence is a time of trying different relationships and roles. Breaking up, making up, and breaking up again can be painful, but this cycle is part of the process of emotional maturing. Staying in a relationship because you do not know how to get out of it gracefully or clinging to a relationship when the other person wants to call it off are two common but very painful situations. In both cases, honesty and open communication are essential. So is realizing that you have control over only your own actions and emotions. You cannot control the behaviors or feelings of others.

These days many teens go out in groups. Others do not date at all. The fact is, dating steadily, dating in groups, or waiting until later to date are all healthy ways of meeting your emotional and social needs.

Peer Pressure

Your peers are people your age or close to your age. They can have great influence over what you think, feel, say, and do. They may exert direct or indirect **peer pressure,** the control and influence people your age may have over you. Peer pressure can occur in many kinds of relationships. The way you handle peer pressure can have a great impact on the decisions you make and, in turn, on your total health.

Peer pressure can be positive or negative. Positive peer pressure may inspire you to pick up and recycle trash, volunteer your time to a worthy organization, exercise, or refrain from drinking or using other drugs. Negative peer pressure, however, may persuade you to take dangerous risks, use alcohol or other drugs, have sex, or cheat on an exam, just for the sake of being accepted by the crowd.

Dating provides an opportunity to feel comfortable with the opposite sex.

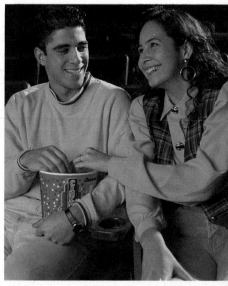

Overcoming The Odds

Chi is 16. He says, "I grew up in a tough place. More like a war zone. Lost more friends to gangs and guns than I can keep track of. Or want to. Anyway, where I grew up your choices were to join a gang and learn to defend yourself or learn to duck the bullets and fight for your life when the outside gangs moved in on you. Giving in just seemed easier. Figured we might not make it down the road anyway, so it was no big deal. It was sort of like, you know, when you get it, you get it.

"They got me started dealing dope when I was 11. Felt like it was the only way to have anything or be anything. It's like the OGs (original gang members) welcomed me and gave me power. At least, that's what I thought. By age 12 I was using pretty heavily and by 13, I didn't really care what happened to anybody else. We got into this rival gang thing then and I actually knifed a guy, or 'made my bones,' as the members would say. We trashed places, gave graffiti warnings, and stole for fun. Some of the members even did drive-by shootings—on a regular basis. For a while, it was a kind of high. I felt like somebody for a change. We even ate out in fancy restaurants. One time, I got my arm twisted and then

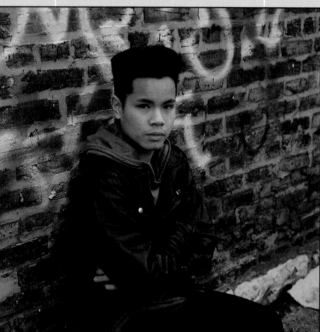

broken. I have scars on my back and face. I just figured that came with the turf. Besides, I was proud of my slices.

"When I was 14, I got into the corrections system. That didn't stop anything. I was really heading down a hole, deep into drugs, thinking about suicide or letting somebody else have it. Then they put me in this program with prisoners. First I thought it was stupid, almost cool. You know, some guys go out to the country for the weekend, I go to prison. Cracked me up. But then I saw what it was like. The conditions and everything. They paired me up with this guy who was there for life for killing a couple of people when he was in a gang and

doing drugs. I realized I didn't want to end up there like he did. He's a huge guy with big tattoos and a big smile. His name is Rajiv. He's in this program where he calls me every week, really talks to me about stuff, lets me know he cares. I go to visit him one Saturday a month. He's tough on me, too. And he tells me how it is when you go from the streets to the cells. He says I don't have to live out his ugly story, he's done it for me. He really listens. Let me put it to you this way: I never thought anybody was there for me. I was dead wrong. This beats being dead, which I almost was—more than once."

1. What kind of self-esteem do you think Chi had when he joined the gang? How did the gang appear to promise that they would make him feel better about himself? How did this promise backfire? Was it worth the cost?
2. What might Chi's story teach teens about self-esteem?
3. Have you ever done something dangerous because you didn't feel you measured up? How might you have boosted your self-esteem in healthier ways?

Manipulation

Manipulation is one way that people exert peer pressure over others. **Manipulation** is an indirect and often sneaky or dishonest means of trying to control another's attitudes or behavior. The person who manipulates another does so to get what he or she wants without respect for the well-being of the person being manipulated. Some means of manipulation include

- mocking or teasing the person in mean or hurtful ways;
- bargaining, or offering to make a deal to get what one wants;
- bribing, or promising money or favors if the person will do what another asks of him or her;
- using guilt trips to get desired results;
- making threats, or using words that show a person intends to use violence or some other negative means to get his or her way;
- using blackmail, or threatening to tell someone else some damaging information if the person does not conform;
- using flattery or undeserved praise to influence another person.

Prejudice

One of the more negative aspects of peer pressure that many high school students face is prejudice. **Prejudice** is a negative feeling toward someone or something that is based not on experience but, rather, on stereotypes. A **stereotype** is an exaggerated and oversimplified belief about an entire group, such as an ethnic group, a religious group, or a certain sex. Stereotypes may hold some truth but are in great part untrue. Prejudice, then, is a kind of ignorance. It denies each member of a group the right to be judged as an individual.

Prejudice prevents healthy relationships from forming. It is always a power relationship in which the victimizer wants to feel or appear superior to the person or group he or she is victimizing. In the process, the person exhibiting prejudice inflicts mental, social, and sometimes even physical damage. Discrimination is a form of prejudice in which people are singled out and often treated negatively as a result of one factor, such as age, sex, race, ethnicity, or even some physical trait.

LESSON 1 REVIEW

Reviewing Facts and Vocabulary

1. Define the term *role,* and state some of the different roles a person may play.
2. Define the words *prejudice, stereotype,* and *discrimination* in a paragraph in which you discuss their relationship to one another.
3. List and explain at least five techniques some people use to manipulate others.

Thinking Critically

4. **Analysis.** Compare your roles as student, son or daughter, and best friend.

5. **Evaluation.** What do you think are some of the advantages and disadvantages of telling everything to your best friend?

Applying Health Knowledge

6. Tell about a friendship you have had or know about that has not worked. Explain why you think the friendship failed.

THE EFFECTS OF VIOLENCE

Violence is the use of physical force to injure or abuse another person or persons. In addition to harming victims physically, acts of violence can leave victims with deep emotional scars. Violence is now a major public health problem in the United States.

Violence in Society

Americans are constantly exposed to violence. From television and music lyrics to so-called "slasher movies," images of violence influence lives and minds. We hear the words *murder, assault, battery,* and *mugging.* We read about increases in domestic abuse, child abuse, elder abuse, rape, and suicide. Now the new words in our "vocabulary of violence" are *drive-by shootings, carjackings,* and *hate crimes.* Many Americans no longer feel safe in their schools, on the streets, or even in their own homes.

Random Violence

In the past, most violent crimes were committed with specific intent—for a reason decided ahead of time and with a specific victim or property targeted. Today, violence has become more vicious and more random. **Random violence** is violence committed for no particular reason and/or against anyone who happens to be around at the time. Innocent people are the usual victims of random violence.

Teens and Violence

More teens than ever before are committing violent crimes and being arrested for serious crimes. They also are more likely to be tried as adults for these crimes and to be given stiffer "adult" sentences.

At the same time, more teens are also becoming the victims of violent crimes—often at the hands of their peers. Teens are three times more likely to be the victims of violent crime than adults.

Violence in Schools

There has been a dramatic increase in both the amount and the seriousness of violence in our schools. According to the United States Justice Department's National School Safety Center, as many as 3 million cases of assault, theft, robbery, and rape occur in United States schools every year. Stories of guns, knives, threats to both teachers and students, hostage-taking, and even killings occur in the news. In such stressful environments, students may find it difficult to learn, and teachers find it hard to teach. Many students are afraid to go to school. This violence is occurring in schools across the nation—from rural to suburban to urban school districts. In addition, the seriousness of crimes in our schools continues to increase, and students are performing these violent acts at younger and younger ages.

Schools are taking steps to stop this violence and its effects. Some inner-city schools in the nation's major cities now use metal detectors to stop students from carrying guns and knives into school. Many schools now have security guards, some with gun-sniffing dogs. Some schools enforce more strict dress codes in an attempt to keep certain types of clothing or jewelry out of the schools to prevent thefts and fights. In addition to fire drills, some schools now have "drop drills" to teach students and teachers how to hit the floor when they hear gunfire. Other ways schools are trying to curb violence are presenting violence prevention programs more frequently and at earlier ages, teaching conflict resolution, working to help students build self-esteem, and teaching about the dangers of alcohol, other drugs, guns, and gangs.

Violence on the Streets

Our streets are no longer completely safe. The incidence of homicide, aggravated assault, battery, and rape continues to rise and take their toll on everyone—even law-abiding citizens. **Homicide** is the willful killing of one human being by another. **Aggravated assault** is unlawful attack, often with a weapon, and having the intent to hurt or kill. **Battery** is the use of physical force to control someone through the use of power. Battery often includes frightening and humiliating a person over time. In our society, battery is the most common form of injury among females. Males also can be victims. Battery is one technique used to pressure teenagers into drug use and/or gangs. Rape, or sexual intercourse by force or threat, is another crime of violence. It is one of the fastest-growing yet least reported crimes.

Guns

Firearms, or guns, claim the lives of about 3,000 young people a year in the United States. Many other teens are left permanently disabled. Along with automobile crashes, gunfire is a common cause of death among teens aged 15 to 19. Guns are readily available. Unfortunately when bought for self-protection by adults or teens, guns too often are used on impulse during arguments or are set off accidently. Many people who own guns keep them loaded, and many do not lock them up for safekeeping.

Gangs

Gangs were once found only in large cities; now they also are found in smaller cities. Because of gang activity, some cities can seem like war zones. Gang members come from all ethnic groups, both sexes, and all economic classes. Gangs have rules, dress codes, symbols, and mottos.

DID YOU KNOW?

- Each day in the U.S. about 16,000 crimes take place on or near schools.
- According to U.S. Bureau of Justice statistics, in one recent year, 400,000 students between the ages of 12 and 19 were the victims of violent crimes.
- It is estimated that up to 90 percent of young people with guns get those guns from home.
- More than half of all homicide victims are killed by handguns.
- The Center to Prevent Handgun Violence reports that 1 percent of handgun violence in the schools occurs in pre-school, 24 percent in elementary school, 12 percent in junior high, and 63 percent in high school.

Wearing certain colors tipping, one's hat a certain way, or spraying graffiti may all signal the presence of gang members. Gangs stake out their "turf" or territory, and rivalries between gangs over this territory are deadly. Often gangs compete for drug deals and drug money. Gang killings also occur.

Members of gangs are often desperate to belong somewhere and to "be somebody." They get a sense of power from the group and from committing crimes. Members look to the gang as a kind of extended family and as a place to get some control. They may seek short-term thrills—no matter how risky, brutal, or deadly. Persons in gangs may be attracted to the promise of large sums of money from drug deals, fancy cars, and/or gang position. Some teenagers may become part of a gang to stop the pressure and threats to join.

Gangs no longer use just knives for weapons. Gang arsenals include automatic weapons, like high-powered assault rifles and UZI submachine guns. Gang members usually "lose big" over time—first by living in fear and eventually by getting injured, killed, or sent to jail—even Death Row. Being in a gang is a no-win, dead-end situation.

Carjackings

Carjacking is the hijacking, or stealing, of a car by force with a weapon. This occurs when a motorist is stopped at a traffic sign or light or is forced to stop. Victims also may be rammed from behind. When they stop and get out to look at the damage, their cars are forcibly taken from them. Victims of this crime may be chosen because the criminal wants the particular make and model of the car. Stolen cars may be taken to "chop shops" where they are sold for parts or used as transportation to commit other crimes.

Some Causes of Violence

Why has violence increased? The many reasons are complicated including the breakdown of the family, high school dropout rates, drug and alcohol addiction and use, and the availability of guns and other weapons. Other reasons are violence in the media, cultural support for violent behavior, racial and gender discrimination, prejudice, low self-esteem, increases in child abuse and neglect, lack of love, few job opportunities, lack of skills, poverty, idle time, and loss of hope. Not knowing healthy ways to vent and deal with emotions is also a factor.

K E E P I N G   F I T

Fair Fighting

Fighting with fists or weapons is never fair. Fighting with words can also be unfair. To keep a fight fair, remember these tips:
- Stick to one issue at a time, not personalities.
- Avoid name-calling and other put-downs.
- Do not interrupt.
- Do not bring in the names of others who support your side of the argument.
- Do not bring up the past.
- Listen to the other person's point of view. Imagine what it is like for him or her.
- Consider working through the argument at another time.
- If things get abusive or scary, call a time-out. If your safety is in jeopardy, leave.

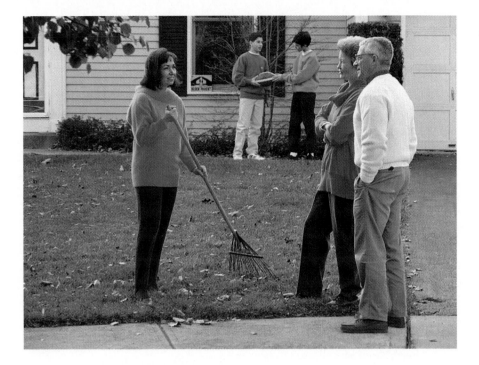

Stopping and Preventing Violence

It is not too late to do something to reduce violence. Many successful programs are being used to teach people ways to solve problems without violence. Conflict resolution and communication skills are being taught in schools. Family counseling, hotlines, shelters for battered and abused people, courses on effective parenting, and rehabilitation of the addicted, juvenile offenders, and former gang members are some of the available programs that exist to help prevent further violence. Prevention programs are now starting in schools with children as young as 6 or 7. Courses in personal safety are on the rise. Programs like Crime Watch, where neighbors look out for neighbors, are spreading. Many communities are now instituting curfews to ban youths under a certain age from city streets late at night. More "storefront" police stations in the middle of high-crime areas are opening. In addition, victims of violence are getting a chance to confront criminals through the legal system. Here victims can let criminals know the effects of their crimes.

What You Can Do

When it comes to violence, certain preventive steps are obvious, such as avoiding alcohol, drugs, guns, and gangs. A person also can learn to keep emotions from erupting into intense anger. Learning basic communication and conflict resolution skills and taking responsiblilty for one's actions are all important steps. A person also can work on building his or her self-esteem. People who feel good about themselves rarely need to lash out at others. Being a person with control doesn't have to mean using force. Reducing exposure to media that promotes and glamorizes violence, prejudice, and aggression can reduce fear and stress.

As individuals, families, schools, and a society, we must recognize that violence cannot be considered an acceptable way of dealing with anger and frustration. We must work together to replace growing fear and violence with growing safety and respect.

DID YOU KNOW?

- A recent study showed that 90 percent of the teens who experience violence either carry guns, have friends who carry guns, or deal drugs.
- One recent study of juveniles in jail indicated that 40 percent of them had been under the influence of illegal drugs and 33 percent under the influence of alcohol when they committed crimes.

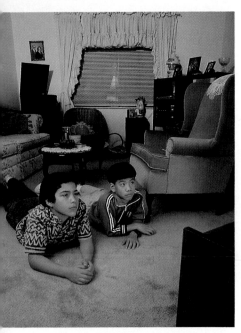

The impact of violence on television and its effect on society is being studied closely.

LOOKING AT THE ISSUES

Violence on Television

Televised violence has been shown to have harmful effects on behavior, relationships, and physical and mental health. One recent report to the American Psychiatric Association suggests that eliminating violence from TV and films could result in 10,000 fewer murders, 70,000 fewer rapes, 1 million fewer car thefts, and 2.5 million fewer burglaries.

Despite these facts, there is heated disagreement in our society about how much violence should be allowed to be shown on television—particularly during prime time when children or young teens might be watching.

Analyzing Different Viewpoints

ONE VIEW. Some people claim that freedom of speech and freedom of the press should ensure people's right to see what they want. Censorship, they claim, denies these rights.

A SECOND VIEW. Others claim that children should not be exposed to television violence, but that it is the responsibility of parents, not the networks, to control their viewing.

A THIRD VIEW. Many parents and organizations feel children should not be exposed to violence in any form, and the best way to ensure this is to keep violence in TV programming to a minimum.

Exploring Your Views

1. Do you think all violence should be banned from television? Why?
2. Do you think TV violence should be allowed if parents control their children's viewing? Until what age?
3. Do you think all TV violence is bad for children, including cartoons where characters are flattened but then get up unharmed and walk away? Why or why not?

LESSON 2 REVIEW

Reviewing Facts and Vocabulary

1. Define *violence, random violence, homicide,* and *aggravated assault* and in a paragraph discuss their relationship to one another.
2. Explain some of the ways in which schools are trying to stop violence and its effects.

Thinking Critically

3. **Evaluation.** Why do you think the number of gangs in the United States has increased?

4. **Analysis.** Analyze this statement: "Violence breeds violence."

Applying Health Knowledge

5. Write a public service announcement about teens and guns. Include information about how to lessen your chances of becoming a shooting victim.
6. In small groups, come up with a plan to try to prevent or stop violence in and around your school. Present your ideas to the class.

BUILDING HEALTHY RELATIONSHIPS

To be a good athlete, you must possess many skills. Skill development takes time and practice. In the same way, to build healthy relationships, you must practice and master a variety of skills, one at a time. Among these are skills in communicating and standing up to peer pressure.

Communication

Communication is a process through which we send messages to and receive messages from one another. With words, gestures, facial expressions, and behaviors, we communicate what we feel, what we need, and what we know. If you want a relationship to be healthy, you must identify and express your expectations—the rules or guidelines by which you are operating. By doing this, you open doors to communication. Then the other person in a relationship can respond or react and share his or her expectations. This type of give-and-take discussion is not easy. It takes practice and lots of energy, but it can be very helpful in preventing misunderstandings. When there is conflict in the relationship, you have already laid the groundwork for constructive communication.

Speaking Skills

When you are speaking, it is important to say what you mean. Do not assume that anyone else can read your mind or know your needs or expectations. It is your responsibility to make them clear. That is the first step to healthy communication.

The inflections, or changes in pitch or loudness, of your voice can also play a large role in how you communicate. Kind words delivered with a sarcastic tone, for example, may not be processed kindly. Talking too loudly can make you seem too bossy or arrogant, even if underneath it all you are actually shy. Saying no too softly may make it seem as if you do not mean what you are saying. So it is not just what you say that is important in communicating, it is also how you say it.

Listening Skills

Listening is an important skill associated with communication. Studies indicate that we may spend 80 percent of our waking hours communicating, with much of that time spent listening. Because listening takes up so much of our time, you would think that most people would be skilled at it—but the opposite is true. The average listener may correctly understand, properly evaluate, and retain only about 30 percent of what was said in a 10-minute presentation. Within 48 hours, memory of what was said drops to an even lower percentage.

People like a good listener. Have you ever noticed that good listeners are often well-liked people? Everyone wants to feel that he or she is being heard and is not going to be judged, corrected, or interrupted.

LESSON 3 FOCUS

TERMS TO USE
- Communication
- Refusal skills
- Passive
- Aggressive
- Assertive

CONCEPTS TO LEARN
- There are many ways to communicate with others.
- Refusal skills help you say no when faced with negative peer pressure.

ATTITUDES AND BEHAVIORS TO EVALUATE
- Self-Inventory, page 114.
- Building Decision-Making Skills, page 115.

GOOD LISTENING RULES

- Give your full attention to the person speaking.
- Eliminate distractions, such as radio or TV.
- Make direct eye contact.
- Do not interrupt. Wait your turn.
- Try to get the general idea of what someone is saying rather than trying to remember every fact the speaker mentions.
- Listen to feelings and gestures as well as to words.
- Do not shift the attention from the other person's problem to your own.
- Indicate your interest. Lean toward the speaker; nod at or encourage the other person by quietly saying "Uh-huh" or "I understand" or "I see."
- Do not decide too early that the subject matter is too hard, too easy, or too upsetting. Give the speaker a chance.
- Ask questions only when it seems necessary.
- Avoid making judgmental or closed responses that might stop or hinder the conversation, such as, "That was dumb!"
- Do not spend so much time concentrating on what you will say next that you miss what the other person is saying.
- Remember what the speaker has said. To be sure you heard it correctly, repeat the idea back so that the person can correct you if necessary.
- When it is your turn to speak, recap the highlights of what the other person has said, using a phrase like, "As I hear it, you were saying. . . ."

Body Language Skills

Communicating without words is nonverbal communication. Expressions on your face and movements of your hands and body are examples. If your words and your face or body seem to be saying two different things, you may be misunderstood. People may get your nonverbal messages rather than your verbal ones. Consider these cues:

- People who are lying often nod their heads at the end of a lie, rub their bodies, rub their hands together, or stop moving altogether.
- Moving the hand to the nose or lips can be a way of showing shame.
- Putting the hands behind the head while talking may show an attitude of superiority.
- Standing with head or shoulders down may be communicating that the person is passive and will not stick up for him- or herself.
- Placing hands into pockets may indicate that the person is afraid.

K E E P I N G   F I T

How to Say NO

Add these tips to your storehouse of refusal skills:

- Buy time. Say you'll get back to the person.
- State exactly how you feel. Be direct and honest.

- Don't apologize for your decisions or values.
- Use direct eye contact to show that you mean what you say.
- Use a firm and friendly tone of voice.
- Use the other person's name.

- Offer an alternative, healthier, more acceptable-to-you option.
- Avoid compromise if you feel strongly about something. Compromise can be a slow way of saying *yes* when you don't mean to.

Refusal Skills

Refusal skills are those techniques and strategies that you can learn to help you say no effectively when faced with something that you do not want to do or is against your values.

Throughout your life people will make many requests of you. Some of these will call for you to respond with a yes, others with a firm and unapologetic no. How you respond can directly affect your mental, social, or physical health—or even your life.

Some styles of refusing are more effective than others. Those that are most effective generally show that you have respect both for yourself and for the other person. Find the way that is best for you to say no.

The Passive Way.   Being **passive** means giving up, giving in, or backing down without standing up for your own rights and needs. People who are passive "go with the flow" and may find themselves in situations they do not want to be in, not knowing how to get out. They may think they are making friends by going along with peer pressure but, in fact, they may be viewed by their peers as pushovers, not worthy of much respect.

The Aggressive Way.   Being **aggressive** means being overly forceful, pushy, hostile, or otherwise attacking in approach. The aggressive approach to saying no might involve punching, yelling, shouting insults, or displaying other kinds of physical or verbal force. The aggressive way violates the rights of others. Though aggressive people may think they will gain their own way and perhaps be seen as powerful and popular, their approach usually backfires. In the long run, people either stay away from aggressors or jump in and fight back. Either way can leave aggressive people hurting.

The Assertive Way.   Being **assertive** means standing up for your own rights, in firm but positive ways. You state your position, acknowledge the rights of the other individual, then stand your ground. You do not bully or back away. You directly and honestly state your case and show that you mean what you say. Assertive people often become role models for other teens. Teens respect people who have the personal power to be true to who they really are.

CONFLICT RESOLUTION

A recent study found that most of our arguments are with relatives, and the negative results of fighting often exceed the benefits of pleasant encounters. Females, especially, tend to be unfavorably affected by family feuding, sometimes becoming depressed after quarrels. Researchers advise following a middle course when a relative makes you "see red"— don't hide your feelings, but if you do argue, try to resolve the conflict quickly and put it behind you.

Consider the most recent argument you had with a relative.

How would things have gone differently if you had followed this advice for conflict resolution?

LESSON 3 REVIEW

Reviewing Facts and Vocabulary

1. Define *verbal* and *nonverbal communication*.
2. List five skills needed for good listening.

Thinking Critically

3. **Evaluation.** Do you think there are situations that call for passive or aggressive behavior, instead of assertive behavior? Explain.

4. **Synthesis.** Write the script for a skit in which a person role-plays passive, aggressive, and assertive ways of saying no.

Applying Health Knowledge

5. Think of an issue, a project, or a person you care a lot about. How might you communicate your caring without using words?

Self-Inventory

Are You a Good Listener?

HOW DO YOU RATE?

Number a sheet of paper from 1 through 10. Read each item below and indicate whether each statement describes you *most of the time, some of the time,* or *never.* Total the number of each type of response. Then proceed to the next section.

1. When listening, I assume I know what the other person is going to say.

2. I interrupt others when they are talking.

3. I find myself thinking about what I am going to say while the other person is talking.

4. I avoid eye contact when listening to the other person.

5. I do several things while I listen, such as doodle, watch TV, or play music.

6. I find that my mind is wandering while someone else is talking.

7. I make judgments on what is being said.

8. I have to ask for things to be repeated.

9. I carry on several conversations at one time.

10. I avoid asking questions if I am not sure I understand what was said.

HOW DID YOU SCORE?

Give yourself 4 points for every *most of the time* answer, 2 points for each *some of the time* answer, and 0 points for each *never* answer. Find your total and read to see how you scored. Then proceed to the next section.

0 to 4
Excellent. You have very good listening skills.

6 to 10
Good. You have some good listening skills but could develop your skills more.

12 or more
Needs Improvement. You have poor listening skills and need to improve them. Doing so may help improve your relationships.

WHAT ARE YOUR GOALS?

If you scored 11 or more, identify an area in which your score is low, and use the goal-setting process to begin making a change. If your listening skills are weak in several areas, set several specific goals for improving them, but do so one at a time.

1. The listening skill I most need to change or improve to better my communication is ____.

2. If this behavior were completely changed, the reaction I would probably find in the people trying to communicate with me would be ____.

3. The steps involved in making this change are ____.

4. My timetable for improving this listening skill is ____.

5. People I can ask for support, assistance, and gentle reminders in trying to develop this skill are ____.

6. The benefits I will receive are ____.

7. The benefits to my relationships will be ____.

8. My reward after identifying, working on, and improving each listening skill on which I need to concentrate will be ____.

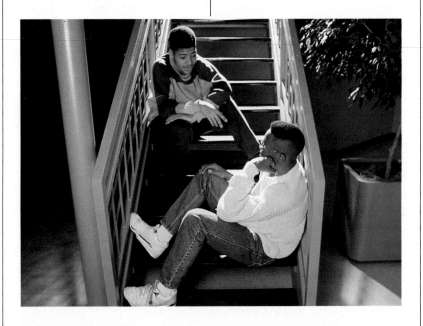

Building Decision-Making Skills

Drew works hard at school, is in a few school clubs, and works for neighbors some Saturdays. He knows the neighborhood he lives in is not considered the best, but it is home to him.

On Drew's way to and from school, he walks by an abandoned building. Some kids from school have kind of claimed this building as theirs. They seem to hang out there a lot, especially before and after school. This group considers itself a gang. They dress alike and have written graffiti on the building. On some occa-sions, Drew has seen adults he didn't know talking to the kids there. Because of this, people at school think the gang does drugs.

Recently Drew's friend, Ron, has begun hanging out at the abandoned building. Ron has even showed Drew a small gun he said he was carrying for a gang member. Ron said he really likes being a part of the gang and wants Drew to be a part too. Ron told Drew that if he joined, he would always have protection in case he ever needed it. What should Drew do about Ron's invitation to join the gang?

A. Tell Ron he doesn't want to join the gang. Tell him he is not into that kind of thing.

B. Try going to the building a few times and see if it's fun. He will still have time to do his homework in the evening.

C. Ask Ron how he sees his friendship with the gang affecting his goals for the future.

WHAT DO YOU THINK?

1. **Choices.** What other choices does Drew have?

2. **Consequences.** What are the effects of each choice?

3. **Consequences.** How might Drew's self-esteem be affected by each choice?

4. **Consequences.** What might Drew's parents say about each choice?

5. **Consequences.** In what way might other people be affected by Drew's decision?

6. **Consequences.** What effect could going to the building have on Drew's total health?

7. **Decision.** What do you think Drew should do? Explain your answer.

8. **Evaluation.** Have you ever been asked to be a part of a gang or clique? For what reason(s) did or didn't you join? How did your decision affect your self-esteem?

Melanie is a very good student, and she has just completed a tough science assignment. Rob, her next-door neighbor and good friend, went away with his family over the weekend to visit his uncle. Late Sunday night, Rob knocks on Melanie's door and asks if he can copy her answers to the science assignment.

WHAT DO YOU THINK?

9. **Choices.** Can you think of five or more choices that Melanie has?

10. **Choices.** Which of the above choices are positive and appropriate ones?

11. **Choices.** Which of the choices are inappropriate? Explain your answers.

12. **Consequences.** What are the advantages of each choice?

13. **Consequences.** What are the disadvantages of each choice?

14. **Consequences.** What risks are involved in this decision?

15. **Decision.** What do you think Melanie should do?

16. **Evaluation.** Have you ever faced a similar situation? If so, how did you handle it? How would you handle a situation like this now? Would it depend on the kind of relationship you had with the other person? Explain.

REVIEW

Using Health Terms

On a separate sheet of paper, write the term that best matches each definition given below.

LESSON 1

1. A bond or connection between people.
2. The control and influence people your own age may have over you.
3. An indirect and often dishonest means of trying to control another's attitudes or behavior.
4. A method of manipulation in which a person promises favors to another person in order to influence his or her behavior.

LESSON 2

5. Violence committed for no particular reason against anyone who happens to be around.
6. The use of physical force to control someone through the use of power.

LESSON 3

7. A process by which people receive and send messages.
8. Techniques that help a person say no when faced with negative peer pressure.

Building Academic Skills

LESSON 1

9. **Writing.** The following lines appear in Shakespeare's play *As You Like It:*
   All the world's a stage,
   And all the men and women merely players;
   They have their exits and their entrances;
   And one man in his time plays many parts.
   Write a paragraph giving your own interpretation of this quote.

LESSON 3

10. **Math.** Pilar gets 8 hours of sleep each night. If she spends 80 percent of her waking hours communicating and 60 percent of that time listening, how many hours a day does Pilar spend listening?

Recalling the Facts

LESSON 1

11. What are some advantages of platonic relationships with members of the opposite sex?
12. What are some advantages and disadvantages of dating one person exclusively?
13. Give two examples of possible results of positive peer pressure.
14. Give two examples of possible results of negative peer pressure.
15. Why is manipulation an unhealthy way for people to fulfill their needs?
16. List five methods of manipulation.
17. What is the cause of prejudice? What may often be its effect?

LESSON 2

18. Why do some teens join gangs?
19. What are some disadvantages of belonging to a gang?
20. Explain what can happen to stolen cars after a carjacking.
21. List several reasons violence has increased in our society.

LESSON 3

22. What can be an unwanted effect of speaking too loudly? Too softly?
23. How can you show your interest in what another person is saying?
24. What is a good way to verify that you have correctly understood a speaker?
25. What is body language?
26. List three examples of body language that might indicate that a person is lying.
27. Why is it important to learn refusal skills?

Thinking Critically

LESSON 1

28. **Analysis.** What is the difference between platonic and dating relationships?

LESSON 2

29. **Evaluation.** If you were the mayor of your town or city, what steps would you propose

to stop violence in the community? Include ways you would carry out your plans.

30. Evaluation. Write a report for or against gun control. Support your position with current information.

LESSON 3

31. Analysis. Compare and contrast *passive, aggressive,* and *assertive* behavior.

32. Synthesis. Kim's father is criticizing her last performance on her grade card, which contained three *C*s and a *D*. Kim's father is threatening to cut off her allowance and ground her for two weeks. Kim put her head and shoulders down and shoved her hands into the pockets of her jeans. What emotions do you think Kim is probably feeling based on her body language?

33. Analysis. Classify each behavior as *passive, aggressive,* or *assertive.*

- Every morning Elizabeth asks Sarah if she can copy her geometry homework. Sarah feels this is wrong, but she always gives Elizabeth her homework to copy.
- Nick wants to take Anita to a party where beer will be served. Anita explains to Nick that although she would like to go out with him, she does not want be around people who may be drinking.
- Anne is unkind to her sister Patti. She often yells at Patti when she forgets to clean up the room they share. Anne also loudly insults and embarrasses Patti at school. Anne does not have many friends.

Making the Connection

LESSON 2

34. Language Arts. Use the library to research the effect of television violence on child development. Is there a connection between what children watch on television and how they interact with others? After you have gathered information, write an editorial to your local newspaper to express your viewpoint.

Applying Health Knowledge

LESSON 1

35. Think about the relationship you have with your closest friend. What does each of you contribute to this relationship?

36. What types of prejudice, stereotyping, and discrimination are problems in your school? Why do you think the problems exist? What could students do to reduce the problems? What might teachers and administrators do to help the situation?

37. Is it possible to eliminate prejudice? Explain your answer.

LESSON 3

38. Review the rules for good listening. Divide a sheet of paper into two columns. Label one column "I usually do this"; label the other column "I need to work on this." Then write each rule in the column that applies to your listening skills. Concentrate on improving one skill every day.

Beyond the Classroom

LESSON 1

39. Community Involvement. Explore what opportunities there are in your community for people who live alone to make new friends.

LESSON 2

40. Parental Involvement. Ask your parents about violence that occurred when they were in high school. What did they see as the causes of this violence? What solutions, if any, were used?

LESSON 3

41. Parental Involvement. Ask your parents to give their opinion of what they think good communication skills are. Which skills do they feel they use in the course of their day?

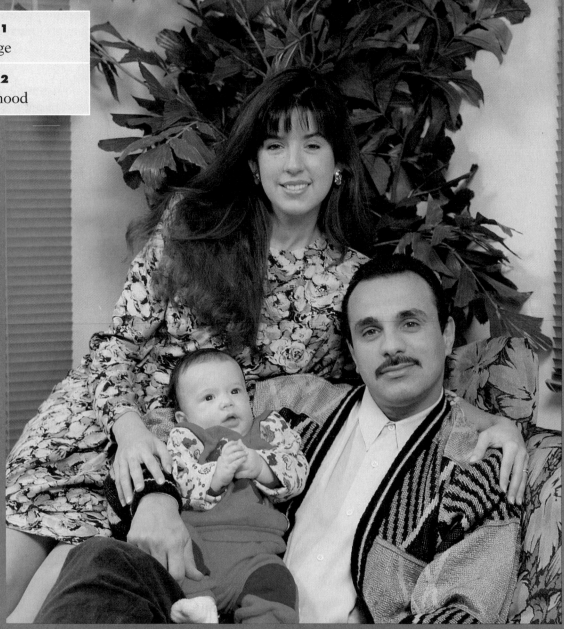

MARRIAGE

Getting married is deciding to spend the rest of your life with some-one else. Marriage is a long-term, ongoing commitment. It is a very serious decision.

Marriage in the Past and Marriage Today

In ancient times a woman was often considered property belonging to her father. A prospective husband had to get permission from the father of his bride-to-be before a marriage could take place. Often there was an exchange of gifts or property in the marriage transaction. The union, which did not take into account the notion of romantic love, was both a business and a social contract. It represented the economic merging of two families.

Today in the United States few marriages are arranged. People choose their own mates. People meet and decide to marry for many reasons, including mutual attraction and affection. Romantic love is often the driving force behind a couple's decision to marry, but it is seldom the reason two people remain married.

Marriage and the Law

In the legal sense, marriage is the joining of a man and a woman according to custom or law. It is a legal agreement between two people to live together and share their lives.

Most states in the United States require a marriage license; some require that both parties have a blood test and undergo medical exami-nations. Most states also require a waiting period of 3 to 5 days during which either party can back out. Almost all states allow people to marry at age 18 without parental consent. More than half the states allow cou-ples to marry with parental permission at 16.

Marriage Trends

Each year about 2.5 million couples are married in the United States. About 95 percent of all Americans marry by the age of 40. Yet there are many new trends in marrying practices today.

Marrying Later

According to the 1990 United States Census, Americans are marrying later now than at any other time during the past 100 years. In 1950 men married at an average age of 23; women, at 20. The average age for first marriages now, however, is 26 for men and 24 for women. Several social factors help explain this trend. High divorce rates may make

LESSON 1 FOCUS

TERMS TO USE
- Marital adjustment
- Divorce

CONCEPTS TO LEARN
- There are many reasons people get married.
- Marriage is an arrange-ment between two peo-ple to face the realities of life as a couple.
- Teen marriages face many risks.

ATTITUDES AND BEHAVIORS TO EVALUATE
- Self-Inventory, page 132.
- Building Decision-Making Skills, page 133.

some people marriage-shy. Young people with divorced parents may be wary about walking down the aisle.

These are also difficult economic times. Jobs are sometimes difficult to secure, and the cost of housing and raising families is high. Young people who want to finish their education or establish careers are also delaying marriage until they achieve their personal goals.

Two-Career Marriages

In 1940 only 15 percent of all married women worked outside the home. Today, about half of all married women in the United States have full-time or part-time jobs outside the home. Two-income households, particularly those without children, may have more money and more social contacts. For some couples, however, two partners working may add fatigue, stress, and competition to the marriage.

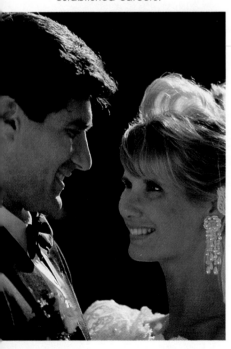

Many people today choose to delay marriage until they have completed their education and established careers.

Staying Single: The Other Option

Staying single has also become more popular. In 1990 there were fewer married couples in the United States in relation to the rest of the population than in previous years. Married couples, with or without children, presently make up 55 percent of the country's 92 million households. That is down from about 60 percent in 1980.

Reasons for Getting Married

Most people say they are marrying because they are "in love," and this may be true. Often, however, there are other motives hidden deep inside. People may decide to marry because they are lonely or they want to escape a bad situation at home. They also may marry because a pregnancy is involved or because they want financial security. Without close self-examination, couples may not even be aware of the motives driving them. If there are serious doubts or questions about reasons for marrying or about the intended spouse, the best time to face them and reconsider is before the marriage.

Factors Affecting Marital Adjustment

Sociologists have conducted extensive research to develop measures of **marital adjustment**—how well people adjust and adapt to marriage and to each other. Researchers have concluded that a well-adjusted marriage is one in which the husband and wife

- agree on critical issues in their relationship,
- share common interests and activities,
- demonstrate affection and shared confidences,
- have few complaints about the marriage,
- do not have feelings of loneliness or irritability.

Researchers have also identified some factors related to social background that were associated with successful marital adjustment. Some of the more significant factors they found included the following:

- similarity in family backgrounds
- domestic happiness of parents
- lack of conflict with parents
- educational achievement of both partners
- friends of both sexes
- participation in organizations
- close association prior to marriage
- security and stability of occupation

The more positive factors involved, the better the marital adjustment. In addition, the ability to be intimate, feel trust, give mutual respect, and be good friends have all been cited as important factors in healthy marriages. In a healthy marriage each partner needs to learn to accept the other person. That means not trying to change the person, not constantly judging him or her, and supporting the person in his or her pursuits. It means accepting that no relationship will ever be perfect.

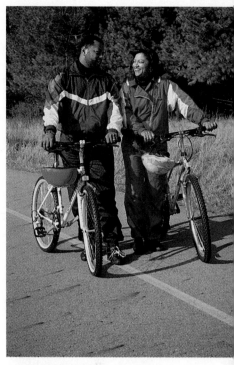

This couple illustrates long-lasting marital happiness.

Marriage and Maturity

Unfortunately, many young couples make a decision to get married based on only the romantic phase of their relationship. To be successful, however, a marriage requires emotional and social maturity. Maturity can be difficult to define, but it can be described in these ways:

- A mature person has the ability and skill to establish and maintain relationships.
- A mature person has the ability to give as well as receive.
- A mature person can perceive and process others' feelings.
- A mature person can compromise and accept not always getting his or her own way.
- A mature person can be flexible.
- A mature person accepts responsibility for his or her feelings and actions and does not blame them on someone else.
- A mature person is personally stable.
- A mature person has established values by which he or she lives. He or she has goals and plans for achieving those goals.
- A mature person is aware of his or her emotional needs and how to meet them in healthy ways. He or she does not expect the spouse or the marriage to meet all these needs.

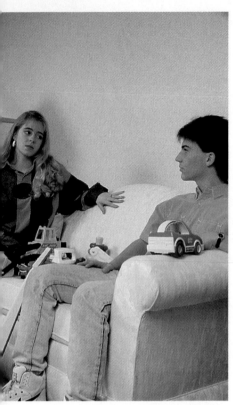

Early marriage and parenthood presents many problems for teens.

Teen Marriages

Adolescence is a time to get to know oneself. This happens through participating in a variety of activities and relationships. During these interactions teens develop a sense of who they are and what they want out of life and a life partner. Unfortunately, teens who choose to marry or feel forced to marry because of unexpected pregnancies often choose their mates before they have any idea who they themselves are or what they want. The results can be disastrous. Consider these facts:

- Females between the ages of 14 and 17 who marry are twice as likely to divorce as females who wait until they are 18 or 19 and three times as likely to divorce as females in the 20-to-24 age group.
- About 80 percent of teenage couples who get married because of pregnancy are divorced within six years.
- Couples with low incomes and couples with little education are more likely to divorce than other groups. Teens who marry often fall into both categories.
- Couples in which neither spouse has a high school diploma are more likely to divorce than couples in which both have college degrees.

In other words, the odds for a successful teen marriage are not good. Teen marriages often deteriorate as the excitement wears off and the responsibilities increase.

Married teens often feel like social outcasts. They are not sure where they fit in. They are neither children nor adults. They are neither carefree teens nor settled married couples. Often they feel isolated from their peers, as if they are missing out on a normal social life. They may be jealous of social contacts outside the marriage. Not yet aware of effective ways to resolve conflicts, they may begin to blame each other for their unhappiness.

Conflicts in Marriage

Marriage takes work. Part of that work is learning to resolve conflicts fairly and without damaging one's own or one's partner's self-esteem. Among the issues that sometimes cause problems in marriages are differences in spending and saving habits, conflicting loyalties involving friends and families, intimacy or sexual problems, jealousy or infidelity, lack of attention, housework, decisions about having children, and child care. Unexpressed, ongoing anger over any of these issues can turn into rage. Unresolved rage can result in name-calling, belittling, ignoring, fighting, living separate emotional lives, or even attacking the partner physically. In some cases, a marriage that began with romantic visions of hope can deteriorate into a constant nightmare.

Developing skills in communication and resolving conflicts before they escalate or get out of hand are essential in dealing with the issues and conflicts in any marriage.

Divorce

A **divorce** is the legal dissolution, or ending, of the marriage contract. During the past two decades, the number of divorces in the United States tripled. The divorce rate for couples marrying today is about 50 percent. About 1 million couples in the United States divorce each year. Though the overall divorce rate has fallen in the last 3 years and is beginning to level off, the rate for teen divorces continues to increase.

The breakup of a marriage can be a highly charged emotional event. It can feel like a death. Dealing with the loss of a marriage may take time. Newly divorced people often display a wide range of physical and emotional reactions. They may suffer from hostility, guilt, rage, or jealousy. They may also suffer from symptoms like sleeplessness, headaches, or ulcers.

Divorce Prevention

During the 1970s and 1980s marriage counselors and other therapists often counseled couples in trouble to take an honest look at themselves and their spouses before deciding whether or not to split up or stay together. They still do. But these days some therapists are counseling people to try harder to stay together. New findings from a 10-year divorce prevention study funded by the National Institute of Mental Health show that couples in training for handling conflict have 50 per-

K E E P I N G   F I T

If Your Parents Are Going Through a Divorce

Living in a home where parents are divorcing can be difficult. If you are in such a situation, keep these tips in mind:

■ Remind yourself that you did not cause the problem.
■ Ask your parents not to fight in front of you.
■ Ask your parents not to ask you to take sides.
■ Remember to take good care of your own health.
■ Find someone to talk to. It may be a friend, adult, or a teacher or counselor.
■ Consider joining a support group for children of divorce. Doing so will help you realize that you are not alone.

- When Richard Biddenstadt of Iowa pulled a strangely shaped beet from his garden, he noticed something doubly strange. Not only was the beet shaped like a figure eight, but there was a ring around its middle. On closer examination, Bidden-stadt discovered it was the wedding ring his father had lost in the garden some 50 years before.
- The custom of having a best man and ushers at a wedding was probably first used to prevent bride-stealing, a common practice in earlier times. Attendants were cho-sen for their strength rather than for their friendship.

cent fewer divorces and one-third the verbal and physical abuse rates of married couples who do not undergo such training. Of course, some-times staying in a marriage can be an unhealthy, even lethal decision—for example, where there is continual physical abuse. However, with help, destructive behaviors can be stopped and marriages can be made healthier than before.

Remarriage

Out of every 10 people who divorce for the first time, 4 remarry. About 50 percent of these do so within 3 years after the divorce is final. Women without children are more likely to remarry than women with children. Remarriages often occur between people more different in background, education, or age than those who marry for the first time. Some people view a second marriage as a solution to all their problems. However, too often, they repeat the same patterns in choosing a partner. They may also repeat the same patterns of emotional responses and actions as in their first marriages. In fact, of those divorced people who remarry, 44 percent divorce a second time.

Marriage and Health

At least half of all couples who marry do not divorce. Many married people who have matured together, weathered life's ups and downs as a team, and become deep friends say there is nothing like it. To have a life partner with whom to share one's goals, dreams, plans, home, children, and old age can be an enriching adventure.

Recent surveys show that many adults believe that being in a happy and intimate relationship is the most important thing in life. Other stud-ies suggest a link between being married and having better health and living longer. Marriage is a major life decision that can affect both part-ners' physical, mental, and social health for many years.

LESSON 1 REVIEW

Reviewing Facts and Vocabulary

1. Name three factors that are important for good marital adjustment.
2. List two reasons Americans may have for marrying later.
3. What are some of the characteristics of matu-rity that are important for achieving a suc-cessful marriage?

Thinking Critically

4. **Analysis.** Analyze this statement, "Love may be enough to start a marriage, but it is not enough to keep it together."

5. **Synthesis.** Write a short story about a teen couple who marry and then divorce. Within the story dramatize some of the reasons for the failure of their relationship.

Applying Health Knowledge

6. Consider the characteristics of a mature per-son. Which of these characteristics describe you? Do you think you are ready for mar-riage? Why or why not?
7. Think of a couple you know who seem to have a successful marriage. What factors seem to play a part in their success?

PARENTHOOD

Having a child can be a wonderful experience. It can be thrilling to love someone so much and have someone love you in return. It can be rewarding to provide a nurturing environment for a child and watch that child grow and develop within it. However, parenting is a huge, ongoing responsibility. Like marriage, it is not something to be taken lightly.

Parenting in the Past and Parenting Now

In early America children were expected to work and contribute to the family's economic well-being by the time they were 6 or 7. Even in the 1800s most people were independent, working, and married by the time they were teens. But today childhood has been extended. Young people often do not reach economic independence until well into their 20s. In addition, in the past parents could often rely on an extended family to help with the raising and care of their children. Today, however, only an estimated 5 percent of families in the United States have an extra adult on whom they can rely in the raising or care of their children. Raising children in isolation and for longer periods of time has made childrearing today particularly demanding.

In the past when people got married, it was assumed they would have children. Today this is not always the case. Changing social attitudes, economics, the importance of education and careers, and new advances in reproductive medical technology have made it possible for parenthood to be a delayed or a deliberate choice.

Trends in Parenting

There are many current trends in parenting. Delayed parenthood, working mothers, father involvement in childrearing, and single parenthood are all more common these days than in the past.

Delayed Parenthood

At one end of the age scale, there are more teen pregnancies than in earlier times. At the other end, more couples are delaying childbearing until their 30s or 40s so that they can complete their education or establish careers before starting families. In fact, particularly among college-educated couples, delaying childbearing has increased in popularity.

More Working Mothers

There are more mothers working outside the home than ever before. According to government statistics, 53 percent of mothers of children

LESSON 2 FOCUS

TERM TO USE
- Adoption

CONCEPTS TO LEARN
- The costs of raising children are complex and demanding.
- Some of the responsibilities of parenthood are maintaining parent health, providing discipline, and giving love.

ATTITUDES AND BEHAVIORS TO EVALUATE
- Self-Inventory, page 132.
- Building Decision-Making Skills, page 133.

Brooke is really proud of her mom. After having three kids, her mom went back to college, graduated from law school, and now works in one of the best law firms in the city. Brooke's dad worked hard for 16 years in a steel factory, financed his wife's education, and then retired when his wife started practicing law. Now he describes himself as a "domestic engineer," meaning he takes care of everything at home. Brooke loves her dad and knows he's happier now than when he worked in the factory, but she's embarrassed by her friends' comments about his "Mr. Mom" role. Brooke knows her dad is no different now than when he worked in the factory.

How can she convince her friends?

aged 5 and under now work outside the home, and about 66 percent of mothers of children 6 to 17 also have outside employment.

A report from the National Commission on Working Women states these facts:

- 75 percent of women return to their jobs within a year of giving birth.
- 75 percent of working mothers work full-time.
- 80 percent of divorced mothers work outside the home.
- 62 percent of married mothers work outside the home.

The report also points out that most mothers who work outside the home do not do so to buy luxuries, as is sometimes thought, but to help make ends meet. Making ends meet can be even more difficult when the cost of day care is high.

More Single Parents

According to the Census Bureau, some 50 percent of all children born now will spend some time in a one-parent household before the age of 18. Of the 10.6 million women who head households, two-thirds are single mothers. Most unmarried mothers in the United States now choose to keep their babies. Today an increasing number of fathers are also raising their children alone.

Many single parents do a good job of raising their children, but raising children alone is not easy. Single parents do not have partners with whom to share decisions, chores, disciplining, financial burdens, or even the joys of parenthood. With no one to relieve them, they often suffer from burnout or depression. Without relief, they may also be more likely to take out their frustrations on their children. They may find it difficult to find time for themselves and may feel they have no life besides their children and their jobs. Single parents with two or more children may also have a hard time finding a partner willing to take on the responsibility of several children.

Single parenthood may also prove stressful for children. One recent study showed that of children who were in trouble in school, more came from single-parent households than from households with two parents. New studies indicate that children from one-parent families are much more likely to live in poverty than children from two-parent households. Another study that followed the progress of 25,000 students for a year showed that children from single-parent families often perform less well in school than children from 2-parent families.

KEEPING FIT

Using Parenting "Warm Lines"

Hotlines, which offer free information and advice, are often for emergency or crisis situations. Recently, lower-key "warm lines" are being made available for parents or other caregivers who need information and support in some daily area of parenting. Right now about 40 agencies across the United States have set up warm lines to assist and support parents. Warm-line workers are either childcare or counseling professionals or have received training from such experts. They help to educate and support struggling parents about issues such as discipline. For more information about such a helpline in your area, consult a local counseling center or librarian.

Because isolation and decreased time for socializing are common complaints of single parents, it is important for them to develop support systems. This may be done through relatives, friends, or organizations such as Parents Without Partners. In addition, providing positive role models of the opposite, absent sex is important for their children. Nearly every community has organizations that can offer advice and support for single parents.

More Father Involvement

Many fathers play a more active role in raising their children than they did in the past. New studies confirm the importance of fathers' roles in child rearing. One study showed that children whose fathers spent time alone caring for them were more capable of showing sympathy and compassion for others as adults. Father involvement also has been linked to children's higher self-esteem, greater sociability, and higher grades.

Some men become househusbands and stay home to take care of the house and children. The decision to do this may be based on many factors. Perhaps the mother's job pays more than the father's, and he stays home to care for his children to avoid day-care costs. Or the father's job may be flexible, allowing him to work from a home office. Regardless of need for income, some fathers choose to spend this time at home with their children.

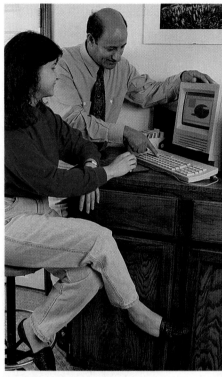

Many fathers play an active role in their children's lives.

Planned and Unplanned Pregnancy

The decision to have a child can be a very complex and private decision for a couple. It is often affected by religious, economic, career, emotional, cultural, and social considerations. Planned pregnancy is making a decision to get pregnant before the baby is conceived. Many couples deliberately decide when to conceive. They may wait until their marriages, careers, or finances are established. They may even put off having babies for years, waiting until they are in a financial and psychological position to parent. Though many babies who are unplanned, or conceived unexpectedly, become welcome additions to families, some of these unplanned children do not. Couples who are not ready to have children may resent new additions to the family. Shaky marriages may be further shaken by unwanted pregnancies. Marriages that take place because of pregnancy are more likely to fail than other marriages. A carefully planned pregnancy between two people ready to nurture and support a child to adulthood remains the route with the best chance of success for both the parents and the child.

Adoption

Some couples who are infertile (and some who are not) adopt children. **Adoption** is taking a child into one's family and legally assuming responsibility for that child, agreeing to raise him or her to adulthood. Adopted children are usually very much wanted and planned for as family additions. Adoptive parents often must go through a lengthy screening process and wait long periods before getting their adoptive children.

Currently there are about 2 million adopted children under age 18 in the United States, many of whom might otherwise be raised in institutions or in foster care situations. About 150,000 children are adopted in the United States annually. Today there are also increasing numbers of adoptions of babies from other nations. Fewer babies are available in the United States than in the past, partly because of contraceptive practices and partly because more single mothers are keeping and raising their children. There are also campaigns to encourage people to adopt disabled, older, and other hard-to-place children. In the past children were usually placed with two parents that matched them in terms of physical characteristics, religion, race, and so on. Increasingly, however, the major requirements for placement of an adopted child are that he or she will be given a healthy, caring home where the child's physical and emotional needs will be met. Today some children are even adopted by single parents.

What Children Need to Be Healthy

According to the National Mental Health Association, to be physically healthy, children need nutritious food, shelter, clothing, sleep, exercise, immunizations, and a healthy and safe environment. To be mentally and emotionally healthy, children need loving and firm parenting. They need to feel loved and wanted. They need to feel there are people nearby who care what happens to them. They need to feel accepted and valued as human beings even if their parents or other caretakers do not approve of particular behaviors.

The Responsibilities of Parenthood

Parents must provide food, clothing, shelter, education, medical care, and protection from harm for their children. They are responsible not only for their children's physical care but also for the emotional, social, and intellectual upbringing of their offspring. Perhaps most important, they must provide unconditional love.

Caring for a child from infancy to young adulthood is expensive. Recent estimates say that to raise a baby born today through the age of 18 will cost between $150,000 and $180,000. Just the first year of a baby's life costs an average of $5,774. There are other costs that are not financial. Having a child requires a tremendous marital adjustment. The original couple now has a third party demanding time, attention, and resources that might have been used instead for only two people. If there were marital problems before the birth of a child, these problems are likely to increase with the birth of a baby.

In helping meet children's needs, parents play many roles. At different times in different situations, they act as teachers, disciplinarians, and counselors. Parents have many responsibilities in addition to the financial ones.

Maintaining Parental Health

Parents need to give their children lots of attention, but a parent should not neglect his or her basic health needs in the process of caring for children. Maintaining one's own health is part of the responsibility of parenting, since a parent cannot function well if he or she is tired, irritable, hungry, or always pressed for time. Parents also need to get away by themselves for short periods of time to relax and enjoy a day or an evening out. A parent must work to keep his or her mental and physical stamina at a high level and keep the relationship between the parents alive and healthy. Taking care of oneself means being a role model for children's future health habits. If children see physical, mental, and social health as parental priorities, they will be more likely to model such behavior in their own lives.

Setting Limits

Parents need to set limits and establish a clearly defined set of rules. Children need to learn restrictions and limitations on behavior. They need to learn to control their impulses. Children also need to learn the consequences of not following rules. When children learn these limits, they become self-directed. A self-directed child is one who can make correct decisions about behavior when adults are not there to enforce rules. Parents should follow these guidelines in disciplining their children:

- Parents should act quickly. Particularly with small children, it is important that misbehavior be dealt with soon after the fact. If children do not understand the link between their misbehavior and the consequences, they may feel they are being punished for no reason. As a result, children's self-esteem may suffer.
- Parents should be consistent. A consistent approach is different from random punishment. Children should come to expect that certain behaviors will result in certain consequences. Discipline should be structured. The children should know what the expectations are and they should know what will happen if they disobey. It can be helpful, especially as children get older, to explain reasons for limits or rules. This helps children develop an understanding of cause and effect. The goal of discipline should be to teach children appropriate behavior, not just to punish, shame, or get revenge. Physical abuse is never warranted; besides, it is not an effective teacher. It only teaches children to be angry and hurt.
- Parents should distinguish between the behavior and the child. Parents should try to make a distinction between actions (behaviors) and the person doing those behaviors. If parents do not make this distinction, children may develop low self-esteem and think of themselves as bad rather than as people who occasionally do bad things.
- Parents should try to ignore minor annoyances and save discipline for larger issues, such as those involving safety or respect.
- Parents need to praise positive behavior. Words of encouragement and pats on the back can do more to help children's self-esteem and promote good behavior than any disciplinary action.
- Parents should remain friendly, fair, and firm, even when disciplining. Parents should not jump into arguments and stoop to children's emotional levels. They should try not to act angry or out of control. They should remember who the adults are and who should be in control of the situation. They also should be unapologetic about exercising discipline but should do so in a positive manner.
- Parents should give children choices in some situations. Providing choices makes children feel they have some control in solving their problems. If parents give children two or more acceptable behavior

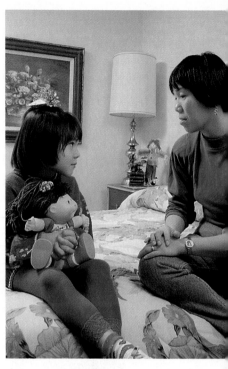

A parent acts as teacher, disciplinarian, and counselor.

Gloria Falanga is 15. She loves softball, drawing, and films. She's always wanted to be a filmmaker, she says, and she's always wanted to be part of a big family—until she got one. "The way I got a big family isn't the greatest," she says. "My father died and my mom went to work in a store in town about 25 miles from our house. It was really hard for her—and for me. We didn't have as much time together, and money was tight.

"When I was around 15, she started to see this man named Jack. He owned the store where she worked. He was divorced and he had three kids. After about six months, I could tell things were getting really serious for my mom, and I could tell she was beginning to prepare me for the news. Then the news hit: they decided to get married. I love my mom and wanted her to be happy and not alone, but I have to say I hated the idea. Nobody could ever take my dad's place. I felt like somehow she was betraying him or something—and me.

"So the next thing you know, they get married and we moved into Jack's house just outside of town. All of a sudden I'm

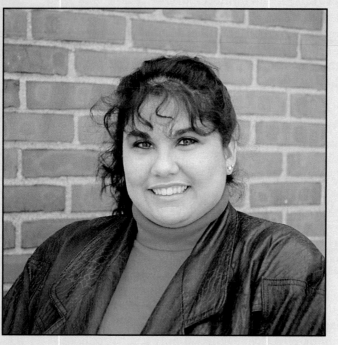

not the only 15-year-old in the house. There's Frank, who's my age, Angee, who's 16, and Kevin, who's 13.

"Jack came on too strong, too, at first, trying to take my dad's place. I finally told him he wasn't my dad and never would be and he backed off. But after a while—a long while—we all started to get adjusted. I think one of the things that helped the most was that this spring we all started playing on a family softball team in our town. We were good. We started really rooting for each other and getting better.

"We also got some family counseling. That helped. And then my mom and Jack decided that we should do something for other people as a family. We had a family meeting about it. So we started—all six of us—volunteering in a soup kitchen every other Friday night. And it has felt good. It also makes me realize that I don't have it so bad, that I'm lucky to have a home, and food, and a group of people who care—even if it's not a group I chose. I guess one of the ways I've learned to deal with it all is to accept what I can't change, then work like heck to make the best of the rest. And I'm even starting to feel closer to Jack."

1. What kinds of adjustments has Gloria had to make in her family life?
2. What philosophy has helped Gloria to adjust to her new stepfamily? What activities have helped family members adjust to one another?
3. Are there relationships in your family that cause you stress? What kinds of activities, outside help, or changes in attitude might you use to handle the situation with less stress?

options, the children are less likely to choose misbehavior as an option.

- Parents should set good behavior examples. What parents *do* is a more effective teacher than what they *say*.

Giving Love, Attention, and Guidance

Children can do without expensive toys or fancy clothes. What they cannot do without is love, attention, and guidance. Parents need to express their delight in their children and their existence whenever possible. They should praise their children for their efforts rather than the results of their efforts. They should give encouragement through words, letters, hugs, and facial expressions. They can show they care by giving their time. Such attention gives internal rewards to children. Children who are well-parented know they are loved not for what they do but for who they are.

Regardless of whether children are planned or unplanned, biological or adopted, or raised in one- or two-parent families, once they arrive, they all have certain basic needs that parents must work hard to meet. In addition to the basics of physical care and unconditional love, children need opportunities to learn and develop independence, responsibility, and competence while being protected and kept secure. They need to develop skills for getting along with others and handling problems. They need to learn how to make healthy decisions that demonstrate respect for themselves and others. They need to develop independence, responsibility, and capability in a variety of areas. They need to develop a sense of pride in their studies or work and recognize that they, more than anyone else, are responsible for their success or failure in life. As the old saying goes, parents must give a child "roots and wings"—a strong and secure family base and the right eventually to lead their own healthy, productive, and independent lives.

DID YOU KNOW?

- Raising children is costly. Just the cost of a college education can put families over the edge. According to The College Board, a child entering college in the year 2000 will need from $33,000 to $45,000 to complete 4 years at a state college and $120,000 to complete four years at a private institution.
- According to the Children's Defense Fund, yearly average costs of child care in New York City are $8,944; in Boston, $5,668; and in San Francisco, $4,264.

LESSON 2 REVIEW

Reviewing Facts and Vocabulary

1. Summarize some current trends in parenting.
2. What basic needs must be met by parents if children are to be healthy?
3. Write a paragraph about planned and unplanned pregnancy. Include the word *adoption* in the paragraph.

Thinking Critically

4. **Synthesis.** Summarize the major responsibilities that you will have to face as a parent.

5. **Synthesis.** Write a skit that illustrates three ways parents can use discipline both to punish and to teach.

Applying Health Knowledge

6. Find out about resources for children of divorce, pregnant teens, or teen parents. List books, articles, and local support groups. Post this information on a school bulletin board.

Self-Inventory

Will You Be an Effective Parent?

HOW DO YOU RATE?

Studies show a relationship between the kind of parenting a person receives and the kind of parent he or she may become. Number a sheet of paper from 1 through 20. Read each statement below, and respond by writing *yes* or *no*. (If you were not raised by a parent, respond for your primary caregiver.) Total the number of *yes* responses. Then proceed to the next section.

1. My parent(s) give me love and affection.
2. My parent(s) give me lots of attention.
3. My parent(s) provide guidance.
4. My parent(s) often praise my efforts.
5. My parent(s) rarely yell at me.
6. My parent(s) distinguish between my misbehavior and me as a person.
7. My parent(s) never abuse me.
8. My parent(s) respect my privacy.
9. My parent(s) set rules and limits.
10. My parent(s) enforce rules and limits consistently.
11. My parent(s) communicate well with me.
12. My parent(s) try to meet my basic physical needs.
13. My parent(s) take good care of themselves and me.
14. My parent(s) make me feel valued.
15. My parent(s) accept me for myself and not for what I accomplish.
16. My parent(s) encourage me to make my own decisions.
17. My parent(s) teach me the value of money.
18. My parent(s) teach me to value and respect others.
19. My parent(s) teach me to take responsibility for my own health.
20. My parent(s) teach me to respect myself.

HOW DID YOU SCORE?

Give yourself 1 point for each *yes* answer and 0 points for each *no* answer. Find your total and read below to see how you scored. Then proceed to the next section.

14 to 20
Good. You are likely to be an effective and caring parent. You have experienced positive parenting.

6 to 13
Fair. You, too, have the potential to become an effective parent, but you may need to work a bit harder at developing positive parenting skills.

Below 5
Caution. You, too, have the potential to become an effective parent. However, you probably need to learn more about parenting before becoming a parent.

WHAT ARE YOUR GOALS?

Choose one or more statements to which your answer was *no*. Use the goal-setting process to start working to achieve improvement for the future.

1. The area related to parenting in which I would like to improve is ____.
2. One specific goal I would like to achieve is ____.
3. The steps involved in achieving this goal are ____.
4. My timetable for achieving this goal is ____.
5. The support materials, groups, and people I will rely on in trying to achieve this goal are ____.
6. My reward for achieving this goal will be ____.
7. I plan to share my information with others by ____.

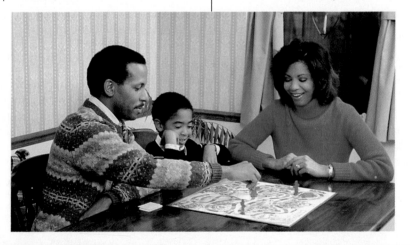

Building Decision-Making Skills

*E*rin is committed to becoming a special education teacher, in part because of her love for her little brother, who is developmentally disabled. This summer she worked in a special school for such students, which strengthened her career interest. She has been disturbed, however, that some of the teachers do not encourage these students to prepare themselves for marriage and parenthood. In fact, some even discourage it or promote the single life. They've explained that there is honest disagreement about this idea both within the profession and in society at large. Erin believes this is discriminatory. She believes that marriage and parenthood are the cornerstones of society for all people, and that marriage and parenthood should be encouraged for all. What should Erin do?

A. Recognize that there are problems of parenthood with which some developmentally disabled people may not be able to deal. Realize that discouraging parenthood is a realistic approach to promoting happiness.

B. Defer to more experienced people and accept their viewpoint.

C. Accept that some people believe one thing but that she is free to hold and promote her own beliefs.

D. Try to change people's minds.

E. Consider each case on its own merits, and encourage marriage and parenthood for some, but not for others.

F. Recognize that her opinion may be affected by personal feelings for her brother and that all people are not like he is.

WHAT DO YOU THINK?

1. **Situation.** Why does a decision need to be made?

2. **Choices.** What other solutions are there to Erin's dilemma?

3. **Consequences.** What are the pros and cons of each solution?

4. **Decision.** How should Erin proceed?

5. **Evaluation.** How do you handle a situation in which you disagree with someone who has more experience than you in dealing with an issue?

*M*elissa's 16-year-old friend has confided that she's pregnant. At least that's what her at-home pregnancy test showed. She's scared, and hasn't told anyone else yet.

WHAT DO YOU THINK?

6. **Situation.** What are the issues with which Melissa and her friend must deal?

7. **Situation.** Where might Melissa take her friend for information on the options available to her?

8. **Choices.** What are some of the solutions that Melissa can offer her friend?

9. **Choices.** Whom should the friend tell about her situation (parents, boyfriend, counselor, others)?

10. **Consequences.** What are the costs and benefits of each solution?

11. **Consequences.** Will the timing of when people are told (and in what order) affect the end result?

12. **Decision.** What advice do you think Melissa should give her friend?

13. **Evaluation.** Have you been in a situation similar to Melissa's in which you have had feelings of both happiness and sorrow for a friend? How did you handle the problem?

REVIEW

Using Health Terms

On a separate sheet of paper, write the term that best matches each definition given below.

LESSON 1

1. The joining of a man and a woman according to custom or law.
2. A marriage in which both spouses work outside the home.
3. A word used to describe a person who remains unmarried.
4. The legal ending of a marriage.

LESSON 2

5. A family with one or more children but only one parent.
6. A husband and father who stays home to care for the house and the children.
7. Waiting to have children until 30 to 40 years old.
8. Taking a child into one's family and legally assuming responsibility for that child.
9. The setting of restrictions on the behavior of children.

Building Academic Skills

LESSON 1

10. **Reading.** Read the following paragraph. Which of the details does not support the main idea?

    Several factors help explain the trend toward later marriages. High divorce rates make some people wary of early marriage. Many young people want to finish their education before marrying. People with established careers have more time to devote to making a marriage work.

LESSON 2

11. **Writing.** Assume that someday you will have a child. Write a three-to-five paragraph composition describing the goals you would have for your child and how you would help your child achieve those goals.

Recalling the Facts

LESSON 1

12. How big a factor is romantic love in the decision to marry and in the success of a marriage?
13. What aspects of a person's health triangle can marriage affect?
14. List five factors present in a well-adjusted marriage.
15. How can divorce affect a person's physical well-being?
16. What percent of divorced people remarry?
17. What are the advantages and disadvantages of two-career marriages?
18. According to 1990 Census figures, how many United States households are there and how many consist of married couples?
19. Name six characteristics related to social background that can have an effect on marital adjustment.
20. Why are teen marriages more likely to end in divorce than adult marriages?

LESSON 2

21. What are the basic responsibilities of parenthood?
22. What is the average estimated cost of raising a child from birth to age 18?
23. How can having a child affect the relationship in a marriage?
24. Write *yes* or *no* to indicate which of the following are problems faced by single parents:
    a. no help in disciplining children
    b. burnout or depression
    c. financial burdens
    d. plenty of free time for dating
    e. difficulty in finding another spouse
    f. fewer housekeeping responsibilities
25. How can single parents get help?
26. Why is it important for a parent to maintain his or her own physical health?
27. What are eight guidelines for disciplining children?
28. How can parents show love to their children?

REVIEW

Thinking Critically

LESSON 1

29. Synthesis. Create a test that you would administer to anyone considering marriage.

30. Analysis. What is behind the thinking in setting state laws that have minimum age requirements for marriage?

31. Evaluation. What is the purpose of requiring couples who want to marry to have blood tests and medical examinations?

32. Evaluation. Should an HIV test be required in order to obtain a marriage license?

33. Evaluation. Why is it important for married couples to develop skills in communication and resolving conflicts?

34. Evaluation. Do you think that "getting out of the house" is a valid reason for teens to get married? Explain your answer.

35. Synthesis. Outline a 5-minute presentation to junior high students on why teen marriage is "risky business."

36. Analysis. Analyze the factors contributing to the increasing number of mothers working outside the home.

37. Evaluation. What are your views on the topic of househusbands?

38. Evaluation. Why do you think parenthood is one of the most serious decisions a person makes?

Making the Connection

LESSON 1

39. Music. Choose a popular song about love. How do you think love depicted in the song compares with love in a marriage?

40. Social Studies. In ancient times marriages were arranged by the couple's parents. What might be some advantages and disadvantages of arranged marriages?

LESSON 2

41. Language Arts. Assume the role of a parent of a physically disabled child. Write a letter to a good friend describing the emotional burdens you carry as well as the special joys of parenthood you experience.

Applying Health Knowledge

LESSON 1

42. Two of your friends, Monica and Pedro, are thinking about marriage. At 18, what problems do they face that would not be problems if they wait 5 years to marry?

LESSON 2

43. Twenty years ago fewer than half of all married mothers worked outside the home. Today 62 percent do. Interview several mothers you know who work outside the home and several who do not. Find out why these women do or do not have outside employment. Categorize their responses and try to draw a conclusion based on their responses.

Beyond the Classroom

LESSON 1

44. Community Involvement. Survey the people living on your block or in your apartment building. Find out how many households are headed by a married couple and how many are headed by a single person. How do your neighborhood's statistics compare with national statistics?

45. Parental Involvement. Ask your parents what they have learned about each other since they got married. Find out what they have learned about marriage that they did not already know before their wedding.

46. Further Study. Investigate the laws regarding marriage in your state. Is a blood test or medical examination required? What are the age requirements with and without parental permission? Are certain persons not allowed to marry in your state?

LESSON 2

47. Further Study. Research and report the views of two child psychologists on the matter of spacing children. What do these doctors suggest as the best age for the first child to be before the next child is born? Do you agree or disagree?

CHAPTER 8

THE BEGINNING OF THE LIFE CYCLE

LESSON 1
Before Birth

LESSON 2
Heredity and
Genetics

LESSON 3
Birth to Late
Childhood

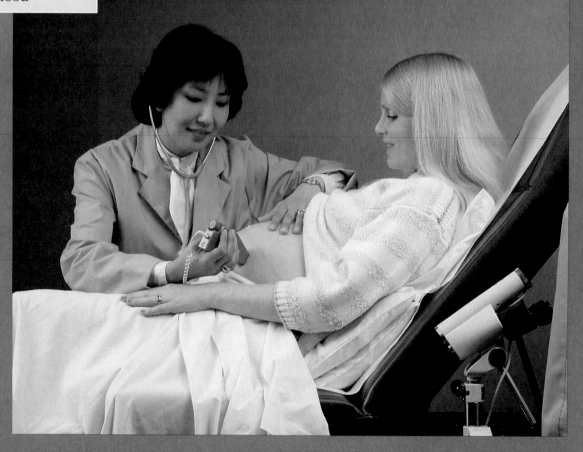

BEFORE BIRTH

Each of us began as a single microscopic cell, much smaller than the tip of a pin. Over a nine-month period of time, this cell divided millions of times and developed the tissues, organs, and systems that make up our complex bodies.

Cells: The Basic Unit of Life

The **cell** is the basic unit of structure of all living things. Your body is made up of trillions of cells. With the exception of the cells that make up the nervous system, each cell has the ability to divide, reproduce, and repair itself.

Cells with similar structure and that do similar work make up a tissue. For example, muscle is a tissue, and blood is a tissue. Organs are two or more tissue types that perform a specific job. The heart, brain, liver, and lungs are examples of organs.

A group of organs that work together to perform a common function form a body system. Examples of body systems include the digestive system, cardiovascular system, and reproductive system. Your body systems work together and are dependent upon one another. You will learn more about the function and care of your body systems when you study Unit 5.

Fertilization

The entire complex human body begins as one cell that is formed by the union of an egg cell, or ovum, from a female and a sperm cell from a male. These two cells are microscopic in size. The union of these cells is called **fertilization** or conception. Fertilization usually occurs in the Fallopian tube. Refer to the illustration on page 138.

As soon as the ovum is fertilized, it is called a **zygote.** A protective membrane forms to surround the zygote and prevent any more sperm from entering the ovum. The zygote divides into two cells, then four cells, and so on, and begins to move through the Fallopian tube to the uterus. This takes about three days.

Implantation in the Uterus

By the time the zygote reaches the uterus, it has divided many times to form a cluster of cells that has a hollow space in the center. It is now called a **blastocyst.** As the cells divide, they begin to implant, or attach, to the lining of the uterus. This process is called implantation. The lining of the uterus is made up of layers of tissue that will protect and nourish the fertilized egg throughout pregnancy. Once implantation has occurred, the cluster of cells is called an **embryo.** At this time the embryo is about the size of the dot over this letter *i.*

LESSON 1 FOCUS

TERMS TO USE
- Cell
- Fertilization
- Zygote
- Blastocyst
- Embryo
- Placenta
- Umbilical cord
- Fetus

CONCEPTS TO LEARN
- A male and female both contribute significantly to the characteristics of the unborn.
- Growth before birth is a gradual process, much like growth after birth.

ATTITUDES AND BEHAVIORS TO EVALUATE
- Self-Inventory, page 154.
- Building Decision-Making Skills, page 155.

As an ovum is released from an ovary, it moves through the Fallopian tube toward the uterus. If the ovum is fertilized by a sperm, it will attach to the lining of the uterus.

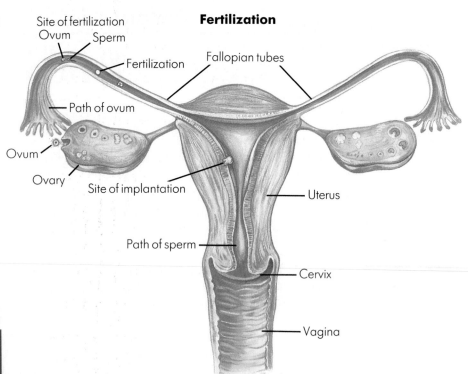

Fertilization

Site of fertilization
Ovum
Sperm
Fertilization
Fallopian tubes
Path of ovum
Ovum
Ovary
Site of implantation
Uterus
Path of sperm
Cervix
Vagina

Development of the Placenta and Umbilical Cord

The cells of the embryo continue to divide, forming three layers of tissue. One layer becomes the respiratory and digestive systems. Another layer develops into muscles, bones, blood vessels, and skin. The third layer becomes the nervous system, sense organs, and mouth.

At the same time, a thin membrane called the amniotic sac forms and surrounds the developing embryo. Fluid in this sac acts as a shock absorber that protects the embryo from jarring and bumping. It also helps insulate the embryo from temperature changes.

An outer layer of cells of the embryo with tissue from the mother develops into the **placenta.** The placenta is made of blood-rich tissue. The embryo is connected to the placenta by the **umbilical cord.** The cord contains blood vessels through which blood flows between the embryo and the placenta. The mother's blood vessels also extend into the placenta. Here nutrients and oxygen pass from the mother's blood into the embryo's blood. The nutrients and oxygen are carried by blood in blood vessels in the umbilical cord to the embryo.

Waste products from the embryo are carried through these same blood vessels to the placenta where they diffuse into the mother's blood. These wastes are then removed from the mother's body.

Fetal Development

During the first 6 weeks of pregnancy, the embryo grows rapidly in length and gains weight. At the start of the third week, it is about one-half to one inch long (2 to 2.5 cm), or 10,000 times the size of the original egg cell! At 8 weeks the embryo measures about an inch and one-half in length (3.5 to 4 cm). From the end of the eighth week until

TEEN PREGNANCY

Over 1 million American teens become pregnant in the United States each year. Of these, about 500,000 give birth. This number is twice what it was just 25 years ago. That means that of every 100 teenage females, 10 will get pregnant and 5 will give birth to their babies before the age of 20. This rate for teenage pregnancy is twice that of European countries.

Pregnancy during adolescence has special risks. Before the age of 20, a young female is still growing. Her pelvis may not be large enough for the passage of a full-grown fetus. Her growing body may not be ready for the physical stress of pregnancy. Since her own nutritional needs are high, she may not consume enough nutrients for herself and her baby. Teenage mothers are more likely than other age groups to have low birth weight babies, who in turn, have a high mortality, or death, rate.

It has been estimated that five out of six of all teen pregnancies in this country are unplanned. They might happen because either the male or the female was unknowledgeable about how to get pregnant, was careless, or simply didn't consider that pregnancy could happen.

About one-sixth of these pregnancies, however, are planned. Teens who plan to get pregnant may not recognize how stressful the pregnancy might be. Combined with the normal anxieties of adolescence, the hormonal and physical changes of pregnancy can be difficult to cope with. Some teens assume that by having a child of their own, they will feel more fulfilled and have something all their own to love. What they don't take into consideration are the financial, emotional, social, and educational costs to themselves and their children, who will need care for the next 18 years of their lives.

Between 50 and 80 percent of teen mothers do not finish high school. A large percentage of the babies born to unmarried parents are born to teens, and many single-parent families where the mother is the head of household live in poverty. Females who have babies by the time they are 15 and 16 are highly likely to have a second child before the age of 20. Because of the poverty and other frustrations associated with teen parenting, many children of teen parents end up in foster care, or are abused or neglected.

Increasingly, there are programs within schools for pregnant teens or teens with young children. In fact, studies show that teen mothers who manage to stay in school after the birth of their babies are less likely to have more children while they are still teens.

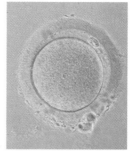
a.

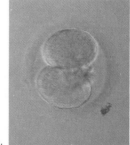
b.

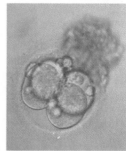
c.

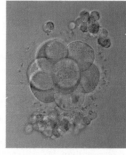
d.

A fertilized ovum divides rapidly to form a cluster: (a) an unfertilized ovum; (b) two-cell stage; (c) eight-cell stage; (d) a blastocyst, a mass of cells that form a hollow ball.

birth, the embryo is known as a **fetus.** The skin of the fetus is clear and hairless and covered with a waxy protective coating. The fetus contains millions of cells that will arrange themselves into tissues and organs.

The brain is one of the first organs to develop. The nervous system grows rapidly, and at 9 weeks the head develops. All the body systems are now present.

Growth of the fetus is rapid during the fourth month, but it slows down in the fifth month. During this time the mother can feel the fetus move. It may begin to suck its thumb. By the end of the sixth month, the fetus is about 14 inches (36 cm) long.

During the last 3 months of pregnancy, the weight of the fetus more than triples. The fetus moves freely within the amniotic sac. The eyes open during the seventh month. During the ninth month the fetus usually moves into a head-down position and is ready for birth. The fetus is now 18 to 20 inches (46 to 51 cm) long and weighs about 7 to 9 pounds (3 to 4 kg).

Prenatal Care

As soon as a female confirms her pregnancy, she should begin prenatal care. This is important because the female's health choices affect the health and well-being of the developing baby. A pregnant female should have regular visits with an obstetrician, a doctor specializing in the care of a female and her developing baby.

The obstetrician gives the pregnant female a complete physical, including blood tests and a pelvic examination. Possible problems may be identified and corrected early. The doctor also helps educate the mother-to-be in important health behaviors. Her dietary choices, for example, are of special concern. She needs a well-balanced diet to ensure proper nourishment for herself and her developing child.

The doctor will monitor the female's weight during her pregnancy and discuss the importance of exercise. An exercise program will be recommended depending on the female's health and level of fitness. Prenatal care also gives the parents-to-be chances to ask questions about pregnancy and the birth process.

Medicines, Drugs, and Pregnancy

A pregnant female must be very careful about what substances she takes into her body. Any medicines should be taken only with her doctor's approval.

No illegal drugs should be taken. Illegal drugs present a very serious threat to the mother and her baby. Babies can be born physically dependent on the drugs their mothers used while pregnant. Use of certain drugs during pregnancy can cause serious birth defects, including mental retardation.

Alcohol and Pregnancy. Females who drink alcohol during pregnancy run the risk of giving birth to babies with birth defects. These babies may be physically, mentally, or behaviorally abnormal. This condition is called fetal alcohol syndrome (FAS).

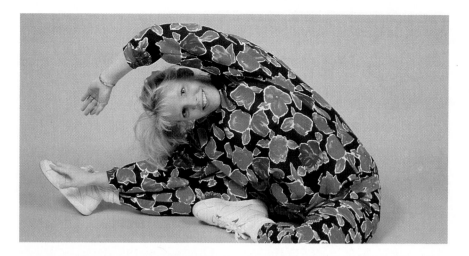

Babies born with FAS are often shorter and weigh less than babies of mothers who did not drink alcohol. FAS babies may have a variety of problems, including impaired speech, a cleft palate, slow body growth, facial abnormalities, poor coordination, and heart defects. Mental retardation, poor attention span, nervousness, and hyperactivity are also common in these children.

When a pregnant female drinks alcohol, the alcohol in her blood flows through the vessels in the umbilical cord into the baby's bloodstream. Unfortunately, the developing baby's body cannot rid itself of the alcohol like an adult body can. A baby born to a female who drinks alcohol during her pregnancy can be born addicted to alcohol.

It is important to remember that fetal alcohol syndrome and all the problems associated with it are completely preventable. These problems do not occur in babies born to females who avoid the use of alcohol during pregnancy.

Tobacco and Pregnancy. A pregnant female also must avoid using tobacco. Babies born to females who use tobacco have a greater chance of being born prematurely with low birth weights. Babies born weighing $5^{1}/2$ pounds (2.5 kg) or less often develop serious health problems early in life. Low birth weight is a leading cause of death in a baby's first year of life.

Females who use tobacco during pregnancy are about two times more likely to have a miscarriage or stillbirth, the birth of a dead fetus, than females who do not use tobacco. As with FAS, the problems associated with tobacco use and pregnancy are preventable.

DID YOU KNOW?

- A female who is infected with HIV can pass the virus to her baby if she becomes pregnant. Most children infected with HIV got the virus from their infected mothers during pregnancy or at birth. During pregnancy, the virus can be transmitted to the unborn through the mother's blood system. At birth, the virus can be transmitted in the vagina. The virus also can be transmitted through breast-feeding.

K E E P I N G F I T

Babies as Intelligent Beings

When you see a baby, how do you react? Do you marvel at the way it responds to the world around it, or do you see it as an as-yet undeveloped person oblivious to its surroundings?

The fact is that babies are highly developed beings. They can see, hear, and even learn while still developing in the uterus.

The next time you see a baby, pay careful attention to its behav-ior. What information does it seem to be taking in? How aware does he or she seem of the surroundings? Spend some time with the baby, keeping in mind that babies are people, too.

End of First Month
- About one-quarter inch (6 mm) long
- Heart, brain, and lungs forming
- Heart starts beating on about the twenty-fifth day

End of Second Month
- About 1½ inches (4 cm) long
- Muscles and skin developing
- Arms, hands, and fingers forming
- Legs beginning to form, along with knees, ankles, and toes
- Every vital organ starting to develop

End of Third Month
- About 3 inches (8 cm) long
- Weighs about 1 ounce (28 g)
- Can open and close mouth and swallow

End of Fourth Month
- 8 to 10 inches (20 to 25 cm) long
- Weighs 6 ounces (170 g)
- Movement can be felt

End of Fifth Month
- About 12 inches (30 cm) long
- Weighs 1 pound (454 g)
- Eyelashes appear
- Nails begin to grow
- Heartbeat can be heard

End of Sixth Month
- Can kick and cry
- Can hear sounds
- Might even hiccup
- Has fingernails

End of Seventh Month
- Weighs 2 to 2½ pounds (910 to 1100 g)
- Can move arms and legs freely
- Eyes are now open

End of Eighth Month
- About 16½ inches (42 cm) long
- Weighs about 4 pounds (1800 g)
- Hair grows
- Skin gets smoother as a layer of fat develops under it

End of Ninth Month
- 18 to 20 inches (46 to 51 cm) long
- Weighs 7 to 9 pounds (3 to 4 kg)
- Organs have developed enough to function on their own

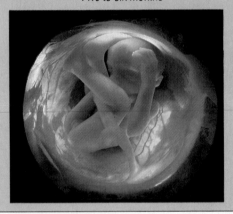

Six weeks

Five to six months

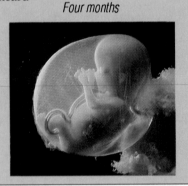

Four months

K E E P I N G   F I T

Being Prepared

Babysitting can have serious consequences if you are not prepared. When you babysit for young children, you should have the following phone numbers:
- where the parent(s) can be reached
- police and fire departments, ambulance, pediatrician, and Poison Control Center
- the nearest neighbor(s)

Do not allow children under 4 to eat foods that they might choke on, such as hard candies.

Do not allow them to put small objects in their mouths.

Keep the children within your sight at all times until they are safely asleep. Then be sure that you can hear them if they should awaken.

The Three Stages of Birth

Babies usually are born headfirst. In the last few weeks of pregnancy, the baby's head moves to the lower part of the uterus. During the birth process the baby is pushed out of the uterus and passes out of the mother's body. There are 3 stages in the birth process. The first stage is dilation, the stretching of the cervix. The cervix is the round, muscular neck, or bottom part, of the uterus. During the 9 months of pregnancy, it remained tightly closed, keeping the fetus inside the uterus. Now it opens to a diameter of about 4 inches (10 cm). This is about the width of your hand. Dilation begins with mild contractions of the muscles of the uterus. These contractions, called labor, shorten the uterus and pull the cervix open. The dilation stage is the longest, most difficult part of the birth process.

When the cervix is fully dilated, the muscles of the uterus continue to contract, moving the baby through the cervix and birth canal. This is the second phase of the birth process. The umbilical cord continues to connect the baby to the placenta during the birth process. Once the baby is born, the umbilical cord is clamped and cut near the baby's abdomen. Any part of the cord that is left will dry up and fall off.

After the baby is born, the contractions of the uterus continue for another 10 to 15 minutes. These contractions push the placenta, now called afterbirth, out of the mother's body. This is the third and final stage of birth.

The Apgar Test

Almost all American hospitals administer a routine test to determine an infant's physical condition at birth. It is named after the late Dr. Virginia Apgar. The Apgar test measures the baby's condition in five significant areas: appearance or coloring, pulse, grimace or reflex irritability, activity, and respiration. Any significant differences from the normal response in each of these areas may require further testing and observation.

> **DID YOU KNOW?**
> - The Apgar test is usually given 1 minute after and repeated at 5 minutes after birth.
> - In each of the 5 areas evaluated, the infant is given a rating of 0 to 2.
> - A total score of 7 to 10 is considered normal.
> - A lower score can be a sign that the baby needs special medical attention.

LESSON 1 REVIEW

Reviewing Facts and Vocabulary

1. Use the following terms in a paragraph to demonstrate your understanding of their meanings: *embryo, fetus, zygote, blastocyst.*
2. List the main events of pregnancy in the order that they occur, beginning with fertilization and ending with birth.
3. Why is prenatal care important?
4. What are the risks involved in drug use during pregnancy?

Thinking Critically

5. **Analysis.** How is proper nutrition an example of good prenatal care?
6. **Analysis.** Compare and contrast an embryo and a fetus.

Applying Health Knowledge

7. Design a poster that warns of the dangers of using tobacco, drinking alcohol, or using illegal drugs during pregnancy.

HEREDITY AND GENETICS

LESSON 2 FOCUS

TERMS TO USE
- Heredity
- Chromosomes
- Genes
- Fraternal twins
- Identical twins

CONCEPTS TO LEARN
- Heredity is a complex process.
- There are many types of genetic disorders.
- Scientists are continuing to explore the causes of many genetic disorders.

ATTITUDES AND BEHAVIORS TO EVALUATE
- Self-Inventory, page 154.
- Building Decision-Making Skills, page 155.

Perhaps no other area of health and the human body is as fascinating as heredity. **Heredity** is the passing of characteristics from parents to offspring. It is heredity that determines what makes you *you*.

Chromosomes and Genes

The process of heredity begins in complex structures called chromosomes. **Chromosomes** are tiny structures within the nuclei of cells. Chromosomes are found in all body cells, except mature red blood cells, which have no nuclei.

Genes are small sections of chromosomes that control hereditary characteristics. Through the genes, characteristics of the mother and father are passed to the offspring. For example, your genes determine your resemblance to your mother or father, the color of your hair, and the color of your eyes. This happens because genetic information merges when an ovum and sperm unite.

Structure of the Chromosomes

Every living organism has a certain number of chromosomes. Human body cells, with the exception of sperm and ova, contain 46 chromosomes. Ova and sperm have half that amount—23 chromosomes each. After fertilization the zygote has 46 chromosomes (23 from each parent), and the hereditary traits of the mother and the father are passed on to another generation.

As you know, the zygote divides, eventually producing trillions of cells that make up the human body. In between each cell division, each chromosome in the cell nucleus duplicates itself. As the cell divides, the two sets of 46 chromosomes separate and each new cell contains 46 chromosomes, identical to those in the first cell. This process continues throughout life.

Girl or Boy? Will the baby be a girl or a boy? Of the 46 chromosomes in a zygote, 2 are specialized sex chromosomes. In females, these two chromosomes look exactly alike and are called X chromosomes. In males, one chromosome is shorter and does not match the other. This smaller one is the Y chromosome. The larger one is the X chromosome.

Remember that sperm and ova contain only half the number of chromosomes as other cells. This means that these cells contain only one sex chromosome, not two. Sperm may contain either an X or a Y chromosome. The ovum can have only an X chromosome. If an ovum is fertilized by a sperm carrying an X chromosome, the baby is a girl because, as the chromosomes pair, the combination is XX. If the sperm is carrying a Y chromosome, the pairing forms an XY combination, resulting in a boy. So the determination of the sex of a child is based on the father's sperm.

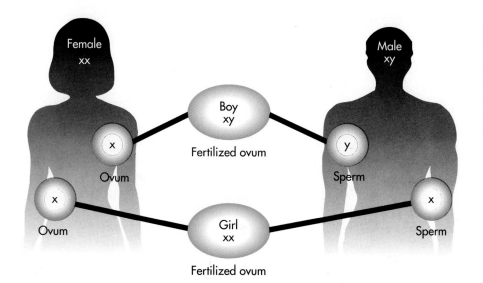

A female produces egg cells that all have the X chromosome. A male produces sperm that have either an X chromosome or a Y chromosome . Whichever sperm fertilizes the egg cell determines the sex of the offspring.

The Genetic Code

As in the case of almost all other body cell activities, the process of heredity involves complex chemical activity. The special chemical compound necessary for the process of heredity is deoxyribonucleic acid (DNA). The DNA code is also called the genetic code.

Each gene consists of a part of a DNA molecule. The DNA molecule resembles a twisted ladder, the rungs being made up of chemical compounds called *bases*. There are four kinds of bases that can be paired in only certain combinations according to their size, much like a jigsaw puzzle.

You have thousands of genes in every cell, and they all contain the same four bases. The variation among genes is a result of the arrangement of these bases along the DNA molecule. Since several hundred pairs of bases are in each gene, a countless number of arrangements is possible.

Cells will make proteins when they interpret the order of these bases, or DNA code. Proteins help build and maintain body tissues. Cells make different proteins when they interpret different orders of bases. Different kinds of proteins will result in individual traits.

Dominant and Recessive Genes

As you can see, the process of heredity is extremely complicated. What determines whether you have blue eyes or brown eyes, straight hair or curly hair? Every person inherits two genes for every trait—one from the mother and one from the father. As the chromosomes divide and separate, the two genes for a particular trait line up next to each other.

Let us take the trait of eye color as an example. The gene for brown eyes (B) is dominant over the gene for blue eyes (b). The gene for blue eyes is recessive.

In the case of many traits, one gene is dominant and the other recessive. This simply means that when the pair of genes lines up, the dominant gene overpowers the recessive one and determines that particular trait.

DID YOU KNOW?

- One in every 2,000 infants is born with cystic fibrosis. The disease, which makes breathing and digestion difficult, is caused by two abnormal genes, one coming from each parent. There are about 8 million Americans who carry this gene, and many are not aware of the fact. If both parents are carriers, their offspring have a 25 percent chance of having the disease.

If each parent has one dominant gene and one recessive gene for eye color, their children will have a 75 percent chance to be brown-eyed and a 25 precent chance to be blue-eyed.

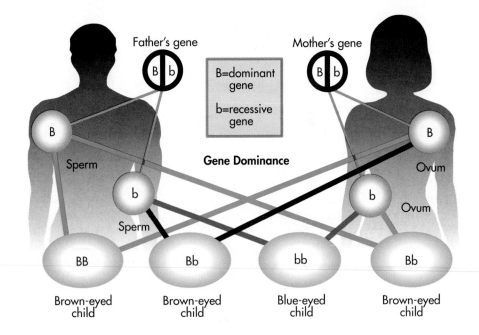

Consider, however, the possible combinations. If both parents have one dominant gene and one recessive gene for eye color, they both have brown eyes. Since both parents have a dominant gene for brown eyes, there is a one in four chance that they will have a blue-eyed child. There are three chances in four that they will have a brown-eyed child.

Genetic Disorders

When you consider the countless number of divisions and processes that must take place to form a fully developed baby, it truly is amazing that most babies are born healthy and normal. However, it is estimated that as many as 250,000 children may be born in the United States every year with major hereditary conditions and disorders that will seriously impair their health.

According to the National Institute of Health, 15 million Americans have some kind of genetic condition or birth defect. At least 40 percent of all infant mortality is the result of genetic factors. Millions of Americans are healthy themselves, but are carriers of defective genetic information. Many do not know it until they have a child born with a birth defect.

DOMINANT AND RECESSIVE TRAITS

Dominant	Recessive
curly hair	straight hair
black or brown hair	blonde or red hair
full lips	thin lips
dimples	smooth cheeks
straight nose	turned-up nose
brown eyes	blue eyes
long, full eyelashes	short, thin eyelashes
freckles	no freckles

THE MYSTERY OF TWINS

In most cases of twins, a female's ovaries release two mature ova instead of one. If a separate sperm fertilizes each ovum, two embryos develop. The two embryos, called **fraternal twins,** have different genetic makeup and therefore do not look any more alike than brothers and sisters normally do. Fraternal twins can be the same sex or different sex.

In about one-third of the cases of twins, identical twins result. In this situation, a single ovum that has been fertilized divides and two embryos develop. These embryos have the same genetic information. These twins will be the same sex and look almost exactly the same. They are **identical twins.**

Research on twins has been expanding greatly. Researchers now use twins to study a variety of physical health problems, as well as questions about psychological development and adjustment.

Twins and Genetic Research

Researchers are currently using twins to study
- genetic influence on temperament;
- genetic and environmental influence on fears and phobias, language development, and intelligence;
- genetic influence on antisocial behavior;
- the onset of alcoholism and affective emotional disorders;
- the causes of cancer and multiple sclerosis;
- the genetic components of coronary heart disease.

Researchers got an unexpected boost from the discovery of identical twins who had been separated from each other at birth. Neither twin nor his adoptive family knew about the other until the twins were reunited at age 39. The similarities in Jim Lewis and Jim Springer were startling. Researchers will try to determine how much was coincidental and how much was the result of being identical twins. What do you think?

- In school they both liked math and disliked spelling.
- Their first wives were both named Linda.
- They had both divorced and remarried, and their second wives were both named Betty.
- Both had a son named James Allen (one spelled Alan), and a dog named Tag.
- Both had gained weight at the same time, and had had the same kind of surgery.
- Both had a white seat around a tree in his yard.

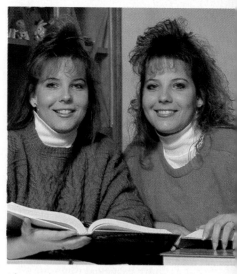

Identical twins have the same genetic makeup. They are always the same sex.

Types of Genetic Disorders

There are more than 4,000 known types of genetic conditions and birth defects. In the broadest definition, any quality an individual inherits is a genetic condition. As used here, however, *genetic condition* refers to genetic diseases and disorders, illnesses, or other conditions of malfunction with which an individual is born.

Any disease, disorder, or other problem present at birth can impair an individual's health. Only a few of the disorders occurring at birth have a known genetic cause. Some are the result of environmental factors. Thus, the term *birth defects* includes not only genetic conditions but many other types of diseases and disorders that are caused by a variety of other factors.

Some birth defects are immediately observable at birth. These include physical malformations, such as cleft lip, cleft palate, and clubfoot.

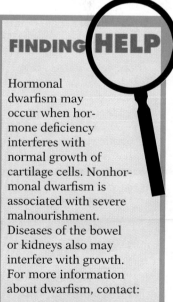

FINDING HELP

Hormonal dwarfism may occur when hormone deficiency interferes with normal growth of cartilage cells. Nonhormonal dwarfism is associated with severe malnourishment. Diseases of the bowel or kidneys also may interfere with growth. For more information about dwarfism, contact:

- Little People of America
7238 Piedmont Drive
Dallas, Texas
75227-9324

Jackie is a typical teen in many ways: she likes to spend time with her friends, has a crush on her favorite rapper, and is excited about her future. Jackie, however, has Down syndrome. Because her parents have helped her maximize her potential, Jackie's achievements have exceeded everyone's expectations. Yet, many of Jackie's peers can see only her disability. Their attitudes range from being overly protective to feeling uncomfortable around her. She wishes people would just accept her as she is.

How do you think Jackie can convince her peers that in many ways she's no different from them?

What would convince you?

While other congenital defects may be present at birth, testing is required to confirm their presence.

Some conditions that may be present at birth do not generate observable symptoms until the infant is several months to a year or more old. Among these are Tay-Sachs disease—a disorder causing the destruction of the nervous system, cystic fibrosis—a disorder that affects the mucous-secreting glands and the sweat glands, sickle-cell anemia—an inherited blood disorder, phenylketonuria (PKU)—an inherited enzyme deficiency, and hearing loss.

Various types of mental retardation, and minimal brain dysfunction cannot be observed until the infant begins, or fails to begin, progressing through the normal stages of physical development.

Identifying Genetic Disorders

In spite of many years of advanced research, medical scientists still are uncertain about the exact causes of many human congenital defects. Scientists do know, however, that a principal cause of birth defects is chromosomal abnormality.

Since chromosomes contain genes responsible for inherited characteristics, even the slightest abnormality can cause severe developmental problems in a fetus. Most miscarriages in early pregnancy are the result of chromosomal abnormalities.

The most serious chromosomal abnormalities are the result of fetal cells that contain more or less than the usual number of chromosomes. Down syndrome is an example. Down syndrome is a condition that results when an individual has 47 chromosomes instead of 46. Down syndrome results in abnormalities of the face and other parts of the body and physical and mental retardation.

Severe birth defects can also occur when parts of chromosomes break off and join onto other chromosomes. This interferes with the normal transmission of genetic information.

There are several methods used to investigate the health of a fetus:

- Amniocentesis, in which a syringe is inserted through the pregnant female's abdominal wall into the amniotic fluid surrounding the developing fetus. The physician removes a small amount of the fluid to examine the chromosomes, study the body chemistry, and determine the sex of the fetus. Amniocentesis is performed usually 16 to 20 weeks after fertilization.

KEEPING FIT

Dealing with Disabilities

Think of someone you know or have seen or read about who has a disability. Ask yourself the following questions, vowing to see the "differently abled" as complete human beings and to concentrate from now on on their abilities rather than on their disabilities.

- Do I see the person's disabilities first?
- What special abilities might I instead focus on seeing and appreciating?
- How would I feel if I were seen only in terms of a disability?
- What steps can I take to help others see that disabilities does not mean inabilities?

Overcoming The Odds

Jeff Barnett is 14. He is a good athlete, a good student, a good son. Some people think he is an only child, but Jeff knows better. The family photos around his house show 3 boys, not 1. Jeff is the only son who has survived. Jeff's 2 brothers, Chuckie and Michael, died of a rare genetic disorder called Leigh's disease. Jeff was 2 and 6 when his brothers died.

Chuckie Barnett became ill first. He developed fevers, muscle weakness, motor and eye problems. He gained a lot of weight. No one could figure out what was wrong—even medical specialists. Then, on a family trip, Chuckie suddenly became ill and died a short time later.

Brain tissue samples sent for testing after Chuckie's death indicated that he had Leigh's disease. For the first time, the Barnetts had a definite diagnosis.

Soon after Chuckie's death, Michael began to show the same symptoms, and for over two years, the Barnetts watched him get worse.

Jeff says, "I don't feel guilty that I'm alive. I just feel it's not right that two of the three kids in my family had this disease when it is so rare.

"I never feel low or totally down because my brothers died. I think my self-esteem is pretty high because I know I can accomplish a lot. My parents haven't treated me as if I'm their only son, either, and they haven't been as overprotective as they might have been. They've given me all the

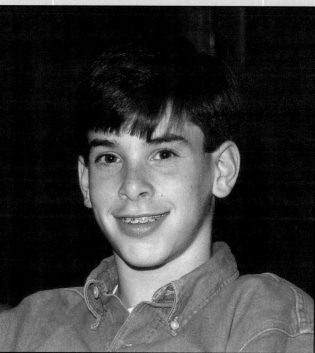

space I've needed, and that's been just great for me."

Jeff and his parents have done a lot to pay tribute to Chuckie and Michael and to turn their double tragedy into positive action and caring for others. Jeff says, "At the preschool that Chuckie attended, there is a dogwood tree planted in his memory with a plaque next to it. At Michael's school, a greenhouse was built in his memory with a plaque and a tree was planted for him, too. Then my mother decided she wanted to do something more about all of this."

In 1990, the Michael and Charles Barnett Center was opened at St. Christopher's Hospital for Children in Philadelphia. The Center's goals include early diagnosis and treatment for those affected by the disease.

With the help of a company called Child's Play Touring Theater, the Barnetts continue to raise funds for the Center. They have developed a program called "Child's Play" in which local school children write poems and stories, the theater company dramatizes them, and the money raised at performances goes toward their cause. In the process, they bring joy to a great many children.

Jeff understands that individuals and their families can make a difference. He says, "This project makes me feel great. Now I know that other people who have Leigh's disease may have a better chance of surviving it."

1. Many people who lose relatives feel survivor's guilt. For what reasons do you think Jeff hasn't suffered from this feeling?
2. Jeff seems to have high self-esteem. What factors in his life might have contributed to this?

- Ultrasound, in which sound waves are used to project light images on a screen. The sound waves are directed at the pregnant female's abdomen and reflected onto a screen. The reflected waves act like an echo and form an image of the fetus. Ultrasound is used to determine the position of a fetus, and if there is more than one fetus in the uterus.
- Chorionic villi sampling (CVS), in which a small piece of membrane is removed from the chorion, a layer of tissue that develops into the placenta. This matter is examined for possible genetic defects. The procedure takes place around the eighth week of fetal development, so it is a procedure that can be done earlier than amniocentesis. In many cases, the results of a CVS are later confirmed by amniocentesis.

Passing on Genetic Disorders

Genetic disorders are passed on much like other physical traits; that is, there are dominant and recessive traits. The mother is the carrier of X-linked conditions. While the mother is not affected, she carries one abnormal gene and one normal gene in her sex chromosomes. There is a 50 percent risk that each male child will be affected by a disease and a 50 percent risk that each female child will be a carrier. Among the more common X-linked conditions are certain forms of color blindness, hemophilia, and muscular dystrophy.

Advances in Human Genetics

Medical professionals have gained much knowledge about genetically related diseases and disorders, and about new research techniques for diagnosing, preventing, and treating such conditions. This knowledge has produced a wide expansion of programs to deal with genetic conditions and birth defects.

One way to help prevent genetically caused birth defects is to identify carriers. Genetic counselors can advise families about the probability of having a child with a genetically related disease. They also can guide families of children with genetic disorders about possible treatment options.

LESSON 2 REVIEW

Reviewing Facts and Vocabulary

1. Define *heredity*, *chromosomes*, and *genes*.
2. List two means of identifying genetic disorders, and describe the processes involved.

Thinking Critically

3. **Analysis.** Compare fraternal to identical twins.

4. **Evaluation.** What are your views regarding the use of amniocentesis as a means of diagnosing disorders or of finding out the sex of a baby before birth?

Applying Health Knowledge

5. Write a one-page descriptive paper about the work of a noted genetic scientist.

BIRTH TO LATE CHILDHOOD

Throughout life you grow and develop physically, socially, emotionally, intellectually, and culturally. Your growth and development is predictable; it follows certain general patterns. However, you will grow and develop at a rate that is unique to you. Your growth and development are affected by your heredity, your environment, and your health decisions.

Several noted scientists have presented theories, or models, of how people develop. These models are helpful in knowing what to expect at different stages in your life.

Developmental Tasks

Experts who have studied growth and development have identified certain basic stages. For each stage, developmental tasks are identified. A **developmental task** is something that needs to occur during a particular stage for a person to continue his or her growth toward becoming a healthy, mature adult. Developmental tasks in adolescence, for example, include forming more mature relationships with peers and achieving emotional independence from parents.

A child learns to trust a parent or other adult as the needs of the child are met and satisfied by the adult.

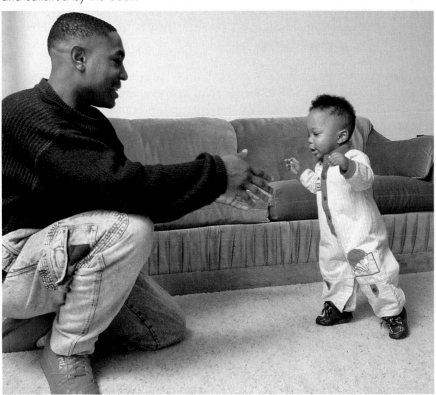

LESSON 3 FOCUS

TERMS TO USE
- Developmental task
- Autonomy

CONCEPTS TO LEARN
- Every person experiences developmental tasks.
- Specific developmental tasks are associated with each stage of growth.

ATTITUDES AND BEHAVIORS TO EVALUATE
- Self-Inventory, page 154.
- Building Decision-Making Skills, page 155.

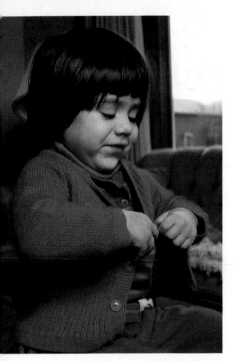

Early childhood is a time of learning new skills and gaining independence.

One of the most widely accepted theories of development is presented by psychoanalyst Erik Erikson. He describes stages of development from birth through old age. Our success in each stage has much to do with our experiences during that stage. Erikson believes, however, that failure at one stage can be overcome by successes in following stages.

Stage 1: Infancy—Trust versus Mistrust

From birth to one and one-half years, you experienced the fastest period of growth in your life! Your weight tripled and your height doubled.

The developmental tasks of an infant include learning to eat solid food, beginning to walk, and learning to talk.

In the first year of life, according to Erikson, one of a child's main tasks is that of developing trust. If a child's needs are met promptly and lovingly, he or she learns to view the world as being a safe place and people as being dependable. If a child's needs are inadequately met or rejected, he or she learns to be fearful of the world and people. As you can see, a child's environment plays a major role in his or her development at this stage.

Stage 2: Early Childhood—Autonomy versus Shame and Doubt

During the second and third years of life, children develop many new physical and mental skills. They master walking, learn to climb, and can push and pull. They increase their vocabulary and even begin talking in sentences. Another important developmental task at this age is learning to control the elimination of body wastes.

Children at this age are proud of these accomplishments and personally try to do as many things as possible. Have you ever been around a 2- or 3-year-old who insisted on putting on his or her own shoes or clothes? This behavior is very typical of children's increasing desire for independence.

If parents accept the child's need to do whatever he or she is capable of, then the child will develop a sense of **autonomy,** the confidence that one can control one's own body, impulses, and environment. However, if parents insist on doing everything for the child or are critical when the child attempts things and fails, then the child will develop doubts about his or her abilities.

KEEPING FIT

Modeling Healthy Behavior

Be a positive role model to the children in your life.
- Teach them safety.
- Encourage them to eat nutritious food.
- Talk to them about the importance of sharing their feelings.

- Share some of your own feelings with them.
- Discuss with them the importance of treating people of all ages, races, and backgrounds with respect.
- Share with them some healthy

ways to resolve conflicts other than through violence or the use of bad language.
- Talk with them about how smoking, drinking, and drug use can harm them.

Stage 3: Childhood—Initiative versus Guilt

During the fourth and fifth years of life, physical abilities develop to the point where a child can initiate play activities rather than merely follow other children. Children at this age often play make-believe, imagining themselves in a variety of adult roles. They copy what they see adults do. They also begin to ask many questions, a sign of intellectual growth.

If parents show approval of these new abilities and activities and encourage questions, children learn initiative, the ability to start something on their own. They also learn to be creative and explore new ideas. If, however, the parent is impatient with all the questions or makes the child think the activities are wrong, the child will likely develop a sense of guilt about self-initiated activities.

Stage 4: Late Childhood—Industry versus Inferiority

Between the ages of 6 and 11, children experience a major part of their social development—school. The developmental tasks at this age reflect social, emotional, intellectual, physical, and cultural growth.

Children learn physical skills necessary for games and activities. They develop basic skills in reading, writing, and calculating. An important task during this stage is building wholesome attitudes toward themselves. Children learn to get along with peers and learn appropriate roles in society. During this stage of development, children develop a conscience. They learn right from wrong. They also develop attitudes toward social groups and institutions.

As children in this stage begin to acquire new skills, they also develop a sense of industry. They begin to make things—cookies, kites, model planes, and the like. The child's sense of industry is reinforced if parents and teachers praise and reward these creative efforts. If, however, an adult scolds the child for making a mess or getting in the way or not following directions, feelings of inferiority and self-doubt may develop.

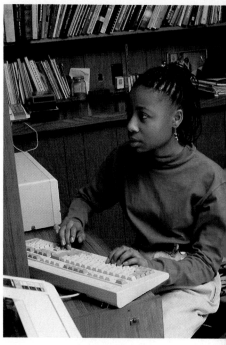

Late childhood is a time of expanding interests and curiosity about the environment.

LESSON 3 REVIEW

Reviewing Facts and Vocabulary

1. Define the term *developmental task,* and give two examples.
2. What are the main developmental tasks during a child's first year?

Thinking Critically

3. **Analysis.** Compare and contrast the development during the first year of life with the development from 2 to 3 years of age.

Applying Health Knowledge

4. What are some things a parent might say or do to encourage a sense of autonomy in their 3-year-old?
5. Research Jean Piaget's theory of development. How does it compare with Erikson's theory? Summarize in a one-page paper which theory you support and why.

Self-Inventory

Development During the Early Years: Are You in Touch?

HOW DO YOU RATE?

Number a sheet of paper from 1 through 15. Read each item below and respond by writing either *agree* or *disagree* for each. Total the number of *agree* and *disagree* responses. Then proceed to the next section.

1. A pregnant female has a responsibility to make good health choices for her unborn child.
2. A female should seek prenatal care as soon as she discovers she is pregnant.
3. I have younger brothers, sisters, cousins, or neighbors that I have taken care of.
4. I would like to be a volunteer with an elementary school program.
5. I think any question a child asks deserves an answer.
6. I have visited a day-care center within the last year.
7. Children have a valuable contribution to make to society.
8. The way I treat a younger child has an impact on that child's self-concept.
9. I avoid picking on or teasing younger children.
10. I occasionally enjoy fun-filled, quality time with younger children.
11. Children with special needs can experience a healthy development.
12. I agree with the old saying that children should be seen and not heard.
13. If a baby was crying for no apparent reason and was not hurt, I would just let him or her cry.
14. If a toddler was throwing a tantrum in a store, I would give the child what she or he wanted just to stop the tantrum.
15. If I were taking care of a child who was struggling with a page of simple addition problems, it would be easier for me to do them than to help the child do them independently.

HOW DID YOU SCORE?

For items 1 to 11, give yourself 2 points for each *agree* answer and 0 points for each *disagree* answer. For items 12 to 15 give yourself 2 points for each *disagree* answer and 0 points for each *agree* answer. Find your total, and read below to see how you scored. Then proceed to the next section.

24 to 30
Excellent. Your understanding of child development and attitudes toward children is commendable.

16 to 23
Good. You have a general understanding of child development and the needs of children.

10 to 15
Fair. You might increase your experiences around children to better understand their developmental needs.

0 to 9
Poor. You might be missing out on some enjoyable experiences and an opportunity for a better understanding of children.

WHAT ARE YOUR GOALS?

If your score was between 16 and 30, complete the statements in Part A. If you scored 15 or below, complete the statements in Parts A and B.

Part A

1. I plan to learn more about the developmental needs of children in the following ways: ____.
2. My timetable is ____.
3. I plan to share what I've learned with others by ____.
4. The personal benefit I will receive from accomplishing this goal is ____.

Part B

5. The attitude or behavior toward children I would like to change most is ____.
6. The steps involved in making this change are ____.
7. My timetable for making this change is ____.
8. My reward for making this change will be ____.
9. I will check my progress toward this goal by ____.

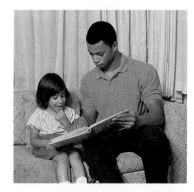

Building Decision-Making Skills

Paula has just found out that her best friend is pregnant. Her friend is the star of the softball team and no one knows about the pregnancy. Her athletic activity has kept her from gaining much weight, and loose clothing helps her hide her secret from her parents, boyfriend, and others. She hopes to finish the season in the next two weeks. She has already accepted a college scholarship. She says she will tell everyone and go to the doctor right after graduation. She wants Paula to help her keep the secret.

WHAT DO YOU THINK?

1. **Choices.** What choices does Paula have?
2. **Consequences.** What are the consequences of each choice?
3. **Decision.** What do you think Paula should do?
4. **Evaluation.** How do you handle situations when people say "I have a secret to tell you, but you have to promise not to tell anyone?" How do you feel afterwards?

Jack is coaching the soccer team his 10-year-old brother plays on. At practice one day Jack overhears his brother mocking another team member because of his ethnic background.

WHAT DO YOU THINK?

5. **Choices.** List three possible choices for Jack.
6. **Consequences.** What are the possible consequences for each choice?
7. **Decision.** What should Jack do? Explain your answer.

Everyone at your table in the cafeteria is making fun of a student who has a disability. They all look at you as if to say, "Come on, join in."

WHAT DO YOU THINK?

8. **Choices.** What are your choices?
9. **Consequences.** What are the probable consequences of each choice?
10. **Decision.** What would you do in this situation?

Sheila is seven months pregnant. She and her husband Tom are very excited about her pregnancy. Tom is hoping for a son, Sheila just wants a healthy baby.

When Sheila and Tom visit Tom's parents, they go out to dinner to celebrate Tom's mother's birthday. In the restaurant the waiter asks if they want anything from the bar. Because of her pregnancy, Sheila declines. Her father-in-law orders a glass of wine for her anyway.

WHAT DO YOU THINK?

11. **Choices.** What are Sheila's choices?
12. **Consequences.** What are the probable consequences of each choice?
13. **Decision.** What should Sheila do?
14. **Decision.** Would your decision be different if you knew Sheila was aged 21? Under 21?

Using Health Terms

On a separate sheet of paper, write the term that best matches each definition given below.

LESSON 1

1. Thin membrane that forms around an embryo that insulates the embryo from temperature changes.
2. What the embryo is called from the eighth week of pregnancy until birth.
3. Doctor who specializes in the care of a female and her developing baby.
4. The stretching of the muscular neck of the uterus.
5. The placenta expelled after the birth of a baby.
6. The process that occurs when an ovum and a sperm cell unite.
7. Contractions preceding the birth of a baby.

LESSON 2

8. The passing on of characteristics from parents to offspring.
9. Tiny protein molecules that control the passing on of characteristics from parents to offspring.
10. Controlling or more powerful gene.
11. An X-linked genetic condition.
12. Two infants that develop at the same time in the same female from two different fertilized ova.

LESSON 3

13. The confidence that one can control one's self and environment.
14. A sense of right and wrong.
15. The ability to start something on one's own.

Building Academic Skills

LESSON 1

16. **Reading.** Read an article about pregnancy. List five to ten words that are unfamiliar to you. Using the information in the article, write definitions for each of the words on your list. Include the title, author, and source of the article.

Recalling the Facts

LESSON 1

17. What do the three layers of tissue that form in an embryo develop into?
18. What does each cell in the human body, except those that make up the nervous system, have the ability to do?
19. Define *tissue* and give two examples. Define *organ* and give two examples. Define *body system* and give two examples.
20. What is the function of the placenta?
21. How do a female's health choices affect the health of her developing baby?
22. What is the leading cause of death in an infant's first year of life in the United States?
23. Describe the three stages of birth.
24. What is the function of the umbilical cord in a developing baby?
25. What five characteristics of an infant's physical condition are assessed by the Apgar test?
26. What are three substances that are best for a pregnant female to avoid? Explain why.
27. What are some problems an infant suffering from fetal alcohol syndrome might experience?

LESSON 2

28. What will happen if a fertilized ovum divides and forms two embryos?
29. What causes most early pregnancy miscarriages in the United States?
30. What is meant by an X-linked condition?
31. How does the male determine the sex of the baby?
32. What is the relationship between dominant and recessive genes?
33. List seven genetic disorders.

LESSON 3

34. State two developmental tasks for each of Erik Erikson's first four stages of development.
35. What causes an infant to learn mistrust?
36. What leads to autonomy in childhood?

REVIEW

Thinking Critically

LESSON 1

37. Analysis. Which of the following questions would be important ones for a pregnant female to ask her doctor? Explain why you chose the answers you did.
   a. Can I take something for my headaches?
   b. Do you think it is a boy or a girl?
   c. Is it all right to continue with my aerobics class?
   d. What should I do when I think I'm in labor?

38. Evaluation. If a pregnant female goes into a bar or restaurant and orders an alcoholic beverage, should her server refuse to bring it to her? Support your answer.

39. Synthesis. What advice might you give a pregnant female who says that smoking calms her worries over giving birth?

40. Synthesis. What advice might you give a friend who tells you she wants to get married and her parents won't give their consent so she's trying to get pregnant?

LESSON 2

41. Synthesis. How would you explain the similarities given for twins Jim Lewis and Jim Springer?

LESSON 3

42. Synthesis. For each of Erikson's first four stages of development, write two comments parents could make to their child to help him or her progress successfully through that stage.

Making the Connection

LESSON 3

43. Science. Research one of Erik Erikson's stages of development. Develop a report on how an individual might develop healthy or unhealthy characteristics based on experiences in the stage you're studying. You may wish to interview parents of young children to determine if they are aware of these stages. Draw conclusions on what people do to promote healthy development.

Applying Health Knowledge

LESSON 1

44. Give at least two examples of cells repairing themselves.

45. Immediately after a baby is born he or she is given an Apgar score. What might you say about a baby with a score of 8?

46. Since cigarette smoke can be harmful to a developing baby, what advice would you give to a pregnant female who finds herself in a situation where she is forced to inhale passive smoke?

LESSON 2

47. Select four traits you possess. Find out if each of these traits is dominant or recessive.

48. Sometimes DNA testing is done to identify persons accused of crimes. What is it about DNA that would make this possible?

49. How could you tell if a set of twins had developed from one fertilized egg or two?

50. Can two brown-eyed parents have a child with blue eyes? Can two blue-eyed parents have a child with brown eyes? Explain.

LESSON 3

51. Think back on the developmental tasks you have successfully completed so far. List each developmental task and give the age you were when you completed each one.

Beyond the Classroom

LESSON 1

52. Community Involvement. Find out what services your community provides for pregnant teenagers.

LESSON 2

53. Further Study. Research different tests that can be done to investigate the health of a fetus. Find out the risks, benefits, and procedures of each.

LESSON 3

54. Parental Involvement. Have your parents tell memories they have of you during various developmental stages.

CHAPTER

9

ADOLESCENCE

LESSON 1
A Time of Growth and Change

LESSON 2
A Time for Understanding Yourself

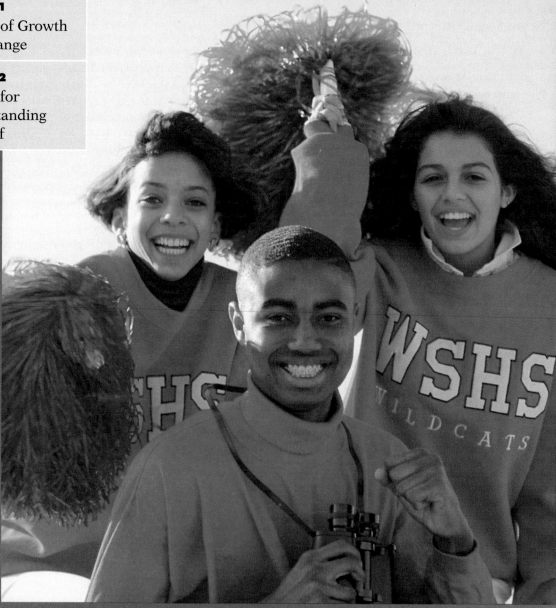

A TIME OF GROWTH AND CHANGE

During the first year of your life, your weight may have tripled and your height may have increased by as much as 50 percent! It was the most rapid growth period you will ever go through. The second fastest growth period takes place near the beginning of **adolescence**— the stage between childhood and adulthood. Growth is rapid and uneven at this time—a sign of puberty and its changes.

Puberty to Young Adulthood

Between the ages of 9 and 13, children begin to go through puberty, which is Erikson's fifth stage of development. **Puberty** marks the beginning of adolescence and is the period of time when males and females become physically able to reproduce. During puberty secondary sex characteristics begin to develop. **Secondary sex characteristics** include body hair and the development of breasts in the female and muscles in the male.

Physical Change

During puberty the feet and hands grow first and are often large in proportion to the rest of the body. This growth can cause a feeling of awkwardness and clumsiness until the arms and legs catch up. Then the muscles grow to fill out the body's framework.

Up to this stage of development, there is very little difference in the size and shape of males and females. As individuals enter puberty, and for the next four to five years, there is great variation in the size and shape of people who are all about the same age. This variation causes concern for many individuals because this is a time of comparison with others. It is important to remember that these differences are perfectly normal.

Puberty is a result of the release of hormones, chemical substances that are released into the bloodstream and travel to other organs and tissues, where they stimulate growth. The male hormone, **testosterone,** and the female hormones, **estrogen** and **progesterone,** are responsible for the physical and emotional changes that take place during puberty.

Mental Change

During adolescence the brain reaches its adult size and weight. Capacity to think and reason increases. At this age, males and females are able to predict the outcomes of many situations. Whereas during childhood they saw only one solution to a problem, during adolescence they begin to look at different ways of solving problems and making decisions. Adolescents' ability to think logically, or reason things out, increases. They begin to be able to solve more complicated problems.

LESSON 1 FOCUS

TERMS TO USE
- Adolescence
- Puberty
- Secondary sex characteristics
- Testosterone (te•STAHS•tuh•rohn)
- Estrogen (ES•truh•juhn)
- Progesterone (proh•JES•tuh•rohn)
- Personal identity

CONCEPTS TO LEARN
- Puberty is a time of physical, mental, emotional, and social changes in adolescents.
- Mastering developmental tasks is a significant step toward maturity for the adolescent.

ATTITUDES AND BEHAVIORS TO EVALUATE
- Self-Inventory, page 170.
- Building Decision-Making Skills, page 171.

Many changes occur during puberty.

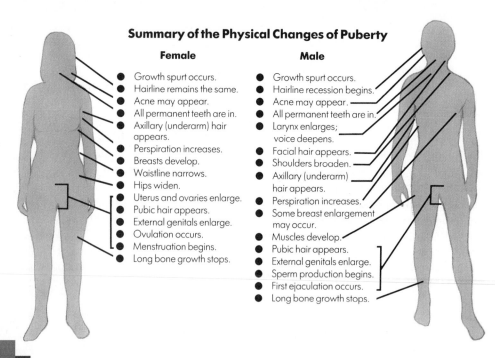

Summary of the Physical Changes of Puberty

Female
- Growth spurt occurs.
- Hairline remains the same.
- Acne may appear.
- All permanent teeth are in.
- Axillary (underarm) hair appears.
- Perspiration increases.
- Breasts develop.
- Waistline narrows.
- Hips widen.
- Uterus and ovaries enlarge.
- Pubic hair appears.
- External genitals enlarge.
- Ovulation occurs.
- Menstruation begins.
- Long bone growth stops.

Male
- Growth spurt occurs.
- Hairline recession begins.
- Acne may appear.
- All permanent teeth are in.
- Larynx enlarges; voice deepens.
- Facial hair appears.
- Shoulders broaden.
- Axillary (underarm) hair appears.
- Perspiration increases.
- Some breast enlargement may occur.
- Muscles develop.
- Pubic hair appears.
- External genitals enlarge.
- Sperm production begins.
- First ejaculation occurs.
- Long bone growth stops.

Culturally Speaking

Rites of Passage

Many cultures publicly recognize a person's change in status. One such change is the movement from childhood to adult status. The Mbuti of Africa have a special rite that recognizes passage to adulthood. For the first time, boys and girls are separated from each other by the society. Girls are joined by friends and live in a special elima house. A festival is given by the village. Each afternoon the girls sing to the boys who sit outside. The boys respond with their own songs, and the ritual is a type of flirtation where future marriage partners may be chosen.

How does your family or culture recognize the transition to adult status?

During adolescence memory skills improve and memory span increases. This aspect of mental growth assists a person in retaining larger and lengthier bodies of information. As with other skills, mental skills improve with use. Each time teens try out new ways of thinking, reasoning, and making decisions, they gain experience that will help in making later choices. In addition, their thinking becomes more flexible.

As they begin to mature, adolescents discover that they are able to look beyond themselves to understand someone else's point of view. These new thinking skills affect a teen's life both in and out of school. Many will develop new interests and hobbies. Career goals begin to come into focus.

Remember, all of these changes do not just happen overnight; they develop over time. As you try out these new abilities, you are likely to make mistakes—everyone does. What is important is that you learn from those mistakes. For example, ask yourself: What could I have done differently? What might have happened if . . . ? By doing this simple mental exercise, you are practicing your new thinking skills and learning for the future. This skill will last you for life.

Emotional Change

Along with spurts of physical and mental change come spurts of energy and strong emotional feelings. Many teens feel that puberty is like being on a roller coaster—with emotions and feelings that go up and down quickly. It is common for teens to sometimes feel on top of the world one day and down in the dumps the next.

Friendships and family love and support are important, yet adolescents may feel unable to let others know what they are feeling and thinking. This difficulty in communicating thoughts and feelings is a normal part of development.

These extra surges of energy and emotion are caused by changes taking place in the body. The very high level of hormones that stimulate growth in the physical body cause emotional change as well.

Social Change

Social change is another important aspect of the development that occurs during puberty and the rest of adolescence. For instance, friendships and peer acceptance become very important. A growing ability to feel more deeply and to consider others' needs is also part of social development. So is the completion of a set of developmental tasks.

Developmental Tasks

Adolescence has been studied by psychologists and sociologists for more than 50 years. They have identified certain developmental tasks that can be considered basic to adolescence. A developmental task is something that needs to occur during a particular age period for a person to continue his or her growth toward becoming a healthy, mature adult. Robert Havighurst, a well-known sociologist in the field of adolescence, suggests that there are nine such tasks facing teens and, often, people in their 20s. These tasks are as follows:

- forming more mature relationships with people your age of both sexes
- achieving a masculine or feminine social role
- accepting one's physique and using one's body effectively
- achieving emotional independence from parents and other adults
- preparing for marriage and family life
- preparing for a career
- acquiring a set of personal standards as a guide to behavior
- developing social intelligence, which includes becoming aware of human needs and becoming motivated to help others attain their goals
- developing conceptual and problem-solving skills

As you can see, there is quite a lot involved in growing up. Each of these tasks is important and must be achieved before reaching maturity.

Personal Identity

Some researchers group a number of the developmental tasks into a general task of achieving a personal identity. A **personal identity** consists of the factors you believe make you unique, or unlike anyone else. The task of establishing your own personal identity has a great impact

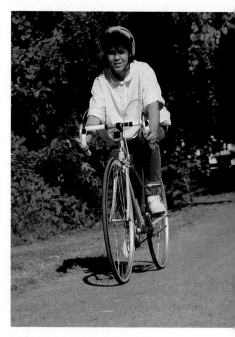

Developing problem-solving skills and learning to use one's body effectively are two developmental tasks for teens.

K E E P I N G   F I T

Facing Acne

Acne is a common problem for adolescents. In fact, 4 out of 5 teens have it. It may last for only a year or 2 or for 10 years or more. Acne is not caused by eating chocolate or greasy foods. It is usually caused by male sex hormones called androgens, which are present in both males and females. If you have acne, consider these tips:

- Avoid oil-based makeup and greasy lotions.

- Keep your face and hair clean.
- Change washcloths every day.
- Don't squeeze or scratch acne.
- Avoid sunlamps.
- For severe acne, consult your family doctor or dermatologist.

Overcoming The Odds

My name is Roselyn. I'm 15. Not too long ago somebody in my neighborhood was interviewed for this book. I thought it was great, and all, that he had been able to overcome his tough situation. I'm not knocking it. But the more I thought about it the more I thought it was important to say there are lots of teens out there—lots and lots of us—who don't have to face awful tragedies, who don't get into trouble, who just go to school and do their thing and basically do what they're supposed to do. So I called up my friend and found out who to call for this book, and here I am, telling it like it is for many of us."

Roselyn continues with great energy, her hands waving as she speaks. "I have to tell you, if you read the papers, see movies, and watch the news, if you listen to all the talk about how troubled all of us teens are, well, it can get pretty depressing. And it makes me flaming mad, sometimes, too. Sure I know kids who are in trouble with drugs, kids who have sex, people who get into other kinds of trouble now and then. But that's not everybody who's a teenager. I think all those constant messages

that there's Trouble in Teenland do a lot of damage to kids' self-esteem. Do you know what I mean?

"Now if you're asking me why I'm saying all this, I say, 'cause I think it's important to

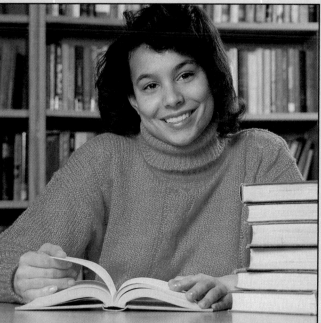

make it known that not all teens are messed up, pot-smoking, window-smashing rejects. I'm 15. I go to school every day. I have a part-time job. I study whenever I can. I'm not a dropout. I don't own a handgun. I don't smoke dope. I don't even smoke cigarettes, for that matter. I'm not pregnant and feel pretty strongly about finishing my education and traveling a lot before I ever settle down."

"Sure, there is arguing sometimes in my family. Sure, there are things I'd change about my body if I could. I'd like to have one main guy in my life and I don't yet. I'd like to be better at algebra and sports and other things. But nobody's perfect. I know that. My parents love me. I know that, too. And I mostly like my brother and sisters, even though they annoy me at times. What I'm trying to say is that you could say I've overcome the odds just by being a quasi-normal, functioning teenager in this crazy, troubled world. And I know there are lots of other teens out there like me, too."

1. How does Roselyn feel about the media's portrayal of today's teens?
2. Is your self-esteem ever affected by the media's messages about teenagers in general? If so, in what ways?
3. If the effects of these messages are damaging to your self-esteem, what steps can you take to ignore, change, or overcome them?
4. What are the dangers in portraying the members of any group—including teens—as uniform, or completely alike?

on all the other developmental tasks and is centered on your self-concept. Questions such as Who am I? and What do I want to be as a person? are common during this search for identity.

Here are some questions you can ask yourself as you form your own personal identity:

- Am I carrying out my responsibilities on my own, without needing someone to remind me of them?
- Do I get my schoolwork done on time?
- Can I make decisions without my peers influencing me?
- Am I thinking about what I want to do after high school?
- Am I thinking about what I want to do after I finish my education?
- Have I examined my beliefs about what types of behavior are appropriate for males and females?
- Am I aware of the image I project as a male or a female?
- Does my behavior reflect a personal set of values and standards by which I live?
- Do I know what people like and do not like about me?
- Do I expect to work for what I want, rather than just having things done for me?

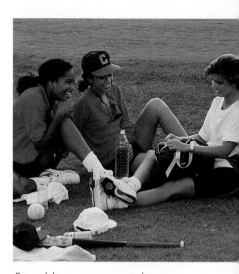

Friendship is important during adolescence. Good friends will not challenge you to do something that goes against what you believe and value.

Friends and Peers

Friendship and peer acceptance are important during adolescence. However, in the process of developing into a healthy adult, it is important for you to establish your own identity, separate from the group.

During adolescence others occasionally will challenge what you stand for, what you believe, and what you think is right or wrong. Good friends, however, will not challenge you to do something that goes against what you believe. They will not try to talk you into doing something that you do not want to do. This is one important guideline for evaluating friendships.

LESSON 1 REVIEW

Reviewing Facts and Vocabulary

1. What is puberty? What are some of the changes that take place during this stage of development?
2. Write a one-page composition about a day in the life of an adolescent. In the composition use the terms *puberty, secondary sex characteristics,* and *hormones.*
3. Define *personal identity,* and describe the actions of someone you know who has a strong personal identity.

Thinking Critically

4. **Synthesis.** Point out the physical changes occurring during puberty that you believe are the most difficult for many teens to accept. Explain the reasons for your choices.

Applying Health Knowledge

5. Select an empty cereal or detergent box to package yourself. Create a design on the outside to represent your personal identity. On the box, list ingredients, features, and other information to tell about the unique you.

A TIME FOR UNDERSTANDING YOURSELF

When someone asks who you are, how do you answer? Do you say something such as, "I'm Kip Martin," "I'm Maria's brother," or "I'm the class president?" Each of these may be an important part of who a person is, but none of them alone truly describes an individual.

You probably have classmates who define themselves according to their friends, their appearance, or their accomplishments. This means of establishing an identity can be a big mistake. These factors may well be important, but they are only a fraction of what makes someone tick. There is much more to understanding an individual.

The Inner You

Adolescence is often a difficult and confusing stage of life. Teenagers can be hard on themselves, and they can be hard on parents, teachers, and friends. The more you know about what is happening during adolescence, the less anxious you will be about what is going on within yourself. What you learn about yourself can assist you in making decisions and in achieving personal goals now and later in adulthood.

Your Goals

The definite plans you have in life are your **goals.** Goals help provide a mental picture of where you plan to go with your life and what you must do to get there. They guide you in the use of time, energy, and other resources.

Goals stem from dreams or hopes that you have. For instance, you may dream of becoming famous, traveling to a foreign country, or managing a business. You may also have dreams that include owning a home, having a family of your own, and helping those less fortunate.

Your dreams and goals are based on what is important to the inner you. Your values determine the kind of person you are. They affect your health practices, how you spend your time, what you decide to buy, and what friends you choose.

Some examples of values are honesty, family, religion, freedom, knowledge, health, respect for others, and respect for the environment. Examining your values will make it easier to understand your feelings and take action that is in line with those values.

Some people go through life avoiding decisions and just letting things happen. Others are pressured by their peers to make choices that are not always the best ones for them. They seem to be unable to set their own goals and to act on their dreams. Goals are rarely achieved by accident. If you want something to happen, you have to be willing to think about it, to make your own choices, and to act on those choices.

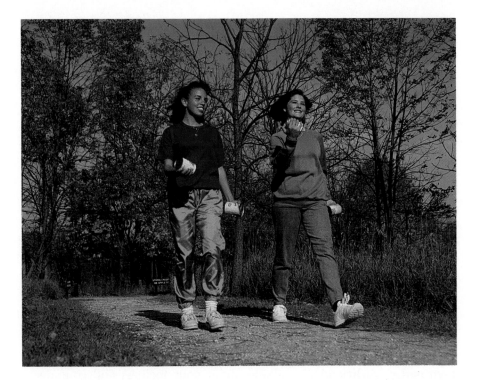

Choose friends whose influence will benefit your health.

Peer Pressure

Pressure from **peers,** or people your own age, is a very common part of adolescence. Peer pressure can include pressure to be like others or to do things they do.

Both peer pressure and popularity are concerns of most adolescents. Teens usually look to their peers for approval and for a measure of their success. It is normal for adolescents to depend on friends to learn more about the kind of people they are. They tend to see themselves through the eyes of their peers. Teens often judge their personalities as well as the way they look by how popular they are. Unfortunately, they can get a wrong view of themselves this way. Your peers may give you the wrong information about yourself. Peers may pressure you into making decisions that can be harmful in the long run.

Making Your Own Decisions.   Everywhere you look, it seems that teens are called on to make decisions. For example, people your age usually have many interests. These may include music, sports, friends, family, school functions, movies, fashion, and dating. Each interest involves various types of decisions—some easy, some more difficult.

During adolescence many teens face decisions related to their sexual feelings. Just as hormones cause physical changes in the body, they also cause changes in feelings and in how the body begins to respond to sexual stimulation. Such stimulation could be a picture or a movie scene, or it could be holding hands or kissing. The body responds in a variety of ways. The face gets hot and flushed, the heart beats faster, the hands get clammy, and there is a fluttery feeling inside. You cannot keep this response and these feelings from happening. They are normal and healthful. However, you can and must decide what to do about these feelings. An important point to keep in mind is that these feelings do not have to be acted on.

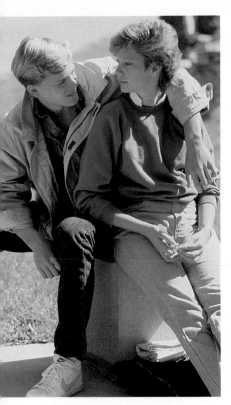

Make responsible decisions about sex before you become too involved to think clearly.

One factor that makes situations involving sexual stimuli difficult is the confusion surrounding one's feelings. A person may be experiencing new feelings—physical feelings of attraction to another person. If a person has not decided on a code of behavior before getting into a situation in which these feelings start to build, he or she will find it difficult to make a responsible decision. People do not think clearly when these feelings begin to build. It is much easier, and a whole lot smarter, to think through a decision about sexual behavior before getting into the situation in the first place. It is helpful to have alternatives in mind—to know just how far you are willing to go. Each person must decide what he or she wants. This decision is not an easy one, nor is it a one-time-only decision. It is a choice that people are faced with many times.

Sexual responses in the body should not be confused with love. You may have heard people say, "I have never felt this way before," "He excites me," or "Because I feel this way, I must be in love." These physical feelings of excitement have nothing to do with being in love. The feelings come about because of hormones in the body.

If you know what sexual feelings are, you can make more responsible decisions concerning them. It is easier to decide clearly about what you want for yourself—now and in the future—before you are in a situation in which these feelings have built up. Talk about them with your boyfriend or girlfriend. By talking about your feelings and your decisions, both of you can learn to understand and to respect each other.

There is nothing wrong with young people who decide that they are not ready for sex. Regardless of what you hear, not all teens are sexually active. Many teens recognize the serious risks associated with sexual activity. Many have made the decision to wait until marriage to become sexually active. These teens have chosen abstinence. **Abstinence** is choosing not to be sexually active. These teens are concerned about their futures. They have made the most healthy decision. Anyone who is thinking about being sexually active should consider the following:

- Do I feel any pressure to have sex?
- Where is the pressure coming from?
- Am I trying to prove something to someone?
- Am I trying to save this relationship by having sex?
- Have I talked with my boyfriend or girlfriend about our expectations from this relationship and how having sex might change it?
- Am I ready to deal with the possibility of being a parent?
- Have I completed my education or training for employment?
- Do I have a job and adequate finances to rear a child?
- How would being a parent affect my goals and dreams for the future?
- What would I do if I found out I had symptoms of a sexually transmitted disease (STD)?
- What would I do if I found out my partner had symptoms of an STD?
- What would my parents or family say if they knew I was having sex?
- Am I willing to accept the consequences of my decision?

Communicating Your Decisions.   Once you have decided what is right for you, you must communicate your decisions clearly.

Before getting in a sexual situation, talk to your date about your decisions and your goals and dreams. Sex is probably on both your minds. It is not easy bringing up the topic of sex and discussing it. Yet both of you are much more likely to reach an understanding and grow closer by talking about this concern.

How do you know when to say yes and when to say no? What do you do if your decision goes against what an individual or group is doing? How do you follow your values and not lose face with peers?

If your decision is no, then say no, without feeling you need to justify yourself. Be aware that others may ask you to justify why you have refused. This line of questioning should alert you that the person asking you has not really accepted your decision, so any explanation will be challenged. Again, you can repeat no. In situations like this, tell yourself that this is a good decision for you, that you will feel better when the pressure is over, and that you will not have to worry about selling yourself out because of others.

In some situations you may need to repeat yourself several times; if the person persists, leave. Avoid compromise if you feel strongly about something. Compromise can be a slow way of saying yes. Remember, good friends will not challenge you to do something that goes against what you believe. They will not try to talk you into doing something you do not want to do.

Facing Adolescence

Adolescence can be a time of joy as well as pain. Sometimes it is a period of special friendships, activity, and fun. At other times there may be loneliness, sadness, and confusion. Usually, there is a mixture of both the good and the painful during this stage of getting to know who you are and how you relate to others. Most teens turn to their family members, friends, religious leaders, and favorite teachers to lend support and comfort during good times and bad. Unfortunately, other teens sometimes turn to destructive behaviors such as drug use, casual sexual activities, or vandalism. These actions result in harm not only to the teens involved but also to others.

Teen Suicide

A much smaller number choose a more desperate action—suicide—in an attempt to deal with the troubles and challenges of adolescence. People commit suicide when they feel completely hopeless. Most are suffering from extreme depression. The depressed person sees no way out of what seems to be an impossible situation. Suicide is the eighth leading cause of death among all ages and the second leading cause of death among teens.

K E E P I N G   F I T

Five Dangerous Lines

If a teen is being pressured to have sex, one of the following lines may be used:

- Everyone's doing it.
- I'll break up with you if you don't.

- If you really love me, you'll do it.
- It will make you a real man or a real woman.
- You won't get pregnant. It will be safe.

Not everyone is having sex. Real love and caring mean getting to know someone and respecting that person's limits and rights. Even protected sex can result in pregnancy or a sexually transmitted disease.

Why do young people try to kill themselves? Several contributing factors have been identified. One is a greater than normal sense of social turmoil. Competition and pressure to succeed in an increasingly complex social environment can become overwhelming.

Another factor is the loss of a love relationship. This type of loss is most often the event that leads to a suicide attempt. Other kinds of

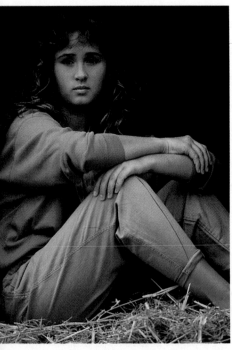

Adolescence can be a time of unhappiness.

HEALTH UPDATE

LOOKING AT THE ISSUES

What Should Be Done About Weapons in Schools?

A 1990 survey of high school students showed that 1 in 5 sometimes carries a weapon to school. As many as 135,000 guns are brought to schools every day in the United States, and in one recent 5-year period, at least 65 students were killed by them.

What can be done to stop students from bringing arms to school? What can be done to make students feel safe enough in school that they do not feel a need to carry weapons?

Analyzing Different Viewpoints

ONE VIEW. One of the ways schools have faced this dilemma is by increasing adult security. In New York City, a majority of schools have security-guard patrols in school halls and on school grounds.

A SECOND VIEW. A second method of cutting down on weapons in schools is to stop students from entering schools with them. Some school districts have random student searches for weapons. In other schools students are not allowed to wear baggy clothing that might conceal weapons. Other schools use metal detectors, and some have removed lockers or required see-through backpacks.

A THIRD VIEW. The approach in some schools has been to educate students about the dangers of guns and other weapons and to teach new strategies for conflict resolution and self-defense. In some schools, students trained in mediating disputes have proved effective in keeping such disputes from becoming violent.

A FOURTH VIEW. Some civil rights groups oppose student searches, claiming they infringe on people's right to privacy. Others claim that concentrating on weapons in schools is the wrong approach—that society needs to concentrate instead on the causes of violence.

Exploring Your Views

1. Which of these approaches or combination of approaches do you think might prove most effective in stopping students from bringing weapons into schools? What additional steps might be needed to protect those students who are unarmed?
2. If there are weapons in your school, what steps do you think your school should take to deal with the problem?
3. What forces in society do you think cause this problem of weapons and violence in the schools?

losses, such as loss of health or loss of status because of academic or social failure, can also make a young person vulnerable to suicide.

Many teens who attempt suicide really do not want to die. They are making a plea for help. Unless you are an expert, you probably cannot tell when a depressed person is likely to commit suicide. That is why when someone you know is depressed, it is critical to get help for that person. It is also important for the entire family to receive help. People who are in danger of suicide need the love and support of family members and friends.

Teen Pregnancy and Parenthood

Adolescence is a full-time job. Add pregnancy—and the birth and care of a child—and life can become very complicated. Becoming a parent is a serious responsibility that changes a person's life. For many teens it is a consequence they did not plan.

Most teens face the pressures and decisions about having or not having sexual intercourse at some time in their lives. The only way to be absolutely certain to avoid pregnancy is not to have sexual intercourse.

From Adolescence to Adulthood

Adolescence is a time of growth. It is the next step to adulthood. Sometimes this growth is painful, and at other times it is exciting and fun. Remember, you do not have to let growth just happen. You can continue to learn about how you are changing and what to expect. Learning more about these changes will help you do the following:

- understand your own behavior and why people react to you as they do
- make appropriate decisions about who you are and who you will be in the future
- behave in ways that reflect your personal values and goals
- achieve your goals and dreams.

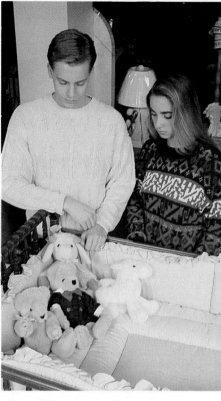

How will these teens' lives be affected by early parenthood?

LESSON 2 REVIEW

Reviewing Facts and Vocabulary

1. What are goals? List three goals you have set for yourself.
2. Define *peer pressure*. What is its effect on someone your age?

Thinking Critically

3. **Synthesis.** Create a skit contrasting successful and unsuccessful ways of communicating yes or no when making decisions.
4. **Synthesis.** Why is it important to have a code of behavior established before getting into a situation that will require you to make a serious decision?

Applying Health Knowledge

5. Survey several teen parents who are in school to learn how their lives and responsibilities changed after having a child.
6. For a week keep a list of all the times you communicate a decision and whether you communicate the decision successfully. During the following week try to increase the number of times you are successful in your communication.

Self-Inventory

Developmental Tasks

HOW DO YOU RATE?

Number a sheet of paper from 1 through 18. Read each item below and respond by writing 3 for *definitely*, 2 for *somewhat*, or 1 for *hardly* or *not at all*. Total the numbers. Then proceed to the next section.

1. I have a picture in my mind of what kind of person I want to be as an adult.

2. I think through problems I face, looking at several possible solutions.

3. I have one or two very close friends with whom I can discuss almost anything.

4. I know of several jobs I think I would be good at as an adult.

5. I am aware of the activities of some of the civic groups in my community.

6. I have more discussions with my parents or other adults than I used to.

7. I am concerned about national and world problems in the news today.

8. I can list the four most important beliefs I have.

9. I know some of the qualities I would look for in a marriage partner.

10. People who know me know I act in a way that supports what I believe in.

11. I am usually comfortable with my behavior as a male or female in social settings.

12. I can describe some ways my life-style would change if I were married and if I had children.

13. I listen to other people's ideas, even though they may differ from my own.

14. I usually have success in making male and female friends with my peers.

15. I know and accept my physical strengths and weaknesses.

16. I do some things alone or with my friends that I used to do with my family.

17. I have several interests I would consider pursuing as career possibilities.

18. I make choices that promote my overall health and well-being.

HOW DID YOU SCORE?

Look below to see how you scored. Then proceed to the next section.

45 to 54
Excellent. You are well on your way to becoming a healthy, mature adult.

23 to 44
Good. You are making good progress on your way to becoming a healthy, mature adult.

17 to 22
Fair. You are working on some of the developmental tasks, but you need to try harder.

Below 16
Poor. You need to get serious about growing up and setting goals to achieve specific tasks.

WHAT ARE YOUR GOALS?

If your score was between 37 and 54, complete the statements in Part A. If your score was between 1 and 36, complete the statements in Parts A and B.

Part A

1. I plan to learn more about each of the developmental tasks in the following ways: ____.

2. My timetable for accomplishing this is ____.

3. I plan to share my information with others by ____.

Part B

4. The developmental task that I would like to work on the most is ____.

5. The steps involved in working on this task are ____.

6. My timetable for achieving this goal is ____.

7. The people or groups I will ask for support and assistance are ____.

8. My rewards for making this change will be ____.

Building Decision-Making Skills

K elly is a freshman cheerleader. She really enjoyed her participation in the first football game and the dance afterward, at which the captain of the team—a senior—asked her to go with him to a party the next night. Her parents said, "Sorry, you're too young to date, and especially a senior." They say Kelly can attend school functions, go out with mixed groups, or perhaps even attend school functions with boys her own age. Kelly feels her parents are treating her like a baby. She tells them all her friends date and she thinks she should be allowed to do so, too. She is thinking of sneaking out to go to the party in spite of her parents' objections.

WHAT DO YOU THINK?

1. **Situation.** Why might this be a difficult situation for Kelly?

2. **Situation.** What immediate decision needs to be made?

3. **Situation.** What other decisions need to be made later?

4. **Situation.** How much time does Kelly have to make the first decision?

5. **Situation.** What risks are involved in this decision?

6. **Choices.** What are Kelly's choices? Which of these choices is totally inappropriate? Why?

7. **Consequences.** Who will be affected by this decision and in what ways?

8. **Consequences.** How might Kelly's health triangle be affected by this decision?

9. **Consequences.** What might happen if Kelly chose to sneak out to the party?

10. **Consequences.** How might her date react if she chose to sneak out to the party?

11. **Consequences.** How might the football captain react if she tells him she can't go to the party?

12. **Consequences.** How might her parents react if she goes to the party without their permission?

13. **Consequences.** How might Kelly's self-esteem be affected by this decision?

14. **Consequences.** What reasons might Kelly's parents have for not giving her permission to attend this party?

15. **Consequences.** How might Kelly feel if she chooses not to attend the party? Might these feelings change if trouble developed at the party?

16. **Consequences.** How might Kelly convince her parents she is ready to date?

17. **Decision.** What immediate decision do you think Kelly should make?

18. **Decision.** What long-term decisions should Kelly make? Explain your answer.

19. **Evaluation.** Have you ever known someone who faced a similar situation? How was it handled? What was the outcome?

20. **Evaluation.** Many teens say they are glad their parents provide some controls on their activities. Do you agree or disagree? Why?

21. **Evaluation.** Someday you may be a parent. What rules would you establish for your teenagers in regard to dating? Would you have the same rules for your daughters as for your sons? Explain your answer.

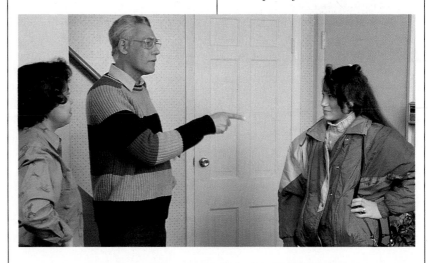

REVIEW

Using Health Terms

On a separate sheet of paper, write the term that best matches each definition given below.

LESSON 1

1. The period of time between childhood and adulthood.
2. Traits such as body hair, breasts in a female, and muscles in a male.
3. Chemical substances in the body that stimulate growth, such as testosterone, estrogen, and progesterone.
4. Something that needs to occur during a particular period of life for a person to continue to grow toward becoming a healthy, mature adult.

LESSON 2

5. Other people of one's own age.
6. The intended taking of one's own life.

Building Academic Skills

LESSON 1

7. **Reading.** Tell whether each statement below expresses a fact or an opinion.
   a. During puberty males and females become physically able to reproduce.
   b. Puberty is like being on a roller coaster.
   c. Good friends are the most important thing in life.
8. **Writing.** Rosa made the following notes. She wants to combine her ideas in one sentence. Help her by writing a grammatically correct sentence that includes all of Rosa's ideas. You may need to add some words of your own.
   Puberty begins.
   between the ages of 9 and 13
   ability to reproduce
   Secondary sex characteristics develop.

LESSON 2

9. **Writing.** Write a paragraph describing one of your goals and how you plan to achieve it.

Recalling the Facts

LESSON 1

10. What is the most rapid growth period in a person's life?
11. At what age does puberty begin?
12. Why do some teens feel awkward and clumsy during the early stages of puberty?
13. Classify each of the following hormones as male or female: estrogen, progesterone, testosterone.
14. What happens to the brain during adolescence?
15. Why should adolescents be able to learn more quickly and more easily than younger students? Give three reasons.
16. What two questions can you ask yourself in order to learn from your mistakes?
17. What causes emotional changes during puberty?

LESSON 2

18. How can having goals help you in life?
19. How can peer pressure and a longing to be popular affect a teen's decisions?
20. What do the following physical signs indicate is happening to the body: the face becomes hot and flushed, the heart beats faster, the hands get clammy, there is a fluttery feeling inside?
21. Why can it be difficult to make a responsible decision while you are experiencing strong feelings of physical attraction for a member of the opposite sex?
22. What might be some unwanted outcomes of having sex to save a relationship?
23. How might becoming a parent while still in high school affect a person's plans for the future?
24. Why is it a good idea to discuss decisions about sex with your boyfriend or girlfriend before you get into a serious situation?
25. List three factors that may contribute to suicide among young people.
26. What is the only absolutely sure way to avoid pregnancy?

REVIEW

Thinking Critically

LESSON 1

27. **Analysis.** Here are several physical changes that occur during puberty. Select two and analyze the impact on one's self-esteem.
    a. acne
    b. growth spurt
    c. appearance of facial hair
    d. development of breasts
    e. increase in perspiration
    f. widening of the hips
    g. narrowing of the waistline
    h. broadening of the shoulders

28. **Evaluation.** Write *strong* or *weak* to describe the personal identity of each of the following students.
    a. One day Consuela hopes to own a hair styling salon. She attends a vocational high school. In addition to courses in hair styling, she is taking business and accounting courses.
    b. Harry never begins to do his homework until one of his parents tells him to get busy.
    c. Chang wants a special set of stereo components. He is working at Burger Barn after school and mowing lawns on Saturdays to earn money to buy the set.

LESSON 2

29. **Evaluation.** Do you think there is too much sex shown on television and in the movies? Why or why not? In what ways might sex on television and in the movies influence the behavior of young people?

Making the Connection

LESSON 2

30. **Social Studies.** Compare adolescence in the 1960s with adolescence today by interviewing people who were teens during that time. What were their concerns? What were their favorite songs ? Who were their role models?

Applying Health Knowledge

LESSON 1

31. Think of several possible ways in which Juan, who is 6′ 2″ tall and weighs 210 pounds, and Rich, who is 5′ 2″ tall and weighs 120 pounds, might react to being different in size from their peers?

LESSON 2

32. Zoe and Jim are seniors. They have been dating for more than a year. Zoe wants to get married after graduation, but Jim wants to go to college. Zoe feels she is ready to add sex to their relationship. Read the dialogue below, and then answer the questions that follow it.

    Zoe: Jim, I want to have sex with you.

    Jim: I don't think that's a good idea, Zoe.

    Zoe: Why not?

    Jim: You might get pregnant.

    Zoe: You could use something. Besides, I'm willing to take that chance.

    Jim: Zoe, you know I want to go to college. It's just too big a risk.

    Zoe: But, Jim, I love you so. It would bring us closer together.

    Jim: Zoe, you're putting too much pressure on me. I think we'd be making a big mistake.

    a. What motives might Zoe have for wanting to have sex?
    b. What mistake is Jim referring to?

Beyond the Classroom

LESSON 2

33. **Parental Involvement.** Talk to your parents about peer pressure they experienced when they were your age. Ask for examples of ways they were pressured. How did they respond to the pressure?

34. **Further Study.** Read an article about a famous sports figure or entertainer. Describe the goals this person set as a youth and what he or she did to achieve them.

CONTINUING THROUGH THE LIFE CYCLE

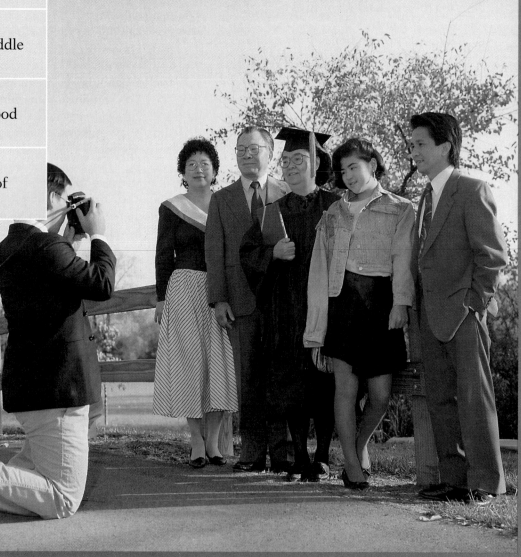

GROWTH FOR A LIFETIME

When compared with the entire life cycle, the stages of infancy, childhood, and adolescence last only a short time. You and your friends may feel that the years of growing up will never end, but these years are only a small part of the rest of your life. With an average life expectancy of 76 years, you truly do have a lifetime ahead of you.

Considering the Entire Life Cycle

The study of all the years of the life cycle, beginning with a person's birth to that individual's death, is a relatively new area of research. In the past, few scientists studied life as a whole. Instead, they focused on the early years because development during infancy and childhood is so rapid. It easily falls into specific stages and is so important to later life. In fact, some scientists believed that human development ended with childhood or early adolescence. They believed there was no growth and development during adulthood. Many researchers saw the progression from birth to death much like hiking up a hill to reach adulthood and then walking across a level plateau that finally headed downward toward the end of life's journey.

Today we know that life is more dynamic than that. Even though human development is very dramatic in early life, it does not end at the age of 6 or 16. Instead, development occurs in every age group.

Developmental Tasks During Adulthood

In Chapter 9 you read about the major developmental tasks for adolescence. A **developmental task** is something that needs to occur during a particular stage for a person to continue his or her growth toward becoming a healthy, mature adult. Failure or difficulty with a task may lead to personal dissatisfaction, disapproval by society, and difficulty with later tasks.

Many of life's early developmental tasks, such as learning to walk, come about mostly as a result of physical maturation. Others, such as learning to read or learning ways to get along with others, are developed primarily from the cultural pressures of society. Still other tasks, such as choosing and preparing for a career, grow out of personal values and goals of the individual. Most developmental tasks originate from all of these factors working together.

Just as infants, children, and adolescents must complete various developmental tasks in order to grow, adults also face certain tasks that lead to maturity. These tasks focus on five major aspects of people's lives:

- occupational role
- individual identity and personal independence
- relationships with other people

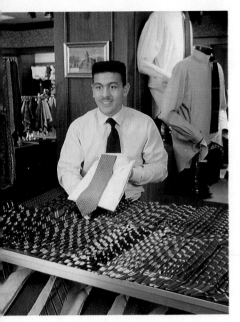

Choosing an occupation is part of establishing identity and personal independence.

- relationship to society
- acceptance of growing older and of the reality of death

Each of these developmental tasks represents lessons that adults must learn to adjust to the world around them.

Establishing an Occupational Role

During adolescence many people start to form ideas about the kind of life they want as adults. An occupation or career is usually a large part of that idea or dream of the future. As they become young adults, people begin to see themselves more clearly in an occupational role. This role may occur through on-the-job training or through education beyond high school as preparation for a career. Making an occupational choice, although it may not be the final one, is one of the major developmental tasks that must be achieved on the way to adulthood.

Establishing an Individual Identity and Personal Independence

The desire for independence during adolescence is preparation for establishing an individual identity as an adult. It also is part of a continuing process, called **self-actualization,** that involves developing one's capabilities to their fullest. If people have a good understanding of their own abilities and goals and feel secure about themselves, they are able to work toward self-actualization and the establishment of an adult identity.

Until young people leave home, at least part of their identity is based on family membership. Comments such as, "He's John's son," "She's Fay's youngest," or "She's still in high school" show family ties and dependence.

Leaving home or starting to work full-time are ways that young adults can begin to achieve self-actualization. At first, they may substitute the emotional support of friends for the support they once received from parents. As their development continues, however, young adults will become more self-sufficient. In so doing, they will be continuing on the developmental path that will lead to the establishment of an individual identity and personal independence.

K E E P I N G   F I T

Making a Family Fitness Contract

Consider the case of Vikki and Jason Scott, a mother-son rowing team who in 1991 competed in the Pan American Games in Cuba. Just a few years ago, Vikki Scott was an overweight, cigarette-addicted mother with no exercise routine. Inspired by her son, she took up the sport. Now they are both on the national team, rowing their way to fitness and closer family bonds.

Why not draw up a family fitness contract? Choose an exercise or sport in which everyone in your family can take part. Make up a contract that spells out when, where, and how you will exercise together and the benefits and rewards.

Establishing Close Relationships

This developmental task involves the ability to build close relationships with people of both sexes while still maintaining a sense of self. During this time there may be several successive romantic relationships. More time may be devoted to romantic relationships than to peer relationships. Some people give romantic relationships a sense of permanence through marriage. Others develop romantic relationships but prefer to remain single. Still others are occupied with establishing a career or defining their own identity, and the ability to develop and maintain close relationships comes later or not at all.

Establishing a Place in Society

One of the tasks of adulthood includes determining where and how a person fits into society. Political ideas, religious views, and a sense of community responsibility contribute to finding a place in society and feeling comfortable with it. Because mature adults have developed an individual identity, they find ways to share their interests in their community. They may, for example, do volunteer work, promote recycling, or join a neighborhood sports team. They take responsibility for what they are doing and what they are becoming.

Establishing an Acceptance of Growing Older and of the Reality of Death

For most people this dual task is perhaps the most difficult of all. However, individuals who have had success in their earlier developmental tasks tend to accept the inevitability of aging, physical and mental decline, and death. These individuals can be found in every community, making each day a rewarding one for themselves and others.

LESSON 1 REVIEW

Reviewing Facts and Vocabulary

1. Why is the study of the entire life cycle a relatively new area of study?
2. Define the term *developmental task;* give an example of a developmental task in adulthood.

Thinking Critically

3. **Synthesis.** Point out one or more developmental tasks that a young adult you know has achieved. Give reasons to show that the individual has worked through the task(s).
4. **Evaluation.** Rewrite the developmental tasks of adulthood in your own words. Place them in the order in which you believe they will occur in your life.

Applying Health Knowledge

5. Write a radio or television script about several adults who are dealing with some of the developmental tasks of adulthood. Share your completed script with your class.
6. Interview people of various ages. Explain the adult developmental tasks to them. Ask them to evaluate the progress they feel they are making on these tasks. Share your findings with the class.

LESSON 2

YOUNG AND MIDDLE ADULTHOOD

LESSON 2 FOCUS

TERMS TO USE
- Transitions
- Empty-nest syndrome
- Cluttered-nest syndrome

CONCEPTS TO LEARN
- Changes after childhood and adolescence occur at certain stages.
- Crucial decisions are made during early adulthood.
- Many transitions occur during middle age.

ATTITUDES AND BEHAVIORS TO EVALUATE
- Self-Inventory, page 192.
- Building Decision-Making Skills, page 193.

Legally, in many states, people are considered to be adults when they reach the age of 18. Physically, they become adults when their physical growth has been completed, around age 25. To many, adulthood is the best time of their life. To others, it is a time of stress and painful struggle. For most individuals, it is both.

Although the stages of life follow one another in a regular order, they occur at different ages in different people. Erikson's sixth and seventh stages of development are young adulthood and middle adulthood.

Young Adulthood

Young adulthood may begin as early as age 17; for most people, however, it starts at about the age of 20 and continues through the 30s. This stage of adulthood begins when individuals do not have to depend on their parents or other adults all of the time. These young adults no longer see themselves as being ruled by their parents. They are able to support themselves financially by holding down a job. Basically, they are aware of what they want from life. They tend to express their emotions in acceptable ways and know how to get along with people. They can deal with everyday situations without becoming easily upset.

Most young adults are at the peak of their physical abilities; they are stronger, quicker, and more alert than ever. Most young adults find they have an increased capacity to learn and to adjust to new situations. Their self-confidence grows as they learn to gather information and put it to use in their own lives. During this time people continue perfecting skills that make them more self-supporting and independent. They are accepted by society as full-fledged members and, in turn, are offered numerous chances to make contributions to the work force and community.

Because the years of young adulthood are the years of choice, a number of crucial decisions are made during this time. Most young adults decide what work to do. This choice may be one that was considered in adolescence or a new one.

Erikson's stage of development, intimacy versus isolation, occurs during young adulthood. This stage involves committing to another person. Many people choose to marry during this time, and the majority of these couples decide to have one or more children. Their new families bring on new responsibilities and additional lessons to learn. However, if fear of intimacy is greater than one's need for it, loneliness and isolation are more likely to occur.

At various stages during the life cycle, adults may feel as they did during adolescence. This is especially true during young adulthood. Young adults may question who they are and what they want from life. If the developmental tasks of adolescence have not been achieved, these young adults may have problems dealing with the changes that come with young adulthood: a career, marriage, or a family. They may not be willing or able to make the adjustments needed.

Middle Adulthood

For most of human history, and in many areas of the world today, only a tiny segment of any population has ever lived much beyond the age of 40. In many parts of the world where short life expectancy is combined with poverty, middle adulthood almost seems to disappear as a stage of the life cycle. In such situations, when people must labor unceasingly for survival, life changes very little between the beginning of adulthood and old age. In more developed parts of the world, however, people live much longer and reach the middle and later years. They come face-to-face with middle adulthood. At the age of 40, 45, or 50, people can see for themselves that they have arrived at a midpoint in the adult years. More than half of their life is gone. For some adults facing middle age, life is seen in terms of time left to live rather than time since birth. For most others, mid-life brings new insight and self-understanding. Such fresh perspectives generally come as the result of conscious self-reflection.

Some middle-aged adults tend to be concerned not only with survival and making a living, but also with thinking seriously about what they want to do with this second half of their lives. In contrast to early adulthood, in which orientation tends to be focused on a person's relationship to others, the middle years are marked by self-evaluation. This can be a period of confusion or a time for asking questions, such as Where am I going? Is this what I want to do with my life? Should I do something different? Is it too late to change direction?

The feeling that time is running out is common during middle adulthood. This feeling often surfaces as a result of the aging or death of a parent, the untimely death of a friend, the realization that children are growing up, or simply because of an increased awareness of the passage of time. All of these events emphasize the limits that time places on life. Sensing these limitations, many people may feel pressured to make changes before it is too late.

Career change, divorce, marriage or remarriage, and other changes in previously established ways of life are common during this stage. Some changes may be beneficial; others may be harmful.

You may have observed people who find it difficult or impossible to accept the passage of time. They may try to deny change by behaving as

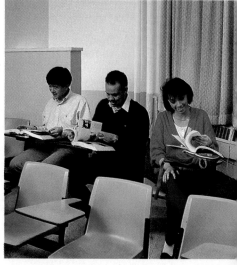

Mid-life brings new challenges and opportunities.

K E E P I N G   F I T

Eating an Anti-Aging Diet

Though there is no known cure for aging, and no Fountain of Youth has yet been found, there are some dietary guidelines that you can follow that can help keep you healthy over time. According to the U.S. Department of Agriculture's Human Nutrition Research Center on Aging, the following anti-aging dietary guidelines might help.

- Eat foods rich in vitamin E, vitamin C, and beta carotene.

- Do not get more than 30 percent of calories from fat.
- Eat low-fat foods rich in calcium.
- Get at least 25 to 40 grams of fiber every day.

- Your chances of living to be 100 or older are best in Arizona, Florida, Hawaii, Idaho, Iowa, Kansas, Minnesota, Nebraska, North Dakota, and South Dakota.
- If you think that senior citizens are confined to bed because of old age, think again. The average number of days they spend ill in bed or with their activities seriously curtailed is only 23 per year, while for those in the 45 to 64 age bracket, the average number of days infirmed is 34.

if nothing is different. Their attitudes, dress, and tastes remain the same. Some may even refuse to recognize the growing independence of their children. Refusing to recognize inner changes during middle adulthood sometimes results in emotional or physical difficulties, which may cause problems in relationships with others.

Some adults who find it difficult to accept the passage of time make drastic changes in their behavior and way of life. Sometimes this is referred to as going through a mid-life crisis. People experiencing these difficulties may imitate youthful or immature ways of living or may wear clothes designed for younger people. Since these middle-aged adults have not recognized and dealt with changes within themselves, they often find they still are not happy.

Most people progress through middle adulthood without serious problems. They adjust their hopes and dreams and adapt their life-styles to their newly experienced feelings of being in touch with themselves. Some make career changes that are more personally satisfying.

Parent-Child and Adult-Child Relationships

Many children reach adolescence at the same time one or both parents or other important adults in their lives are going through the process of self-evaluation. Because middle adulthood can be as difficult for adults as adolescence is for teens, tension and conflict may increase. Both adults and adolescents are working through stages in which many changes are taking place. As a result, the personal needs of the adult and the teen often come into conflict. An understanding of developmental tasks and an awareness of the needs of others can help keep conflicts and tensions between adolescents and adults to a minimum.

Transitions

There are a number of **transitions,** or changes, in all stages of life. A major transition during middle adulthood is based on Erikson's stage of development called generativity versus stagnation. This stage focuses on helping others, especially young people. Generativity involves a commitment to the future. This can include active concern for young people and for the society in which young people will live and work as adults. Refusal to accept and deal with changes during middle adulthood can result in self-absorption, or preoccupation with meeting only one's own needs.

K E E P I N G   F I T

Becoming a Walking Encyclopedia

Many older adults get vigorous exercise by becoming mall walkers, track walkers, or sidewalkers. Walking is a kind of exercise that promotes maximum cardiovascular benefit with minimum risk of injury. And walking is an exercise that can benefit all ages.

Choose an older adult as a walking buddy. Exercise with the person regularly. As you walk, share your thoughts, opinions, histories, and experiences. Learn what you can from the person's life experiences. In the process, you may find that you not only become more fit, but you may become a walking encyclopedia!

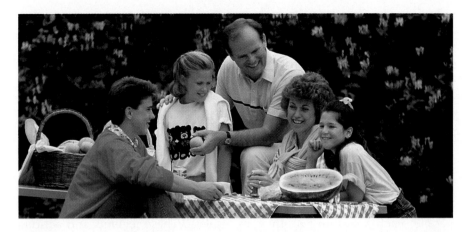

Another transition facing the middle-aged adult involves children leaving home and entering adulthood. This is sometimes called the **empty-nest syndrome.** If children have been the reason for a couple's staying together, divorce may take place when the couple discovers that the only factor they had in common is no longer there. However, coming to terms with themselves and aligning their dreams with reality allows many couples to reestablish close relationships as well as to grow as individuals. Single people may marry for the first time or remarry if they have been divorced or widowed. Women who have devoted their lives to home and family often go back to paid employment or begin a new career.

A recent transition involves the return of adult children to the home of their parents. The term **cluttered-nest syndrome** is often used to identify the situation in which parents must adjust, once again, to the presence of children in their lives. Many adult children return to their parents' home for economic reasons, such as insufficient income to afford both college and a place of their own or to rent or purchase housing on their own. Still others return after a divorce or the birth of a child for whom they cannot afford care.

DID YOU KNOW?

- According to researchers at the Philadelphia Geriatric Center, people who care for invalids need breaks. New programs offer respite care— breaks from the daily caretaking. These breaks allow care-givers to do chores, get rest and, in the long run, be refreshed for future caregiving.

LESSON 2 REVIEW

Reviewing Facts and Vocabulary

1. Summarize the signs indicating that a person has reached young adulthood.
2. Define the term *transition,* and give two examples of transitions people face during middle adulthood.

Thinking Critically

3. **Analysis.** Write a paragraph analyzing a crucial decision made by a young adult you know or have read about.
4. **Synthesis.** Develop two corresponding lists: concerns facing middle-aged adults who are experiencing the empty nest syndrome and concerns middle-aged adults feel as they face the cluttered nest syndrome.

Applying Health Knowledge

5. Find examples on television, in magazines, or in newspapers to illustrate people going through the stage of generativity versus stagnation.
6. Create a cartoon, bulletin board, or other illustration to show a family experiencing the empty-nest syndrome or the cluttered-nest syndrome.
7. Prepare a skit, with follow-up questions, based on someone who may be going through a mid-life crisis.

LATE ADULTHOOD AND AGING

Erikson's eighth stage of development is late adulthood. Old age is often treated more as a disease than as a stage in human development. Because our society tends to emphasize youth and economic productivity, the wisdom and experience of age are sometimes ignored. Often there is a lack of respect for the elderly and a feeling that once people reach a certain age, they are useless. These feelings and actions sometimes make it difficult for older adults to feel worthwhile.

Chronological age does not necessarily make a person old. There are many "young" people well past 70. Some 80-year-olds are in better physical condition than some much younger people. In our society age 65 was selected as the cutoff point between middle and later adulthood. This age was adopted primarily for social purposes, such as eligibility for retirement and various pensions, discounts, and services reserved for those often referred to as "senior citizens." Age 65 does not, however, indicate a magic age at which there is a decline in individual capabilities, productivity, or potential.

Late Adulthood

The trend toward better health and the resulting longer life expectancy has reshaped people's ideas of old age. The potential human life expectancy averages about 85 years of age with a maximum life duration of about 115 years. With the advances in diagnosing and treating illnesses and by practicing a healthy life-style, people can increase both their quality of life and their anticipated life expectancy.

Measures of Age

Aging, like all phases of growth and development, is predictable but very individual. **Gerontologists,** people who study and work in the area of aging, cite three measures of age. The first is **chronological age.** This is simply the number of birthdays one has had.

The second, **biological age,** is how well different parts of the body are functioning. Fitness standards for various chronological ages include how fast a person recovers from running up a flight of stairs or how fast blood clots. The rate of biological aging is influenced by heredity, life-style, and health habits, especially diet and exercise. Poisons taken in from the environment over a lifetime and the illnesses a person has had also influence biological age.

The third measure of age is **social age,** which involves a person's life-style. For example, at each phase of development, there are some general **age norms,** things a person is expected to be doing at a particular chronological age. For example, our society expects a 16-year-old to be going to high school, meeting and socializing with a variety of people, possibly working part-time, or preparing for a career after finishing high school. These norms, which are imposed by the society in which one lives, give people a timetable, but they do not always reflect what people want to do or are able to do.

The Physical Process of Aging

You have learned that certain body cells are replaced continually. The life of a blood cell is about 120 days; that of an intestinal cell is about 1.5 days. As a person ages, this process of cell division slows. The cells that are capable of dividing and producing new cells gradually decrease activity.

As cells grow older, their nuclei change and age pigment collects in the cells. Age pigment is thought to be the result of cells becoming less efficient in processing and ridding themselves of cell wastes. With the gradual buildup of age pigment, cell function slows and cells gradually deteriorate.

As part of the aging process

- skin loses its elasticity and begins to wrinkle;
- hair turns gray;
- nails become brittle;
- hearing and vision problems may develop;
- bones gradually lose calcium, becoming more brittle;
- basal metabolism slows;
- kidney function slows;
- the endocrine system decreases its secretion of hormones;
- the body's immune system becomes less efficient;
- a loss of lean body mass occurs, often accompanied by an increase of fat tissue;
- joints become less mobile; muscular strength weakens;
- vital capacity, the total amount of air that can be exhaled from the lungs after a deep breath, lessens;
- the heart pumps blood less efficiently;
- the body's ability to use glucose diminishes, lessening the body's available energy.

Although all of these physical characteristics of aging are inevitable if a person lives long enough, they are very individual and directly related to a person's overall life-style. If people continue to be active, eat a nutritious diet, and take good mental and physical care of themselves, the function of these body parts remains more efficient.

Culturally Speaking

Not Older, But Better

In Japan, the older one is, the wiser one is thought to be. Young people seek the advice of older people, and the aged are treated with great respect. The Amish also recognize that older members of society have valuable experience to share. Because the Amish limit the use of new technology, older people greatly contribute to their culture.

In societies where technology changes rapidly, the elderly may not become familiar with "new" ways of performing tasks, and their experience may not be valued. In societies that value age, older people are an active part of life. However, in societies where the elderly are considered "outdated," older people are frequently separated from daily group life.

What value does your culture place on aging? How can you tell?

KEEPING FIT

Developing Friendships Across the Ages

In our society, the young and old are too often segregated, or kept apart. If you have a good relationship with a senior citizen, continue to nurture it; you both have lots to gain from knowing one another. If you don't have a significant relationship with a senior citizen, develop one. Spend more time or correspond with a grandparent or other elderly relative. Get to know an elderly neighbor. Or volunteer in an organization that pairs teens with older adults. Put some time and effort into enriching the life of a senior and, in turn, have your own life enriched.

Overcoming The Odds

Noel Johnson is 92 years young. He is a glowing example of how old age does not have to mean illness, dependence, or lack of fitness. He has run in marathons seven times and is now preparing to run in his eighth. "I ran my first New York marathon when I was 80 years old," he says. "I was the first 80-year-old ever to have completed the 26-mile run. I've even run two marathons just seven days apart."

Johnson works out daily and with great dedication. He says, "I just got off the exercise bike. I was on that for one hour. Then I'll be on my rebounder (trampoline) for one hour. I think that's more beneficial than running because you're going up and down every second, and it vibrates every cell in your body." He continues, "I have my light weights that I work out with 10 or 15 minutes 2 or 3 times a day." He also works out on a treadmill daily. "I'll be running the New York Marathon in November," he continues. "I run about 3 or 4 miles right now, but soon I'll run 10 miles twice a day in preparation for the race."

Noel Johnson also loves to box. He is the World Senior Boxing Champion.

Johnson was not always so

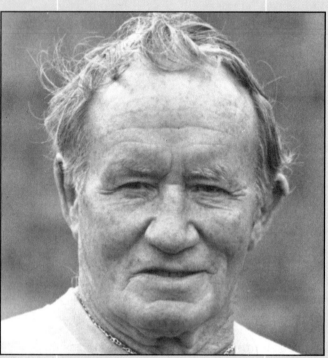

healthy or committed to fitness. At 72, he was 40 pounds overweight. He smoked cigarettes and drank alcohol, and he had a heart condition. His doctor gave him 6 months to live. In fact, he was in such bad shape that his life insurance was canceled. "My son said I should go into a retirement home, and I said that wasn't necessary. Then he said, 'Well, will you show me you can walk?' I started walking and walking and then running, too. And that's when I began my athletic career—at age 72!"

Johnson's amazing achievements and overall fitness have been studied by health scientists. Since 1971, he has been part of an ongoing study of master athletes over age 40 at the University of California at Davis. He is now also being studied at the University of Florida at Gainesville, where tests again show he is in superb shape. He says, "They told me in Florida after a bone scan from ankle to head that my structure was as strong and clear as anything they had examined." On a treadmill test, his pulse was 63, and researchers got it to over 200, a pulse rate that Johnson says would make the "average person drop dead."

Noel Johnson has written 2 books and is already planning his third. He has traveled and lectured in 21 countries around the world. Among his other goals: running a marathon when he reaches 100—an age, he says, "when I know I'll be in better condition than I am now."

1. Noel Johnson is an example that it is never too late to make changes to improve your health and self-esteem. Do you believe it is never too late? Explain.
2. What steps can you take right now to begin improving your overall fitness?

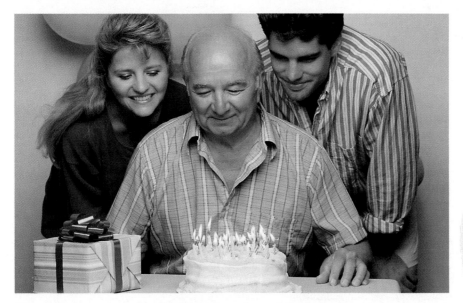

There are three measures of aging: chronological, biological, and social.

The Needs of the Elderly

Just like everyone else, the elderly have basic emotional needs. They need to love and be loved, to feel they are making a contribution, and to feel they are worthwhile individuals.

A variety of factors affects a person's ability to adjust to aging. For example, looking at aging as a lifelong process contributes to a better understanding and acceptance of later adulthood as a vital stage in life. People who have coped with changes all of their lives are better able to cope with the changes resulting from aging. Their attitude toward aging and their activity level have a great influence on how they adjust to getting older. People who remain active and involved tend to adjust better. Flexible policies for retirement and educational and counseling services help older adults prepare for and adapt to this stage in their lives.

Family relationships are a very important factor in helping individuals successfully adjust to aging. In some families grandparents not only care for young children but also prepare meals and do other chores so that other family members can go to work. Because older people need to feel useful and wanted, those who do not have relatives living with or near them often face the greatest difficulty in adjusting to old age.

K E E P I N G   F I T

Finding a Mentor

Having a mentor—an older person who is an expert in an area in which you are trying to excel—can be a great source of knowledge and encouragement. Famous artists and musicians over the ages have had mentors. These days, there are mentor programs in businesses and schools.

Think of a talent or craft that you would like to learn, improve, or develop. Locate an older person who is considered competent in that area. Ask the person if you can learn from him or her. Offer to be an unpaid assistant or run errands for the person in return for his or her time and guidance.

- The Fifty-Plus Runners Association based at Stanford University has about 2,000 members who frequently take part in research on exercise and aging, such as the effects of running on bone composition and on joints.
- Hulda Crooks at age 91 became the oldest woman to climb Mt. Fuji in Japan.
- Thelma Tulane of Washington, D.C., is 80. She has arthritis and sometimes uses a walker. But she also dances with a troupe called Dancers of the Third Age, a group of elderly people who perform in hospitals and schools.

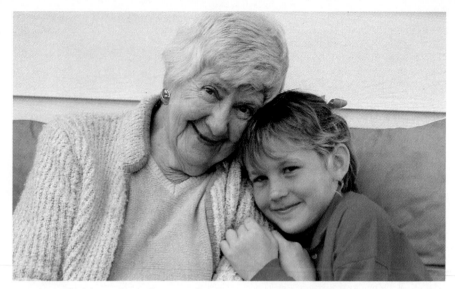

Young and old can learn from each other.

Elderly people who maintain friendships and contact with other people after retiring cope better with aging. Programs, such as Adopt-a-Grandparent, have been started in many communities to keep the elderly involved with others, especially with young people. The rewards for such involvement are twofold. The elderly feel needed and useful, and the young people get enjoyment from sharing and learning from the elderly.

Whether living alone or with others, the elderly need to be as independent as possible. They need privacy and time to be alone to take care of their own needs, hobbies, and other interests. They need a place to keep their personal items. They need money of their own to spend without having to account for it.

Services that enable elderly people to maintain their own homes are available in some communities. These services make it possible for many elderly people to remain independent and to still make their own decisions.

LESSON 3 REVIEW

Reviewing Facts and Vocabulary

1. Define and describe the three measures of age.
2. Give examples of six physical changes that people experience as they age.

Thinking Critically

3. **Analysis.** Analyze how a person's age might measure differently based on chronological, biological, and social age scales.

4. **Synthesis.** Develop an activity program for the elderly. Discuss your reasons for each aspect of the program.

Applying Health Knowledge

5. Visit a senior citizen center and write a report on positive aspects of your visit.

DEATH—PART OF THE LIFE CYCLE

Facing death, whether it be one's own or that of a loved one, is always difficult. People often avoid talking or even thinking about the subject of dying because of the emotions it brings up. A primary response to the prospect of dying is fear. It is quite natural to fear the unknown, and, despite the greater strides in our understanding of the process of dying, death is a subject on which no one can speak from firsthand experience. However, understanding and accepting one's feelings about death are important parts of mental health.

Clinical Death and Brain Death

Death is defined in many ways. **Clinical death** occurs when a person's body systems stop working. Sometimes clinical death can be reversed, life can be restored, and the person can make a full recovery. For example, a person could be a victim of drowning and be revived through cardiopulmonary resuscitation (CPR), a procedure to restore normal breathing and force the heart to pump blood after a cardiac arrest. If resuscitation is not successful, the brain cells do not receive the oxygen they need. Brain death can occur. **Brain death** is the loss of function of the entire brain, including the brain stem. When that happens, the person cannot be revived.

Stages in Brain Death

Among the first brain cells to die are those in the cerebral cortex. This area of the brain controls sensation and voluntary action, stores memory, and directs complex thought and decision-making processes. The victim may continue to live, but without any of these functions.

If the brain continues to be cut off from oxygen, cells in the midbrain die. This part of the brain controls emotions, alertness, and consciousness. The victim lapses into a coma, although heart function and breathing may continue.

If lack of oxygen continues, the brain stem dies. It is this area of the lower brain that stimulates the action of the heart and lungs.

Understanding and Accepting Death

Although it is often said with humor that "no one gets through this life alive," very few people know how to deal realistically with this fact. Many people do not experience the death of a loved one until late in life. Even though a large proportion of the population used to die before age 40, many more now live past age 70.

As death becomes a more foreign or distant experience, there is less opportunity for passing along lessons of how to cope with it, either to the person who is dying or to the family and friends who live afterward.

LESSON 4 FOCUS

TERMS TO USE
- Clinical death
- Brain death
- Thanatology

CONCEPTS TO LEARN
- Death is part of our life cycle.
- There are five stages in accepting death.
- Stages of grief are similar to the stages of accepting death.

ATTITUDES AND BEHAVIORS TO EVALUATE
- Self-Inventory, page 192.
- Building Decision-Making Skills, page 193.

At the same time, an increasing proportion of deaths occur as a result of illness such as cancer or AIDS, in which the process of dying is prolonged and emotionally painful.

Several factors influence one's understanding of and attitude toward death, including personal experience, spiritual beliefs, family attitudes and values, and one's age. Children's understanding of death increases in developmental stages. Infants up to two years have no real concept of death other than the fact that someone may be present at one moment and gone the next.

From ages 2 to 5 years, children recognize death but do not understand that it is permanent. Children may see death as being like sleep. Many children at this age have a great deal of faith in their own ability to make things happen simply by wishing.

From ages 5 to about 9, children may see death as a personification, that is, in the form of a real or imaginary person, such as an elderly man, a fairy princess, an angel, or a skeleton. They may begin to see death as being permanent, but cannot see it as something that could happen to them.

By about age 10, children may see death as final and inevitable. They are ready to deal with the reality of death, but have difficulty accepting that it can happen anytime to anyone. Such an understanding develops as children enter adolescence.

Each of these stages is general and will vary from person to person. Each stage depends on what other people have told the individuals about death and what experiences they have had with it.

Stages in Accepting Death

In recent years studies by scientists in the field of **thanatology,** from the Greek word, *thanatos,* meaning "death," have led to an understanding of what dying people go through. Their studies can greatly help the dying and their loved ones deal effectively with the situation. These researchers have learned that dying, like living, is a process. While there are different styles of dying, there are common elements and problems that all people experience as they prepare for death.

A pioneer in understanding the psychology of dying is Elisabeth Kübler-Ross, a psychiatrist, who identified five emotional stages that dying people typically pass through. For several decades she has worked with hundreds of dying patients and their families to better understand what a person goes through in coming to grips with his or her own death.

KEEPING FIT

Dealing with Grief

Losing someone that you love can be devastating. Watching someone you are close to grieve can also be very difficult.

Keep in mind the following tips:
- There is no one way to grieve. Each person has his or her own individual style and timetable for recovering from the loss of a loved one.
- Tears, anger, depression, guilt, fear, or having physical symptoms or anxiety attacks are all normal reactions to grief.
- The grieving process cannot be rushed. It generally takes years, not months.
- Talking about the person who has died rather than avoiding the subject helps everyone cope with the death.

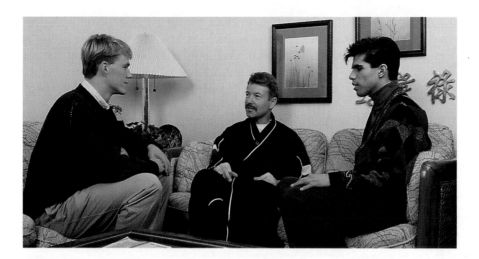

These five stages in the acceptance of death are similar to those we all experience when faced with any significant loss. However, each person's reactions are individual and will vary in degree. The stages are simply a general guideline for understanding and accepting the process of dying and death.

Stage 1: Denial. Denial is a person's initial reaction to any loss. It is the "No, not me; it can't be" stage when the patient cannot accept the fact of his or her fatal illness. This stage is an attempt to avoid reality by saying or thinking, "It is all a bad dream and will go away." During this time people often have a feeling of isolation or helplessness.

Stage 2: Anger. A person moves from denial to the second stage, anger, which is the "Why me?" stage. Anger is a natural reaction, an outlet for resentment at being a victim. Since customs often stand in the way of people's being able to vent their anger, it is often expressed in other ways. There may be an envy of others who still have life ahead of them. The patient may become hard to handle, critical, demanding, or unco-operative. Family members and friends may see this as an expression of ingratitude and respond by making their visits shorter and less frequent. As a result, the patient may possibly feel even more isolated and rejected and may become even more unpleasant to relatives, friends, and medical practitioners.

Stage 3: Bargaining. As the anger subsides and the patient begins to accept the reality of the situation, a stage of bargaining frequently follows. The dying person often tries to bargain for more time with good behavior. This stage may include attempts to postpone the end by praying, seeking better medical treatment, and promising to mend his or her ways.

Stage 4: Depression. This stage is a time of grieving for what the patient has already lost and for what will be lost. Commonly a period of silence and withdrawal, the dying person tries to become separate from all that he or she has known and loved. The patient worries about family and money. The feelings of numbness, isolation, anger, and rage felt previously are now replaced with a sense of great loss. Rather than attempting to comfort the dying person by saying that everything will be all right, loved ones should encourage him or her to grieve.

A child's first experience with death may be when a pet dies.

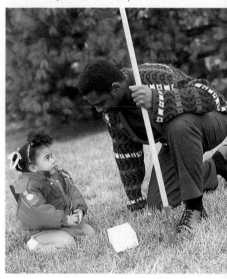

- Hospice care is family-centered health care for the terminally ill. Through team effort of loved ones, hospice nurses, home healthcare workers, and a participating physician, a dying patient can live out the rest of his or her life at home or in a home-like setting. Some hospitals even have hospice units.
- Three-quarters of women will become widows. The average length of their widow-hood will be 12 years.

Stage 5: Acceptance. The fifth stage of dying is that of acceptance. While the previous stage, depression, involves facing reality, it leaves a person feeling helpless. Although acceptance is not a happy or an unhappy stage, it is not a time of helplessness or resignation. Instead, it allows for action and for facing reality in a constructive way. Personal and financial matters often are taken care of during this stage.

Kübler-Ross identified another emotion that operates throughout all the stages just described. That emotion is hope. There usually is hope that there will be a cure or a remission and that death will not occur.

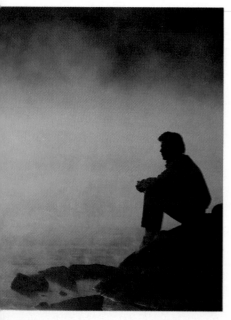

Dealing with the loss of a loved one takes time.

HEALTH UPDATE

LOOKING AT THE ISSUES

Medical Ethics

One well-known medical ethics case is that of Nancy Cruzan, who, as the result of an auto accident in Missouri, was in a coma from 1983 until 1990. In that year, the U.S. Supreme Court ruled that the family could remove her feeding and water tubes. They did so, and she died 11 days later.

In another case, 87-year-old Helga Wanglie lies in a coma in Minneapolis with no chance of recovery. The doctors want to remove life support, but her spouse refuses, saying he has no right to decide when and if she should die. Who should make life and death decisions?

Analyzing Different Viewpoints

ONE VIEW. Opinion surveys indicate that between 75 to 90 percent of the population would not want to be kept alive on life support systems if these systems could not return them to normal life.

A SECOND VIEW. Some people feel that no one has the right to terminate another's life, no matter how hopeless the medical condition of the patient.

A THIRD VIEW. Many people want to specify while they are healthy what their specific treatment requests would be should they be rendered helpless and unable to communicate their wishes. By signing a living will or a more detailed document that offers a range of choices in various medical situations, they make their wishes known.

A FOURTH VIEW. Other people argue that people without medical training cannot fully understand the choices of medical treatment and their implications. Therefore, they say, neither patients nor their families should make life and death decisions because they are unqualified to do so. Such decisions, they argue, should instead rest with medical professionals.

Exploring Your Views

1. Do you think that life support equipment should be removed in the event of irreversible brain damage or permanent coma? Why or why not?
2. Should a doctor be allowed to bring about death if the person is suffering in pain from an incurable illness?
3. Should a doctor provide the means by which an individual can take his or her own life?

Grief Experienced by Others

The family and friends of the dying person also must cope with death. Grief and mourning can develop through a series of stages much like Kübler-Ross's stages of dying. According to Kübler-Ross, survivors of a person who has died go through a stage of denial or disbelief, then a stage of anger. This anger may be directed toward the dying person or toward friends or others in the family. If there is forewarning of the death, the grieving person may bargain to prolong the dying person's life. As the grieving person realizes the futility of this, depression sets in. Later the survivors pass to a stage of acceptance as they understand that the death of the person is a reality.

When the stage of acceptance has been reached by those who are dying and by their loved ones, the process of grieving is usually shorter and less painful. Accepting the impending death of a loved one does not mean you do not care. Instead it means you care enough to make the end as pleasant as possible for all concerned, especially the person who is dying.

Experiencing grief may not be as distinct as previously defined. J. W. Worden has identified tasks of grief, in which a person can move back and forth through tasks and experience positive and negative emotions at the same time. These tasks also can overlap. The tasks include accepting the reality of the loss, experiencing the pain of the loss, adjusting to an environment in which the deceased is missing, and withdrawing emotional energy and reinvesting it in another relationship.

The death of someone you love is one of life's most shocking, and even shattering, experiences. Encouragement and comfort from others is needed to help survivors pass through their grief and mourning. In the event of sudden death, there has been little or no time for preparation. Thus, grief tends to last much longer. The real impact of the death may not surface until months later.

In order to regain physical, mental, and emotional health, the survivors need to be able to talk about what has happened and to express their feelings. Through such conversations, people can come to accept the death of their loved one and continue with their lives.

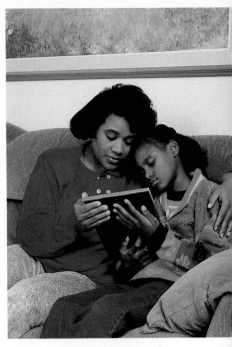

Grief is a part of life that will pass as people come to accept the death of a loved one and realize that their own lives must go on.

LESSON 4 REVIEW

Reviewing Facts and Vocabulary

1. Define *clinical death* and *brain death;* explain the difference between the two.
2. Describe the stages in brain death.

Thinking Critically

3. **Analysis.** Write a short paper pointing out how people's perceptions of death may vary with their stage in life, life experiences, and family influences.

4. **Evaluation.** Who should make the decision whether one lives or dies? Explain your reasoning.

Applying Health Knowledge

5. Using community resources, complete a course in cardiopulmonary resuscitation.
6. Write a two-page paper comparing the customs and attitudes toward death of another culture with those of your society.

Self-Inventory

Are You Up-to-Date About the Elderly?

HOW DO YOU RATE?

Number a sheet of paper from 1 through 20. Read each item below and respond by writing *yes* or *no* for each item. Total the number of *yes* and *no* responses. Then proceed to the next section.

1. Do you think young people should have a general understanding of the emotional and physical changes of aging?

2. Do you feel that most people who live to their 70s, 80s, and 90s can still contribute to society?

3. Do you think that older people can learn new things?

4. Do you believe that older people can change or readjust their lives?

5. Can you name at least five older people whose personal qualities you admire and would like to share?

6. Do you agree to allow older people to work as long as they wish?

7. Do you believe that the elderly are vital human beings?

8. Do you spend time with an elderly relative, neighbor, or friend?

9. Do you have one or more friends who are elderly?

10. Do you enjoy talking with older people?

11. Would you be willing to accept an older relative living in your home?

12. Can you name one or more older adults who lead a physically active life?

13. Have you ever volunteered your services to the elderly?

14. Have you ever experienced the death of a close friend or relative who was elderly?

15. Have you ever visited a nursing home?

16. Do you enjoy television programs, short stories, and books written about or by elderly people?

17. Can you state the major purpose of the Gray Panthers organization?

18. Do you believe that older people should continue to exercise regularly in their later years?

19. Do you occasionally take time to listen closely to an elderly person's memories of earlier times?

20. Do you avoid listening to or telling hurtful jokes that stereotype the elderly?

HOW DID YOU SCORE?

Give yourself 1 point for every *yes* answer and 0 points for every *no* answer. Add the total and read below to see how you scored. Then proceed to the next section.

15 to 20:
Excellent. Your attitudes and behaviors related to the elderly are commendable and up-to-date.

10 to 14:
Good. Your attitudes and behaviors related to the elderly are positive, but limited in scope.

5 to 9:
Fair. You need to update your attitudes and behaviors and to increase your experiences related to the elderly.

Below 5:
Needs Improvement. You're missing out on some great experiences and good friends among the elderly.

WHAT ARE YOUR GOALS?

If you received a score of 10 to 20, complete the statements in Part A. If your score was 9 or less, complete Parts A and B.

Part A

1. I plan to learn more about aging and the elderly by ____.

2. My timetable for accomplishing this is ____.

3. I plan to share my information with others by ____.

Part B

4. The attitude or behavior toward the elderly I would most like to change is ____.

5. The steps involved in making this change are ____.

6. My timetable for accomplishing this is ____.

7. The people or groups I will ask for support and assistance are ____.

Building Decision-Making Skills

K rista has made a commitment to visit her grandparents in another city over the weekend. She has always been the "apple of their eye" and has enjoyed doing things with them throughout the years. This time they are house-bound, because her grandmother is recovering from surgery. They hope Krista's visit will cheer them up. Today the boy Krista has been dating for a few months asked her to take part in a series of fun activities his family is planning for the weekend. This is appealing, not only for the fun, but because she has been trying to get to know his parents. What should Krista do?

A. Explain the commitment to her boyfriend and his parents and tell him that she doesn't want to disappoint her grandparents.

B. Ask her parents to change plans and spend only part of the weekend at her grandparents so that she can spend at least part of it with her boyfriend.

C. Ask her parents to go without her and to tell her grandparents that she is with her boyfriend and his family.

D. Tell her grandparents the situation and let them decide what she should do.

WHAT DO YOU THINK?

1. **Situation.** What decision needs to be made?

2. **Situation.** Why does a decision need to be made?

3. **Situation.** How much time does Krista have to make this decision?

4. **Choices.** What other possible choices might Krista make?

5. **Consequences.** What are the costs and benefits of each choice?

6. **Consequences.** How might Krista feel about each choice?

7. **Consequences.** How might her boyfriend feel about each choice?

8. **Consequences.** How would her parents probably feel about each choice?

9. **Consequences.** How would her grandparents probably feel about each choice?

10. **Consequences.** How might Krista's health triangle be affected by this decision? Explain your answer.

11. **Decision.** What choice do you think is best for Krista? Explain your answer.

12. **Decision.** How might Krista carry out her decision?

13. **Evaluation.** Have you found yourself torn between doing something you really want to do and something you feel committed to doing? Describe the situation, how you handled it, and what you learned from it.

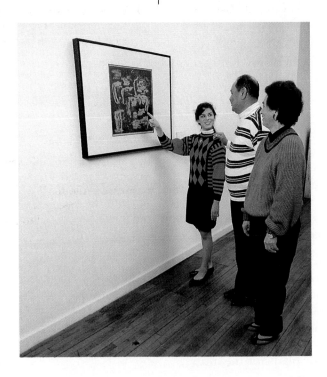

REVIEW

Using Health Terms

On a separate sheet of paper, write the term that best matches each definition given below.

LESSON 1
1. Preparation for a career.
2. Realization that one has developed in all ways to one's fullest.
3. Need to be accomplished in order for one to become a healthy, mature adult.

LESSON 2
4. The stage that may begin as early as age 17.
5. Changes.
6. A stage experienced by adults about 40 to 50 years old.
7. Being completely involved with one's own wants or needs.
8. A change caused by children leaving home and entering adulthood.

LESSON 3
9. People who study aging.
10. The number of years one has lived.
11. Acceptable behaviors of a certain age group.

LESSON 4
12. Type of death that occurs when one's heart stops beating.

Building Academic Skills

LESSON 1
13. **Writing.** Write several paragraphs describing skills you have developed through the years that have depended on your physical maturation.

LESSON 2
14. **Writing.** As you approach young adulthood, you are probably making plans and setting goals for your future. Write a letter to yourself that you will read when you turn 40. Include your thoughts about aging and your plans for the future.

Recalling the Facts

LESSON 1
15. Explain why developmental tasks need to occur.
16. What three factors influence the completion of developmental tasks?
17. Before a young person leaves home, on what is his or her identity usually based?
18. Life is like a journey beginning with what and ending with what?
19. In what ways might adults show an interest in their community?

LESSON 2
20. What is the approximate age range of young adulthood?
21. What stage of development did Erikson identify as occurring in young adulthood? Describe this stage.
22. What are two changes that may occur in middle adulthood?
23. Name at least two circumstances that might cause a person in middle adulthood to begin to feel that life is coming to an end.
24. What are the three stages of life that follow childhood and adolescence?

LESSON 3
25. What type of aging is determined by the functioning of body parts?
26. List at least three factors that affect a person's ability to adjust to aging.
27. Who are gerontologists?
28. What is social age?
29. How might one's biological aging process be slowed down?

LESSON 4
30. List in order and explain the five stages of dying as identified by Elisabeth Kübler-Ross.
31. How do the stages of dying differ for the person dying and his or her loved ones?
32. What is needed for survivors to be able to work through their grief and mourning?

REVIEW

Thinking Critically

LESSON 1

33. **Synthesis.** Self-esteem increases as one experiences success. What are some successes you have had in your life?

LESSON 2

34. **Analysis.** Compare concerns one might have in young adulthood to concerns in middle adulthood.

35. **Analysis.** What are some advantages of deciding not to marry in young adulthood? What are some disadvantages?

36. **Evaluation.** What advice would you give to someone who is suffering from the empty-nest syndrome? What advice would you give someone experiencing the cluttered-nest syndrome?

LESSON 3

37. **Analysis.** Review some of the ways your body changes as you approach old age. What could you be doing now to help slow down your body's aging process?

38. **Synthesis.** What needs do all age groups share?

LESSON 4

39. **Analysis.** Think about how you and your family deal with the issue of dying. What factors affect the way you view death in your family?

40. **Evaluation.** Some people feel that a person's bodily functions should not be sustained by machines once the brain is dead. What is your opinion of this?

Making the Connection

LESSON 3

41. **Science.** Volunteer to help conduct exercise classes at a retirement or nursing facility. Differentiate between a program designed to meet the physical health needs of the elderly and one designed to meet the physical health needs of a teenager.

Applying Health Knowledge

LESSON 1

42. Being unable to successfully complete developmental tasks can lead to difficulty in later stages in life. Discuss what might get in the way of an adolescent being able to complete developmental tasks.

LESSON 2

43. You notice that your dad has started to dress like you and your friends. How do you feel about this? What do you think is causing this behavior? What would you do about it?

LESSON 3

44. Your grandmother is going to live with you. What do you think you could do to make your grandmother comfortable?

45. Many older people are placed in nursing homes when they need a great deal of care. Visit a nursing home and describe what you saw. Do you feel this is a place you would someday want to call home? Why or why not?

LESSON 4

46. Imagine that a classmate has just been killed in a car crash. What would you say to that person's parents and siblings? In what way could you help them cope with their grief?

Beyond the Classroom

LESSON 2

47. **Parental Involvement.** Interview your parents, asking questions about the dreams, hopes, plans, and goals your parents set for themselves when they were your age. Find out why they made the plans they did and how they feel about what they have actually accomplished.

48. **Further Study.** Research Erik Erikson's stages of development. Give examples of feelings one might have at each stage.

CHAPTER

11

INTEGUMENTARY, SKELETAL, AND MUSCULAR SYSTEMS

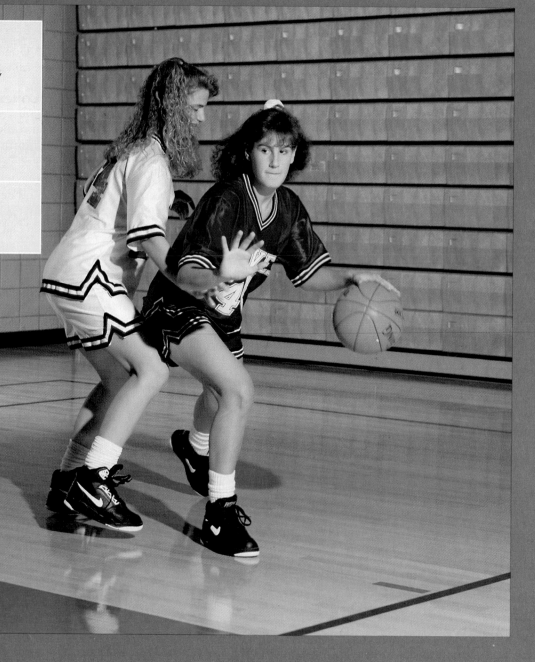

THE INTEGUMENTARY SYSTEM

Your **integumentary system** includes your skin, hair, nails, and sweat glands. Your skin is the primary organ of your integumentary system. Besides being the largest organ of the body, it probably has the greatest number of functions. Your skin also has a great effect on your overall appearance because so much of it is visible.

Functions of Your Skin

Your skin's main function is to serve as a watertight covering. It helps protect internal tissues and organs and is the body's first line of defense against invading pathogens. It provides protection against the ultraviolet rays of the sun.

Another important function of the skin is the regulation of body temperature. Your skin has an enormous supply of tiny blood vessels just beneath the surface. When your internal temperature rises, circulation to these blood vessels increases. As internal heat is circulated through these surface vessels it is lost by the process of radiation. Increased internal heat causes the sweat glands in the skin to become more active, releasing perspiration through pores onto your skin. As perspiration evaporates, your skin cools. If the internal temperature of the body drops, circulation to the blood vessels in the skin slows down, sweating stops, and body heat is conserved.

The skin is also a major sense organ, serving as a means of communication with your outside environment. Nerve endings in your skin are responsive to pain, pressure, changes in temperature, and texture.

Structure of the Skin

Your skin has two main layers. The outside layer is the epidermis; the inner layer is the dermis. Below the dermis is tissue called the hypodermis. The hypodermis is not part of your skin, but it attaches your skin to bone and muscle.

Epidermis

The **epidermis** is the outer, thinner layer of skin and is made up of both dead and living cells. Most cells of the epidermis contain a protein called keratin. Keratin helps waterproof and protect the cells.

There are many levels of cells in the epidermis. Dead cells make up the outermost level. These cells slough off or shed when clothing rubs your skin or when you wash. Through this shedding, your outer skin is replaced about once a month. New cells rise to the surface to replace the old ones.

LESSON 1 FOCUS

TERMS TO USE
- Integumentary system
- Epidermis (ep•uh•DUR•mihs)
- Dermis (DUR•mihs)
- Sebaceous (sih•BAY•shuhs) glands
- Sweat glands
- Follicle
- Athlete's foot

CONCEPTS TO LEARN
- Every living organism is protected from the environment by a protective covering.
- The skin has functions that are important to your health.
- Problems of the skin require varying degrees of attention.
- Healthy skin can be promoted by following healthy habits.

ATTITUDES AND BEHAVIORS TO EVALUATE
- Self-Inventory, page 216.
- Building Decision-Making Skills, page 217.

Skin color in humans is determined largely by the amount of the pigment melanin in the skin. The melanin in dark skin absorbs most of the sun's ultraviolet rays in tropical areas where the sun's rays are intense. However, enough of the rays still get through so the body can produce vitamin D. Vitamin D is necessary for proper bone growth and to prevent rickets. In areas with less intense sun rays, such as in northern latitudes, light skin allows sufficient amounts of ultraviolet rays into the body so it can produce vitamin D. The melanin in dark skin in northern latitudes may absorb too much of the ultraviolet rays, and the body is not able to produce vitamin D. People with dark skin who live in northern areas need to drink vitamin D-enriched milk or eat foods rich in vitamin D to avoid rickets.

The skin is a waterproof shield, a regulator of body temperature, and a barrier to pathogens.

The new cells are produced in the inner level of the epidermis. It is here that cells containing melanin are found. Melanin gives the skin its color—the more melanin, the darker the skin—and helps protect it from the sun's radiation. The production of melanin is increased when you are out in the sun, causing the skin to tan. Freckles are small spots of melanin.

The epidermis on your fingers, palms of your hands, toes, and soles of your feet contain ridges that form a unique pattern. Your footprint may be on your birth certificate. Footprints are used for identification of newborn babies. Your unique fingerprint identifies you. No two people, not even identical twins, have the same print. If you cut or injure your toes or fingers, the skin will heal, forming the same print.

Nails. Your fingernails and toenails are dead cells that grow out of the epidermis. Living cells extend from the root of the nail, below the epidermis, to just above the base of the nail. As living cells die and are replaced, they are pushed up forming the rest of the nail. The nail is surrounded by the cuticle, the nonliving epidermis surrounding the edges of your fingernails and toenails. If you have ever lost a nail, you probably grew another one. New nails will grow as long as the root is still alive.

Dermis

The **dermis** is the inner, thicker layer of skin. Differences in total skin thickness are due to the thickness of the dermis. For example, skin on your back has more dermis than skin on the back of your hand.

The dermis has protein fibers that give the skin its elasticity, or spongy, flexible quality. As a person ages, the skin loses some of its elasticity, resulting in wrinkles. Nerve endings, glands, and hair follicles extend into the dermis.

Glands. There are two main kinds of glands in the skin, sebaceous glands and sweat glands. **Sebaceous glands** connect to hair follicles and produce an oily secretion called sebum. Sebum oils the skin and

Layers of Skin

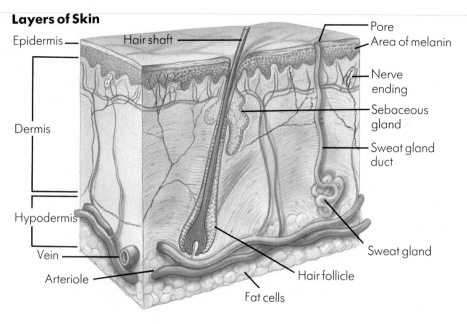

Epidermis, Hair shaft, Pore, Area of melanin, Nerve ending, Sebaceous gland, Sweat gland duct, Dermis, Hypodermis, Vein, Arteriole, Fat cells, Hair follicle, Sweat gland

hair, preventing drying and helping protect against some pathogens. Overactive oil glands, however, can result in oily skin and hair. Oil glands prevent the skin from absorbing too much water.

Sweat glands secrete perspiration through ducts to pores on the surface of your skin. Sweat glands are found in most areas of your body, but they are most numerous in the soles of your feet and the palms of your hands. When your body gets hot, pores in your skin open up and perspiration is released. Perspiration is a mixture of water and waste products. Some sweat glands are affected by emotional stress, such as fear, anxiety, or pain. At such times, they produce more perspiration than usual.

Many people think perspiration causes body odor. Perspiration itself does not cause an odor. Bacteria acting on perspiration cause an odor. Sweat glands are numerous under the arms, which is the reason body odor tends to be a problem in that area.

Hair. Humans have hair present on almost all skin surfaces of their bodies. You have between 100,000 and 200,000 hairs on your head! The roots of hairs are made up of living cells and grow out of the dermis. A hair root grows out of a **follicle,** which is a small pocket that holds the root in the dermis.

Through the follicle the root is supplied with blood and nerve tissue. As new hair cells are made, old hair cells are pushed up and out of the hair follicle and die. The hair visible on your head is made up of such dead cells.

Hair normally grows at a rate of about 6 inches (15 cm) per year. Each hair on your head grows for about 4 years, rests a few months, and then falls out. You lose between 25 and 100 hairs a day.

Hypodermis

The hypodermis attaches your skin to bone and muscle. Blood vessels and nerves that supply your skin pass through the hypodermis. This layer is made up of fatty tissue and serves as the body's natural insulation against heat and cold. It also acts as an inner cushion to protect internal organs from injuries.

Problems of the Integumentary System

Many problems of the integumentary system are not life-threatening. Nevertheless, they can affect how a person looks and how a person feels about him- or herself. Some of these problems are temporary. Following healthy habits may help eliminate some of these problems.

Skin Problems

Acne, which is a clogging of the pores of the skin, is the most common skin problem during adolescence.

During adolescence the increase in hormone production causes oil glands to enlarge and produce more sebum. Excess sebum makes the skin oily, providing an ideal place for bacteria to grow. Since there are more oil glands in the area of the face than in other parts of the body, acne occurs there.

It takes many years and extra care to grow and maintain long hair.

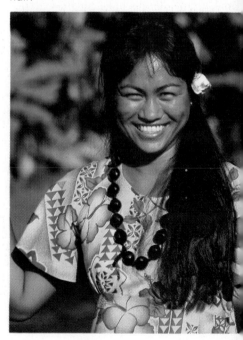

FINDING HELP

Commercial suntanning parlors began to appear in the U.S. in 1978, and the tanning business has been booming ever since. If you or your friends are tempted to try out a tanning business, do your skin a favor. Take the medical experts' advice and stay away from artificial—as well as the sun's—tanning rays.

For more information about healthy skin, write to the Skin Cancer Foundation 245 Fifth Avenue Suite 2402 New York, NY 10016

Ringworm sores usually have a circular or ringlike appearance.

The oil secreted by the oil glands moves out through pores in the skin. Excess sebum can clog these pores and cause the following conditions:

- A whitehead results when sebum gets trapped in a pore and plugs it.
- A blackhead develops if this plug of sebum becomes exposed to air and dead skin and sebum become dark.
- A pimple is formed if bacteria get into the clogged pore and infect it. The infected pore fills with pus.

Picking or squeezing pimples can spread the infection, possibly leaving the skin scarred. There is no cure for acne at this time. Keeping the skin clean is most important. Washing with warm water will help rid excess oils from the skin.

Another skin problem can be caused by ringworm. Ringworm is a common fungal infection that affects different parts of the body. It gets its name from the fact that it appears as a whitish ring. The ringworm fungus causes **athlete's foot,** which is an infection of the skin between the toes. The redness and itching can be treated with talcum or antifungal powders. Athlete's foot is very contagious. That is the reason it is important to wear a foot covering in locker rooms and showers.

Jock itch is another common skin infection caused by the ringworm fungus. Jock itch mainly occurs in the groin area.

Washing, drying carefully, and dusting with talcum or an antifungal powder will usually clear up the condition. Avoid using ointments, because they can make the condition worse by holding in moisture. To help relieve the discomfort of jock itch, wear loose cotton clothing to allow proper ventilation. Since jock itch can be spread easily, always use your own soap and towels.

Boils are skin infections that result in swelling, redness, and the formation of pus. They are caused by bacteria and can destroy skin tissue. Boils can be serious infections and should be treated by a doctor. Like acne, boils should not be squeezed. They are infections, which means that the bacteria that cause them can spread and form other boils on the body. Keeping skin clean helps prevent boils.

Warts are small growths caused by viruses. Warts appear as raised growths on the outer layer of the skin. Most warts are painless and harmless, but the virus that causes them can spread and form more warts. If that happens, or if there is any change in the size or color of a wart, see your doctor immediately. Color change may indicate a more serious problem.

Moles are small, round, slightly thick places on the skin. They may be black or brown and are present from birth. Moles are not usually dangerous, but if they start to change color, a doctor should be consulted immediately.

Psoriasis is an ailment in which red patches appear on the skin, followed by the skin's turning white and flaking off. Psoriasis should be treated by a doctor and is usually lessened with the use of medicinal creams. The cause is not known.

Vitiligo is probably caused by an absence of melanin in certain patches of skin. This skin turns whitish to pinkish. There is no cure for vitiligo, but it appears to be harmless. The affected area should be kept away from direct sunlight.

Blisters are raised areas that are filled with a watery liquid. They are usually the result of skin being rubbed, injured, or burned. Blisters can form anywhere on the body. A blister should be protected so that it will not break. A broken blister can become infected.

A callus is a hard, thickened layer of skin that forms as a result of continued friction or rubbing. Calluses are common on the soles of the feet. Many musicians have calluses on their fingers from playing string instruments. Calluses are annoying, but not harmful. They can be reduced by using a pumice stone, which is a porous stone.

Friction can also form a corn. A corn usually has a hard inner core that can be painful. Corns usually appear on or between toes. Corns may be softened by soaking them in water. Wearing shoes that fit properly is the main way to prevent calluses and corns on the feet.

Hair Problems

Dandruff is one of the most common hair and scalp problems. Dandruff is caused by the flaking of the outer layer of dead skin cells covering the skull. It is noticeable on the head because the flakes of skin can cling to the hair. Regular, thorough washing of hair can control ordinary dandruff. However, special shampoos also are available. Sometimes what appears to be dandruff is actually a skin infection. If itching and scaling persist, a health professional should be consulted.

Head lice are insects that attach themselves to human hair and skin and feed off blood. Lice make the scalp itchy and uncomfortable and can cause infection. Lice can usually be killed by medicinal shampoos.

Head lice can spread from one person to another. Therefore, it is wise not to use other people's combs, brushes, towels, or hats.

Nail Problems

Hangnails are bits of loose cuticle around the base or side of the fingernail. If hangnails are not removed, they can become infected. Do not pull or bite a hangnail. Cut off the major part and cover with a bandage. Hangnails can be prevented by pushing the cuticle back gently each time you wash your hands.

An ingrown toenail results when the nail pushes into the skin and cuts it. Trimming your toenails carefully will prevent this condition.

Care for the Skin, Hair, and Nails

Caring for your skin, hair, and nails is a lifelong process. You can promote your health by following healthy grooming habits.

Warts are common viral infections. Treatment depends on the area of the body where they appear.

K E E P I N G F I T

Avoiding Toenail Torment

An ingrown toenail occurs when your toenail—often the one on your big toe—begins to rub on and cut into the surrounding skin. The result can be very painful. Sometimes, the irritated or swollen area can even become infected. To prevent ingrown toenails:
- Don't wear shoes that are too tight.
- Try not to "put the brakes on" too much when you play sports by screeching to a halt and shoving your toes against the tips of your shoes.
- Keep your toenails clipped, but don't clip them too short.
- Keep them cut straight across rather than rounded.

Healthy Skin

CONFLICT RESOLUTION

Andrew has tried repeatedly to get his parents' permission to go to a tanning salon. He's not convinced by their claim that the radiation is harmful. Andrew has heard that the new tanning beds mostly use UV-A radiation, which causes the skin to burn more slowly than UV-B rays.

As Andrew's friend, what comments would you make to him about this topic?

Every morning and evening wash your face with soap and water. If your face is very oily, wash it once more during the day. Pat your skin dry with a clean towel. If you use creams and cosmetics, select them carefully and avoid greasy preparations. Eat a well-balanced diet. Vitamin A helps promote healthy skin. Milk, egg yolks, liver, green and yellow vegetables, and yellow fruits are good sources of vitamin A. Get plenty of rest and exercise. Try to keep your hands away from your face.

Thorough washing with soap and water on a daily basis slows bacterial growth and helps control body odor. Deodorants and antiperspirants can help mask body odors or reduce the amount of perspiration.

Skin and the Sun.   Understanding the sun's effect on the skin and knowing some protective steps to take can help you better care for your skin. The sun does not have the same effect on everyone. Some people tan more easily than others. Some people with fair skin may never tan; they may just burn.

Ultraviolet rays are light rays that come from the sun. Two types of ultraviolet rays are important in considering the sun's effects on the human body. The shorter rays, most intense in the middle of the day, are the main cause of sunburn. The longer rays, in the morning and late afternoon, are less strong in terms of sunburn.

Do not be fooled on a hazy or cloudy day. Up to 80 percent of ultraviolet rays can penetrate haze, light clouds, or fog. Ultraviolet rays can also be reflected upward from the ground, sand, and water. Snow is an excellent reflector, sending back more than 85 percent of the rays.

Do not judge a sunburn by how red you look while you are still out in the sun. It takes about 2 to 8 hours after exposure for a sunburn to show. The pain from the burn is greatest about 6 to 48 hours after exposure.

In addition to causing sunburn, exposure to the sun's ultraviolet rays can permanently destroy the elastic fibers that keep the skin tight. The sun causes the skin to age prematurely, that is, before its time. The layers of skin cells also thicken with repeated sun exposure. This gives the skin a hard, leathery texture.

KEEPING FIT

Sunscreens

Follow these guidelines in regard to sunscreens.
- Wear a sunscreen that is water-resistant and waterproof.
- Apply liberally 15 to 30 minutes before you go out into the sun.
- Reapply at least every 2 hours.

- Don't forget places like ear lobes, nose, and balding spots.
- Wear a sunscreen with an SPF of 15 or higher. *SPF* stands for *sun protection factor*. Sunscreens are rated by number from SPF 2 to SPF 50. The

numbers indicate the sunscreen's ability to screen out the sun's harmful ultraviolet rays, which are known to cause skin cancer.
- Stay out of the sun between 10 A.M. and 3 P.M. if possible.

Ultraviolet radiation also damages the deoxyribonucleic acid (DNA), the genetic material in skin cells. Accumulated DNA damage can result in the formation of cancerous cells. Excessive sun exposure is the primary cause of certain types of skin cancer. Therefore, you should protect your skin. Use a sun block if you are going to be in the sun for a prolonged period of time. Sun blocks stop the sun's rays by reflecting them.

The effects of the sun on your skin may not show up for years and cannot be stopped by any cosmetic ointments. These effects are cumulative, or increasing, and the damage is irreversible. The healthiest behavior is prevention. Avoid overexposure to the sun's ultraviolet rays.

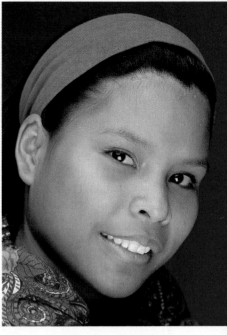

Taking care of your skin takes time and effort but it will contribute to your overall appearance.

Healthy Hair

Your hair has a great impact on your appearance. Wearing a style that fits your features and type of hair and taking proper care of your hair are important aspects of total health.

Brushing your hair helps keep dirt from building up and helps evenly distribute the natural hair oils. These oils keep the hair soft and give it its shine. Overbrushing can cause hair to pull out or break off. A good brushing once a day is enough. Massaging the scalp along with brushing helps increase circulation in the scalp.

Washing your hair regularly is necessary for healthy hair. If possible, let your hair dry naturally. Try to avoid using blow dryers because the heat can damage your hair. Heat from electric curlers or curling irons also dries out hair, causing the ends to break or split.

Healthy Nails

Good nail care includes keeping nails clean and evenly trimmed. Keep cuticles pushed back and clip hangnails with a nail clipper. You should cut toenails straight across, leaving the nail just at or slightly above skin level. If you cut the nails too low, you increase your risk of skin infection and ingrown nails.

Fingernails should be slightly rounded. Use a nail file or emery board to shape the nails. Always file in the same direction, rather than using a sawing motion. Clean, trimmed nails add to your overall appearance.

LESSON 1 REVIEW

Reviewing Facts and Vocabulary

1. What are the functions of the skin?
2. Explain the unique characteristics of the epidermis.
3. What effect does the sun have on skin?

Thinking Critically

4. **Analysis.** Analyze the following statement: "I look healthier with a good tan."

Applying Health Knowledge

5. Think of the healthy grooming habits you have established. Which are the most important to you? What are your least favorite grooming activities? What changes might you make in your routine to make these activities less bothersome?
6. Design a poster about the dangers of the sun's ultraviolet rays and their effects on the human body.

LESSON 2

THE SKELETAL SYSTEM

You might think of the skeletal system as the girders and cross-beams that make up the framework of a building. The muscular system is like the bricks and mortar that cover the framework.

TERMS TO USE

- Axial (AK•see•ul) skeleton
- Appendicular (ap•en•DICK•u•lar) skeleton
- Cartilage
- Ossification (os•seh•fuh•KAY•shun)
- Ligaments
- Tendons

CONCEPTS TO LEARN

- Bones have four main functions.
- The skeleton gives stability to the body.
- A healthy diet is essential to maintaining healthy bones.

ATTITUDES AND BEHAVIORS TO EVALUATE

- Self-Inventory, page 216.
- Building Decision-Making Skills, page 217.

Functions of Your Skeletal System

Unlike a building, which cannot move, your skeletal and muscular systems work together to allow you to walk, run, jump, bend, lift, and carry. The skeletal system not only allows movement, it also provides a supporting framework for your body. This system protects delicate, internal organs. Bones are the principal storage place for essential body minerals, such as calcium and phosphorus. Calcium is one of the minerals that promotes strong bones. Another important function is the production of red and white blood cells in the red marrow of bones.

Structure of the Skeletal System

Your skeletal system is divided into two main parts. The **axial skeleton** includes the bones of the skull, the sternum (breastbone), the ribs, and the vertebrae (spine).

The bones of the skull protect the brain and form the shape of the face. The 12 pairs of ribs attach to the sternum in your chest area and to vertebrae in your back. These bones protect your lungs and heart. The 33 small bones that make up your spine are called vertebrae. Vertebrae protect your spinal cord.

The **appendicular skeleton** includes the 126 bones of the shoulders, arms, hands, hips, legs, and feet. The appendicular skeleton helps you perform a wide range of movement. Refer to the illustration on page 205 to identify the two main divisions of the skeleton.

Your body's framework is made up of both bone and **cartilage,** a strong, flexible material that provides a smooth surface that makes movement at a joint smooth. Cartilage supports the nose and ears, connects the ribs to the sternum, and acts as a cushion between adjoining vertebrae.

A baby's skeleton is mostly cartilage. As the body grows, cartilage cells are replaced by bone cells and minerals through a process called **ossification.**

The periosteum is a tough membrane that adheres tightly to the outer surface of bone. This living membrane is richly supplied with blood vessels that branch into the bone at various points. The periosteum is vital in nourishing the bones and in producing bone cells. It contains bone-forming cells called osteoblasts, which are important in bone growth and repair.

Adults have about 206 bones in their skeletal system. Bones range in size from the smallest bone, the stapes in the middle ear, which is about

0.1 inch (3 mm) long, to the longest bone in the body, the femur, or thighbone, which is usually about 27 percent of a person's total height.

Types of Bones

Bones are grouped according to their shapes. There are four basic types in the human body.

■ Long bones, like the femur, are found in the arms and legs. The shafts of a long bone are called the diaphyses. The ends of long bones are called epiphyses. Long bones are very strong. The inner cavity of long bones contains yellow marrow, which is a fatty tissue. The epiphyses of long bones form joints with other bones. Epiphyses are composed mainly of spongy bone tissue. The enlarged ends give stability to joints. Muscles attach to the epiphyses. The inner parts of the epiphy-

The axial skeleton is shown here in yellow. The appendicular skeleton is shown in green.

The Two Divisions of the Skeletal System

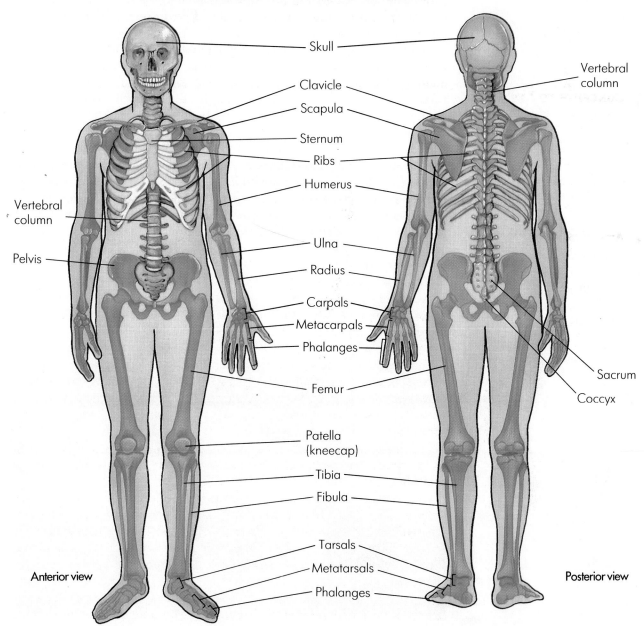

Skull

Vertebral column

Clavicle

Scapula

Sternum

Ribs

Humerus

Vertebral column

Ulna

Pelvis

Radius

Carpals

Metacarpals

Phalanges

Sacrum

Coccyx

Femur

Patella (kneecap)

Tibia

Fibula

Anterior view

Tarsals

Metatarsals

Phalanges

Posterior view

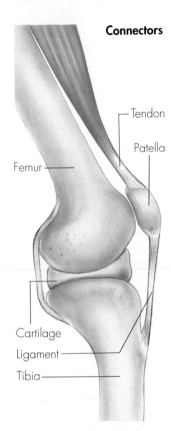

Connectors

Femur

Tendon

Patella

Cartilage

Ligament

Tibia

Ligaments, tendons, and cartilage are types of connective tissue. Ligaments connect bones to bones. Tendons connect muscles to bones.

ses contain red marrow. Red marrow produces red blood cells and most of the white blood cells in the blood.

■ Short bones, like those in the wrists and ankles, are as broad as they are long. Over half of all the short bones in the body are in the hands and feet.

■ Flat bones, like the ribs and skull bones, have a thin, flat shape. These bones generally serve to protect vital body organs.

■ Irregular bones, like vertebrae, have a shape that does not fit with the other types of bones.

Joints

The point at which two bones meet is called a joint. Most joints allow movement of the body framework. Imagine that you did not have a joint at the point where your arm bones meet at your elbow. What kinds of activities would be restricted?

Bones in the skull form immovable joints. The joints that are formed by vertebrae are slightly movable. However, most of the joints in the body are freely movable.

Ball-and-socket joints, such as the shoulder joint, allow you the most range of movement. Hinge joints, such as the knee joint, allow movement back and forth in one plane. Pivot joints occur when one bone rotates around another, such as your head turning on your spine. In gliding joints, such as in the hand and foot, bones are able to slide over one another.

At joints where movement occurs, bones are bound together by ligaments and muscles. **Ligaments** are strong bands or cords of tissue that connect the bones to one another at a moveable joint. Ligaments hold the bones in place. **Tendons** are bands of fiber that connect muscles to bones. Drum your fingers on your desk. The movement you see in the back of your hand is from the action of tendons.

Problems of the Skeletal System

Skeletal system disorders and injuries to bones can be the result of many factors, including sports and recreational mishaps, viral infections, poor diet, and poor posture.

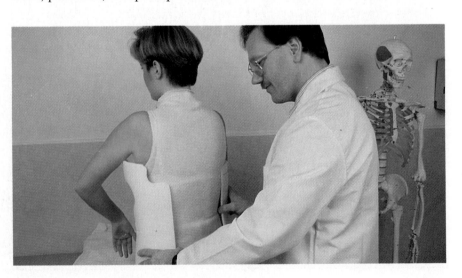

Body braces can be used to halt and correct a curvature of the spine.

Bone Fractures

Fractures are any type of break in a bone. Following are descriptions of some types of fractures.

- closed fracture—the broken bone does not protrude, or stick out, through the skin
- open fracture—the broken bone protrudes through the skin
- complete fracture—the bone is broken in two or more fragments
- incomplete fracture—the fracture is not completely across the bone
- hairline fracture—the fracture is incomplete, and the two parts of the bone do not separate

Scoliosis

Scoliosis is a lateral, or side-to-side, curvature of the spine. It usually develops during puberty. Most schools have scoliosis screening programs, usually conducted by the school nurse. Depending on the severity of the curvature, treatment may include exercise, a special brace, or surgery. If left untreated, a person may experience serious back problems in adulthood.

Osteoporosis

Osteoporosis is a condition that results from a loss of calcium in the bone. The bones become weakened and can break easily. In addition, the back may become hunched. Osteoporosis is most commonly found in older females. Exercise and a diet high in calcium can help prevent osteoporosis.

Osteomyelitis

Osteomyelitis is a term given to inflammation of the soft inner surface of the bones. Many times this inflammation is caused by bacteria. Antibiotics, such as penicillin, are used to treat the infected bones. Surgery is sometimes necessary to remove damaged bone tissue.

Injuries to Joints

Sprains are the most common injury to joints. A sprain occurs when tissue around a joint is twisted or receives too much pressure. The ligaments around the joint are stretched or torn, resulting in swelling and pain

KEEPING FIT

Too Much of a Good Thing

Practicing the same sport and the same motions within that sport every day for at least two hours can greatly increase your risk of injuries from overuse. The repeated motions that some sports require—such as throwing in baseball—can wear down both your ligaments and your tendons. This can cause tissues to tear and even cause bones to break. So don't overdo it.

around the joint. If blood vessels are injured, too, there may be discoloration of the skin. Sprains occur most often in the joints with a wide range of movement, like the wrist and ankle. Although sprains usually heal by themselves, it is a good idea to see a doctor.

A dislocation results when a bone slips from its normal position at a joint. A doctor must put the bone back in place and immobilize the joint so that the tissue can heal.

You have probably read of athletes who have torn a cartilage in the knee. A torn cartilage is a serious joint injury. It can result from a sharp blow or severe twisting of a joint. Doctors can now repair some cartilage tears with arthroscopic surgery.

A bunion is a painful swelling of the bursa in the first joint of the big toe. The cause of bunions is wearing tight or high-heeled shoes, which cram the toes and cause them to bend in an abnormal way. It is important to wear shoes that fit properly. Special exercises may also be recommended by a doctor. In severe cases, surgery may be required.

Bursitis is a painful condition that occurs when the bursa in a joint becomes inflamed. It is common in the shoulder and knee joints. Bursitis may result from an injury, or an infection or from overuse of the joint. Mild cases of bursitis are treated by resting the joint.

HEALTH UPDATE

LOOKING AT TECHNOLOGY

Arthroscopic Surgery

Until the early 1970s when the arthroscope was developed, knee surgery involved a large incision, lengthy hospitalization, and a long recovery time. Now advances in knee surgery are making prospects better for knee-injured athletes, particularly for those without major knee damage.

Arthroscopic surgery is the name of the procedure now often used to repair these injuries to the knee. The arthroscope, a tiny fiber-optic camera, allows the surgeon to look inside the knee and perform the needed procedure. *Arthro* means "joint" and *scope* means "to view," and the device does just that— allows the surgeon to view the damaged joint. The arthroscope actually has three parts: a fiber-optic light source, a tube, and magnifying lenses.

Before the procedure, the patient is given local or general anesthesia. Then a few small incisions, called portals, are made around the knee. A sterile saline solution is injected through one of these portals to expand the joint, while the surgeon inserts the arthroscope into the others to examine the knee completely. Looking through the eyepiece or at a TV monitor, the doctor has a clear view to most areas of the knee. Tiny instruments can be inserted through separate portals to perform the operation. A biopsy may be taken, tissues can be examined, and repair to or removal of damaged ligaments and cartilage can take place.

Arthroscopic surgery rarely takes more than an hour and recovery time is greatly reduced. Though rest is recommended after the procedure, many athletes who have the procedure are back on the playing field in no time at all.

DID YOU KNOW?

- The thigh bone is the longest bone in your body.
- The stapes bone, which is in your middle ear, is the smallest bone in your body.
- Bones are lightweight; they comprise about 14 percent of your total body weight.
- At birth, everyone has 350 bones. Many of these join, as you grow. By adulthood, you have 206 bones.

Arthritis is an inflammation of the joints. Its cause is not completely known, and it affects people of all ages. Arthritis can be very painful and can restrict movement.

Care of the Skeletal System

Like other cells of the body, bone cells get the nutrients and oxygen they need as blood circulates in bones. With proper health care, bones can be strong and healthy.

Essential Minerals for Bones

In order to grow, harden, and repair, bones must have an adequate supply of minerals, especially calcium and phosphorus. Bones store these two minerals. If you have enough calcium and phosphorus in your daily diet, your body does not use the deposits in bones.

However, if you have a mineral deficiency in your diet, your body takes away some of the mineral supply in the bones to provide minerals to the blood, muscles, and nerves. This can cause weakening of the skeleton and increases a person's chance of bone fractures.

Caring for your bones and joints means including in your diet foods that contain minerals and vitamins that promote bone growth. The mineral calcium is a building material for bones. Sources of calcium include dairy products and leafy vegetables. Phosphorus combined with calcium gives rigidity to bones. Sources of phosphorus include peas, beans, milk, liver, meat, cottage cheese, broccoli, and whole grains. Vitamins A and D work to utilize calcium and phosphorus in bone formation. Sources of vitamin A include milk and other dairy products, green vegetables, carrots, and animal liver. Sources of vitamin D include fish oils, cream, butter, egg yolks, milk, and liver. Vitamin D is produced in the skin with exposure to ultraviolet rays in sunlight.

Regular physical activity, especially weight-bearing exercises, increases bone mass. While exercising, make sure that you use proper equipment and wear shoes and clothing for the particular activity you choose. Doing so can help prevent injuries and protect the skeletal system.

FINDING HELP

Too many people think that because there is no cure for arthritis, nothing can be done to treat it. That is a false assumption. The Arthritis Foundation has many programs including some self-help courses and exercise classes. For free information on how to cope more effectively with arthritis, contact the Arthritis Foundation, P.O. Box 19000, Atlanta, Georgia 30326

LESSON 2 REVIEW

Reviewing Facts and Vocabulary

1. What are the two main divisions of the skeletal system?
2. What are three functions of bones?
3. Describe two injuries or diseases of the skeletal system.
4. Classify and give examples of four freely moveable joints.

Thinking Critically

5. **Analysis.** What might happen if a young person did not include enough minerals, especially calcium, in his or her diet?

Applying Health Knowledge

6. At the grocery store ask the butcher for soup bones. Try to get a long bone. Ask the butcher to saw it in half for you. Identify the periosteum, yellow marrow and epiphyses, spongy bone tissue, and red marrow.

THE MUSCULAR SYSTEM

LESSON 3 FOCUS

TERMS TO USE
- Smooth muscles
- Skeletal muscles
- Flexors
- Extensors
- Cardiac muscle

CONCEPTS TO LEARN
- Muscles are responsible for or involved in many body functions.
- Muscles are responsible for movement.
- Exercise is vital to the health of the muscular system.

ATTITUDES AND BEHAVIORS TO EVALUATE
- Self-Inventory, page 216.
- Building Decision-Making Skills, page 217.

Bones form the body's framework. Bones alone, however, cannot produce movement without the muscles that are attached to bones.

Functions of Your Muscular System

All body movements depend on characteristics of muscle tissue—the ability to contract, or shorten; the ability to extend, or stretch; and the ability to return to the original shape after contraction or extension. Muscles in your body are responsible for moving bones, pumping blood, moving food through the digestive system, and controlling air movement in and out of your lungs.

What Makes Muscles Contract?

Muscle contraction is started by the triggering action of nerve impulses. Nerves supplying most of the skeletal muscles that provide movement originate at the spinal cord. At the point where the nerve enters a muscle, it breaks up into numerous nerve endings, which, in turn, stimulate muscle fibers by means of tiny buttonlike endings called motor end plates. A neuron may branch to supply many muscle fibers.

Muscle Tone

All muscle fibers do not contract at the same time. While some are contracting, others are relaxing. Even when you are sleeping, some fibers are in a state of contraction, bringing about a certain degree of firmness, or tone, to your muscles. In the case of aging or poor health, muscles lose some or all of their tone. When you are in good health, a constant flow of impulses from nerves maintains muscle tone. Tone is essential for maintaining posture. Exercise and good nutrition improve muscle tone.

Structure of the Muscular System

A muscle consists of a mass of fibers grouped together. Almost all of the individual muscle fibers a person will ever have are present at birth. General muscle growth is an increase in the size rather than the number of the muscle fibers.

Muscle fibers are made of smaller fibers called myofibrils. Thick and thin filaments make up each myofibril. The thick filaments are made up of the protein myosin. The thin filaments are made up of the protein actin. Myofibrils are divided into sections called sarcomeres. When a muscle fiber receives an impulse from a nerve, actin filaments slide over the myosin filaments and move toward the center of the sarcomeres and toward each other during contraction. When the muscle relaxes, the actin filaments return to their original positions.

Types of Muscles

Your body has three basic types of muscle tissue. These types are smooth muscle, skeletal muscle, and cardiac muscle.

Skeletal muscles give shape to the body and are essential in performing physical movements.

The Skeletal Muscles

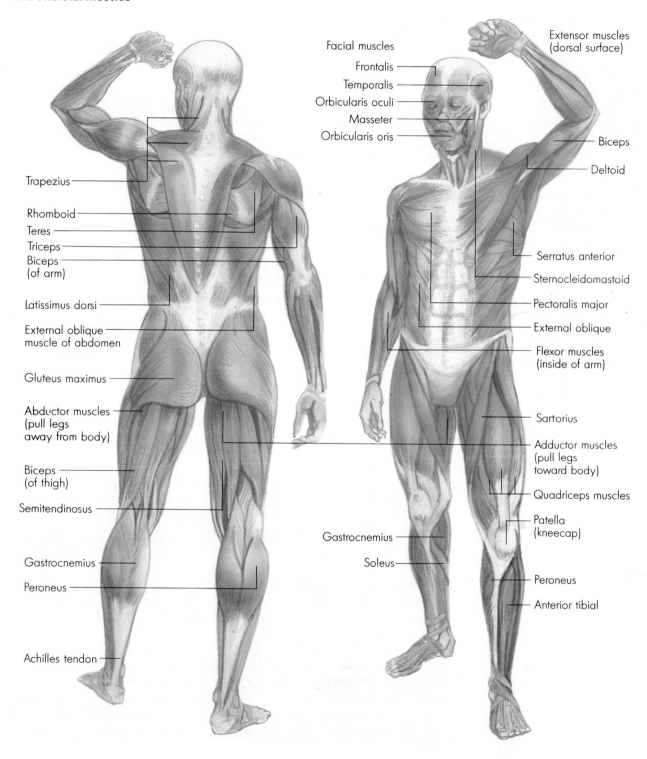

Facial muscles
Frontalis
Temporalis
Orbicularis oculi
Masseter
Orbicularis oris

Extensor muscles (dorsal surface)

Biceps
Deltoid

Trapezius

Rhomboid
Teres
Triceps
Biceps (of arm)

Latissimus dorsi

External oblique muscle of abdomen

Gluteus maximus

Abductor muscles (pull legs away from body)

Biceps (of thigh)

Semitendinosus

Gastrocnemius

Peroneus

Achilles tendon

Serratus anterior
Sternocleidomastoid
Pectoralis major
External oblique
Flexor muscles (inside of arm)

Sartorius

Adductor muscles (pull legs toward body)

Quadriceps muscles

Patella (kneecap)

Peroneus

Anterior tibial

Gastrocnemius

Soleus

FINDING HELP

Although muscular dystrophy often strikes young adults, treatment can help them live a relatively normal life. For more information about this disease, contact the local or national office of the Muscular Dystrophy Association, 3561 East Sunrise Drive, Tucson, AZ 85718. You may wish to find out about current research efforts as well as about what activities the association sponsors in your community.

Smooth muscle, sometimes called unstriated muscle, is located in such places as the intestines and blood vessels. Smooth muscles are involuntary because they work without a person's conscious control.

Skeletal muscles are attached to bones and cause body movement. Skeletal muscles are voluntary. They are under conscious control. Skeletal muscles account for about 40 percent of body weight.

Skeletal muscles work in pairs. While one contracts, its counterpart extends. When a skeletal muscle contracts, bones are pulled by tendons, which attach muscles to bones. The tendons that connect a muscle to a bone must be connected to another bone, so that there is something to pull against when the muscle contracts. Muscles that bend a limb at the joint are called **flexors;** those that straighten a limb are called **extensors.** If the flexors and extensors both contracted at the same time, they would work against each other, and there would be no movement.

Cardiac muscle is a special type of striated tissue that forms the walls of the heart. This muscle pumps blood through your cardiovascular system. Cardiac muscle is involuntary muscle.

Your heart is the most important muscle in your body. It works continuously, day and night. Just like other muscles, the more exercise the heart gets, the stronger it becomes. A strong heart works more efficiently; that is, it does the same amount of work with less effort.

Problems of the Muscular System

You have probably experienced sore muscles after overworking them. This condition is temporary. Many other conditions of the muscular system are not temporary. They have an impact on a person's health and life-style.

Muscle Strain

A muscle strain is one of the most common injuries to muscles. A strain, or a "pulled muscle," is a sudden, painful stretching or tearing of muscle fibers. Strains usually occur in large muscles and are a result of overexertion. A strained muscle needs to be rested in order to heal. Ice

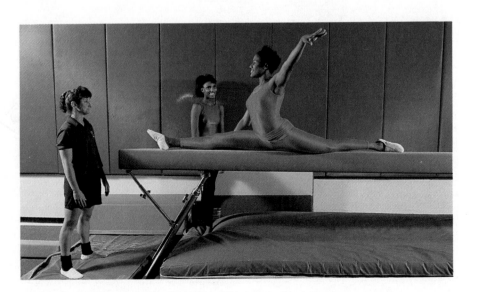

Muscles that are exercised and cared for are flexible and allow extraordinary movement.

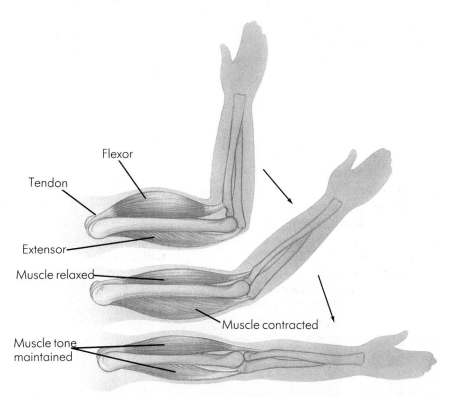

Flexor

Tendon

Extensor

Muscle relaxed

Muscle contracted

Muscle tone
maintained

should be applied to a strain for the first 24 hours. After that, heat should be applied to the strain.

Muscle Cramp

Have you ever been swimming and had a muscle cramp? A cramp occurs when a muscle contracts spasmodically and involuntarily. The muscle feels tense, knotted, and painful. A cramp may occur from using certain muscles for too long a period of time. Have you ever been writing for a long time and had your hand develop a cramp? Cramps also result from overworking in the heat. Cramps can be treated by gently stretching the muscle and firmly massaging the knot out of the muscle. Heat may also be used to help the muscle relax.

Myasthenia Gravis

Myasthenia gravis is a disease that is characterized by muscles that are weak and easily fatigued. The most commonly affected muscles are

K E E P I N G   F I T

A Foot Massage

A foot massage relaxes the muscles of your foot and relieves stress.
- Wash your hands and your feet.
- Place your right foot on your left knee.
- Hold your foot there with your right hand.

- Place your thumb on the sole of your foot.
- Place your fingers up toward your toes.
- Put firm pressure on your foot.
- Moving your thumb in a circular motion, massage from the

heel up toward your toes.
- Rub each toe with a circular motion between the thumb and the index finger.
- Repeat the process, working from the toes to ankle.
- Now switch feet.

Overcoming The Odds

Jill Eshleman is 23. She has a very rare form of muscular dystrophy. She says, "When I was born, there was no indication of a problem. Then, at age 4, I had heart failure from the disease, but they didn't know why. At 6, I had pneumonia. That's when I had surgery that made an opening into my trachea. I called it my 'trach'. They knew I was a very sick child, and they gave me 2 months to live. My spine had curved because the muscles were not strong enough to hold it straight. I had scoliosis, and my mom and dad designed a special walker. I was too sick to go to school, so I was tutored at home until 8th grade.

"Then my health stabilized and I tried four classes a day in the public school. I still had my trach. School was tough. In ninth grade it was better than being tutored at home, but it was not a good experience. I was painfully shy. The kids were hesitant, so they didn't really approach me. I had one good friend and the rest of the time I stayed by myself. I felt very self-conscious of what other kids thought."

After high school, Jill went to a community college and then completed a computer program for the disabled. "That's when I blossomed—when I got around people who were just like me," she says.

"Recently, I moved out on my own permanently. I love living alone," she says. "I was able to buy a house right up the road from my mom. I've

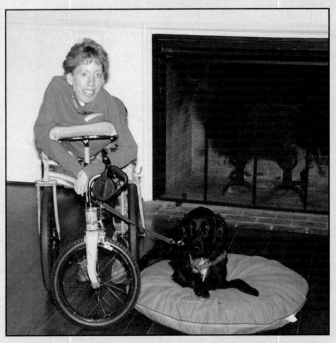

been working for three years. I started out in customer service and now I do bookkeeping for a company that imports Australian coats. I'm still using my special homemade walker. I have my driver's license. I'm learning to play an electric keyboard. My kitchen counters are low so that I can cook for myself. And I have friends now."

Jill is 4 feet 8 inches tall and weighs 52 pounds. Yet, she says, laughing, "My current health problem is pimples."

Jill has signed up with an organization called Canine Partners for Life, Inc. in Cochranville, Pennsylvania. Soon they will provide her with a special canine friend to help her. "They train dogs for your special needs," she says. "My dog will be able to pick up things off the floor, open heavy doors, retrieve a cordless telephone, and help me with steep ramps. He's an Australian sheep dog named Money. The dogs are trained for a year with a family, then at the Canine Partners kennel for a second year."

Jill concludes, "These days I feel good about myself. I would say to other people, set a goal so that when you feel frustrated you can think about it and get inspired. I really feel you have to inspire yourself. No one else is going to do it for you."

1. In what ways has Jill achieved independence? In what ways has she been willing to get help when she needs it?
2. Jill says that in high school other students felt hesitant about approaching her and she about approaching them. Do you ever have such reactions to people who are different from you? How can you overcome such hesitancy?

the eye muscles, which may result in drooping eyelids and double vision. Symptoms can be relieved with medicines.

This disease can affect anyone, but for reasons unknown, it is most common in women of childbearing age. The disease may occur during pregnancy or following an infection.

Muscular Dystrophy

Muscular dystrophy is a crippling disease characterized by a progressive wasting away of skeletal muscles. Muscular dystrophy is usually inherited.

With this disease the muscle cells are unable to function properly and are replaced by fatty tissue. The symptoms of muscular dystrophy vary depending on the part of the body that is affected. A person may experience muscle weakness, difficulty standing or walking, or frequent falls. Early detection of muscular dystrophy is crucial because, even though the disease cannot be cured, muscle weakening can be delayed. Exercise can help maintain flexibility.

Care for the Muscles

The more you use your muscles, the more efficient and strong they become. A program of regular exercise with stretching, warm-up, and cool down increases muscular strength and flexibility. Exercise increases muscle mass and stamina. By including an activity that promotes balance and coordination, falls and injuries can be reduced. Proper equipment and clothing can help protect muscles during exercise. Practicing good posture can help strengthen back muscles. Remember, your heart is a muscle and benefits from exercise just as other muscles do. Regular exercise strengthens the heart and makes it work more efficiently by increasing the amount of blood pumped in a single beat. As a result, the heart can pump fewer times and has more time to rest between beats. As with all other body cells, a healthy diet is important to the health of all your muscles.

LESSON 3 REVIEW

Reviewing Facts and Vocabulary

1. What are two important characteristics of muscle tissue?
2. What are the three types of muscles?
3. Describe two injuries or diseases related to the muscular system.

Thinking Critically

4. **Synthesis.** What possible benefits to muscles may be derived from warming up and stretching before exercise?

5. **Synthesis.** Suggest ways that a person can prevent injury to skeletal muscles.

Applying Health Knowledge

6. Get a chicken drumstick and thigh that are still attached. Pull back the skin and flex the leg. Watch which muscles contract and flex. Cut through the tendons at the base of the leg and separate the muscle groups. How many muscle groups are there? Can you identify the large blood vessels and the ligaments?

Self-Inventory

Care of Your Integumentary, Skeletal, and Muscular Systems

HOW DO YOU RATE?

There are many things you can do to promote these three body systems. Take the following self-inventory, and rate yourself on your health behaviors. On a separate sheet of paper, answer *always*, *sometimes* or *never* to the following questions.

Integumentary System

1. I keep my hair clean, cut, and styled in a way that fits my features and type of hair.
2. I keep my nails clean and evenly trimmed.
3. I avoid prolonged exposure to the sun.
4. When I am in the sun, I use an appropriate sunscreen.
5. I wash my face twice daily and use only creams and cosmetics appropriate for my skin type.
6. I avoid picking at acne.
7. I eat a well-balanced diet that includes an adequate source of vitamin A.

Skeletal System

8. My diet includes food sources of calcium and phosphorus.
9. My physical activity includes weight-bearing exercises.
10. I wear proper equipment for the activities I participate in.
11. I know how to care for a sprain.

12. I wear proper shoes for the activities I participate in.

Muscular System

13. I exercise three to five times a week.
14. I warm up and stretch before beginning to exercise.
15. I work to increase my muscular strength.
16. I know how to care for a muscle cramp.
17. I practice good posture in order to strengthen my back muscles.
18. I cool down after exercising.
19. I participate in activities that increase my balance and coordination.
20. I choose a healthy diet.

HOW DID YOU SCORE?

Give yourself 2 points for each *always* response, 1 point for each *sometimes* response, and 0 points for each *never* response. Total your score. Then proceed to the next section.

31 to 40
Excellent. Your health choices show you are taking care of these systems.

21 to 30
Good. However, there are some things you could do better to promote these systems.

Below 21
Look out! You may be taking unnecessary risks that could affect your health.

WHAT ARE YOUR GOALS?

Identify an area in which your score was low, and use the goal-setting process to begin making a change.

1. The behavior I would like to change or improve is ____.
2. If this behavior were completely changed, I would look, feel, and act differently in the following ways: ____.
3. The steps involved in making this change are ____.
4. My timetable for accomplishing this is ____.
5. People I will ask for support or assistance are ____.
6. The benefits I will receive are ____.
7. The rewards for making this change will be ____.

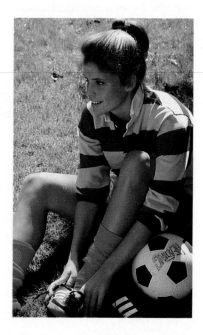

Building Decision-Making Skills

N ick has had close family members die of muscular dystrophy and feels very strongly about raising funds for the muscular dystrophy telethon. He is forming an organizing committee in his homeroom for a dance at his school to benefit the charity. A couple of friends start making jokes about "Jerry's kids" and suggest that any fund-raising dance should benefit the students of their school, not people they don't even know. What should Nick say to his friends?

WHAT DO YOU THINK?

1. **Situation.** Why does Nick need to make a decision?

2. **Choices.** Should Nick respond to these students? If so, what are his possible approaches?

3. **Choices.** Should Nick relate his response to his personal situation? Explain your answer.

4. **Consequences.** What will probably happen if Nick does not make a decision?

5. **Consequences.** What will probably happen if Nick changes his plan and organizes a dance to raise money for the senior class trip or some other school activity?

6. **Consequences.** How might Nick's self-esteem be affected by this decision?

7. **Consequences.** How might Nick's health triangle be affected by this decision?

8. **Consequences.** How will Nick's family be affected by this decision?

9. **Consequences.** Should school fund-raising activities benefit only students?

10. **Consequences.** What are the benefits of participating in an event that benefits a particular charity?

11. **Decision.** What do you think Nick should do? Explain your answer.

12. **Evaluation.** Have you ever been in a similar situation? If so, how did you handle it? Would you handle it differently now?

S cott's friends on the football team have grown considerably in the past year and have earned spots on the varsity football team, which is one of the most successful in the state. In addition to status in school, some varsity players on this team are virtually assured of college scholarship opportunities. Scott is very talented and dedicated, but just not big enough. His friends have told him the answer is simple—just do as they did and use steroids, which they got from older players. Scott knows the dangers of using steroids and he doesn't want to take those risks. What should he tell his friends?

WHAT DO YOU THINK?

13. **Situation.** If Scott didn't know the facts about steroids, where could he find them?

14. **Situation.** What difference does it make what he tells his friends?

15. **Situation.** What might make this a difficult decision?

16. **Choices.** What choices does Scott have?

17. **Consequences.** What are the costs of each choice?

18. **Consequences.** What are the benefits of each choice?

19. **Consequences.** How can Scott accept the fact that he's too small to get a college football scholarship?

20. **Consequences.** If money is a problem, how might Scott go to college if he doesn't get the football scholarship?

21. **Consequences.** How might Scott's parents help him accept the fact that he won't get a football scholarship?

22. **Consequences.** Are there any circumstances under which you would suggest that Scott take the steroids? Explain your answer.

23. **Decision.** What do you think Scott should do? Explain your answer.

Rᴇᴠɪᴇᴡ

Using Health Terms

On a separate sheet of paper, write the term that best matches each definition given below.

LESSON 1

1. The outer, thinner layer of skin made up of both living and dead cells.
2. The inner, thicker layer of skin.
3. Water and other waste products secreted from the sweat glands.
4. Disease of the skin caused by a fungus and symptomized by a whitish ring.
5. A common hair and scalp problem symptomized by flakes of skin.

LESSON 2

6. A strong material that gives support and flexibility to the body's framework at the joints.
7. A process by which cartilage becomes bone as the body matures.
8. The point at which two bones meet.
9. A curvature of the spine that may develop during puberty.
10. A condition that results from a loss of calcium in the bones.

LESSON 3

11. A mass of fibers grouped together.
12. Kind of muscle that forms the walls of the heart.

Building Academic Skills

LESSON 1

13. **Reading.** Use the context clue in the following sentence to define the word *cumulative*. The increasing effect of the sun on your skin is cumulative, and the damage is irreversible.

LESSON 2

14. **Math.** Four bones make up the human leg: the femur, the patella, the tibia, and the fibula. The bones in both legs make up what percentage of the 206 bones found in the adult skeletal system?

Recalling the Facts

LESSON 1

15. What is the largest organ in the body?
16. Explain the process by which your skin helps regulate body temperature.
17. What eventually happens to dead cells in the epidermis?
18. In what part of the skin are new cells formed?
19. What causes body odor?
20. Name two functions of the hypodermis.
21. What can be a serious result of excessive exposure to the sun over a period of time?
22. How does regular brushing benefit your hair?
23. What causes athlete's foot and how can it be avoided?
24. What are some basic procedures to follow for good nail care?

LESSON 2

25. What is the smallest bone in the body? The longest?
26. Name the four kinds of bones in the human body and give an example of each.
27. In what part of the population is osteoporosis most common?
28. What two minerals are important for your bones to grow, harden, and repair?
29. For each condition below, write *yes* if it affects a joint. Write *no* if the condition affects some other part of the skeletal system.
    a. sprain
    b. dislocation
    c. fracture
    d. torn cartilage
    e. bursitis
    f. arthritis
    g. osteoporosis

LESSON 3

30. What are the three types of muscles?
31. What is the most important muscle in the body?
32. What is the best way to keep your muscles strong and working efficiently?

REVIEW

Thinking Critically

LESSON 1

33. Analysis. Why is it not possible for two people to have the same fingerprints?

34. Analysis. Compare the results of too much and too little sebum being produced by the sebaceous glands.

35. Synthesis. Jackie has ringworm. Sandra borrows Jackie's comb every morning before school. What problem is Sandra likely to develop and why?

36. Synthesis. Sally was at the beach from 4 o'clock to 6 o'clock on Tuesday afternoon and did not get a sunburn. On Wednesday, she was at the beach from 11 o'clock in the morning to 1 o'clock in the afternoon and did get a sunburn. Why did she burn on Wednesday and not on Tuesday?

37. Analysis. Review this statement: "To avoid the sun, I'm going to a tanning booth."

LESSON 2

38. Synthesis. Devise and write out a plan for a person who has a deficiency in calcium and phosphorus.

39. Analysis. How are ligaments and tendons alike? How are they different?

LESSON 3

40. Analysis. Compare flexor and extensor muscles.

41. Synthesis. Compare and contrast the three basic types of muscles.

Making the Connection

LESSON 2

42. Language Arts. Interview several people who work in the sports or exercise field. Examples include a physical therapist, a trainer, or a dance instructor. Write a two- to three-page report that describes the academic preparation necessary for that career and the individual's personal characteristics that would be necessary to be successful in that field.

Applying Health Knowledge

LESSON 1

43. What phrases in skin product ads should be viewed with skepticism?

44. John spends a lot of time working on his tan. What can you tell him about the harmful effects of the sun on skin?

45. You have a mole on the left side of your neck. Recently you noticed that it has changed color from light brown to black. What should you do?

46. You have noticed white flakes in Ted's hair and on the shoulders of his dark shirts. What might Ted's problem be?

47. Duane shoveled snow for two hours on Friday afternoon. The day was bright and sunny. Now Duane appears to have a sunburn. How could Duane get a sunburn in the winter?

48. Explain how your overall appearance makes a statement about how you feel about yourself.

LESSON 2

49. Celia, who is 8, and her grandmother, who is 63, went roller skating together. They both fell down. Celia's grandmother broke her wrist, but Celia was uninjured. Why do you think Celia's grandmother broke a bone?

LESSON 3

50. Julio strained a muscle during wrestling practice. What should he do for it?

51. Shirley sometimes experiences muscle cramps during swimming practice. What advice would you give her for the next time this happens?

Beyond the Classroom

LESSON 3

52. Community Involvement. Contact your local chapter of the Muscular Dystrophy Association. Find out what this organization is doing to help people who have this disease.

THE NERVOUS AND ENDOCRINE SYSTEMS

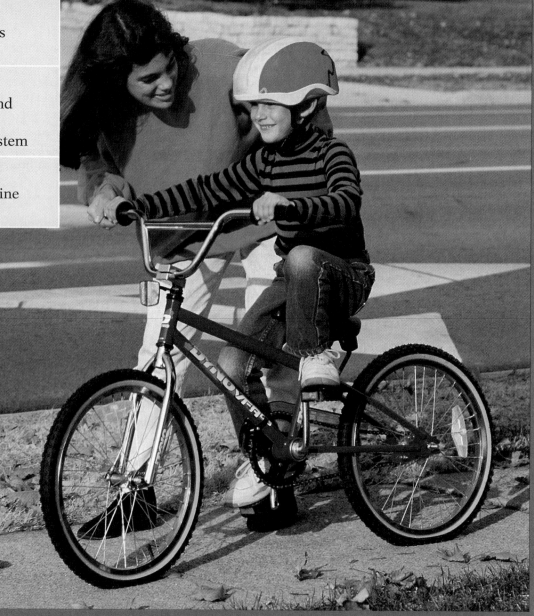

THE NERVOUS SYSTEM

Think of the series of events that take place when you eat a meal. Your eyes register that food is on your plate. Your hands move to pick up a utensil. You pick up the food. You then raise the food to your mouth, which opens at just the right time. You put the food in your mouth and start chewing. Your mouth has already begun secreting saliva to begin the digestive process.

You perform this act so regularly that it may seem automatic, but it is not. Eating is just one of many body functions that require coordinated responses and movements. The nervous system, along with the endocrine system, controls the coordination of all body functions. These two systems work together in such a way that the body is regulated and integrated and acts as a unit.

Functions of the Nervous System

Your nervous system is your body's communication network and control center. This system transmits information by nerve impulses from one nerve cell to another throughout your body. Your nervous system senses changes not only within your body but also outside your body in your environment. Those changes are interpreted and you respond to them. This happens in split seconds so that your body adjusts quickly to any internal or external changes. For example, when you touch a hot object in your external environment, how quickly do you respond?

Functions of Neurons

Nerve cells, which are called **neurons,** are the functional and structural parts of the nervous system. Neurons are classified according to their functions. There are three main types of neurons: sensory neurons, interneurons, and motor neurons.

- Neurons that have specialized receptor ends and are located in the skin and other sensory organs are called **sensory neurons.** Sensory neurons receive stimuli, such as sounds, and send impulses to your spinal cord and brain. You have sensory receptors for heat, cold, pain, hearing, taste, sight, smell, touch, and balance.

- Neurons within the brain and spinal cord that relay impulses from sensory neurons to motor neurons are called **interneurons.**

- Neurons that carry impulses from interneurons to muscles and glands are called **motor neurons.** When you touch a hot object you lift your hand away. When you are in an emergency situation your adrenal glands release adrenaline and you have extra energy. You will learn more about neurons later in this chapter.

LESSON 1 FOCUS

TERMS TO USE
- Neurons
- Sensory neurons
- Interneurons
- Motor neurons
- Cerebrum
- Cerebellum
- Brain stem
- Reflex

CONCEPTS TO LEARN
- Your nervous system is your body's communication network and control center.
- Damage to neurons is permanent.
- Your brain is a complex, computer-like center of your nervous system.

ATTITUDES AND BEHAVIORS TO EVALUATE
- Self-Inventory, page 244.
- Building Decision-Making Skills, page 245.

The central nervous system consists of the brain and spinal cord. The peripheral nervous system consists of the cranial and spinal nerves that branch from the brain and spinal cord.

The Nervous System

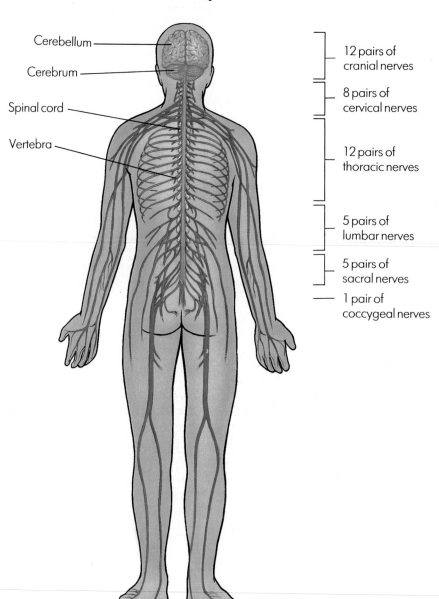

Cerebellum

Cerebrum

Spinal cord

Vertebra

12 pairs of
cranial nerves

8 pairs of
cervical nerves

12 pairs of
thoracic nerves

5 pairs of
lumbar nerves

5 pairs of
sacral nerves

1 pair of
coccygeal nerves

Structure of the Nervous System

Two main divisions of the nervous system are the central nervous system (CNS) and the peripheral nervous system (PNS). The CNS includes the brain and spinal cord. The PNS connects the CNS to other parts of the body by 43 pairs of nerves that extend from the CNS. The PNS consists of nerves and ganglia, which are groups of nerve cell bodies.

Structure of Neurons

Neurons are the structural parts of both the CNS and the PNS. Neurons have three basic parts: a cell body, dendrites, and an axon.

The Cell Body. The cell body has a nucleus and is the center for receiving and sending nerve impulses. It also is the center for making proteins and using energy for the maintenance and growth of the neuron. The shape of the cell body varies according to the type of neuron. Some sensory neurons are round, those on the surface of the brain are diamond-shaped, and motor neurons are star-shaped.

Dendrites. Dendrites are threadlike extensions of the cell body. They are usually short and have many branches. Dendrites receive and carry impulses toward the cell body. Some neurons may have many dendrites, others may have only one dendrite, while some may have no dendrites.

Axons. Each neuron has only one axon. An axon is a threadlike extension of a cell body that carries impulses away from the cell body. An axon of one neuron may have enough branches to make contact with as many as 1000 other neurons. Axons vary in length from a few millimeters to more than 1 meter. In the PNS, however, axons are longer. Some axons extend from the spinal cord to muscles in the fingers and are as long as 40 inches (102 cm).

Many axons in the PNS have a whitish coating or sheath of fatty material, called myelin, around them. The myelin sheath insulates the nerve fiber and speeds the transmission of impulses.

The Nerve Impulse

Neurons are unique body cells. Unlike other cells, neurons cannot replace themselves. Damage to neurons is permanent. Neurons are unique also in that they are very sensitive and can react to even the slightest stimulus. Once excited, a neuron can rapidly send an electrical charge from the point of stimulation to the brain or spinal cord. This charge can travel as fast as 248 miles (399 km) per hour!

A nerve impulse is an electrical charge that races along neurons from the point of stimulation to the brain or spinal cord. The more myelin a neuron has, the faster the impulse travels. Suppose you are walking home with a friend. At an intersection the "Don't Walk" sign lights up. You stop, wait for the "Walk" sign, and proceed. But during this time,

The Nerve Impulse

Skin
Receptors
Axon
Sensory neuron
Axon
Cell body of sensory neuron
Spinal cord
Dendrites (receptors)
Interneuron
Cell body of interneuron
Dendrites of motor neuron
Dendrites of interneuron
Synapse
Cell body of motor neuron
Dendrites of motor neuron
Motor neuron
Axon
Skeletal muscle

A nerve impulse travels from the receptors of a sensory neuron across an interneuron to a motor neuron to muscle fibers.

you never stop talking with your friend. It sounds simple enough, but the event of stopping and waiting involves millions of nerve cells.

Sensory receptors in your eyes are stimulated by the signal light and translate the stimulation into a nerve impulse. Now each sensory neuron begins a series of electrical and chemical changes to transmit the impulse. The impulse moves from the receptor ends of dendrites to the cell body and along the axon to the dendrites of another sensory neuron. The impulse has to cross a very narrow gap called a synapse, the junction between the axon end of one neuron and the dendrite of another neuron.

The impulse is transmitted in this way to your spinal cord, where interneurons carry the impulse to your brain. Your brain translates the message and sends an impulse back through motor neurons to muscles in your legs. You stop at the corner. The process repeats itself when the sensory receptors in your eyes receive the stimulus of the "Walk" light. This time you start walking across the street.

The Central Nervous System

In one way or another, every body function involves the central nervous system (CNS). Remember, the spinal cord and brain make up this control center, which is one of the two divisions of the nervous system.

The Spinal Cord

The spinal cord is about the same diameter as your index finger, is less than 2 feet (61 cm) long, and contains about 10 billion nerve cells. The spinal cord is protected by the vertebrae, the bones that make up your spine. It is also protected by cerebrospinal fluid that acts like a shock absorber, and by three layers of connective membranes called the spinal meninges.

The Brain

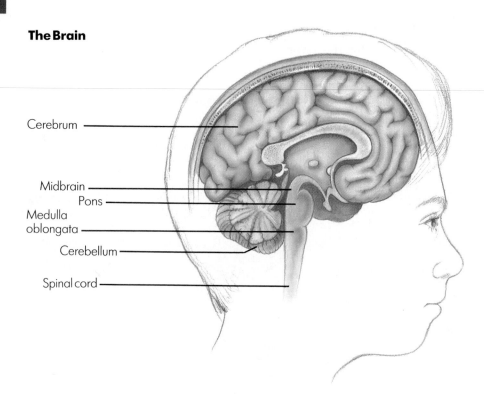

Cerebrum

Midbrain
Pons
Medulla oblongata
Cerebellum

Spinal cord

Your brain has three main divisions: the cerebrum, the cerebellum, and the brain stem.

The Brain

The brain is the largest, most complex part of the nervous system. Your brain helps you receive messages—think, remember, and reason—and coordinates your muscular movement. Your brain is involved in your emotions and everything you sense. It weighs about 3 pounds (1.4 kg) and contains almost 100 billion neurons. At birth, the brain weighs about 1 pound (0.5 kg). In humans, it reaches full size by age 6.

The brain is supplied with the food and oxygen it needs from a vast network of blood vessels. Although the brain makes up only about 2 percent of your total body weight, it uses 20 percent of the oxygen you inhale. The brain can be without oxygen for only 4 to 5 minutes before suffering serious and irreversible damage.

The brain is protected by eight cranial bones which form the skull, and three layers of membranes called cranial meninges. Cerebrospinal fluid between the meninges cushions the brain from injury.

The work of the brain is similar to that of a computer or a chemical factory. Brain cells produce electrical signals and send them along pathways called circuits. These circuits receive, process, store, and retrieve information much like a computer does. Unlike a computer, however, the brain creates its electrical signals by chemical means. The proper functioning of the brain depends on the many complicated chemical substances that brain cells produce.

The brain has three main divisions: the cerebrum, the cerebellum, and the brain stem.

The Cerebrum.   The largest, most complex part of the brain is the **cerebrum.** The cerebrum is divided into two identical halves called the cerebral hemispheres. The right hemisphere controls muscular activity and receives sensory input from the left half of the body. The left hemisphere controls the muscular activity and receives sensory input from the right half of the body.

Each hemisphere has four lobes. Each lobe is named after the bone in the skull that protects it:

- The frontal lobe controls voluntary movements, motivation, mood, and aggression.
- The parietal lobe is involved with a wide variety of sensory information—heat, cold, pain, touch, and body position in space.
- The occipital lobe contains the sense of vision.
- The temporal lobe contains the senses of hearing and smell, as well as memory, thought, and judgment.

K E E P I N G   F I T

Moving Your Body, Moving Your Mind

When you sit in the same position for a long time, a main nerve in your leg gets squeezed and stops sending information to your brain. When this happens, you may feel "pins and needles," and your foot may seem "asleep." If you move around, you will quickly take the pressure off the nerve and "wake up" your leg and foot.

Getting up and changing position may be good for your mind, too. By standing, you increase circulation. One new study suggests, in fact, that just standing up periodically, will help improve your thinking. Taking deep breaths will increase the oxygen supply to your brain, increasing your mental capacity.

Each hemisphere of the brain is divided into four lobes. Each lobe is involved in different functions.

Brain Lobes

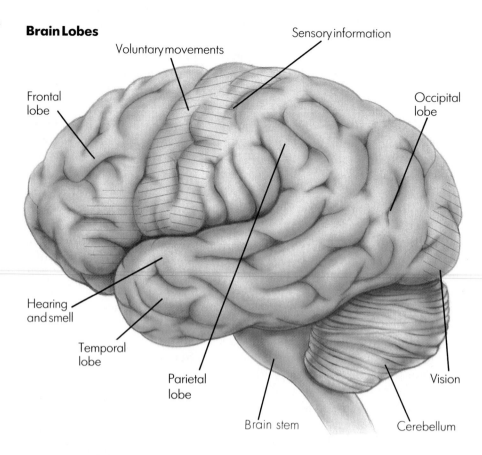

Voluntary movements

Sensory information

Frontal lobe

Occipital lobe

Hearing and smell

Temporal lobe

Parietal lobe

Brain stem

Vision

Cerebellum

The Cerebellum. The cerebellum is the second largest portion of the brain. It is situated beneath the occipital lobes of the cerebrum. The cerebellum is also divided into two hemispheres.

The **cerebellum** functions as a center for the coordination of skeletal muscle movement. It receives impulses from the balancing centers of the inner ear, from muscles, and from the motor areas of the brain. The cerebrum determines what movements the body will make, initiating the nerve impulses that activate the muscles. The cerebellum coordinates these nerve impulses to ensure accurate, controlled, and rapid movements. The cerebellum also maintains equilibrium during movements as it receives information from the sensory organs.

The Brain Stem. The **brain stem** connects the spinal cord to the brain. The brain stem includes the medulla oblongata, pons, midbrain, and interbrain.

K E E P I N G   F I T

Headaches

There are many different kinds of headaches, including tension headaches that throb and occur on both sides of the head; migraines, that may cause severe pain and nausea; and cluster headaches, that may cause pain around or behind one eye. According to one recent survey, the following major causes of headaches were identified: sinus infections, job or school stress, eye problems, weather, allergies, and the use of certain foods.

Getting too much sleep may also result in headaches.

If you suffer from frequent headaches, try to determine what triggers them. If they are very frequent, very intense, or last over long periods, consult a physician.

Overcoming The Odds

Eric Meneely is 21. School, sports, friends, and playing piano were all important to him. Then, he almost lost it all.

Eric was on his motorcycle. Distracted by some girls playing soccer, he didn't see that the car in front of him had stopped. He says, "I swerved and my head went crashing through his back windshield, then I rolled over the roof of the car, and my feet broke the front windshield. Luckily, I was wearing a helmet. If I hadn't been, I'd have been all over the road. It was all my fault.

"Miraculously, I had few external injuries. However, I had a brain injury. I apparently hit the right side of my brain. That affected what the left side of my body can do. Also, my right eye has a palsy of the optic nerve. This makes my eye go off to the right." Doctors have told him that surgery can repair his eye problem. However, there are other enduring problems. Eric says, "I slur my speech a little bit. And I can't drive until my eye is fully functioning again.

"I went against my parents' wishes when I bought the motorcycle. They were quite upset, but I was on the big teen immortal kick. I thought accidents happened only to other people."

Meneely says that after the

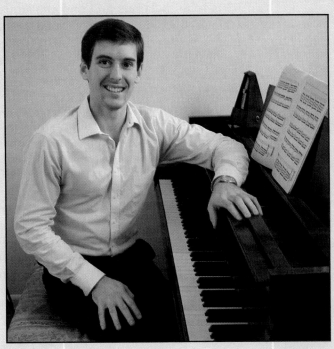

accident, his self-esteem suffered. "I felt like such a fool for buying the motorcycle and going against my parents. And I felt incompetent." These days, however, he is rebuilding his confidence by learning to compensate. "The memory is a little shaky, so I either write things down or tell one of my friends to remember for me.

My running is shaky, too, but I do it. As for playing the piano, I can't explain how I compensate, but I do."

Eric is back in college now. He is studying to become a physical therapist to help people who have injuries like his own. "It's not the way I would have chosen to get on-the-job training," he says, "but my own therapy and rehabilitation have served just that way. Because of what I've been through, I think I'll have greater insight and a more in-depth understanding of what patients go through. I think that most of what we worry about is trivial. You don't realize how important some things are until you almost lose it all."

1. How does Eric plan to put his near-tragic experience to good use in the future?
2. How did the accident affect Eric's self-esteem?
3. What concerns do you have right now that deeply upset you and hurt your self-esteem but might actually prove to be rather trivial?
4. If there are things about yourself that eat away at your self-esteem, what changes can you make? How can you compensate, as Eric learned to do?

DID YOU KNOW?

- People who are right-handed are usually left-brain dominant while people who are left-handed may be right-brain dominant or have mixed dominance.
- People who are left-brain dominant may be more logical and verbal than their right-brain counterparts.
- People who are right-brain dominant may be gifted mathematically, musically, or artistically.
- One in ten persons is left-handed, and the tendency may be inherited.

The medulla is the lowest part of the brain stem. It contains control centers that regulate heartbeat, breathing, and the diameter of the blood vessels. The control centers for vomiting, sneezing, swallowing, hiccuping, and coughing are also located in the medulla.

Just above the medulla, the brain stem enlarges to form the pons. The pons serves mainly as a pathway for nerve impulses passing to and from the cerebrum. It contains nerve fibers that link the cerebrum and the cerebellum. The pons also plays a part in controlling respiration.

The shortest part of the brain stem is the midbrain, which lies just above the pons. The midbrain connects the brain stem with the fibers from the cerebellum. Its nerve centers help control movements of the eyes and the size of the pupils.

Located above the midbrain is the interbrain. The interbrain consists of two parts—the thalamus and hypothalamus. The thalamus is like a relay station for incoming sensory impulses, such as vision. The thalamus also influences mood and movement related to fear or anger.

The hypothalamus has nerve centers that control different body processes and keep body conditions balanced. For example, nerve centers in the hypothalamus regulate body temperature and food and water intake. Neurons from the hypothalamus stimulate the pituitary gland to release hormones that control many body functions, such as metabolism and sexual development. The hypothalamus also plays an important role in emotional responses.

The Peripheral Nervous System

Peripheral means "located away from the center." The peripheral nervous system (PNS) consists of nerves that branch from the central nervous system. The PNS carries messages between the CNS and the rest of the body. The PNS consists of 12 pairs of cranial nerves that branch from the brain, and 31 pairs of nerves that branch from the spinal cord. The PNS is composed of two subdivisions—the somatic nervous system and the autonomic nervous system:

- The somatic system includes cranial and spinal nerves that transmit impulses from the CNS to skeletal muscles. This involves voluntary responses—responses under your control.
- The autonomic system includes nerve fibers that connect the CNS to smooth muscles, such as the intestines, to the heart, and to glands. This system produces responses in involuntary muscles and glands.

KEEPING FIT

The Headache/Food Connection

If you have frequent headaches, try to determine if your headaches are induced, or brought on, by specific foods. Try eliminating these foods from your diet one at a time. The following are common headache triggers: seafood, citrus fruits, milk, caffeine, fatty food, and onions.

Foods that contain MSG, (which is often found in processed food), nitrites, (which are used in lunchmeat), and the amino acid tyramine, (which is found in chocolate), are also common headache triggers. Other foods that contain tyramine include sour cream, yogurt, and vinegar.

The Autonomic Nervous System (ANS)

The autonomic nervous system's constant regulation of internal body processes enables the body to maintain a stable internal environment. There are two divisions of the ANS—the sympathetic division and the parasympathetic division. These two divisions affect the same organs, but basically produce opposing effects.

The Sympathetic Division. The sympathetic division responds to the body's needs during increased activities and in emergencies. For example, when you are excited, the sympathetic division would cause your heart to beat faster and your breathing rate to increase. Sympathetic nerves lead to all of the vital organs and glands, including the liver, heart, kidneys, pancreas, stomach, and salivary, sweat, and adrenal glands.

The Parasympathetic Division. The parasympathetic division generally opposes the actions of the sympathetic system by slowing body functions. It slows down the heartbeat, opens blood vessels, and lowers blood pressure. The balance of activity between the sympathetic and parasympathetic divisions is controlled by the CNS.

ACTION OF THE AUTONOMIC NERVOUS SYSTEM

Organ	Action of Sympathetic Division	Action of Parasympathetic Division
Heart	Increases heartbeat	Slows heartbeat
Arteries	Raises blood pressure by constricting arteries	Lowers blood pressure by dilating arteries
Stomach and intestines	Slows movement	Speeds up movement
Sweat glands	Decreases activity Increases secretion of sweat	Increases activity Decreases secretion of sweat
Muscles of iris	Dilates pupil	Constricts pupil

Reflex Action

A **reflex** is a spontaneous response of the body to a stimulus. It occurs automatically, without conscious thought or effort. You cannot stop or keep some reflex actions from happening. In what ways do these reflex actions serve as protection?

The knee-jerk reflex is an example of a simple reflex. Tapping a ligament just below the kneecap initiates the reflex.

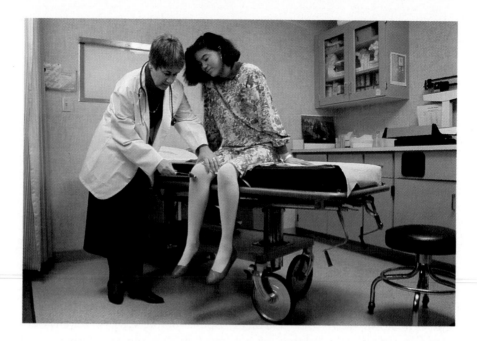

A simple reflex, such as occurs when the doctor taps the ligament below your knee, involves the interaction of only two neurons—a sensory neuron and a motor neuron. The doctor's tap is the stimulus that initiates the nerve impulse. The impulse travels along sensory neurons to the spinal cord. Here the impulse moves across the synapse to the dendrites of a motor neuron. The impulse travels back to leg muscles, causing them to contract and the knee to jerk.

In other reflexes, when a receptor is stimulated (for example, when your hand touches a hot stove), the axon of the sensory neuron makes contact with a connecting neuron in the spinal cord. This neuron, in turn, contacts a motor neuron that sends an impulse down its axon to the muscles. The muscles respond by pulling the hand away from the stove. All of this happens in a split second, even before pain is perceived by the brain.

The nerve chain of sensory and motor neurons involved in the reflex action is called a reflex arc.

LESSON 1 REVIEW

Reviewing Facts and Vocabulary

1. Describe the three types of neurons.
2. What is the difference between the sympathetic and parasympathetic divisions of the autonomic nervous system?

Thinking Critically

3. **Analysis.** How does the central nervous system compare with the peripheral nervous system?

Applying Health Knowledge

4. Make a diagram to show the parts of the brain, listing examples of what each part controls.
5. Test your reflex reaction. Have someone hold a dollar bill above your thumb and index finger. As he or she releases the dollar, trap it using only your thumb and index finger, without moving your arm. Mark where you caught the dollar. Repeat several times. Chart your reaction times.

PROBLEMS AND CARE OF THE NERVOUS SYSTEM

The normal functioning of the nervous system can be disturbed in a number of ways. An infectious disease, such as syphilis, can attack and destroy nerve tissue in the brain or spinal column. Accidents can damage or destroy nerve tissue. Illegal drug use, including alcohol use, can destroy brain cells and lead to a variety of nervous system disorders.

In general, problems with the nervous system can be divided into four categories: injuries, degenerative diseases, communicable diseases, and genetic disorders.

Injuries

Each year many young people suffer brain injuries resulting from motor vehicle accidents, falls, sports, and physical abuse. In addition, many people suffer spinal cord injuries.

Head Injuries

The brain is protected by the skull bones and the fluid that surrounds it. However, any direct blow to the head can lead to possible brain injury. A person may experience a concussion, a temporary disturbance of the brain's ability to function. A concussion is caused by a sharp blow to the head. Concussions are the most common and mildest kind of brain injury.

Concussions usually result in a temporary loss of consciousness and a memory loss of events just before and after the injury. Mild concussions, however, may not result in either loss of consciousness or memory loss.

A more serious injury to the brain is a contusion. A contusion of the brain is a bruise caused by a head injury. This bruising may cause swelling of the brain. In the brain stem, contusions produce severe neurological damage. A severe contusion could result in a coma, a state of unconsciousness resulting from an injury to the brain. A coma indicates that there has been serious damage to nerve tissue.

Depending on which brain cells are damaged, and how serious the injury is, the person will lose the ability to perform certain functions. If the cerebellum is damaged, a person may suffer from lack of balance or lack of muscular coordination. Damage to the brain stem could result in a loss of the sense of pain or in loss of the body's ability to regulate temperature.

Spinal Cord Injuries

The spinal cord is surrounded by protective membranes, shock-absorbing fluid, and the backbone. These defenses protect it from the

---

LESSON 2 FOCUS

TERMS TO USE

- Parkinson's disease
- Multiple sclerosis
- Meningitis
- Poliomyelitis
- Rabies
- Down syndrome
- Epilepsy
- Cerebral palsy

CONCEPTS TO LEARN

- The nervous system can be damaged by injuries, degenerative diseases, communicable diseases, and genetic disorders.
- Any damage to the nervous system disturbs the impulse pathways to and from the brain and spinal cord.
- By following basic rules of safety, many head and spinal injuries can be prevented.

ATTITUDES AND BEHAVIORS TO EVALUATE

- Self-Inventory, page 244.
- Building Decision-Making Skills, page 245.

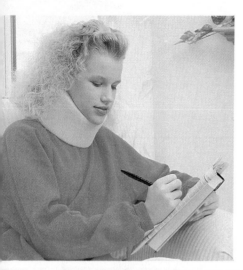

The consequences of a spinal injury will depend on the amount of damage to the spinal cord.

bumps and falls common in everyday life. However, they often are not enough to protect it from more serious accidents.

One of the most common injuries to the spinal cord is a pinched nerve. This occurs when one of the cartilage disks that separates the vertebrae moves slightly as a result of a sudden jerking of the body, a blow, a fall, or a jolt. The disk can press on or pinch a nerve, causing discomfort and often great pain.

Remember that all messages to and from the brain go through the spinal cord. Injury to the spinal cord means that these messages cannot get through. Depending on the severity and location of the injury, this breakdown in communication could be mild or serious, or could result in death. An injury anywhere on the spinal cord could cause paralysis.

In general, injury to the upper part of the cord causes more extensive damage. An injury at the neck level, for example, may cause paralysis in both the arms and the legs. Someone with such an injury is called a quadriplegic. Injury at the chest level or lower affects the legs and lower body. Someone whose lower body is paralyzed is called a paraplegic.

Some spinal injuries require people to wear a neck collar or a special corset to support the back. Other injuries require traction, in which weights are used to balance out parts of the spinal cord, to give relief from pain. Surgery is the last resort to correct spinal injuries.

HEALTH UPDATE

LOOKING AT TECHNOLOGY

New Hope and Better Care

There are many new and exciting medical and technological advances that may offer new hope and better care to people with brain and spinal cord diseases and injuries.

MAPPING THE BRAIN. Through the BrainMap Project, researchers at Johns Hopkins University in Maryland and the Research Imaging Center at the University of Texas Health Science Center in San Antonio are trying to make the first comprehensive map of the brain. Using computers and other imaging techniques, they are compiling data about the brain that may be used by doctors and researchers around the world. Very soon, the project will result in a comprehensive system of information about the brain. A doctor who has a patient with a rare or difficult brain problem can feed information about that problem into the system and learn the latest data and research regarding it.

COMPUTERIZED LEG BRACES. Researchers at the Massachusetts Institute of Technology are studying special computerized leg braces that may prove helpful to people such as those with multiple sclerosis.

STAND-UP WHEELCHAIRS. Newly designed wheelchairs called "standing wheelchairs" are now being made available. They allow a paralyzed person to stand up and say hello face-to-face, reach for things in high places, or even dance cheek-to-cheek.

Degenerative Diseases

Degeneration means a breakdown or deterioration of function or structure. Three common degenerative diseases of the nervous system are Parkinson's disease, multiple sclerosis, and Alzheimer's disease.

Parkinson's Disease

Parkinson's disease, first described in the 1800s by James Parkinson, usually affects people between the ages of 50 and 75.

The exact cause of Parkinson's disease is not known. **Parkinson's disease** is a disease that interferes with the transmission of nerve impulses from the motor areas of the brain. It is a progressive disorder, meaning that it gradually involves more and more nerves. The result is uncoordinated muscular movement. This disease is characterized by slow voluntary movements and tremors.

With the discovery of new medicines, the effects of this disease have been dramatically controlled in many patients.

Multiple Sclerosis

Multiple sclerosis (MS) is the progressive destruction of the myelin sheath that surrounds nerve fibers. This coating is gradually destroyed and scar tissue forms in its place. Neurons become permanently damaged. The scar tissue interferes with the ability of the nerve fibers to send impulses. The impulses may even be blocked completely. Voluntary control of muscles gradually decreases.

The effects of MS depend upon which nerves are involved. MS is quite unpredictable. Symptoms may occur and disappear in random patterns. They may occur once and never reappear. There is no known cure for MS. Therapy is directed at managing the complications. Many patients are able to lead full, productive lives.

Alzheimer's Disease

Alzheimer's disease was first described by Alois Alzheimer in the early 1900s. It is a progressive, degenerative disease that generally affects people over 60 years old. About $2\frac{1}{2}$ million Americans suffer from this disease. It is the fourth leading cause of death in adults, after heart disease, cancer, and stroke.

FINDING HELP

You can get more information about disorders of the nervous system by contacting the following organizations:

- Alzheimer's Association
  70 East Lake Street
  Suite 600
  Chicago, IL 60601

- American Parkinson Disease Association
  60 Bay Street
  Suite 401
  Staten Island, NY 10301

- Epilepsy Foundation of America
  4351 Garden City Drive
  Landover, MD 20785

- National Multiple Sclerosis Society
  205 East 42nd Street
  New York, NY 10017

K E E P I N G   F I T

Rethinking Disabilities

Next time you get caught in the trap of thinking an amputee or a person in a wheelchair can't perform, think of the following trio, all winners of the Victory Awards at the National Rehabilitation Hospital in Washington, D.C.:

- Skip Wilkins had his spinal cord cut in a water skiing accident, but that didn't stop him. He now stars in all kinds of wheelchair athletic events.
- Joni Tada, paralyzed from the neck down after a diving accident, creates her drawings with a pencil between her teeth.
- Bruce Demby had his leg blown off in Vietnam. He now competes and wins in special track-and-field events and also serves as a ski instructor.

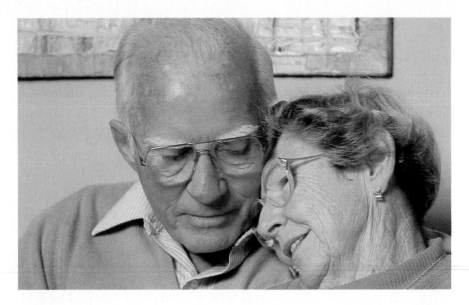

Caregivers are important to a person who has Alzheimer's disease. This man cares for his wife who has Alzheimer's.

Alzheimer's disease causes general mental deterioration. Patients gradually lose their memory and powers of judgment. Speech and body coordination may also be affected. Although there is no cure, researchers continue to search for effective treatment for the symptoms of the disease.

Communicable Diseases

Communicable diseases of the nervous system are caused by pathogens that can enter the brain in several ways. They may enter directly through a fracture in the skull. Others may be spread from ear and sinus infections. They may also be carried from some other part of the body to the brain through the bloodstream. Some, such as the virus that causes rabies, move through a peripheral nerve to the brain.

Encephalitis, meningitis, poliomyelitis, and rabies are communicable diseases that may result in damage to the nervous system.

Encephalitis

Encephalitis is an inflammation of the brain caused by a virus and sometimes by bacteria. Neurons in the brain may be damaged. Symptoms may include headaches, fever, and sometimes convulsions. Although most patients recover from encephalitis, some suffer permanent brain damage.

Meningitis

What word does *meningitis* resemble? What part of the nervous system do you think this disease affects? **Meningitis** is an inflammation of the meninges. It can be caused by bacteria or viruses. Symptoms include severe headaches, high temperature, vomiting, and sore or tight neck muscles. Antibiotic medicines are used to treat meningitis when it is caused by bacteria, making the chances for recovery excellent. Antibiotic medicines are ineffective, however, when the source of the infection is viral.

Poliomyelitis

Poliomyelitis, or polio, is a viral infection that affects motor neurons in the spinal cord and brain stem. The virus enters the body through the mouth, reaches the bloodstream through the stomach and lungs, and then attacks the central nervous system. This infection can result in paralysis of one or more limbs, usually the legs. If nerves controlling the diaphragm become infected, the respiratory system may become paralyzed. Polio epidemics occurred in the 1940s and early 1950s. The development of the Salk and Sabin vaccines in the 1950s has brought this once life-threatening disease under control.

Rabies

Rabies is a viral infection of the brain and spinal cord. Humans become infected if they are bitten by an animal infected with the virus. Symptoms of rabies include restlessness, mental depression, and painful throat spasms. Rabies is a life-threatening disease. There is a vaccination for rabies that consists of a series of injections after a person has been bitten.

Genetic Disorders

Some diseases of the nervous system are hereditary, they are passed from parent to child through inherited genes. These disorders include phenylketonuria and Down syndrome.

Phenylketonuria

Phenylketonuria (PKU) is rare, occurring in about 1 out of every 15,000 babies born in the United States, and is transmitted by a recessive gene. PKU is characterized by an inability of the body to break down a substance found in some foods called phenylalanine. The resulting buildup of this substance in the body interferes with the normal development of the brain. Symptoms of PKU appear in the first few weeks of life. PKU can be detected by a blood test even before any symptoms appear. With early treatment, mental retardation can be prevented. Treatment consists of a special diet that restricts any foods that contain phenylalanine.

CONFLICT RESOLUTION

Jamahl will be 16 next week and has been eagerly waiting to get his driver's permit. Until yesterday, his parents had agreed he could get it on his 16th birthday. Then Jamahl was diagnosed with epilepsy. Now his parents say getting a driver's permit is out of the question because it may not be safe for him to drive. They're afraid he might have a seizure while driving. Jamahl's doctor says that the right dose of medication should keep the seizures under control. Jamahl thinks his parents are overreacting to his disease.

Can you think of a way to resolve the conflict between them?

KEEPING FIT

New Strides for the Disabled

There are about 43 million Americans with disabilities. The Americans With Disabilities Act now requires that hotels offer special telephones with phone flashers, tape-recorded safety instructions, and other features for the speech and hearing impaired. A new hotel in Florida has also included roll-in showers for people in wheelchairs, talking alarm clocks, and special training for employees that gives them a view of what it is like to have a disability.

Is your school user-friendly for people with handicaps? Think of ways that you can help make your school environment better for those people. If you have a disability, why not lead the effort?

Down Syndrome

Down syndrome is characterized by mild to serious mental retardation and short stature. It is the result of a chromosomal abnormality. Humans normally have 46 chromosomes, 23 pairs in each body cell. A child with Down syndrome has 47 chromosomes in each body cell, with the extra chromosome being with the twenty-first pair. The cause of the extra chromosome is not completely understood. The incidence of having a baby with Down syndrome increases with the age of the mother. There is no cure for Down syndrome. Special education can enhance what a Down syndrome child can achieve.

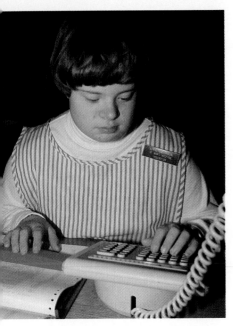

A child with Down syndrome can learn skills that were once thought to be beyond the capacity to learn.

Other Disorders of the Nervous System

Although many disorders of the nervous system have known causes, some may have many possible causes. In some cases, the cause is unknown. Epilepsy and cerebral palsy are two such disorders.

Epilepsy

The term *epilepsy* comes from a Greek word meaning "seizure." **Epilepsy** is a disorder of the nervous system that is characterized by a sudden burst of nerve impulses in the brain. This sudden burst of impulses is transmitted to the muscles and results in a seizure, a physical reaction that may be slight or intense.

The reason for this sudden discharge of nerve impulses is not completely understood. It may be the result of a chemical imbalance in the brain, a tumor, or an injury to the brain before or during birth. There may be other causes, such as a high fever in childhood or an infection. Sometimes children who have epilepsy simply outgrow it as they reach their teenage years.

There are two types of seizures—grand mal and petit mal.

- Grand mal seizures usually last about 2 to 5 minutes, and the person may fall to the floor, losing consciousness. During the seizure, the muscles become tense causing the body to shake. The person may be sleepy after the seizure, but usually has no memory of it.
- Petit mal seizures are so slight that they often pass unnoticed. The person may go into a daze or have a blank stare for about 30 seconds. He or she may experience slight dizziness or faintness.

There is no present cure for epilepsy, even though there are medicines that control most seizures. Persons with epilepsy generally live a normal, healthy life. The disorder does not affect their intelligence or ability to function.

Cerebral Palsy

Cerebral palsy refers to a group of nonprogressive neurological disorders that are the result of damage as the brain is developing. Damage may occur before or during birth if oxygen to the brain is decreased or cut off. Pressure to a baby's head during birth can cause damage to the cerebrum. Accidental injury, lead poisoning, and certain illnesses can also cause cerebral palsy.

The Endocrine System

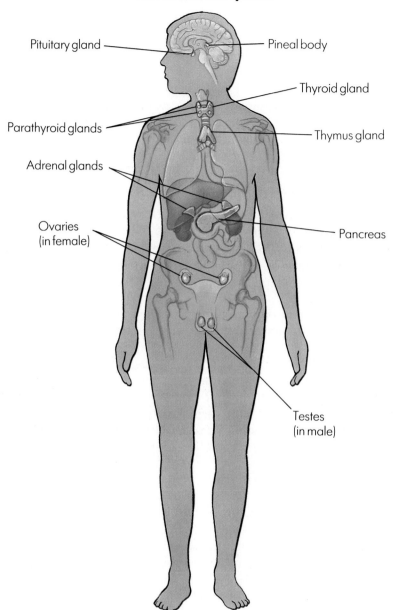

Pituitary gland

Pineal body

Thyroid gland

Parathyroid glands

Thymus gland

Adrenal glands

Ovaries
(in female)

Pancreas

Testes
(in male)

The Pituitary Gland

The **pituitary gland** is about the size of an acorn and is situated at the base of the brain. Because the pituitary gland regulates other endocrine glands, it is often referred to as the master gland.

The pituitary gland has three lobes. The anterior lobe and the posterior lobe secrete various hormones and have a great effect on the other glands. The intermediate lobe is still not completely understood.

The Anterior Lobe of the Pituitary. The hormones released from the anterior lobe control a range of body functions. They regulate metabolic activities of cells and stimulate other endocrine glands. The anterior lobe produces at least five different hormones. They are as follows:

■ The somatotropic hormone, also known as the growth hormone,

DID YOU KNOW?

■ Scientists have identified over 30 different hormones in the human body.
■ Since the 1940s, scientists have been able to create synthetic hormones in the laboratory.
■ The tallest man on record was Robert Pershing Wadlow, who was 8 feet, 11 inches in height.

influences growth in most body tissues. It especially influences the skeleton and skeletal muscles.

■ The thyroid-stimulating hormone (TSH) regulates both the size and activity of the thyroid gland.

■ The adrenocorticotropic hormone (ACTH) controls the manufacture and secretion of hormones produced in the outer layer of the adrenal glands.

■ Two gonadotropic hormones control the growth, development, and functions of the gonads, which is another name for the ovaries and testes. In females, the follicle stimulating hormone (FSH) triggers the development of egg cells, or ova, in the ovary. FSH also stimulates cells in the ovary to produce estrogens, female sex hormones. In males, FSH stimulates the testes to produce sperm cells.

In females, the leuteinizing hormone (LH) is responsible for ovulation, or the release of a mature ovum from the ovary. LH also stimulates cells in the ovaries to produce progesterone, a female sex hormone. In males, LH stimulates cells in the testes to produce testosterone, a male sex hormone.

The Posterior Lobe of the Pituitary. The posterior lobe of the pituitary gland secretes two hormones, antidiuretic hormone (ADH) and oxytocin.

ADH's principal effect on the body is to regulate the balance of water in the body. It stimulates the kidneys to retain water by returning it to the blood. If the kidneys did not return water to the blood, a person would have excess water in the urine and experience a serious internal water shortage. Oxytocin stimulates the smooth muscles in the uterus of a pregnant female causing contractions during the birth of a baby.

The Thyroid Gland

The **thyroid gland** is one of the largest glands of the endocrine system. It is a twin mass, consisting of a left and right lobe, located in the neck at the junction of the trachea and larynx. Thyroxine contains iodine, and is the principal hormone produced by the thyroid gland.

Thyroid hormones regulate the metabolism of carbohydrates, fats, and proteins in body cells. **Metabolism** is the sum total of all chemical reactions within a cell. The metabolism of nutrients within a cell is important in providing the cells with a source of energy.

The Parathyroid Glands

The **parathyroid glands** are the smallest glands of the endocrine system and are situated on the lobes of the thyroid gland. The hormone from these glands, parahormone, regulates the body's calcium and phosphorus balance. These minerals are necessary for normal functioning of muscle and nerve tissue.

The Adrenal Glands

The two adrenal glands are located on each kidney. The **adrenal glands** consist of two parts—the outer portion, called the adrenal cortex, and the inner portion, called the adrenal medulla.

The Adrenal Cortex. The adrenal cortex, which is absolutely essential for life, secretes a mixture of hormones that affects numerous body functions. Hormones from the pituitary gland stimulate the adrenal cortex.

Aldosterone is the principal, most potent hormone that the adrenal cortex produces. Its function is to conserve the body's sodium and water balance.

The inner layer of the cortex produces a group of hormones that affect metabolism. Cortisone affects the metabolism of carbohydrates and proteins. Other hormones secreted from the cortex help a person cope with stress.

The Adrenal Medulla. The adrenal medulla is highly dependent upon the hypothalamus and the autonomic nervous system for regulation. It secretes the hormone epinephrine, more commonly called adrenaline, which increases heart action, raises blood pressure, increases respiration, and suppresses the digestive process.

This hormone is also known as the emergency hormone because it is released into the blood in greater amounts during highly emotional states, such as when a person experiences fear or anger.

The Pancreas

The **pancreas** is a gland that serves two systems—the digestive and the endocrine. This elongated, flattened organ lies behind the stomach, attached to the first section of the small intestine by a duct that transports its digestive juice to the intestine.

Scattered throughout the pancreas are small clusters of cells that are separate from the exocrine portion of the gland. These clusters make up the endocrine part of the pancreas. They are called the islets of Langerhans for Paul Langerhans, a German scientist who first noticed them in 1869. There may be as many as a million of these clusters that produce two hormones affecting the metabolism of glucose (blood sugar).

One hormone, glucagon, helps maintain the sugar level of the blood by stimulating the liver to convert glycogen to glucose, thus raising the blood sugar level. Glycogen is a storage form of glucose in the liver and muscle cells. The other hormone, insulin, tends to decrease blood sugar levels. Insulin stimulates the liver to form glycogen from glucose. Insulin is a complex protein substance and is essential to life.

The Ovaries and the Testes

The ovaries in the female and the testes in the male are part of the reproductive system. The ovaries produce and release ova, and the testes produce and release sperm. Both the ovaries and testes are endocrine glands.

As endocrine glands, the ovaries and the testes produce hormones that are responsible for the development and maintenance of secondary sex characteristics. The secretion of the hormones progesterone and estrogen by the ovaries is stimulated by hormones from the pituitary gland. Hormones from the pituitary gland stimulate the testes of the male to produce and secrete the hormone testosterone.

Disorders of the Endocrine Glands

Most disorders of the endocrine glands are related to the production of too much or too little of a hormone. There are other possible causes, however. Following is a description of some problems associated with endocrine glands.

The Pituitary Gland

If, during the growing years, the anterior lobe of the pituitary gland does not produce enough of the growth hormone, a person does not grow. The person's stature is short because of delayed bone growth. Bones are usually normal in shape, however. If this condition is diagnosed early, proper treatment can be prescribed. With early treatment, a child may reach full height.

If too much of the growth hormone is produced during the growing years, the bones lengthen abnormally, resulting in a condition called giantism. If too much of this hormone is produced after the growing years, the bones thicken instead of lengthen. In this rare condition, called acromegaly, the soft tissue over the bones enlarges, making the face look massive and the hands and feet look large and awkward.

If the posterior lobe of the pituitary does not function, a person will experience a very large increase in the output of urine, a condition known as diabetes insipidus. This disease is rare and is not related to the more commonly known diabetes.

The Thyroid Gland

The metabolic action of thyroid hormones is very important during the growth years. A lack of thyroid hormones during the early growing years results in cretinism. This condition results in arrested growth, mental retardation, slow heart rate, and dry, yellowish skin.

Myxedema is a condition that results from lack of thyroid hormones. The metabolic rate drops, and mental and physical activity becomes sluggish. By administering thyroid hormones, all symptoms of myxedema usually disappear within a few weeks.

A simple goiter is an enlarged thyroid gland. It is caused by a dietary deficiency of iodine. Goiters are not a very common problem in the United States because of the availability and use of iodized salt.

The Parathyroids

Underproductive parathyroids cause the level of calcium in the blood to drop. This results in muscle spasms, called tetany, which can be painful. Overproductive parathyroids cause calcium to be withdrawn from the skeleton, leaving bones weak and susceptible to fracture.

The Adrenal Glands

Addison's disease is caused by underproductive adrenal glands. Persons with Addison's disease lose excessive amounts of salt through the kidneys. They may experience a serious drop in blood pressure. Adrenal cortex hormones are used to treat Addison's disease.

Overproduction of adrenal hormones can result in Cushing's disease. The person may be weak and tired and have an excess of fatty deposits in the face.

The Pancreas

If insulin is not being produced or is not functioning, glucose accumulates in the blood and tissues and is passed out of the body through the urine. The result is a loss of nutrients and energy the body needs to carry out its basic activities. This condition is called diabetes mellitus.

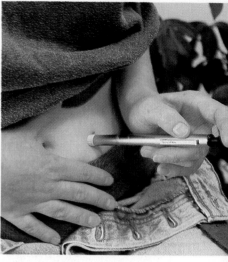

This female is using a pen-like device to inject herself with insulin. This injection helps her keep her blood sugar level within a normal range.

Care of the Endocrine System

The glands of the endocrine system work together to keep your body healthy. This system usually takes care of its own chemical balance. However, as with other body systems, good health habits are important. For example, because the thyroid gland needs iodine, this mineral must be part of your diet. This kind of care is especially important in the teen years because the body is growing and changing so rapidly.

LESSON 3 REVIEW

Reviewing Facts and Vocabulary

1. Why is the pituitary gland called the master gland?
2. Make a chart showing the hormones produced by the pituitary gland. Include what they do.
3. What happens if the thyroid gland does not function properly?

Thinking Critically

4. **Analysis.** Compare the ovaries and testes.
5. **Synthesis.** What endocrine gland would you predict is not functioning properly if the following conditions exist?

a. excess sugar in the urine
b. impaired growth, causing a person to be abnormally small for his or her age
c. muscle spasms
d. vomiting, weakness caused by a serious drop in blood pressure

Applying Health Knowledge

6. Find out which hormones can be made synthetically. For what are these hormones used?
7. Research what an endocrinologist does. Write a narrative report describing this person's work.

Self-Inventory

Care of the Nervous System

HOW DO YOU RATE?

Number a sheet of paper from 1 through 10. Read each item below, and respond by writing *always, sometimes,* or *never* for each item. Total the number of each type of response. Then proceed to the next section.

1. I wear a seat belt when traveling by car.
2. I wear a helmet when riding a bicycle, skateboard, rollerblades, or motorcycle.
3. I wear protective headgear whenever I participate in a contact sport.
4. I follow basic safety rules when cycling.
5. I get at least 8 hours of sleep each night.
6. I exercise regularly.
7. I avoid alcohol and other drugs.
8. I determine the depth of water in a pool or lake before diving.
9. I wear safety goggles when required for class or sports.
10. I avoid injuries to the spinal cord by lifting and carrying objects properly.

HOW DID YOU SCORE?

Give yourself 3 points for each *always* response, 1 point for each *sometimes* response, and 0 points for each *never* response. Find your total, and read below to see how you scored. Then proceed to the next section.

20 to 30
Excellent. Your health choices show you are taking care of your nervous system.

10 to 19
Good. You have a good understanding of ways to protect the nervous system, but you could use more caution.

Below 10
Needs Improvement. You may be taking unnecessary risks with your most vital body system.

WHAT ARE YOUR GOALS?

If you scored between 20 and 30, complete the statements in Part A. If your score was under 20, complete Parts A and B.

Part A

1. I plan to learn more about the care of the nervous system in the following ways: ____.
2. My timetable for completing this is ____.

Part B

3. The behavior I would like to change or improve is ____.
4. The steps involved in making this change are ____.
5. My timetable for making this change is ____.
6. The people or groups I will ask for support are ____.
7. My rewards for making this change will be ____.

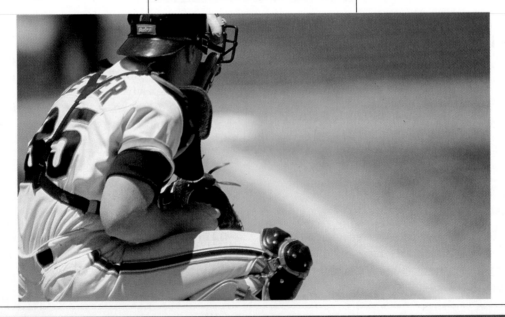

Building Decision-Making Skills

Jenna's brother, Michael, is a mildly retarded Down syndrome child. Michael attends classes for developmentally handicapped youngsters. Lately Michael has talked with Jenna about his desire to join a regular third-grade class. He wants Jenna to help him convince his parents to talk with school administrators about making the switch to regular classes. Jenna is concerned about the social, intellectual, and emotional difficulties Michael might face in a regular classroom. She feels he might be better off staying where he is. What should Jenna do?

A. Support Michael in whatever he chooses to do.

B. Leave the decision up to their parents and the school administrators.

C. Get an opinion from one of Michael's teachers or from a specialist in the field of developmentally handicapped children.

D. Talk with Michael about waiting until next year when he may be more capable of accepting the challenges in a regular classroom.

WHAT DO YOU THINK?

1. **Choices.** What other choices can you think of for Jenna?

2. **Consequences.** What are the costs and benefits of each choice?

3. **Consequences.** Who will be affected by Jenna's decision?

4. **Decision.** What do you think Jenna should do? Explain your answer.

5. **Evaluation.** Have you ever been asked to do something that you knew might not be best for the person who asked? How did you handle the situation?

Your friend, Lauren, has been looking very tired lately. Her grades are dropping, because she falls asleep in class. Her relationships with her family and friends are deteriorating because she is so irritable. Her new job at the pizza shop requires her to work from 8 P.M. to midnight five days a week. You know that she doesn't really need the money.

WHAT DO YOU THINK?

6. **Situation.** Does Lauren need to make a decision?

7. **Choices.** What are her choices?

8. **Consequences.** What are the consequences of each of the choices?

9. **Decision.** What do you think Lauren should do? Explain your answer.

James is caught in a downpour on the way home from school one afternoon. His friend, Will, drives by on his motorcycle and stops to offer James a ride. The only problem is that James doesn't have a helmet. He is getting soaked. What should he do?

A. Tell Will "No, thanks," and hurry on his way.

B. Accept the ride and, just this once, ride without a helmet.

C. Accept the ride, but ask Will if he can wear his helmet.

WHAT DO YOU THINK?

10. **Choices.** Can you help James come up with some other possible solutions?

11. **Consequences.** What are the advantages and disadvantages of each choice?

12. **Decision.** What should James do?

Using Health Terms

On a separate sheet of paper, write the term that best matches each definition given below.

LESSON 1

1. Fatty material that coats axons and speeds the transmission of an impulse.
2. Narrow gap between the axon of one neuron and dendrite of another neuron.
3. Connective membranes surrounding the spinal cord.
4. Connects spinal cord to brain.
5. Spontaneous response of the body to a stimulus.
6. The largest and most complex part of the brain.

LESSON 2

7. The inability to move.
8. A degenerative disease of the nervous system in which the myelin sheath surrounding nerve fibers is destroyed.
9. A genetic disorder of the nervous system in which one has inherited an extra chromosome, resulting in mental retardation.
10. A state of unconsciousness caused by an injury to the brain.

LESSON 3

11. Gland at the base of the brain, often called the "master gland."
12. The sum total of all chemical reactions within a cell.
13. The clusters of cells in the pancreas that produce insulin.
14. A hormone secreted by the adrenal medulla and known as the "emergency hormone."

Building Academic Skills

LESSON 2

15. **Reading.** Read several current magazine articles about people who have suffered paralysis as a result of injuries received in accidents. What generalizations can you make about the quality of life these people have had since their accidents?

Recalling the Facts

LESSON 1

16. What are the two parts of the central nervous system?
17. What does the peripheral nervous system consist of?
18. Explain the action of a reflex.
19. List the three main divisions of the brain.
20. What is the function of the autonomic nervous system?
21. What division of the autonomic nervous system responds to the body's needs during increased activities?
22. Give two examples of the opposing actions of the sympathetic and parasympathetic divisions of the autonomic nervous system.

LESSON 2

23. Name two degenerative diseases of the nervous system. Describe the symptoms.
24. Name two communicable diseases of the nervous system. Describe the symptoms.
25. What is PKU? How is it diagnosed? How is it treated?
26. Tell what a concussion is and what the results of a concussion might be.
27. Tell what a contusion is and what the results of a contusion might be.
28. What causes a pinched nerve?

LESSON 3

29. What are hormones and what is their function?
30. What is the difference between endocrine glands and exocrine glands?
31. Describe why the ovaries and testes are regarded as endocrine glands.
32. Which endocrine gland affects the body's response to stress? How?
33. What is the largest gland in the endocrine system and what does it do?
34. Which gland secretes insulin? What is the function of insulin in the body?
35. Name three disorders associated with an improperly functioning pituitary gland.

REVIEW

Thinking Critically

LESSON 1

36. **Synthesis.** Suppose your frontal lobe was injured and you began to suffer from mood swings. How do you think your life might change?

LESSON 2

37. **Evaluation.** Why do you think people continue to experiment with drugs, knowing the risks to the nervous system?

38. **Evaluation.** In some states, parents are required by law to have their child immunized against polio before the child enters school. Do you think parents should be required by law to do this? Why or why not?

39. **Synthesis.** Summarize reasons for the stigma that has historically been attached to epilepsy.

40. **Analysis.** Think of the different tasks you perform in a day. Decide which of these tasks you think you could still perform if you became a paraplegic. Which tasks would require retraining in order to accomplish them? Which of your daily tasks could you still perform without retraining if you became a quadriplegic?

LESSON 3

41. **Synthesis.** Your friend has not been growing properly and has just found out that her pituitary gland is not producing enough growth hormone. What might happen to your friend? What treatment may your friend receive?

Making the Connection

LESSON 1

42. **Language Arts.** Research scientific discoveries about how the left brain and right brain work. Which of these sides affects writing and other language functions? Of interest may be studies done with individuals who have suffered brain damage.

Applying Health Knowledge

LESSON 1

43. Imagine that you are approaching a busy intersection. When you are about 10 yards away, you notice a 4-year-old on a bike heading right for the street. Which part of your autonomic nervous system will respond? How do you know?

44. You know that to perform even the simplest task your nervous system goes through a series of events. List the events your nervous system goes through when you copy information from the chalkboard.

45. Imagine that your friend recently had a head injury. When you talk with your friend, he tells you that he is having trouble feeling things and that he has already cut himself and didn't know it until he saw the blood. What part of your friend's brain may have been damaged? How do you know?

LESSON 2

46. Find out how each of the communicable diseases discussed in this chapter are transmitted. What can you do to protect yourself from getting each disease?

LESSON 3

47. Find out more about diabetes insipidus. What medical help might a person suffering from this disorder be able to get?

Beyond the Classroom

LESSON 2

48. **Further Study.** Sometimes a disease is named for a famous person who has been affected by it. Lou Gehrig was a player for the New York Yankees. In 1941 he died of a disorder that has since been called Lou Gehrig's disease. Find out what this disease is and how it affects a person.

49. **Futher Study.** Make a report showing medical progress during the past 25 years of any disorder discussed in this chapter.

CHAPTER 13

CARDIOVASCULAR, LYMPHATIC, AND RESPIRATORY SYSTEMS

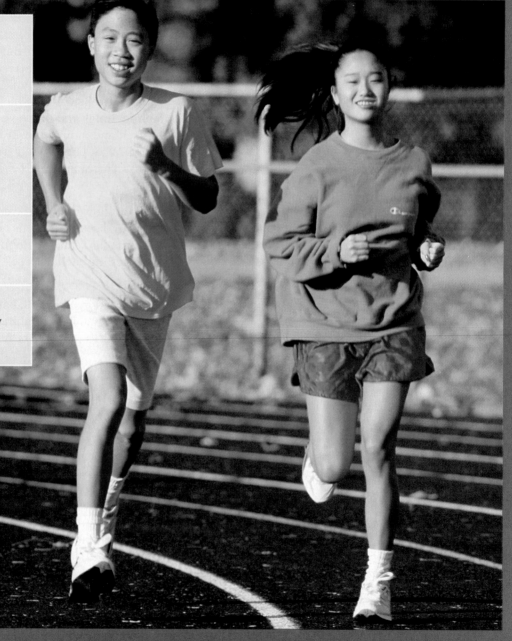

THE CARDIOVASCULAR SYSTEM

Your cardiovascular system moves blood throughout your body. Think of this system as a transport system serving body cells as a delivery and pick-up system.

Functions of the Cardiovascular System

The major function of the cardiovascular system is to maintain an internal body environment in which all body cells are nurtured. As your heart pumps blood, blood vessels carry oxygen and nutrients to body cells. Oxygen and nutrients pass from the circulating blood into cells. At the same time, carbon dioxide and other wastes are picked up by the blood and distributed to the lungs and kidneys where they are released from the body. Your body cells could not function without these two processes occurring.

Structure of the Cardiovascular System

Your cardiovascular system includes your heart, blood, and a network of branching blood vessels.

The Heart

Your heart is one of the most vital organs in your body. It started beating before you were born and it has been beating every minute of your life. Your heart is a pear-shaped muscular organ about the size of your fist. It is enclosed in a loose-fitting sac called the pericardium. The pericardium protects the heart.

Chambers of the Heart. The heart is divided into four chambers, two on the left side and two on the right side. The two upper chambers are called atria. The two lower chambers are called ventricles. The heart chambers are referred to as the left atrium, the left ventricle, the right atrium, and the right ventricle. The two halves of the heart are separated by a wall called the septum. A valve separates each atrium and ventricle. The valves keep the blood flowing in the proper direction.

Your heart is a pump that moves blood through two major pathways. **Pulmonary circulation** is the flow of blood from the heart to the lungs and back to the heart. Two major veins return blood that carries wastes from body cells to the right atrium. As the right atrium fills, it contracts and blood flows into the right ventricle. This ventricle pumps the blood to the lungs through the pulmonary arteries. In the lungs, carbon dioxide and oxygen are exchanged. The blood picks up oxygen from inhaled air in

LESSON 1 FOCUS

TERMS TO USE

- Pulmonary circulation (PUL•muh•NER•ee)
- Systemic circulation
- Plasma
- Hemoglobin
- Platelets
- Arteries
- Capillaries (KAP•uh•LER•eez)
- Veins

CONCEPTS TO LEARN

- The continuous flow of blood through the circulatory system depends on the heart.
- To maintain all the cells that make up the human body, there must be a continuous stream of nutrients from the outside world and a continuous removal of waste products from the cells.

ATTITUDES AND BEHAVIORS TO EVALUATE

- Self-Inventory, page 270.
- Building Decision-Making Skills, page 271.

Blood low in oxygen is pumped from the right ventricle to the lungs through the pulmonary arteries (shown in blue). Blood rich in oxygen returns to the left atrium through the pulmonary veins (shown in red).

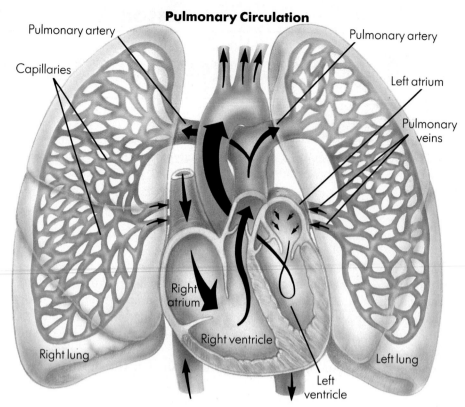

Pulmonary Circulation

Pulmonary artery

Capillaries

Pulmonary artery

Left atrium

Pulmonary veins

Right atrium

Right ventricle

Left ventricle

Right lung

Left lung

the lungs and releases carbon dioxide into the lungs. When you exhale, you get rid of the carbon dioxide. Blood with a fresh supply of oxygen returns to the left atrium in the pulmonary veins.

Systemic circulation moves blood to all body tissues except the lungs. The oxygenated blood flows from the left atrium to the left ventricle. The left ventricle is the most muscular part of the heart. It pumps blood through the aorta, the largest artery, to all of the parts of the body. This blood supplies body cells with nutrients and oxygen. Blood returns to the heart from the body through major veins called the inferior and superior vena cava. The systemic circulation includes circulation through the coronary arteries to nurture the heart muscle.

Blood

Blood is the fluid that transports all of the substances that the body needs to sustain life. Blood delivers oxygen, hormones, and nutrients to the cells and carries away wastes that the cells produce. The blood also contains certain cells that help fight infection. Blood is made up of a liquid called **plasma** in which the other parts—red blood cells, white blood cells, and platelets—are suspended.

Plasma. About 55 percent of the total volume of your blood is plasma, which is about 92 percent water. Plasma transports dissolved nutrients, waste products, and mineral salts as well as hormones, enzymes, and vitamins.

Red Blood Cells. Red blood cells carry oxygen from the lungs to all body cells. The oxygen-carrying substance in red blood cells is known as

The Cardiovascular System

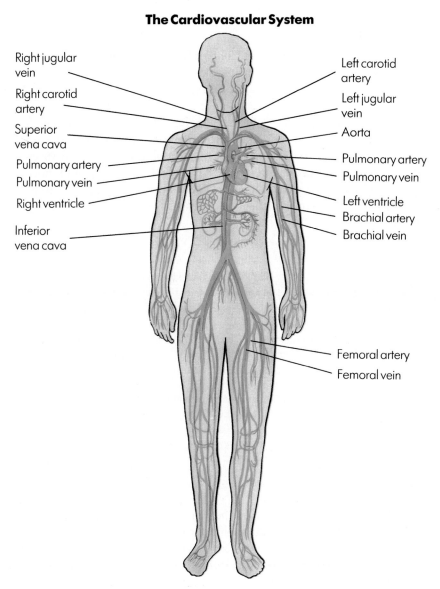

Right jugular vein

Right carotid artery

Superior vena cava

Pulmonary artery

Pulmonary vein

Right ventricle

Inferior vena cava

Left carotid artery

Left jugular vein

Aorta

Pulmonary artery

Pulmonary vein

Left ventricle

Brachial artery

Brachial vein

Femoral artery

Femoral vein

The cardiovascular system is a closed system of vessels through which blood, pumped by the heart, maintains the health of body cells by providing constant oxygen, nutrition, and removal of waste products.

There is no risk of infection when giving blood. New disposable needles are used each time.

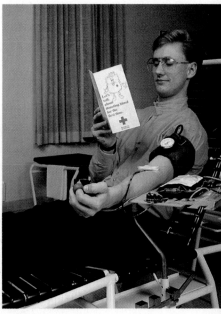

hemoglobin. It is a protein compound that is rich in iron. Hemoglobin is a pigment that gives blood its red color. Red blood cells also carry carbon dioxide, a waste product from body tissues, to the lungs. Red blood cells are the most numerous cells in blood. New red blood cells are continually being produced in bone marrow.

White Blood Cells.   The main function of white blood cells is to destroy invading pathogens. Some white blood cells surround pathogens and ingest them. White blood cells are produced in red bone marrow. Production of white blood cells increases when there is an infection in the body. Normally, there are fewer white blood cells than red blood cells in a person's blood.

Platelets.   Blood **platelets** are the smallest parts of the blood. Platelets are crucial in preventing the body's loss of blood. They initiate a chain of reactions that results in the clotting of blood. Platelets produce small fibers, called fibrin, that trap red blood cells at the site of a cut or a broken surface. These trapped cells form a clot, which helps prevent more blood loss.

Blood Types

Do you know your blood type? This information could be very important if you needed a blood transfusion in an emergency. Tests for human blood types classify red blood cells as type A, type B, type AB, or type O.

A person who has type O blood is referred to as a universal donor because that person can give blood to a person with any blood type. On the other hand, a person who has type AB blood is referred to as the universal recipient because he or she can receive any type of blood.

For transfusions to work, the blood types must match. Hospitals and blood banks take extreme care in checking blood types before giving transfusions.

BLOOD BANKS

Many cities have blood banks where blood is collected from healthy donors and stored. Blood banks store whole blood—blood that still contains both plasma and blood cells. Whole blood can be frozen and kept for long periods of time. When refrigerated, whole blood can be stored for several weeks. Transfusions of whole blood are given most often when a patient has suffered a severe loss of blood.

In some cases, such as those involving burn victims, the need may be for blood volume rather than blood cells. Plasma transfusions are given in these situations. Plasma is separated from whole blood by a centrifuge machine. This machine whirls the blood at a high speed, causing the blood cells to settle to the bottom, leaving a layer of plasma on the top.

Rh Factor. About 85 percent of the United States population has certain proteins in the blood, called Rh factors. These people are said to be Rh-positive. The remaining 15 percent of the population lack these proteins and are Rh-negative. What significance does the Rh factor have for your health?

A person with Rh-negative blood should not be given Rh-positive blood. Mixing the two causes antibodies to be produced. Rh-negative blood containing Rh antibodies causes the red blood cells of the Rh-positive blood to clump together. This mixing can occur when an Rh-negative person receives Rh-positive blood through a transfusion. This can cause serious complications and even result in death.

K E E P I N G   F I T

Knowing About Cholesterol

For people 20 years of age and older, a desirable blood cholesterol level is less than 200. From 200–239 levels are considered borderline high. 240 and above is high. Now, even children are tested if there is a family history of high cholesterol.

Most people can reduce cholesterol levels by taking these steps:
- Reduce the intake of cholesterol-containing foods and fat.
- Increase the intake of soluble fiber.
- Maintain ideal weight; if overweight, lose that weight.
- Get regular aerobic exercise.
- Don't smoke.

Overcoming The Odds

Carmella Garcia is 15. She plays the trumpet, likes soccer, and has a part-time job walking dogs. She is also president of her class. She loves to run, and she has set two track records at her school in the past year. "I've always loved to run," she says. "It's like I was born with running shoes. My dad was the same way when he was younger. But it was what happened to my mom that really got us all more focused on being fit."

What happened to her mom was a heart attack. "Mom is only 52, so it was really a surprise. She was at work when it struck. I'll never forget that call from the hospital. My dad's face turned to stone. The next thing I knew, we were all there. It seemed like we lived at the hospital.

"Later they did coronary bypass surgery on her. When I saw her after the operation, I thought I was going to pass out. She looked so old.

"My mom wasn't fat or anything like that but she was a little overweight and she smoked. She's a nervous type of person like my sister, and I think that's part of what happened. Plus, she loves to cook, and she loves to eat.

"Well, the medical center where she had her operation had this program called Lifestyle II, a program for heart patients and their families. So when my mom was stronger all five of us started to go to the two-hour sessions every week. We all had our cholesterol tested. My mom's

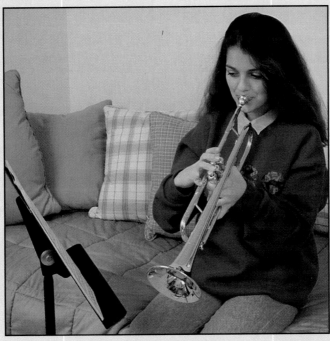

had been real high. Mine was okay. My dad's was a little elevated. My brother's was okay. But my sister's, well, that was the surprise. Hers was over 300. And she's even thin. My sister's cholesterol and my mom's and dad's are being watched really carefully. My sister may even go on medication if our home plan doesn't lower her cholesterol enough.

"They taught us in the classes how changing our life-style as a family could help not just our mom but all of us to live longer and healthier. We had classes about low-fat diets, stress management, and regular exercise. They gave us this chart to keep track of how far and often we walk—as well as our pulse rates. My mom has given up cigarettes and coffee.

"I guess when that phone call came in about my mom, I thought that could be it. It was a low point in my life. But I guess now I am grateful in a funny kind of way that it all happened because it has brought us so close and it has made us all so much more aware of how important family and staying fit are. Lifestyle II is a good name for the program, I think, because it's like we've all been given a second chance. And we're taking it."

1. Carmella's family had to be shaken up by a heart attack to make the necessary life-style changes. Why do you think it often takes a scare for people to begin caring for their cardiovascular health?
2. What steps can you take to improve your cardiovascular health? What steps can you take to help your family members become more fit?
3. How do you think taking such steps might affect your self-esteem? Your family relationships?

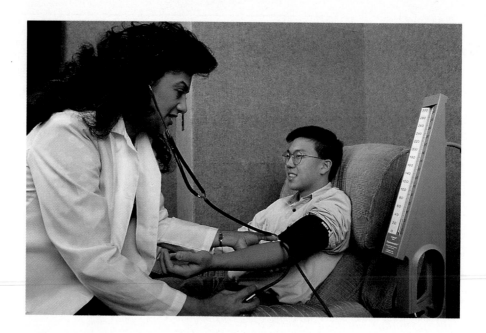

Blood pressure is the measure of the force of blood on the walls of blood vessels.

BLOOD PRESSURE

As blood flows from the arteries into the capillaries, blood pressure lowers. Blood pressure is the force of blood on the walls of blood vessels. By the time blood reaches the venules, it has lost all but about one-twelfth of its pressure. This low pressure is necessary because the thin, tiny capillaries could not withstand the force at which blood is pumped through the arteries. Blood pressure is reduced even more as the veins get larger. Muscular activity is necessary to maintain the blood flow through the veins.

Blood leaves the ventricles under a high pressure. As you might expect, pressure is greater in the left ventricle and aorta than in the right ventricle and pulmonary artery. Blood pressure is greater in the left ventricle because blood must be pumped with enough force to send it throughout the body. The right ventricle sends blood a shorter distance—to the lungs.

Each time the ventricles contract, blood surges through the arteries with such a force that the walls of the arteries bulge. At this point in the cycle of heart action, arterial pressure is at its greatest and is called systolic pressure. As the ventricles relax to refill with blood, arterial pressure is at its lowest and is called diastolic pressure.

A sphygmomanometer is an instrument used to measure blood pressure. You have probably had your blood pressure measured during a checkup. To have this done, a health professional wraps a blood pressure cuff around your arm just above the elbow. The cuff is then inflated with air until circulation in your arm is blocked. As air is slowly released from the cuff, the health professional uses a stethoscope to hear the sound of the blood beginning to move through the constricted area again. He or she listens for the return of a pulse in the artery. The number on the sphygmomanometer gauge at this point represents your systolic blood pressure. It is the upper number of the fraction representing your blood pressure and is usually between 110 and 140.

As air continues to be released, the person taking the reading listens for a change in the tone of your pulse or for the sound of the pulse to disappear completely. The number on the gauge at this point represents your diastolic blood pressure. It is the lower number of the fraction and is usually between 70 and 90.

DID YOU KNOW?

- Men have more blood and more blood vessels than women do.
- The aorta is the largest blood vessel in the body. It is about 1 inch in diameter.
- There are about 10 billion capillaries in your body.
- The average heart pumps about 70 times per minute.
- A well-conditioned athlete can have a resting pulse as low as 45.

Blood Vessels

Your blood vessels make it possible for blood to be distributed throughout your body. There are over 60,000 miles (96,540 km) of blood vessels in your body. They are divided mainly into arteries, capillaries, and veins.

Arteries.   The largest blood vessels, called **arteries**, carry blood away from the heart. As part of the systemic circulation, the left ventricle pumps oxygenated blood through the largest artery, the aorta. As part of the pulmonary circulation, the right ventricle pumps blood that is low in oxygen through the pulmonary arteries to the lungs. Arteries branch into smaller vessels called arterioles. These microscopic branches regulate the flow of blood into capillaries.

Capillaries.   The smallest blood vessels are called **capillaries.** Some capillaries are 50 times thinner than a single strand of hair. Nutrients and oxygen from the blood pass to body cells through capillary walls. Waste products from the cells move into the blood through capillary walls.

Veins.   The system of capillaries leads into tiny branches of veins called venules. These venules lead to **veins**, the vessels that carry the blood back to the heart. Veins become thicker and larger in diameter as they get closer to the heart. The walls of veins are thinner than those of arteries.

Veins do not have to withstand the great pressure the arteries do. Another difference between veins and arteries is that the inner lining of the veins forms valves that help direct the flow of blood. These valves prevent blood from flowing back into the capillaries. Regulating blood flow is especially important in the legs and feet where the blood must flow against the force of gravity to return to the heart.

LESSON 1 REVIEW

Reviewing Facts and Vocabulary

1. In what ways is the cardiovascular system a transport system?
2. Describe the changes in pressure as blood flows through the blood vessels. What is meant by systolic and diastolic pressure?

Thinking Critically

3. **Analysis.** Compare the pathways of pulmonary and systemic circulation.
4. **Analysis.** When might a blood pressure reading be a health concern?

5. **Evaluation.** Why do you think the body has more red blood cells than white blood cells? When would you expect the body to make more white blood cells?

Applying Health Knowledge

6. Write a paragraph describing a typical day in the life of your heart.
7. Have your blood pressure checked in class by the school nurse. What is the average blood pressure for the class? How does the blood pressure of students who exercise regularly differ from those who do not?

PROBLEMS AND CARE OF THE CARDIOVASCULAR SYSTEM

LESSON 2 FOCUS

TERMS TO USE
- Congenital
- Thrombosis
- Embolus

CONCEPTS TO LEARN
- Genetic, environmental, and life-style problems can affect the cardiovascular system.
- Congenital heart disease covers a wide variety of conditions.
- Many of the risk factors related to heart disease are within your control.

ATTITUDES AND BEHAVIORS TO EVALUATE
- Self-Inventory, page 270.
- Building Decision-Making Skills, page 271.

There are a variety of problems that can affect the cardiovascular system. With proper care, some problems can be avoided; others can be treated.

Problems of the Cardiovascular System

In this lesson, you will read about congenital heart disease, heart murmurs, varicose veins, thrombosis, anemia, sickle-cell anemia, leukemia, and hemophilia. In Chapter 29 you will read about other diseases of the heart.

Congenital Heart Disease

Before birth the heart begins as a single tube. It enlarges and divides into chambers. This process involves a progression of developmental steps. A disruption in this process can result in a defect in the heart. Babies born with such a defect have congenital heart disease. The term **congenital** means "occurring at birth."

Congenital heart disease covers a wide variety of conditions. The heart may have a hole between two chambers. The valves may not function properly, or there may be a blockage of the blood flow. The defect may be in the blood vessels leading to and from the heart. Certain types of defects may not be noticed right away. In some cases the defect heals itself as the heart grows following birth. Other defects may require surgery.

There are numerous causes of congenital heart disease. Only a small percentage of these defects have a genetic cause. Some defects result from a viral infection during the early months of pregnancy, illegal drug use, or a vitamin deficiency. Most cases can be treated or corrected with surgery.

Heart Murmurs

Have you ever used a stethoscope to listen to your heart? Blood makes strong, clear sounds as it passes through a healthy heart. If the heart is not functioning properly, other noises may be heard as blood moves through the chambers.

A heart murmur is an abnormal sound. The major cause of heart murmurs is a defective valve in the heart. A valve that is too narrow causes the blood to be pushed through the restricted opening with more force. A valve that does not close properly allows blood to leak back through it. Both situations cause the sound labeled a "murmur". Most murmurs are slight and do not need correction. More serious murmurs may require treatment.

A Congenital Heart Problem

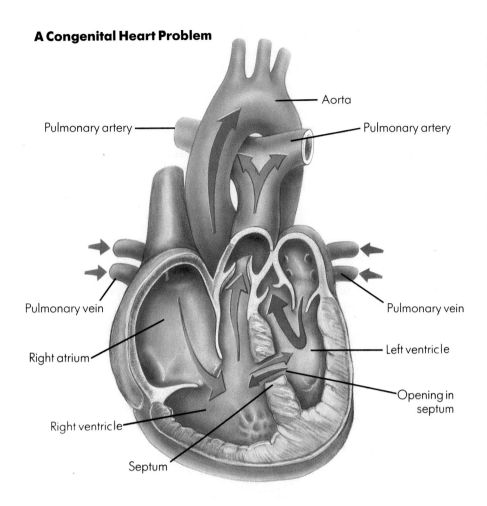

Aorta

Pulmonary artery

Pulmonary artery

Pulmonary vein

Pulmonary vein

Right atrium

Left ventricle

Opening in septum

Right ventricle

Septum

A common congenital heart problem involves an abnormal opening in the septum, the wall that divides the right and left chambers of the heart. The oxygen-rich blood in the left ventricle can mix with the deoxygenated blood in the right ventricle. The result is that blood circulating through the baby's body does not have the level of oxygen it needs. The baby will have a "bluish" appearance. This problem can be corrected surgically.

Varicose Veins

Varicose veins are swollen and enlarged veins, especially in the legs. Varicose veins develop when the valves in the veins are weakened. This condition may affect both sexes and all ages. Some people inherit the tendency to develop varicose veins. Other contributing factors include the following:

- prolonged periods of standing
- obesity
- pregnancy
- wearing very tight clothing
- aging, which can cause veins to lose their tone and elasticity

KEEPING FIT

Blood Donors

Requirements for blood donors vary from state to state. Generally there are minimum age and weight requirements. In addition, general good health is required and donors should not have active colds, sore throats, other infections, or have had recent surgery.

To find out about your state's requirements for donating blood call your local Red Cross chapter, hospital, or blood bank.

Blood flow in the veins from the legs to the heart goes against gravity. When the valves in the veins are weak, they cannot close tightly to prevent the backflow of blood. Blood then collects in the veins. As a result, veins become dilated and valves cannot function efficiently. This condition can be very painful.

Exercise is not only a means of prevention but also a recommended treatment for varicose veins. Through exercise, circulation in the legs and back to the heart is improved. Exercise also massages the walls of the veins and helps them regain their elasticity. If necessary, final treatment is surgical removal, or stripping, of the veins.

Thrombosis

Thrombosis is the presence or formation of a blood clot within a blood vessel. A blood clot, called a thrombus, occasionally occurs in blood vessels, and usually remains attached to its place of origin. Clots can interfere with blood flow through the vessels.

A clot that becomes dislodged from its place of origin is called an **embolus.** An embolus can travel to other parts of the body, blocking important blood vessels. A coronary embolism is the result of an embolus that blocks an artery in the heart. A pulmonary embolism results when an embolus blocks a blood vessel in the lungs. Clots in the arteries to the brain cause a stroke. When the brain's supply of oxygen is blocked, brain cells are damaged.

Anemia

Anemia is a condition caused by a deficiency of red blood cells or by a low concentration of hemoglobin in the red cells. With a low level of hemoglobin, body cells do not receive a sufficient amount of oxygen. Treatment depends on the specific cause. The three main causes are as follows:

- a serious loss of blood
- a decrease in the production of red blood cells because of malfunctioning red bone marrow
- a nutritional deficiency, such as a lack of iron in the diet

Red blood cells are normally round. Sickle cells have a crescent shape because of the action of the hemoglobin they contain.

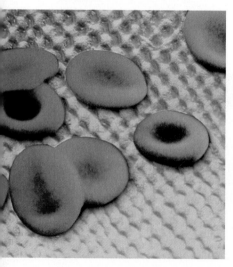

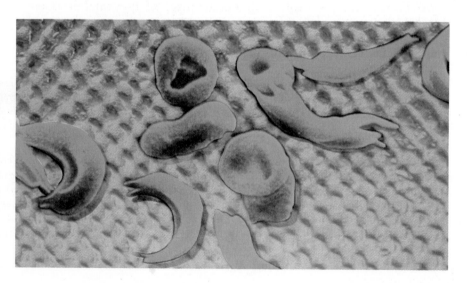

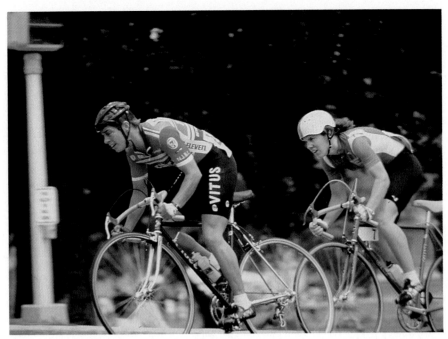

Culturally Speaking

Hemoglobin, Malaria, and Sickle-Cell Anemia

Hemoglobin has a variety of forms. Most variations of hemoglobin occur in areas where malaria is a constant threat. Geneticists suggest that these different hemoglobins provide protection against malaria by making the red blood cells poor hosts for the protozoa that cause the disease. The protozoa enter the blood when a person is bitten by an *Anopheles* mosquito.

Hemoglobin "HbS" causes sickle-cell anemia if a child inherits the gene from both parents. The HbS gene is common throughout Africa.

Sickle-Cell Anemia

Sickle-cell anemia is an inherited condition, resulting from a defect in the hemoglobin within red blood cells. The red blood cells develop a sickle shape and clump together, obstructing blood flow to the tissues. This obstruction leads to the death of tissues because they are deprived of oxygen. The symptoms of sickle-cell anemia are severe joint and abdominal pain, weakness, and chronic kidney disease. There is no cure for sickle-cell anemia. However, it can be treated with blood transfusions and pain-relieving medicines.

Leukemia

Leukemia is a type of cancer that is the result of abnormal production of one or more types of white blood cells. These cells are immature and are not able to help fight pathogens. A person with leukemia is highly

---

KEEPING FIT

Leg Pain: When Calves Speak

Leg pain can be caused by many factors, many of them not serious. However, some leg pain may indicate hardening of the arteries, which can put a person at increased risk of heart attack or stroke. Blocked arteries cannot supply needed blood to the body's extremities, and pain results.

If a parent or grandparent shows the following signs, urge him or her to see a doctor:

- pain that occurs when walking
- pain that occurs after walking
- pain that increases with distance walked
- pain that stops when standing or after a short rest

LOOKING AT TECHNOLOGY

Some Heartening News About Hearts

There are many new technological advances that are now available or are soon to be available to people with heart diseases and disorders.

■ Blood and urine tests are now available to quickly alert doctors to which high blood pressure patients are most likely to have heart attacks.

■ Doppler ultrasound is now being used by cardiologists to show trouble in blood vessels before they develop into major problems. The test, which uses sound waves, is less expensive and faster than other methods of diagnosis.

■ Clotbusters, medicines given to heart attack victims right after their attacks, can prevent much of the damage associated with the attacks.

■ The use of aspirin, given immediately following a heart attack, has been found to be helpful in preventing thrombus formation for some patients. Aspirin decreases the tendency of blood platelet cells to adhere to the blood vessel walls. Some studies show that aspirin therapy may be more effective in men than in women.

■ Heart-defibrillators are now being used in some locations by fire fighters, lifeguards, and police. The devices, which administer electric shocks to heart attack victims on the scene before medical help can arrive, have already saved many lives. New plans to place them in sports arenas, schools, and other public places are now being considered.

■ Atherectomy is a new, less expensive, and less complicated way of removing blockages in arteries and blood vessels. Guided by an X-ray image, a stiff tube is inserted into the blocked area. Then, a small tool similar to a drill is threaded into the blocked area, and the plaque causing the blockage is shaved or chipped away. The procedure may be a better alternative to angioplasty, the balloon technique now used to clean out arteries, which tend to narrow again.

■ The ventricular assist device, now being tested, is a permanently implanted device that mechanically takes on the work of the heart's major pumping chamber.

■ Total artificial heart is a mechanical pump that will be available within 20 years to replace damaged hearts. Unlike earlier heart replacements, this one will not have to be connected to tubes or wires running outside the patient's body. Instead, electrical impulses sent through the skin to implanted receivers will do the work that the heart once was able to do.

susceptible to infection. In addition, the large numbers of white blood cells interfere with red cell and platelet production. Leukemia can result in the following conditions:

■ anemia and a general feeling of being tired resulting from lack of red blood cells

- abnormal bleeding from cuts or bruises, caused by insufficient platelets to help clot the blood
- general openness to infection, since the white blood cells that stimulate antibody production are underproduced

The causes of leukemia, the most common type of cancer in children, are largely unknown. Some subtypes of the disease seem to be genetic; others may be traced to a virus.

Bone marrow transplants have been very successful in treating some types of leukemia. Certain medicines and radiation may slow down the rate of the disease. However, the death rate is still high.

Hemophilia

Hemophilia is an inherited disease in which a clotting factor is absent or abnormal. This causes the blood to clot very slowly or not at all. A person who has hemophilia can bleed to death very easily. Treatment involves giving the patient an injection of the clotting factor. If too much blood is lost, a complete transfusion may be done.

Care of Your Cardiovascular System

Most of the risk factors related to cardiovascular problems are within your control. Your choices and behaviors affect the health of your cardiovascular system.

You probably know that smoking puts added stress on the cardiovascular system. Nicotine in cigarettes increases blood pressure and heart rate. Not smoking as well as avoiding the smoke of others is a healthy choice. Being overweight causes the heart to pump more blood through more blood vessels. It's important to eat a healthy diet. Limiting your intake of foods high in fat, cholesterol, and salt will protect both your heart and blood vessels. In addition, a regular exercise program will strengthen the heart, making it work more efficiently. Exercise will also help circulation. Finally, having regular medical checkups enables your doctor to monitor the health of your cardiovascular system and encourage healthy behaviors.

CONFLICT RESOLUTION

Although heart disease is the number one killer of both males and females, it tends to affect females later in life. This fact often results in a myth that females don't get heart disease. This myth is one reason researchers routinely have omitted females from heart-disease studies.

How does this gender bias in research put females' health at risk?

LESSON 2 REVIEW

Reviewing Facts and Vocabulary

1. Define two problems of the cardiovascular system.
2. Explain how a defective valve in the heart could affect blood flow.

Thinking Critically

3. **Analysis.** Compare a thrombus and an embolus.

Applying Health Knowledge

4. Make a list of health behaviors you practice to promote care of your cardiovascular system. Make a separate list of additional behaviors that you want to practice. Write an essay describing how you plan to care for your cardiovascular system now, in 10 years, and in 20 years.

THE LYMPHATIC SYSTEM

The cardiovascular system moves blood throughout the body to nourish cells and remove waste products. The lymphatic system transports a fluid called lymph. **Lymph** is a clear yellow fluid that fills spaces around cells. Lymph is present in all body tissues.

Functions of the Lymphatic System

Your lymphatic system helps your body maintain your body's fluid balance by carrying excess fluid away from tissues. Lymph moves through lymphatic vessels and returns to your bloodstream. If this fluid were to remain in the spaces around cells, swelling of your tissues would result. This system also helps your body defend itself against pathogens.

Structure of the Lymphatic System

The lymphatic system consists of lymphatic vessels, lymph nodes, lymph, and lymphocytes. The spleen, tonsils, and thymus gland also play a part in the functioning of the lymphatic system.

Lymphatic vessels are distributed throughout the body much the same as blood vessels. Lymphatic vessels form a network that carries lymph to two lymph ducts, one in the neck area and the other in the chest area. These ducts empty into veins of the cardiovascular system.

At certain places in the body, lymph passes through lymph nodes. **Lymph nodes** are masses of tissues that filter lymph before it returns to the blood. They are located along lymph vessels, mostly in the neck, groin, and armpits. **Lymphocytes** are a type of white blood cell that multiply in lymph nodes and lymph tissue to destroy invading pathogens.

Types of Lymphocytes

There are two main types of lymphocytes—T cells and B cells. T cells are produced in bone marrow and are transported to the thymus gland, which is located behind the sternum. T cells can release a toxin that weakens a pathogen so that it can be ingested. T helper cells are a type of T cell. These cells stimulate the other type of lymphocyte, B cells, to produce antibodies that destroy or neutralize invading pathogens. Antibodies help destroy pathogens. They can attach themselves to pathogens so that they can be ingested by white blood cells.

Lymphatic Organs

Have you ever been sick and felt swollen areas just below your ears? You were feeling swollen lymph nodes. They swell when the body is fighting an infection and producing more lymphocytes.

The Lymphatic System

Lymph vessels are present in most body tissues.

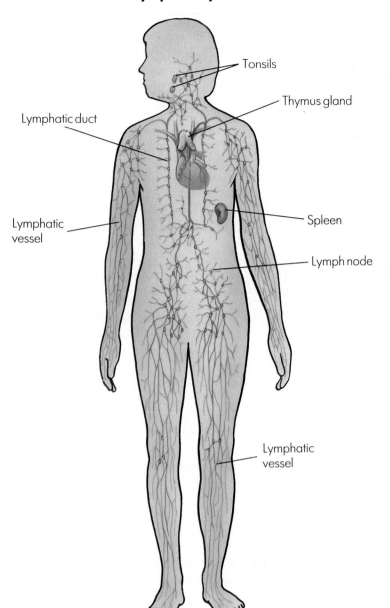

Tonsils

Thymus gland

Lymphatic duct

Lymphatic vessel

Spleen

Lymph node

Lymphatic vessel

The spleen is an organ located slightly behind the stomach on the left side of the body. The spleen plays an important role in keeping the blood free of foreign substances and also in storing B cells.

Tonsils are a mass of lymphatic tissue in the back of the throat. The adenoids are similar masses. Tonsils and adenoids trap and filter out pathogens that enter the body through the mouth and nose. When the body has been invaded by pathogens, the tonsils swell as they produce lymphocytes to kill the pathogens.

The thymus gland produces lymphocytes in infants and children and is important in the development of the body's defense system.

Problems of the Lymphatic System

Several problems can affect the lymphatic system. Some can usually be cured; others have no cure.

DID YOU KNOW?

- A study at the University of Virginia suggests that colds are more likely spread by fingers and hands (skin-to-skin contact) than through sneezes or coughs. Hand washing, then, might be the best preventive measure when someone in your family has a cold.
- A hefty allergic sneeze can throw water particles out across the room at speeds up to 100 miles an hour.

Tonsillitis

Tonsils can become infected even when they are helping to fight infections in other parts of the body. When they are infected, tonsils become inflamed and tender. Symptoms are a sore throat and fever. Infected tonsils may be treated with antibiotics. In some cases, tonsils are surgically removed.

Hodgkin's Disease

Hodgkin's disease is cancer of lymph tissue. The cancer cells spread quickly through the lymphatic system. Hodgkin's disease is treated with radiation for localized areas and chemotherapy when the disease has spread. The cure rate is high for localized areas.

Immune Deficiency

Your body protects itself against anything that might enter it and cause it harm. T cells are an important part of that defense system. T cells stimulate B cells to produce antibodies that fight pathogens and give you immunity to many diseases. If there is any disruption of T cell activity, an immune deficiency results.

For example, HIV, the virus that causes AIDS, destroys T cells. As a result, a person who has been infected with HIV cannot fight other pathogens effectively. An HIV-infected person will eventually develop AIDS. However, in the meantime, he or she will have many infections that would ordinarily be controlled by a healthy defense system. Eventually, one of these infections will cause the person to die.

Care of the Lymphatic System

Taking care of your lymphatic system involves helping your body fight disease. This means making sure that you care for your total health by eating properly, exercising regularly, and getting enough sleep. Having regular medical checkups and staying up-to-date on your immunizations are other important steps you can take.

LESSON 3 REVIEW

Reviewing Facts and Vocabulary

1. Describe the function of lymphocytes.
2. What are the functions of the lymphatic system?

Thinking Critically

3. **Analysis.** Compare the components of the lymphatic system.

Applying Health Knowledge

4. Gather statistics and information about Hodgkin's disease. What age groups are affected? What are the rates of recovery?

THE RESPIRATORY SYSTEM

While reading this paragraph, you will inhale two or three times without even thinking about it. Have you ever counted the number of times you inhale in a minute?

Functions of the Respiratory System

Respiration is the exchange of gases between you and your environment. There are two major parts to respiration. **External respiration** is the exchange of oxygen and carbon dioxide between the blood and the air in the lungs. As you breathe, you inhale air that contains oxygen into your lungs. Oxygen moves from your lungs to your blood. Carbon dioxide moves from your blood to your lungs. **Internal respiration** is the exchange of gases between the blood and the body cells. Oxygen moves from your blood to your cells. Carbon dioxide moves from your cells to your blood. Without the oxygen you could live only a few minutes.

Structure of the Respiratory System

The main parts of the respiratory system are the nasal cavity, pharynx, larynx, trachea, bronchi, and lungs.

The Nasal Cavity

Air enters the body primarily through the nasal cavity, which is the inner nose. Here the air is warmed and cleaned by mucous membranes and tiny hairs called cilia that line the nose. The mucous membranes also secrete mucus, which adds moisture to the air. All the upper air passages are lined with mucous membranes.

The Pharynx and the Larynx

From the nasal cavity, air moves through the **pharynx,** or throat, the **larynx,** or voice box, and into the **trachea,** or windpipe. The larynx contains two pairs of ligaments called vocal cords. As air passes over these cords, the cords vibrate and sound is produced.

The epiglottis is a flap of tissue that covers the larynx. When you swallow, it closes, covering the opening of the larynx. This covering prevents solids and liquids from getting into your larynx and trachea. The epiglottis opens when you breathe to allow air to pass into the lungs.

The Trachea and the Bronchi

The trachea is lined with a mucous membrane and covered with cilia. Cilia are in constant movement, keeping foreign particles from reaching

---

LESSON 4 FOCUS

TERMS TO USE
- External respiration
- Internal respiration
- Pharynx (FAIR•inks)
- Larynx (LAIR•inks)
- Trachea (TRAY•key•uh)
- Bronchi
- Diaphragm (DIE•uh•FRAM)

CONCEPTS TO LEARN
- Respiration takes place at different levels within the body.
- Respiration is the exchange of gases between you and your environment.
- Polluted factors in the environment negatively affect the quality of respiration.
- Respiration is vital to life.

ATTITUDES AND BEHAVIORS TO EVALUATE
- Self-Inventory, page 270.
- Building Decision-Making Skills, page 271.

The air you inhale is cleaned, moistened, and warmed as it moves through the upper respiratory passages.

Upper Respiratory System

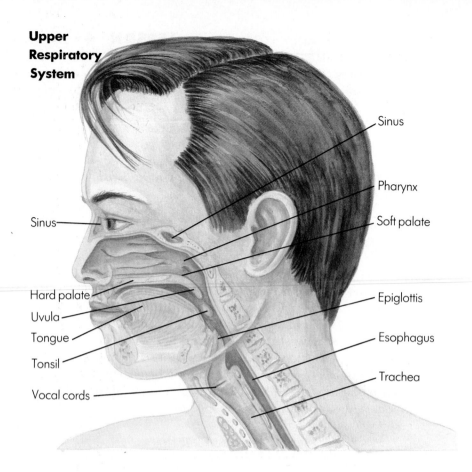

Sinus

Pharynx

Soft palate

Sinus

Hard palate

Uvula

Tongue

Tonsil

Vocal cords

Epiglottis

Esophagus

Trachea

the lungs. The trachea extends into the chest area and divides into two branches called **bronchi,** or bronchial tubes that lead into the lungs.

The Lungs

The lungs are two cone-shaped organs that are enclosed and protected within two layers of membranes, called pleura. Each lung is divided into sections called lobes. There are three lobes in the right lung and two lobes in the left lung. Within the lungs, each bronchus divides and then subdivides, forming a network of tubes that resemble tree branches. These divisions of the bronchial tubes are called bronchioles.

At the end of each bronchiole is a cluster of thin-walled air sacs called alveoli. There are about 300 million alveoli in the lungs.

The alveoli are covered with a vast network of capillaries. Thin capillary walls and equally thin alveolar walls allow the exchange of oxygen and carbon dioxide to take place.

Air is constantly being drawn into and expelled from the lungs by successive changes in pressure within the chest. However, the lungs do not do this work—the diaphragm and chest cavity do. The movement of air into and out of the lungs is regulated by changes in air pressure—both within the lungs and outside the body. Muscles in the rib cage and the diaphragm make this movement possible. The **diaphragm** is a muscle that separates the chest and abdominal cavities.

When you inhale, your rib muscles and diaphragm contract. The diaphragm moves downward and the ribs are pulled upward and outward. This action enlarges the chest cavity, creating lower pressure in

DID YOU KNOW?

- About 44 million Americans suffer from allergies and asthma.
- About 11 million have asthma, including 3 million children.
- About half a million people are admitted to hospitals in the U.S. each year because of asthma.
- Between 50 percent and 90 percent of the people with asthma have asthma that is caused by allergies.
- The number of asthma-related deaths in the U.S. has doubled over the past 20 years.

the lungs. Air rushes into the lungs to equalize the pressure between the lungs and the outside environment.

Just the reverse happens when you exhale. The diaphragm relaxes, moving upward, and the ribs move inward, increasing the pressure within the lungs. Air moves from the higher pressure within the lungs to the outside environment where the pressure is lower.

Problems of the Respiratory System

The respiratory system is a common site of infection in the body. Pathogens have easy access into the body through the mouth and nose. Colds and sore throats are common problems with the upper respiratory tract. More serious respiratory infections are those that affect the lower respiratory tract. These include bronchitis, pneumonia, pleurisy, bronchial asthma, tuberculosis, and emphysema.

Bronchitis

Bronchitis is an inflammation of the lining of the bronchial tubes. Bronchitis can be either acute or chronic.

Acute bronchitis often develops as a result of a severe cold. A person usually experiences fever and coughing. Acute bronchitis can last for several weeks.

Chronic bronchitis is a longer-lasting, recurring disease. It can get progressively worse. A person may experience long coughing spasms, shortness of breath, wheezing, and long-lasting colds. Most important in the treatment of chronic bronchitis is avoiding respiratory irritants, such as dust, fumes, smoke, or other air pollutants.

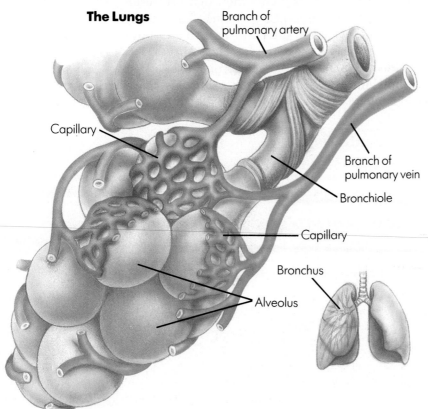

The Lungs

Branch of pulmonary artery

Capillary

Branch of pulmonary vein

Bronchiole

Capillary

Bronchus

Alveolus

The alveoli are surrounded by a network of capillaries. External respiration takes place in the alveoli.

Pneumonia

Pneumonia is an infection of an area of the lungs. Pneumonia can be caused by bacteria or viruses. The infection may involve parts of the lungs, such as the bronchioles or an entire section or lobe.

Pneumonia often affects a person whose resistance is already low because of another illness. Bronchial pneumonia causes difficult and painful breathing. A person may also have a severe cough. Medical care is important because of the risk of complications and the possibility of a recurrence.

Lobar pneumonia is an infection affecting one or more lobes of the lungs. Prior chronic respiratory or heart disease, poor nutrition, alcoholism, and exposure to sudden changes in temperature are all factors that make a person more susceptible to developing this type of pneumonia. Chills, high fever, coughing, chest pains, and difficult breathing are all symptoms of lobar pneumonia. Because this disease can have serious complications, medical treatment is important. Hospitalization is often necessary.

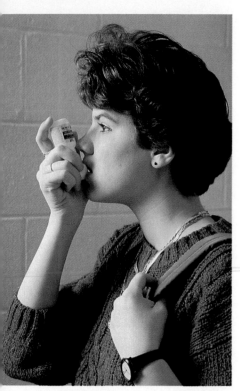

A bronchodilator helps reduce the swelling and production of mucus in the bronchial tubes of someone with asthma.

Pleurisy

Pleurisy is an inflammation of the pleural membrane, a double-wall lining that covers the lungs. Pleurisy usually results as a complication from another disease, such as pneumonia. A person may experience shortness of breath and sharp pains in the chest.

Bronchial Asthma

Bronchial asthma is a condition that can result from a sensitivity to pollen, dust, certain foods, or animal hair. Strong emotional responses also can bring on the attack of bronchial asthma. These irritants and emotional stresses cause the linings of the bronchioles to produce large amounts of thick mucus. The bronchioles constrict and breathing is difficult. An attack of bronchial asthma is characterized by wheezing and coughing as air moves through the narrowed bronchioles.

Tuberculosis

Tuberculosis is an infectious bacterial disease of the lungs characterized by the growth of tubercles, or nodules, on the lungs. Tuberculosis

---

K E E P I N G   F I T

Posture and Breathing

When you stand erect, sit erect, or walk erect, you give the breathing mechanisms in your body the best opportunity to do their work. By slouching, you hinder efficient breathing. Practice sitting with your back straight in a chair that supports your head and back. Stand with your head up, neck straight, shoulders down and back, stomach and buttocks in, but hold yourself naturally, not stiffly. Also try standing with your arms down at your sides, then inhaling deeply as you raise your arms outstretched to shoulder level. Breathe out fully as you lower your arms.

bacteria attack the alveoli and cause inflammation of tissues and organs. Symptoms include fever, weakness, loss of appetite, and severe coughing. Chest X rays detect tuberculosis, which used to be one of the principal causes of death. Most cases of tuberculosis can be treated successfully with antibiotics. However, medicine-resistant forms of tuberculosis have recently become more prevalent.

Emphysema

Emphysema is a disorder that causes the alveoli to disintegrate and to lose their elasticity, making it difficult for air to pass out of the lungs. The normal exchange of carbon dioxide and oxygen in the alveoli is disrupted. This condition cannot be reversed. Emphysema is caused by breathing in foreign matter such as smoke and smog particles over a long period of time. Inhaled smoke from burning cigarettes is the primary cause of emphysema. Symptoms include difficult breathing and coughing.

Care of the Respiratory System

Since the respiratory system is highly susceptible to infection, you should pay close attention to any nasal or sinus condition, or to coughing or wheezing that lasts more than a few days. Hoarseness or loss of voice can also be a sign of a respiratory infection.

Try to keep nasal passages open during a cold or respiratory infection. Keep in mind that respiratory passages are very delicate. Avoid blowing your nose too hard or trying to hold back a cough or sneeze.

A regular program of exercise helps keep the lungs working efficiently. Exercise strengthens the lungs and helps keep the other parts of the respiratory system clear. Avoiding polluted air, as well as never smoking yourself, help promote the health of your respiratory system.

LESSON 4 REVIEW

Reviewing Facts and Vocabulary

1. What function does the nasal cavity serve as part of the respiratory system?
2. Describe the process that takes place in the alveoli.
3. What is the difference between acute and chronic bronchitis?

Thinking Critically

4. **Analysis.** Compare external and internal respiration.

Applying Health Knowledge

5. Interview three smokers and three non-smokers. Ask them how often they experience respiratory infections, sore throats, and colds. Draw some conclusions.

Self-Inventory

Care of the Cardiovascular and Respiratory Systems

HOW DO YOU RATE?

Number a sheet of paper from 1 through 20. Read each item below, and respond by writing *always*, *sometimes*, or *never* for each item. Total the number of each type of response. Then proceed to the next section.

1. I eat a well-balanced diet.
2. I get at least 20 minutes of aerobic exercise 3 times a week.
3. I manage the stress in my life.
4. I avoid foods high in fat.
5. I limit the amount of salt I put on my food.
6. I do not smoke.
7. I avoid breathing in others' smoke.
8. I stay within 5 pounds (2.2 kg) of my ideal weight.
9. I regularly have my blood pressure checked.
10. I know my cholesterol level.
11. I avoid foods high in cholesterol.
12. I eat foods rich in iron (liver, green leafy vegetables, dried fruits, enriched cereals) daily.
13. I study or work in a well-ventilated area.
14. I sleep 7 to 8 hours every night.
15. I keep records of my immunizations.
16. My immunizations are up-to-date.
17. When possible, I avoid pollen, dust, and animal hair.
18. When I have a choice, I ask for a seat in the nonsmoking section in a restaurant.
19. I avoid blowing my nose too hard when I have a cold.
20. I don't try to hold back a cough or sneeze.

HOW DID YOU SCORE?

Give yourself 2 points for every *always* answer, 1 point for every *sometimes* answer, and 0 points for every *never* answer. Find your total, and read below to see how you scored. Then proceed to the next section.

26 to 40
Excellent. Your health choices show you are taking care of your cardiovascular and respiratory systems.

11 to 25
Good. Your health choices are good, but you could work to better promote a healthy cardiovascular and respiratory system.

Below 11
Look out! You may be taking unnecessary risks that could affect the health of your cardiovascular and respiratory systems.

WHAT ARE YOUR GOALS?

Identify an area in which your score was low, and use the goal-setting process to begin making a change.

1. The behavior I would like to change or improve is ____.
2. If this behavior were completely changed, I would look, feel, or act differently in the following ways: ____.
3. The steps involved in making this change are ____.
4. My timetable for accomplishing this change is ____.
5. People I will ask for support or assistance are ____.
6. The benefits I will receive are ____.
7. My reward at the end of each week will be ____.

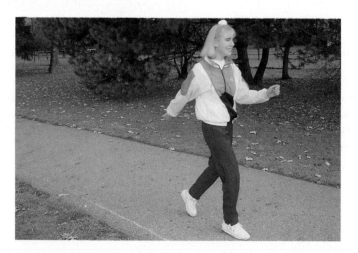

Building Decision-Making Skills

T omorrow is the school blood drive, which is part of a competition between schools in the area to see who can donate the most blood to send to victims of the disaster in the next county. Chung, the captain of the football team, really supports the cause. In fact, he personally knows people who will benefit from the drive. His friends are all signing up and encouraging him to join them. He just turned 17 and this is the first year he is eligible to donate. Although he is really queasy about the whole idea, he feels pressure from his friends to be "macho" and to participate in this blood drive.

WHAT DO YOU THINK?

1. **Situation.** Why do you think Chung feels the pressure to donate?

2. **Situation.** What questions do you think Chung might have about donating blood?

3. **Situation.** Where might Chung find out what it's really like to donate blood?

4. **Choices.** What are Chung's choices?

5. **Choices.** If Chung decides not to participate in the blood drive, what choices does he have for handling the situation?

6. **Consequences.** What are the pros and cons of each choice?

7. **Consequences.** How might Chung's self-esteem be affected by this decision?

8. **Consequences.** How might his peers be affected by this decision?

9. **Consequences.** How might his family be affected by this decision?

10. **Consequences.** What's the worst thing that might happen to Chung if he donates blood? How could he prepare for these possibilities?

11. **Consequences.** What positive outcome can he expect from donating blood?

12. **Decision.** What do you think Chung should do? Explain your answer.

13. **Evaluation.** How will he know if he made a good decision?

B enson knows that his friend has high blood pressure, but every day at lunch his group ends up going to a fast-food restaurant that serves all "the wrong kinds of food." His friend also eats desserts that only add to his weight problem, and thus, his blood pressure problem. Benson wants to help his friend.

WHAT DO YOU THINK?

14. **Choices.** What might Benson do to help his friend? What can't Benson do to help his friend?

15. **Consequences.** What are the advantages of each choice?

16. **Consequences.** What are the disadvantages of each choice?

17. **Consequences.** What risks are involved in this decision?

18. **Consequences.** How might Benson's health triangle be affected by this decision?

19. **Consequences.** How might the friend's health triangle be affected by this decision?

20. **Decision.** What should Benson do? How should he implement the decision?

21. **Decision.** How might Benson handle the situation if he makes a suggestion and his friend refuses to accept it?

22. **Evaluation.** Have you ever been in a similar situation? How did you handle it? What did you learn that could be applied to this situation?

REVIEW

Using Health Terms

On a separate sheet of paper, write the term that best matches each definition given below.

LESSON 1
1. The force of blood on blood vessel walls.
2. Blood component made up of protein and iron and carried in red blood cells.
3. Small fibers produced by platelets that trap red blood cells and form a clot.
4. Circulation through the lungs.

LESSON 2
5. A blood clot that becomes dislodged from its place of origin.
6. Term that means "occurring at birth."
7. An abnormal sound in the heart.
8. Presence of a blood clot in a blood vessel.

LESSON 3
9. Fluid that enters lymphatic capillaries before returning to the blood.
10. Masses of tissues that filter lymph.
11. White blood cells that multiply in lymph tissues to destroy pathogens.
12. Cancer of the lymph nodes.

LESSON 4
13. Membranes that line the nasal cavity.
14. A flap of tissue that covers the larynx.
15. Breathing too quickly, thereby lowering the level of carbon dioxide in the blood.
16. Muscle that separates the chest cavity from the abdomen.

Building Academic Skills

LESSON 1
17. **Math.** If your heart beats 70 times a minute, and pumps 5 quarts of blood each minute, how many pints, quarts, and gallons of blood would your heart pump in 34 minutes? How many in the course of a 7-hour school day? During exercise, if your heart pumps 20 quarts per minute, how many pints, quarts, and gallons of blood would your heart pump in 47 minutes?

Recalling the Facts

LESSON 1
18. What is plasma?
19. What are the functions of the blood?
20. Describe two types of circulation.
21. What are the chambers called in the human heart?
22. Why are platelets important to your health?
23. Why is it important to know your blood type?
24. What are the components of blood and what function does each one serve?

LESSON 2
25. How can one lower his or her risk of heart disease?
26. What causes varicose veins?
27. Describe two conditions that are examples of congenital heart disease.
28. Explain why sickle-cell anemia is a serious condition.

LESSON 3
29. Explain the function of the lymphatic system.
30. List the organs that make up the lymphatic system.
31. How can one care for his or her lymphatic system?
32. Why do lymph nodes swell when a person has an infection?

LESSON 4
33. What are the functions of mucous membranes and tiny hairs in the nose?
34. What are causes and symptoms of hyperventilation?
35. What are some respiratory irritants?
36. Name and briefly describe three serious respiratory infections.
37. What regulates the movement of air in and out of the lungs?
38. Explain why food does not usually get into the trachea.
39. What are the main parts of the respiratory system?
40. What causes sound when you speak?

REVIEW

Thinking Critically

LESSON 1

41. Synthesis. If a person who has blood type B and is Rh-positive needs a transfusion, what types of blood can he or she safely be given? To what types could this person safely donate blood? What if the person is type A and Rh-negative? What types could this person safely be given? To what types could he or she donate blood?

LESSON 2

42. Synthesis. How might suffering from anemia affect your life?

43. Evaluation. When one suffers from leukemia, it is sometimes necessary to have a bone marrow transplant in order to survive. A blood relative is often the best match for a successful transplant. In order to obtain such a match, parents have been known to have a baby to save their other child's life. The hope is that the new baby's bone marrow would exactly match that of the leukemia patient. What do you think about this situation and all the implications for the leukemia sufferer, the parents, and the baby?

LESSON 3

44. Analysis. What is the relationship between the cardiovascular and lymphatic systems?

LESSON 4

45. Evaluation. Some workplaces are smoke-free. What are some advantages and disadvantages of this policy? Judge the appropriateness of such a policy.

46. Analysis. What is the difference between external and internal respiration?

Making the Connection

LESSON 1

47. Math. Compare survival rates of various kinds of leukemia a generation ago with those today. Prepare a bar graph that shows your findings. Interpret these statistics and suggest reasons for the changes.

Applying Health Knowledge

LESSON 1

48. Take your heart rate by counting your pulse for 10 seconds and multiplying by 6. This is your heart rate for a minute. The average heart rate is 72. How does your heart rate compare? What might affect your heart rate?

49. Give three situations in which one's sympathetic nervous system might speed up one's heart rate.

50. What can a person do to keep his or her blood pressure normal?

LESSON 2

51. When might medical personnel type a person's blood?

52. Categorize the following food items as being generally healthy or unhealthy for your heart: potato chips, broccoli, cheese, apple pie, coffee, fish, bagels, butter.

LESSON 3

53. What might happen if one's lymphatic system shut down?

LESSON 4

54. Research the respiratory infection known as walking pneumonia. What is it and why is it called that?

55. When one stops smoking, the lungs begin to improve. What implications does this have for smokers?

Beyond the Classroom

LESSON 1

56. Further Study. Identify a health agency that focuses on some aspect of cardiovascular disease or fitness. Find out what this organization does for public education.

LESSON 4

57. Community Involvement. Interview a number of people to find out what home remedies they have heard of or use to cure hiccups. Compile a report reflecting what you have learned.

CHAPTER 14

DIGESTIVE AND URINARY SYSTEMS

LESSON 1
The Digestive System

LESSON 2
Problems and Care of the Digestive System

LESSON 3
The Urinary System

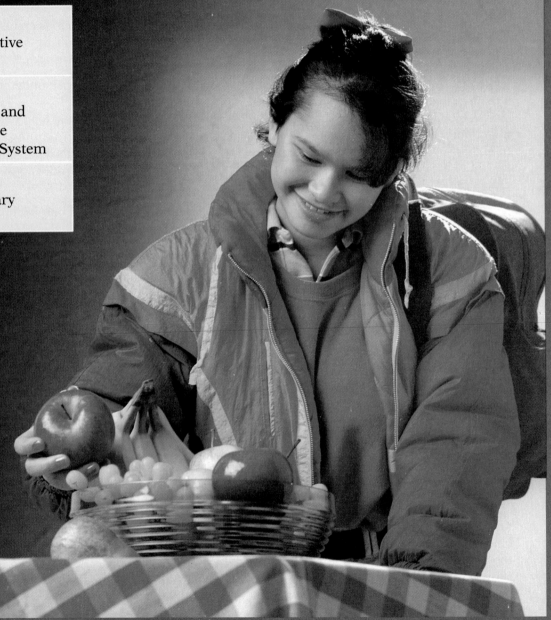

THE DIGESTIVE SYSTEM

Digestion is the breaking down of food into simpler substances to be carried in the blood to body cells. This process is both mechanical and chemical. The mechanical portion involves chewing, mashing, and breaking food into smaller pieces. The chemical portion involves changing food into simpler substances by digestive enzymes. Enzymes are proteins that affect the rate of many body processes. Digestive enzymes speed up the breakdown of food. Many enzymes are produced in the body.

Functions of the Digestive System

The digestive system performs three different functions:

- The first is **digestion**—the physical and chemical breakdown of foods into smaller pieces.
- The second is **absorption**—the passage of digested food from the digestive tract into the circulatory system.
- The third is **elimination**—the expulsion of undigested food or body wastes.

Structure of the Digestive System

Digestion takes place in the gastrointestinal tract, which includes the mouth, esophagus, stomach, small intestine, and large intestine.

The Mouth and Teeth

Food enters the gastrointestinal tract through the mouth, which is lined with many nerve endings that respond to heat, cold, pain, and pressure. The mouth is the only part of the digestive system that has this sensitivity.

What happens when you take a bite of pizza or hamburger? The teeth and the tongue make the first contact. The primary function of teeth is to break the food into smaller pieces. This process of chewing, called **mastication,** prepares the food to be swallowed.

The Salivary Glands

Secretions are added to food as it moves through the digestive tract. This process starts in the mouth. Three pairs of salivary glands secrete saliva. Saliva is a watery solution that contains an enzyme that starts the digestion of carbohydrates.

Saliva softens and moistens food, making it easier to chew and swallow. Saliva cleanses the teeth and helps neutralize acids in the mouth. Saliva also helps keep the mouth moist and flexible, which is important for speech. The autonomic nervous system controls the secretion of saliva.

The Tongue

The tongue is a muscular organ that plays a primary role not only in tasting and speech, but also in chewing and swallowing. In order for you to recognize the flavor of a food, it must be in the form of a solution.

The velvetlike look of the tongue is a result of small projections, called papillae, that cover the tongue's surface. Taste buds, about 9,000 of

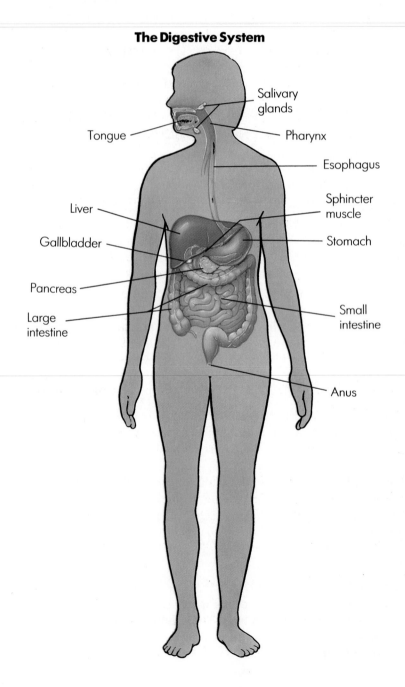

The Digestive System

Salivary glands

Tongue

Pharynx

Esophagus

Liver

Sphincter muscle

Gallbladder

Stomach

Pancreas

Large intestine

Small intestine

Anus

The organs of the digestive system form a continuous passageway.

them, cover the tongue but are most heavily concentrated around the papillae. There are at least four different kinds of taste buds. Each kind is located in a different area of the tongue. The four are sweet, sour, salty, and bitter.

Swallowing.   In your mouth your tongue forms the food into a ball to prepare for swallowing. Swallowing involves numerous muscles in your mouth and pharynx.

As you begin to swallow, the tip of the tongue slightly arches, pushing the food to the back of the mouth. The back of the tongue elevates, and a wave of muscular contractions passes over the tongue, forcing food into the pharynx.

At the same time, the uvula, a small muscular flap of tissue suspended at the back of the mouth, closes the opening to the nasal passages. The epiglottis, the flap of tissue covering the trachea, closes to keep the food from entering the respiratory system. However, if you talk or laugh while swallowing, the epiglottis will open and food may enter the windpipe. When this happens, you have a reflex response. You choke and cough to force the food out of the windpipe.

Your body has another built-in protection system to keep the food from entering the respiratory system. When you are swallowing, the nerve impulses that are responsible for breathing stop, making it almost impossible to swallow and breathe at the same time.

The Esophagus

When you swallow, food enters the esophagus, which is a muscular tube that extends from the pharynx to the stomach and is situated behind the trachea and heart. It is about 10 inches (25 cm) long. A series of involuntary muscular contractions—a process called **peristalsis**—moves food through the esophagus. It takes solid food about nine seconds to move through the esophagus. Food moves through the entire digestive tract as a result of peristalsis.

A sphincter muscle, which is a circular muscle at the entrance to the stomach, allows food to move from the esophagus into the stomach. When the muscle is relaxed, it forms an opening. When the muscle contracts, the opening closes. Sphincter muscles located along the digestive tract prevent food from backing up as it moves through the digestive process.

The Stomach

The stomach is a very muscular organ. Refer to the illustration on page 278 and note the three layers of muscles. The outer layer is longitudinal; the middle layer is circular; the inner layer is oblique, or at an angle.

The three main activities that take place in the stomach are listed below.

- temporary holding or storage of the food until it is ready to enter the small intestine
- mixing of the food and gastric juices together to form a substance called **chyme**
- control of the rate at which food enters the small intestine

- Though amounts may differ from person to person, on average, the human stomach can hold slightly more than one quart (0.9 l) of food.
- Any food that you eat takes a 30-foot (9.1-m) journey.
- The hydrochloric acid in your stomach is strong enough to dissolve razor blades. This acid works to destroy any bacteria in the food that reaches your stomach.

After a meal, food stays in the stomach for about three to four hours. The rate at which the stomach empties varies considerably. Liquids pass through rapidly. Solids remain until they are well-mixed with gastric juices. The stomach's capacity for food is about 1 quart (0.9 l).

The stomach is lined with mucous membranes and glands that secrete gastric juices. **Gastric juices** contain hydrochloric acid, digestive enzymes, and mucus. Gastric juices start the digestion of proteins.

As the stomach fills, muscular contractions churn and mix the food with gastric juices and move it toward the small intestine. The chyme moves into the small intestine as a result of peristalsis. Very little food is absorbed into the blood from the stomach. Food has not been broken down enough for absorption. However, some medicines and drugs, such as aspirin and alcohol, are absorbed into the blood from the stomach.

The Small Intestine

The major part of digestion and absorption occurs in the small intestine, which is about 20 feet (6 m) in length and 1 inch (2.5 cm) in diameter. It consists of three parts: the duodenum, the jejunum, and the ileum. Chyme enters the duodenum from the stomach. The ileum opens into the large intestine.

Peristalsis moves chyme through the small intestine at a relatively slow rate for approximately three to five hours. Chyme that enters the small intestine includes partially digested carbohydrates and proteins and undigested fats. Intestinal juices produced by glands in the lining of the small intestine, along with secretions from the liver and the pan-

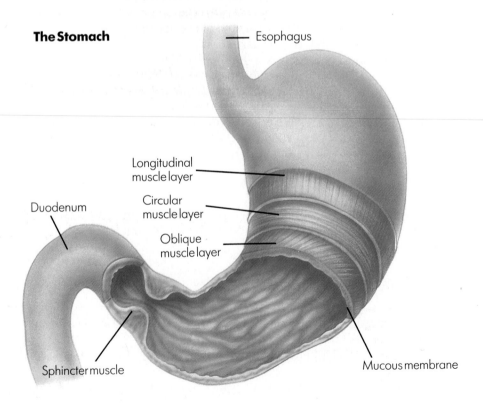

The Stomach

Esophagus

Longitudinal muscle layer

Circular muscle layer

Oblique muscle layer

Duodenum

Sphincter muscle

Mucous membrane

As the muscular wall of the stomach contracts and expands, chyme is formed as food mixes with gastric juices.

creas, complete the chemical breakdown of all food. You will learn more about the liver and pancreas later in this lesson.

The small intestine is lined with millions of fingerlike projections called villi. Each villus has a network of capillaries. Digested food particles are absorbed from the small intestine into the capillaries in the villi. Villi, especially those in the jejunum, increase the surface area for the absorption of digested food particles about 600 times. Food particles enter capillaries in the villi and are then carried throughout the body by the blood. Undigested food materials move by peristalsis into the large intestine.

The Large Intestine

The lower part of the digestive tract is the large intestine, or colon. It is about 2½ inches (6 cm) in diameter and 5 to 6 feet (1.5 to 1.8 m) long. Movement through the large intestine is very slow. The main functions of the large intestine are the absorption of water and the elimination of undigested food.

The undigested food that moves to the large intestine is in a very watery state. The walls of the large intestine absorb most of the water from the undigested food and return the water to the bloodstream. This action is important in maintaining the water balance in the body.

Many harmless bacteria normally live in the large intestine. They serve a useful purpose by acting on the undigested food. The action of the bacteria changes the consistency to a semisolid waste, called feces. Feces pass from the body through the anus, as a bowel movement.

Organs That Help Digestion

The liver, the gallbladder, and the pancreas are organs that contribute to the digestive process. Juices are secreted into the digestive tract that are essential for completing the digestion of carbohydrates, proteins, and fats.

The Liver.   Besides being the largest gland in the body, the liver is perhaps the most versatile. The liver of an average adult weighs about 3½ pounds (2 kg) and is a dark reddish-brown color. Scientists have identified over 500 functions of the liver.

K E E P I N G   F I T

Understanding Fiber

Soluble fiber, which dissolves in water, may lower cholesterol; insoluble fiber, which does not dissolve, may help protect you from colon cancer and other bowel problems. Though most fruits, vegetables, and grain products contain both kinds of fiber, some do not. Among the sources of soluble fiber are barley bran, oat bran, dried beans, and legumes; among the sources of insoluble fiber are wheat bran, corn bran, and nuts.

There are many delicious high-fiber foods and new sources of fiber on the market. To increase your fiber intake, why not try eating more popcorn, dried fruit, nuts, or beans?

When chyme enters the duodenum, the sphincter muscle relaxes and allows bile and pancreatic enzymes to enter the duodenum.

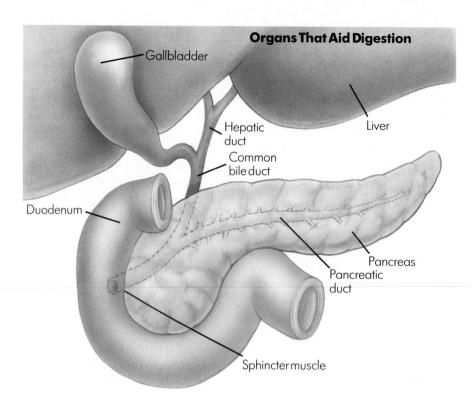

Organs That Aid Digestion

Gallbladder

Hepatic duct

Common bile duct

Liver

Duodenum

Pancreas

Pancreatic duct

Sphincter muscle

Following are six major functions of the liver:

■ The liver produces **bile**, a yellowish-green, bitter fluid important in the breakdown of fats. The liver secretes up to 1 quart (0.9 l) of bile daily. Bile flows to the gallbladder through the hepatic duct where it is stored.

■ The liver converts the sugar glucose to glycogen, which is a form of starch, and stores it until needed.

■ The liver helps maintain the level of glucose in the blood. When the blood glucose level falls, glycogen is converted to glucose and released into the blood.

■ The liver removes worn-out red blood cells as blood circulates.

■ The liver changes toxic waste materials, such as ammonia, into a less toxic substance—urea, the chief substance in urine.

■ The liver stores a variety of substances including vitamins A, D, E, K, and B_{12}, and minerals such as iron.

K E E P I N G   F I T

Medications and the Digestive Process

Americans spend millions of dollars a year for medications to aid in the digestive process. Much of this expenditure is a waste of money. Here is what you can do to help prevent problems and promote healthy digestion:

■ Chew your food thoroughly.
■ Eat slowly.
■ Eat a balanced diet.
■ Try to swallow your food without drinking liquids.
■ Drink five to six glasses of water daily.

■ Limit your intake of carbonated, acidic beverages.
■ Try not to eat too many fried or other greasy foods.
■ Avoid eating as a way of dealing with problems.
■ Stop eating before you feel full.

The Gallbladder. The gallbladder is a small sac 3 to 4 inches (7 to 10 cm) long that stores bile. It is located on the undersurface of the liver. The neck of the gallbladder forms a duct leading to the duodenum, the first section of the small intestine. The gallbladder stores bile until food moves into the duodenum from the stomach. A hormone produced in the small intestine stimulates the release of bile through the bile duct into the duodenum.

The Pancreas. Recall that the pancreas produces the hormone insulin as part of the endocrine system. As part of the digestive system, the pancreas produces three digestive enzymes: trypsin, which digests proteins; amylase, which digests carbohydrates; and lipase, which digests fats. These enzymes are released into the small intestine through a series of ducts.

HOW DO YOU KNOW WHEN TO EAT?

You have read about how food is digested in your body, but what signals you to put food into your body? This is regulated by two sensations—hunger, a craving for food, and appetite, a desire for a certain kind of food. The hypothalamus, which is a small area of the brain, is the control center for hunger.

One theory is that the hypothalamus is stimulated by the glucose level in your blood. Glucose is a kind of sugar. When the glucose level is low, a cluster of nerve cells in the hypothalamus is stimulated and sends out nerve impulses. You respond by eating to satisfy that hungry feeling.

As your stomach fills with food, the glucose level rises and another area of the hypothalamus is stimulated. This time, nerve impulses give you a feeling of fullness. You stop eating.

LESSON 1 REVIEW

Reviewing Facts and Vocabulary

1. Trace the path a bite of pizza follows until it is absorbed into the bloodstream.
2. Describe the three different functions of the digestive system.
3. Define the following terms and use each in a sentence: *digestive enzyme, papillae, saliva, peristalsis.*

Thinking Critically

4. **Analysis.** Support the following statement: "The real work of the digestive system is done in the small intestine."

5. **Synthesis.** Change the names of the different parts of the digestive system to parts of mechanical instruments or machines based on their actions.

Applying Health Knowledge

6. Prepare a chart that shows what happens to food once it leaves the stomach. Describe the function of each organ involved in the digestive process.
7. Select three organs in the digestive system and make a life-size model of each. Make a poster that describes each organ's function in the digestive process.

PROBLEMS AND CARE OF THE DIGESTIVE SYSTEM

LESSON 2 FOCUS

TERMS TO USE
- Indigestion
- Hiatal hernia
- Gallstones
- Peptic ulcers
- Gastritis
- Appendicitis
- Hepatitis

CONCEPTS TO LEARN
- Some digestive disorders are functional and can be prevented by avoiding certain situations or foods.
- A healthy digestive system is related to the practice of good eating habits.

ATTITUDES AND BEHAVIORS TO EVALUATE
- Self-Inventory, page 292.
- Building Decision-Making Skills, page 293.

The complex digestive system usually functions normally, digesting and absorbing food and eliminating undigested material. However, there are problems that are common to many people.

Common Functional Problems

Many digestive problems are related to eating habits and to the kinds of food eaten.

Halitosis

Halitosis, or bad breath, can result from disorders of the teeth or gums, from eating certain foods, and from using tobacco. The most frequent cause is poor oral health care. If daily brushing and flossing do not take care of halitosis, the cause may be a tooth or gum infection. A dentist can check that possible cause. Bad breath can also be the result of poor nutrition or of problems in the stomach or intestines. Contrary to the message given in advertisements, mints and mouthwashes do not prevent or cure halitosis, although they may cover up the odor.

Indigestion

Indigestion occurs when your body does not properly break down foods. It can be caused by stomach disorders, by eating too fast or too much, by eating certain foods, or by indulging in an excess of alcohol. Indigestion can also be caused by stress or can be a result of lactose intolerance. People with lactose intolerance do not have the enzyme that is needed to digest milk sugar, or lactose. Some symptoms of indigestion are cramps in the abdomen, a buildup of gas, and nausea.

Heartburn

Heartburn occurs when acid content from the stomach backs up into the esophagus. This backup can occur if the sphincter muscle between the esophagus and stomach does not close tightly. If a person has a **hiatal hernia,** a condition in which the upper part of the stomach pushes through the diaphragm, he or she may experience heartburn. If heartburn recurs or continues, a medical examination is necessary.

Gas

A certain amount of gas in the stomach or the intestines is normal. When a person has an excess amount of gas, it can be very uncomfortable. Certain foods seem to be gas-forming for some people and not for others.

Nausea and Vomiting

Nausea and vomiting can be caused by motion (such as the rocking motion of a car, boat, or plane), pathogens, medicines, drugs, or other substances in the stomach. Nausea is a feeling of distress, fullness, and weakness. Nausea often precedes vomiting. Vomiting is a reflex response that can be a protection if you swallow a foreign substance. Vomiting is the result of reverse peristalsis, or waves of muscular contractions, in the stomach and esophagus. It is usually accompanied by strong muscular contractions in the chest and abdomen.

Diarrhea

Diarrhea is a condition in which the feces are watery and are expelled frequently. It can occur when food moves through the large intestine too rapidly. Numerous conditions can cause diarrhea, including a change in diet, food poisoning, overeating, emotional turmoil, and nutritional deficiencies. Diarrhea can also be caused by viral and bacterial infections. If water is not being reabsorbed into the bloodstream, dehydration or an excessive loss of body fluids can result. To prevent dehydration, a person should drink plenty of liquids, especially water. Diarrhea usually clears up when the cause of it is eliminated. Medical help is often necessary.

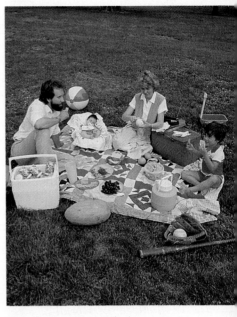

Good company and pleasant surroundings can help the digestive process.

Constipation

Constipation is a condition in which feces become dry and hard and bowel movements are difficult. If feces stay in the large intestine too long, too much water is absorbed out of them. Constipation can be caused by a lack of fiber in the diet, erratic eating habits, drinking too little water, a lack of exercise, or constant use of laxatives. Eating a well-balanced diet, drinking plenty of water, and exercising regularly are the best ways to avoid constipation.

Common Structural Problems

Most digestive problems are temporary and not serious. However, if any problem continues for a long period of time or is accompanied by fever or other symptoms of illness, a medical checkup may be necessary.

Doctors have a variety of instruments and tests that allow them to view the gastrointestinal tract and detect problems.

Gallstones

Gallstones are small crystals formed from bile that can block the bile duct between the gallbladder and the duodenum, which is the first section of the small intestine. Gallstones can be treated either with medicines to dissolve them or by surgical removal of the gallbladder. Some gallstones can be shattered by ultrasound-guided shock waves.

Overcoming The Odds

Corey McManus is 18. He has big plans. Right now he is taking courses at a community college. In the future, he hopes to attend a culinary institute, study in France, and become a chef.

Corey recently graduated from the First State School at the Medical Center of Delaware, the nation's only outpatient school for chronically ill children. He attended the school for four years, taking regular academic courses in a hospital where doctors and nurses are available to give medical care when necessary.

Corey says, "I was born a diabetic. I grew up on fruits, nuts, and juices and no candy. I started giving myself insulin shots when I was 8 or 10 years old. Then, around the age of 14, I got really sick. I spent 5 months in a hospital. I have rapid progressive diabetes, and it started progressing. Besides having high blood pressure, I was diagnosed as having renal failure. I had what is called a kidney biopsy, and was told that I would need a kidney transplant." In the meanwhile, Corey went on CAPD, a portable system that acts as an artificial kidney, cleaning impurities from the blood. "To get a kidney," he says, "you have to get on a list, and it sometimes takes a long time. I was on the list for three years."

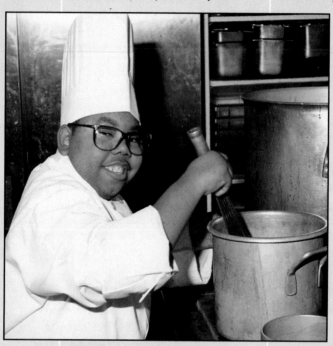

Because of his health problems Corey was a particularly hard match. He not only needed a kidney, he also needed a pancreas. A perfect match was found, and Corey received a new kidney and pancreas. However, after the operation, there were serious complications. He was in a coma for nearly a month, and his medical bill reached a quarter of a million dollars.

Because Corey had such difficulty digesting food, he was restricted from food with salt because of his high blood pressure and because foods high in salt can clog the kidneys. But the outcome of these restrictions hasn't all been bad. It is partly because of them that Corey's love of food and creative cooking has emerged. Now he has turned those restrictions into a promising career.

He continues, "I have side effects from medicines, and I still take insulin. But I feel great about myself. My best friend is me," he says with great energy. "My favorite person is me."

1. How have the restrictions of Corey's medical condition and diet inspired him to move forward and plan his future?
2. What restrictions are present in your life? What creative solutions might you use to work with these restrictions?
3. Corey says that he is his own best friend. If you are your own best friend, how do you think you got that way? If you are not, what can you do to become a better friend to yourself?

Ulcers

An ulcer is an open sore on the skin or in the mucous membrane. As the surface tissue breaks down and dies, it leaves a raw, inflamed area. Ulcers that develop in the digestive system are called **peptic ulcers.** There are two main types of peptic ulcers. Gastric ulcers develop in the stomach, and are caused by an overproduction of hydrochloric acid and pepsin. Pepsin is a digestive enzyme in gastric juice. Duodenal ulcers develop in the duodenum and also result from too much gastric acid secretion.

Peptic ulcers are aggravated by stress and the use of tobacco. Doctors think some people may have a hereditary tendency to develop ulcers. We also know that overuse of aspirin irritates the stomach lining and can promote the formation of ulcers.

A person who has a peptic ulcer will usually experience pain in the upper part of the stomach, usually when the stomach is empty. Peptic ulcers may be treated with medicines that neutralize or reduce stomach acid or with antibiotics. In some cases surgery may be necessary, but because of the development of new medicines, surgery can frequently be avoided.

Gastritis

One of the most common disorders of the stomach is **gastritis,** which is an inflammation of the mucous membrane that lines the stomach. Gastritis can result from the presence of irritant foods, alcohol, or bacteria or viruses. A person suffering from gastritis usually experiences stomach cramps and pain in the upper abdomen. Vomiting usually occurs. Antibiotics cure the condition if bacteria are the cause.

Appendicitis

Appendicitis is the inflammation of the appendix, which is a 3- to 4-inch (8- to 10-cm) extension at one end of the large intestine. As a result of bacteria or foreign matter that gets lodged in it, the appendix becomes swollen and fills with pus. If it bursts, the pus spreads to other body organs, poisoning them.

The symptoms of appendicitis are usually pain and cramps in the lower right portion of the abdomen. These symptoms may be accompanied by fever and vomiting. Under no condition should laxatives be

---

K E E P I N G   F I T

Lactose Intolerance

When people say they are allergic to milk they may mean they are unable to digest lactose, or milk sugar. To digest milk sugar requires the enzyme lactase, and people who cannot digest lactose usually have low levels of the enzyme. When a person's body cannot correctly digest lactose, drinking milk may result in gas, bloating, pain, or diarrhea.

About 70 percent of the world's population is lactose intolerant to some degree. However, Caucasians from northern and western Europe tend to be lactose tolerant. Among the groups with lesser abilities to tolerate lactose are those of Mediterranean, African, and Asian roots.

Cross-cultural Cancer

Researchers from China, Canada, and the United States have been studying why Chinese-Americans have four to seven times more colon and rectal cancer than Chinese who live in China. In fact, the colon cancer risks increase the longer a Chinese immigrant lives in North America.

The study concludes that saturated fats in the Western diet may be the single greatest factor in the high colo-rectal cancer rates here. Also cited as a cause for higher cancer rates is the sedentary life-style of many Americans— particularly the amount of time they spend sitting.

given to a person with these symptoms. Such substances can cause the appendix to burst. A doctor's care is essential. Surgical removal of the appendix may be necessary.

Hepatitis

Hepatitis is a serious inflammation of the liver that is most often caused by a viral infection. The severity of the infection depends on the type of virus involved. The two most common types are hepatitis A, which is sometimes called infectious hepatitis; and hepatitis B, which is sometimes called serum hepatitis. One symptom of hepatitis is jaundice, which is characterized by a yellow discoloration of the skin. The yellow color is the result of a malfunction of the liver.

Hepatitis A is transmitted by direct contact with an infected person or by contact with polluted water. Recovery is slow. Bed rest and a balanced diet are essential.

Hepatitis B results when the virus enters the bloodstream from a transfusion of contaminated human blood, from unclean needles used to administer medicines or drugs, or from surgical or dental instruments that have not been sterilized. Hepatitis B has also been known to be transmitted through sexual contact with an infected person.

Tooth Decay

It may surprise you to see tooth decay listed as a disease of the digestive tract. Teeth help prepare food for proper digestion. Tooth decay weakens a tooth and affects the way a person can bite and chew food. Tooth decay is also perhaps the most preventable disease of the digestive tract. Regular brushing, flossing, and dental checkups are the keys to preventing tooth decay.

Crohn's Disease

Crohn's disease is a chronic disease of the digestive tract. The cause of the disease is not known, but it may be influenced by heredity and environment. As the mucous lining of the digestive tract becomes inflamed, absorption of digested food from the small intestine is severely affected. Symptoms include cramps, diarrhea, and weight loss. Treatment depends on the severity of the symptoms. A diet that avoids raw fruits and vegetables is important. Medical help is essential.

Hemorrhoids

Hemorrhoids are a result of swelling of the veins in the lower rectum and anus. Internal hemorrhoids stay within the rectum. Swellings that push through the anus, however, produce external hemorrhoids. People who sit a lot or suffer from constipation are more susceptible to hemorrhoids. The signs of hemorrhoids includes itching, pain, and bleeding. Sitting in hot baths and using ointment may relieve the discomfort. If the pain and bleeding are severe, the hemorrhoids may need to be surgically removed. Regular exercise and a diet high in fiber can help prevent hemorrhoids.

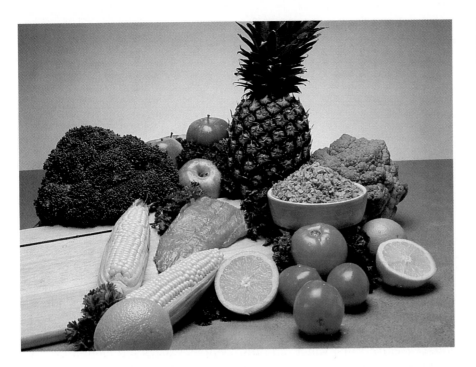

Care of the Digestive System

The main way to care for the digestive system is to practice good eating habits.

- Eat a variety of foods. Make sure your diet is low in fat and high in fiber.
- Eat regular meals. Eat complete meals at regular intervals during the day.
- Make meals a relaxing time. Do not hurry through your meals. Relax and enjoy them.
- Eat enough but not too much. Eat enough food to satisfy your hunger, but not so much as to stuff yourself.
- Drink plenty of water. Your digestive system needs a lot of water to do its job properly.

DID YOU KNOW?

- You can digest food even if your stomach has been removed. This is because most of the digestive process occurs in the small intestine.
- No gastrointestinal problem is listed among the ten leading causes of death among children and adolescents.

LESSON 2 REVIEW

Reviewing Facts and Vocabulary

1. What are two causes of halitosis?
2. What is lactose intolerance?

Thinking Critically

3. **Analysis.** How do diet and exercise contribute to the prevention of many common digestive disorders?

4. **Synthesis.** Develop a plan for an individual who eats too much and eats too fast.

Applying Health Knowledge

5. Make a list of over-the-counter medicines you have heard about for common digestive disorders. Tell what each can be used for. Then suggest a behavior that might eliminate the problem without the need for medicine.

THE URINARY SYSTEM

Three systems work together to regulate and control internal body conditions. The urinary system filters wastes from the circulatory system and eliminates the wastes from the body in the form of urine. The respiratory system removes the waste product carbon dioxide. The digestive system removes solid wastes.

Functions of the Urinary System

Water-soluble waste products are the result of all the chemical changes in the cells. Some of the wastes contain nitrogen and would become toxic if they remained in the body. As blood flows through the kidneys, extra salts, water, and nitrogenous wastes are filtered out into small tubules. The liquid wastes are stored temporarily in the bladder.

Structure of the Urinary System

The urinary system consists of two **kidneys;** the **ureters,** which are tubes that lead from the two kidneys to the bladder; the **bladder,** which stores the wastes in the form of urine; and the **urethra,** the tube that leads from the bladder to the outside of the body.

The Kidneys

The two kidneys are bean-shaped and are about the size of a fist. They lie on either side of the spine in the small of the back. The kidneys are embedded in a mass of fatty tissue that protects them. Within each kidney are as many as one million highly specialized tubules called nephrons. **Nephrons** are the functional units of the kidneys. Each nephron involves a tubule and a cluster of capillaries, called a glomerulus. The section of each nephron that surrounds the glomerulus is called Bowman's capsule.

Blood flows into each kidney through a renal artery that immediately branches into much smaller arterioles. Each glomerulus is an extension of the arterioles.

Because of the sudden change in the size of the blood vessels from arterioles to capillaries, pressure is built up as the blood flows through the glomerulus. Nephrons remove these substances from the blood, return the substances the body needs to the blood, and eliminates the remainder as urine. Urine is constantly being formed and collected in the bladder.

Although they are small, the kidneys do a tremendous amount of work. The kidneys filter every drop of blood in your body about once every hour. They are constantly separating harmful substances from the substances your body can use.

The fluid that passed through the filtering part of the kidney is called filtrate. Your kidneys process about 40 to 50 gallons (152 to 189 l) of filtrate each day. Of this, less than ½ gallon (2 l) is expelled as urine.

The Bladder and Urethra

The bladder is a muscular organ that stores urine. **Urine,** the liquid waste material, collects in the bladder until it is ready to be passed out of the body. The bladder may hold as much as a pint (500–600 ml) of urine. The need to urinate is stimulated as the bladder becomes full. Sphincter, or circular, muscles relax and allow urine to flow through the urethra. Control of the sphincter muscles is voluntary. In babies, lack of control is normal. An infant urinates when the bladder is full enough to cause a reflex stimulus.

Problems of the Urinary System

Because the function of the kidneys is so essential to maintaining the balance of fluids in the body any disruption of this function is potentially serious. Some of the more common disorders are described here.

- Incontinence is the inability of the body to control the bladder and the elimination of waste. Bladder incontinence may occur if the sphincter muscle that closes the urethra is torn, weak, or damaged. This condition is more common in older adults.
- Cystitis is a bacterial infection of the bladder that occurs most frequently in females. Symptoms include a burning sensation and a high frequency of urination. Fever and blood in the urine may be present.

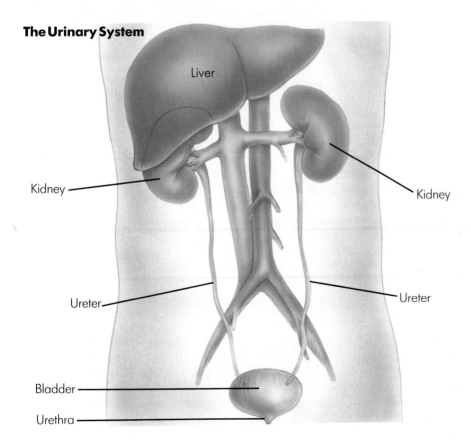

The Urinary System

Liver

Kidney

Kidney

Ureter

Ureter

Bladder

Urethra

The urinary system functions in maintaining constant conditions in the body's internal environment.

- Your kidney is about the size of your fist.
- Your right kidney is probably slightly lower than your left one.
- You can survive with just one kidney.
- Two kidneys filter about 50 gallons (190 liters) of blood each day.
- Each day in the United States, Americans' kidneys filter about 10 billion gallons of liquid.

It is important to seek medical attention. If left untreated, the infection can move to the ureter and kidneys.

- Nephritis occurs when the nephrons of the kidneys become inflamed or infected. Symptoms may include high blood pressure, weakness, fatigue, and swelling of body tissues. Treatment usually involves relieving the symptoms.
- Urethritis is an inflammation of the urethra, the tube leading from the bladder to the outside of the body. The passage of urine becomes painful and difficult.
- When the kidneys are unable to rid wastes from the body, poisonous substances build and the normal function is seriously affected. The result is a series of symptoms called uremia. Dialysis, a treatment that literally cleans a person's blood, is usually required for uremia.
- Kidney stones are stonelike crystals that sometimes form from mineral salts and urea. Small stones may pass out of the body in

CONFLICT RESOLUTION

Carrie's younger sister, Sue, has a serious kidney disorder that requires frequent hemodialysis. The expense of the procedure and the need for the family to stay close to the hospital have put severe limits on everyone in the family. Carrie is starting to feel that she's as restricted by Sue's disease as Sue is. However, whenever Carrie complains, her parents say she should be thankful that she's healthy. Carrie feels more and more resentful toward her sister and can't help feeling guilty about it.

How can Carrie resolve her feelings?

HEALTH UPDATE

LOOKING AT THE ISSUES

How to Get Enough Organs for Transplants

The number of organ transplants is on the rise. For example, between 1983 and 1987, the number of kidney transplants in the United States went from 6,112 to 8,967; the number of heart transplants from 172 to 1,512. Technological advances have made these procedures safer than ever before. However, the problem is that there are many more people in need of new organs than there are organs being donated.

Analyzing Different Viewpoints

ONE VIEW. Some people propose paying donors for their organs. They believe that there is such a need for these organs that payment would provide the necessary incentive for more people to donate. (Presently, in the U.S., it is a felony—a major federal crime—to buy or sell a major body part, so the laws would first have to be changed.)

A SECOND VIEW. Others are horrified by the idea of selling organs. Some state religious or ethical objections. Others point out what has happened in countries like India where the poor often sell their kidneys for small amounts of money and where black market sales of organs flourish. Some people fear that selling organs in the U.S. might result in abuses of the poor or elderly—or even in murder to get organs for profit.

A THIRD VIEW. Another view is to let people with such problems die, unless they can pay for the cost of this procedure.

Exploring Your Views

1. How do you feel about being a living donor—donating a kidney, for example, if someone close to you needed it? What about for a stranger?
2. How do you feel about signing a donor card, requesting that, upon your death, your organs be donated?
3. How do you feel about people being allowed to sell their organs?

urine. Large stones can cause great pain. If a stone blocks the flow of urine, an infection often results. In the past surgery was necessary to remove a kidney stone. Now, however, a procedure called lithotripsy is frequently used. High-intensity sound waves are focused on the area where the stones are located. The sound waves pass through the body and literally crumble the stones. The technique is painless, and the resulting pieces pass out of the body in urine.

■ Kidney failure may be caused by a blockage of urine, a very serious case of nephritis, or loss of blood. Normally a person can survive with one kidney, but if both kidneys fail or have to be removed, the person will die. Three techniques are in use today to help people who suffer from kidney failure.

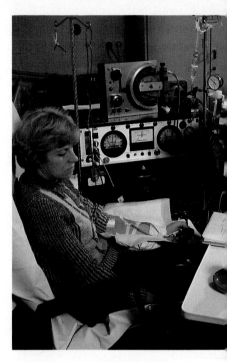

Hemodialysis is a technique in which a person is connected to an artificial kidney machine. The machine, which is about the size of a washing machine, filters wastes from the blood. Dialysis must take place three times a week for approximately four hours each time. This kind of dialysis usually takes place in a hospital or clinical setting.

Peritoneal dialysis is a technique that uses the peritoneum, a thin membrane that surrounds the digestive organs inside the abdomen, to filter the blood and remove waste products through the use of a catheter, a tube that provides a passageway for fluids. Peritoneal dialysis allows the patient to be treated at home.

Another technique is a kidney transplant. A donated kidney is surgically placed within a person's body and functions just as the original kidney did.

An artery in the patient's arm is connected by tubing to the machine. Her blood flows through an artificial membrane that acts as a kidney and filters out waste materials. The cleansed blood then flows back into the patient's circulatory system. This procedure is hemodialysis.

Care of the Urinary System

The main way to care for your urinary system is to drink plenty of fluids. This should include six to eight glasses of water every day. A nutritionally balanced diet also plays a part in the care of the urinary system. Practicing good personal health care will help prevent the risk of infection to urinary organs. Any changes in urine color, odor, or frequency should be discussed with a doctor. Regular physical checkups are necessary to detect changes in urine content.

LESSON 3 REVIEW

Reviewing Facts and Vocabulary

1. Describe the function of the kidneys.
2. Describe the function of two systems, apart from the urinary system, that have a role in ridding the body of waste material.
3. Define the terms *urine, nephrons,* and *hemodialysis.*

Thinking Critically

4. **Analysis.** How does drinking plenty of fluids each day promote a healthy urinary system?

5. **Analysis.** How might kidney dialysis affect a person's life-style?

Applying Health Knowledge

6. Find out what is involved in kidney transplants. How do doctors match a donor and recipient? How long is the wait for a donor? What advancements have been made in the procedure? What is the success rate for this type of surgery?

Self-Inventory

Care of the Digestive and Urinary Systems

HOW DO YOU RATE?

There are many things you can do to promote healthy digestive and urinary systems. Number a sheet of paper from 1 through 25. Read each item below, and respond by writing *always or most of the time, sometimes,* or *seldom or never* for each item. Total the number of each type of response. Then proceed to the next section.

1. I eat a variety of healthy foods every day.
2. I do aerobic exercises for 20 minutes at least three times a week.
3. To reduce stress, I engage in activities that I like.
4. I drink at least six to eight glasses of water a day.
5. I chew each bite of food thoroughly before swallowing.
6. I eat two or more servings of fruit each day.
7. I eat foods that are high in fiber every day.
8. I eat three or more servings of vegetables each day.
9. I avoid overeating.
10. I stop eating before I am full.
11. I have a dental checkup every year.
12. I avoid eating when I am under stress or emotionally upset.
13. I regularly engage in activities that reduce my stress.

14. I brush my teeth after every meal.
15. I floss my teeth daily.
16. I eat foods that have a high water content such as celery, soup, and apples.
17. I take a drink whenever I pass a water fountain.
18. I limit the amount of salt in my diet.
19. I have regular bowel movements.
20. I look for changes in urine color, odor, or frequency.
21. I avoid salty snacks, such as chips, crackers, and pretzels.
22. I use laxatives only when recommended by a doctor.
23. I choose to drink fruit juices instead of soft drinks.
24. I seek medical attention when diarrhea persists for more than 48 hours.
25. I limit the amount of foods that might cause gas, such as carbonated beverages.

HOW DID YOU SCORE?

Give yourself 3 points for every *always or most of the time* answer, 1 point for every *sometimes* answer, and 0 points for every *seldom or never* answer. Find your total, and read below to see how you scored. Then proceed to the next section.

55 to 75
Excellent. Your health choices show you are taking care of your digestive and urinary systems.

35 to 54
Good. Your healthy choices are good but there are some things you could do to promote a healthier digestive or urinary system.

15 to 34
Fair. While you are doing some things to protect yourself from digestive and urinary problems, much improvement is still needed.

Below 15
Poor. You are taking unnecessary risks that could affect the health of your digestive and urinary systems both now and in the future.

WHAT ARE YOUR GOALS?

Identify an area in which your score was low, and use the goal-setting process to begin making a change.

1. The behavior I would like to change is ____.
2. If this behavior were completely changed, I would look, feel, or act differently in the following ways: ____.
3. The steps involved in making this change are ____.
4. My timetable for accomplishing this is ____.
5. People I will ask for help or assistance are ____.
6. The benefits I will receive as a result of making this change are ____.
7. My reward at the end of each week will be ____.

Building Decision-Making Skills

Matt is a junior in high school. His little brother with whom he has a very close relationship has been diagnosed as having kidney damage that can be corrected only by a transplant. Matt has been identified as being the best donor. His parents have already asked him if he is willing to donate one of his kidneys. He is frightened and feels that he has no choice in this situation.

WHAT DO YOU THINK?

1. **Situation.** What do you think Matt is afraid of?

2. **Situation.** What risks are involved in this situation? To Matt? To his brother? To his parents?

3. **Choices.** What choices do you think Matt has?

4. **Choices.** Where might Matt go for more information? Whom might he talk to about this situation?

5. **Consequences.** How might Matt deal with his fears?

6. **Consequences.** How might Matt's health triangle be affected by this decision?

7. **Consequences.** How might his self-esteem be affected by this decision?

8. **Decision.** What do you think Matt should do?

9. **Evaluation.** Have you ever known anyone who faced a decision involving life and death? Describe the situation and your feelings about the courage involved in making that decision.

Jan and Angela, both sophomores in high school, have been best friends since third grade when Jan moved to town. Their families are good friends and periodically join together for an outing or a special occasion. Last spring Angela started being concerned about her weight. She told Jan she was going to lose 15 pounds—for sure this time. When she started eating less and exercising more she began to lose, slowly at first. She was very excited about her progress and Jan was happy for her. However, as time went on, it seemed that all Angela ever talked about was food. She even started showing some interest in cooking and often brought "treats" to school. By fall Angela had lost a lot of weight. In fact, her friends started asking Jan why Angela was still trying to lose more weight when she was already so thin. Jan is beginning to worry about her friend. What should she do?

WHAT DO YOU THINK?

10. **Situation.** What reasons might Jan have for being concerned?

11. **Choices.** What choices do you think Jan has?

12. **Consequences.** What are the advantages of each of the possible choices?

13. **Consequences.** What are the disadvantages of each of the possible choices?

14. **Consequences.** How might Angela's health triangle be affected by Jan's decision?

15. **Consequences.** How might Angela's family react to each of the possible choices?

16. **Consequences.** How might Jan's family react to each of the possible choices?

17. **Consequences.** What risks are involved in this situation?

18. **Decision.** What do you think Jan should do? Why do you think so?

19. **Decision.** How might Jan implement, or accomplish, her decision?

20. **Evaluation.** Have you ever known anyone with an eating disorder? If so, describe what the situation was like and what you learned from it.

REVIEW

Using Health Terms

On a separate sheet of paper, write the term that best matches each definition given below.

LESSON 1

1. The chemical and physical breakdown of food into smaller pieces.
2. The passage of digested food from the digestive tract into the circulatory system.
3. A tube that extends from the pharynx to the stomach.
4. A digestive juice produced in the liver that helps break down fats.
5. The largest gland in the body.

LESSON 2

6. Bad breath.
7. A swelling of the veins in the lower rectum and anus.
8. A condition caused when the stomach's acid backs up into the esophagus.
9. A strong result of reverse peristalsis.
10. An open sore on the skin or in the mucous membrane.
11. An inflammation of the mucous membrane that lines the stomach.

LESSON 3

12. Two bean-shaped organs that excrete the waste products of metabolism.

Building Academic Skills

LESSON 1

13. **Reading.** List the following processes in the order in which they take place in the body: absorption, elimination, digestion.
14. **Math.** If your dentist gives you a shot of a local anesthetic that numbs the lower right half of the mouth, about how many of your taste buds will be "out of order" until the anesthetic wears off?
15. **Reading.** Arrange the following organs of the digestive system in the order in which food passes through them: stomach, esophagus, duodenum, large intestine, ileum, mouth, jejunum.

Recalling the Facts

LESSON 1

16. What are the mechanical processes that take place during digestion?
17. What are the chemical processes that take place during digestion?
18. What functions do the nerve endings in the mouth serve?
19. During swallowing, what happens to breathing activity?
20. What is the role of the sphincter muscles located along the digestive tract?
21. Name two drugs that are absorbed directly into the blood from the stomach.
22. In what part of the digestive system does most of the chemical breakdown of food take place?
23. List three enzymes produced by the pancreas and describe the function of each.
24. What are the two main functions of the large intestine?
25. List three major functions of the liver.
26. What is the function of the gallbladder?

LESSON 2

27. What causes heartburn?
28. What is a hiatal hernia?
29. What can cause gas?
30. List three symptoms that may be present in a person suffering from appendicitis.
31. What medication should never be given to people who may have appendicitis?
32. What body organ is affected by hepatitis?
33. What is the usual treatment for hepatitis?
34. List three ways to prevent tooth decay.

LESSON 3

35. Name the four parts of the urinary system.
36. What is the difference between the ureters and the urethra?
37. In what body organ is urine stored?
38. Why are the kidneys important?
39. Why is it important to seek medical attention if you believe you have cystitis?
40. Name and define four problems that may be associated with the urinary system.
41. Describe the process of hemodialysis.

REVIEW

Thinking Critically

LESSON 1

42. Synthesis. Write a one-page composition that would explain why many gastrointestinal illnesses are stress-related.

43. Analysis. Summarize the work of gastric juices.

44. Synthesis. Develop a plan that would help young people prevent gastrointestinal problems.

45. Analysis. What evidence can you find that might indicate that gastrointestinal problems will increase in the years ahead?

LESSON 2

46. Synthesis. Explain what a person should do if she or he experiences heartburn regularly.

47. Analysis. Compare the conditions known as diarrhea and constipation.

48. Analysis. In what ways are smoking, stress, and digestive problems related?

49. Analysis. What causes appendicitis, and what can be its result?

LESSON 3

50. Synthesis. If you could do so, how would you redesign the urinary system of the human body? Make a drawing or diagram to show how this system would work. Name and label the parts of the system.

51. Evaluation. What are the three most important things you can do to keep your urinary system running smoothly?

52. Synthesis. What ideas can you add to those in the text that might help to keep your urinary system in good working order?

Making the Connection

LESSON 3

53. Math. Calculate the cost to an individual of kidney dialysis for one year based on average costs of treatment in your local area. A hospital billing office or an insurance agency can assist by providing current figures. Share your findings with the class.

Applying Health Knowledge

LESSON 1

54. You may have experienced the sensation of eating something and having it "go down the wrong way," making you choke. What causes this? What usually prevents this?

LESSON 2

55. Derek brushes his teeth after every meal and before he goes to bed, but his brother is always telling him he has bad breath. Which of the following should Derek do?
   a. Start using a mouthwash every morning.
   b. Visit a dentist.
   c. Eat a breath mint every hour.

56. Amanda's parents have recently divorced, and she must decide which one of them she wants to live with. She also broke up with her boyfriend a month ago. These problems have been making her very unhappy and causing her to lose sleep and overeat. Is Amanda more likely to experience diarrhea or constipation? Why?

LESSON 3

57. You notice that your sister has gone to the bathroom six times in the last three hours. She tells you she has found blood in her urine and is experiencing a burning sensation whenever she urinates. You feel her forehead, and it is hot. What urinary infection might your sister be suffering from?

Beyond the Classroom

LESSON 2

58. Parental Involvement. Ask your parents to tell you about any problems with the digestive or urinary system they have experienced. Find out what their symptoms were, what actions they took to correct the problem, and how they evaluated the effectiveness of their actions.

59. Further Study. Research a digestive problem described in Lesson 2. Write a short paper on its causes, symptoms, and cures.

CHAPTER

15

THE REPRODUCTIVE SYSTEMS

LESSON 1

The Male Reproductive System

LESSON 2

The Female Reproductive System

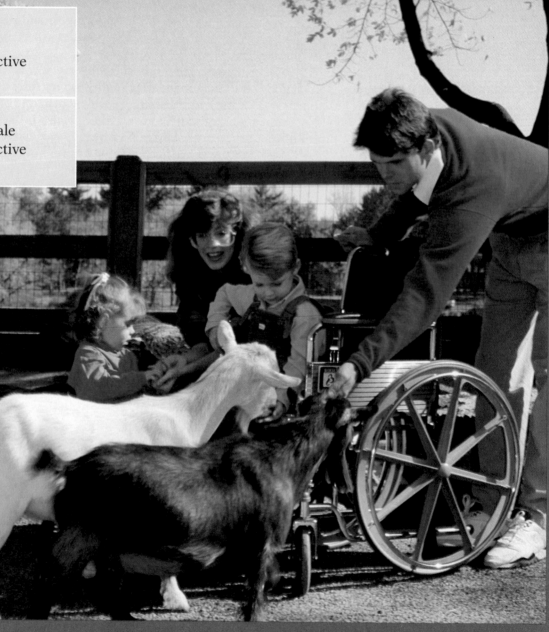

THE MALE REPRODUCTIVE SYSTEM

When a male reaches puberty, hormones released by the pituitary gland stimulate the testes to begin producing testosterone. **Testosterone** is a male hormone that causes the testes to produce sperm. Testosterone is also responsible for other physical changes, such as the enlargement of the external reproductive organs that take place during puberty. In addition, testosterone is responsible for the development of secondary sex characteristics. These include broadened shoulders; facial, pubic, and underarm hair; a deepened voice; and muscular development.

The Function and Structure of the Male Reproductive System

The functions of the male reproductive system are the production of sperm and the transfer of sperm to a female's body during intercourse. As a result of intercourse, a sperm may unite with an egg cell, or ovum. If this occurs, the female is pregnant.

Male Reproductive Organs

The male reproductive system includes the testes, epididymis, vas deferens, seminal vesicles, prostate gland, Cowper's glands, urethra, and penis.

The Testes. The **testes,** or testicles, are two small glands that produce sperm. Both the production and survival of sperm require a temperature that is lower than body temperature. The testes hang outside the male's body in a sac called the scrotum. The **scrotum** protects sperm by keeping the testes at a temperature slightly below the normal body temperature of 98.6°F (37°C). If body temperature rises, the muscles of the scrotum relax, lowering the testes away from the body. If body temperature drops, the muscles contract, pulling the testes closer to the body. If the testes are too warm or too cold, the normal production of sperm does not occur.

Each testis contains several hundred yards of coiled tube that produce sperm and provide a passageway in which sperm move. Each sperm is shaped somewhat like a tadpole, the head containing the nucleus and the tail being the means of movement. Sperm cells are so tiny that 500 of them lined up end to end would measure only 1 inch (2.5 cm). Once a male reaches puberty, he is capable of producing sperm for the rest of his life.

The Epididymis. The tubes in each testis join a larger coiled tube, called the epididymis. The epididymis, located at the outer surface of each testis, stores sperm temporarily. Sperm mature in the epididymis.

LESSON 1 FOCUS

TERMS TO USE

- Testosterone (te•STAHS•tuh•rohn)
- Testes
- Scrotum (SKROHT•uhm)
- Semen
- Urethra (yu•REE•thruh)
- Penis
- Sterility

CONCEPTS TO LEARN

- The male reproductive system consists of the penis and scrotum, the epididymis, vas deferens, seminal vesicles, prostate gland, Cowper's glands, and urethra.

ATTITUDES AND BEHAVIORS TO EVALUATE

- Self-Inventory, page 310.
- Building Decision-Making Skills, page 311.

The Male Reproductive System

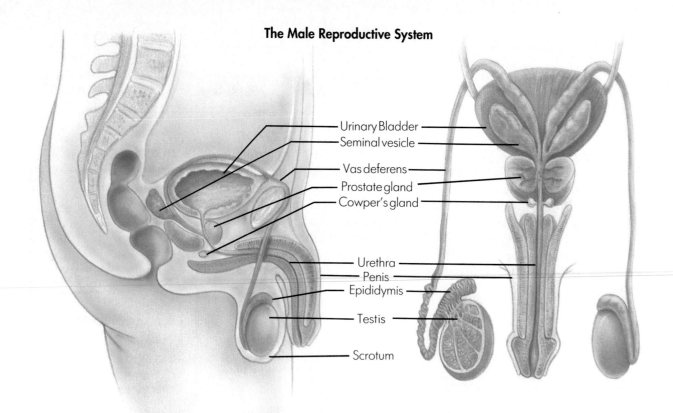

Urinary Bladder
Seminal vesicle
Vas deferens
Prostate gland
Cowper's gland
Urethra
Penis
Epididymis
Testis
Scrotum

The Vas Deferens and the Urethra. The vas deferens is a tube that extends from the lower end of each epididymis and connects with the urethra. Each vas deferens is about 18 inches (46 cm) long. As sperm move through the vas deferens, they are mixed in a fluid produced by the seminal vesicles.

The seminal vesicles are glands about 2 inches (5 cm) long and are attached to the vas deferens near the base of the bladder. These glands secrete a fluid that mixes with sperm to make them more mobile and to provide nourishment. The secretion of the seminal vesicles contains nutrients and is rich in fructose, a form of sugar. The seminal vesicles and vas deferens meet to form the ejaculatory duct, which opens into the urethra.

Sperm are then mixed with fluids secreted from the prostate gland, a small gland that surrounds the urethra, and from Cowper's glands, which are located below the prostate gland. The mixture of the fluids from the seminal vesicles, the prostate gland, and Cowper's glands with sperm forms **semen,** or seminal fluid. When a male ejaculates, he releases semen.

The **urethra** is a small tube that extends from the bladder as well as from each vas deferens through the penis to the outside of the body. The bladder stores urine, which leaves the body through the urethra. Both semen and urine leave the body through the urethra. However, they do not pass through the urethra at the same time. A muscle near the bladder contracts, preventing urine from entering the urethra when semen is present. Because urine is very high in acid, the lining of the urethra tends to be acidic. The secretion from the Cowper's glands (also called bulbourethral glands) lubricates the urethra and neutralizes the acid content before semen is ejaculated. This secretion also causes a small drop of clear fluid to leave the penis before the semen comes out. This fluid is called preejaculatory fluid.

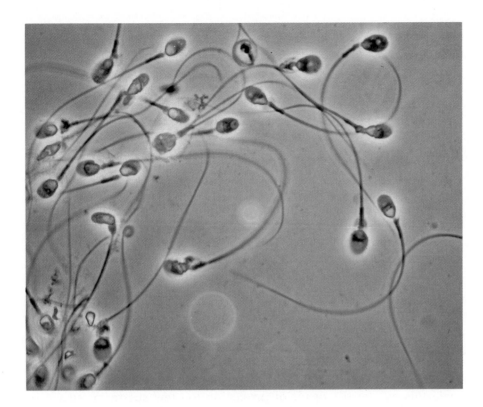

Sperm shown here are magnified 300 times.

The Penis. The **penis** is the external reproductive organ composed of spongy tissue that contains many blood vessels. As a result of increased blood flow, the penis becomes enlarged and erect. When the penis is erect, ejection or ejaculation of semen can occur through the urethra. Sometimes an erection results from the friction of clothing.

Males of every age experience erections. When a male enters puberty, he may experience an erection during the day. The erection may occur for no reason at all. Erections also occur as the result of being sexually aroused. Ejaculation does not always follow an erection.

When a male begins to produce sperm, he may experience a nocturnal emission, or "wet dream," which is an erection and an ejaculation during sleep. This is a normal occurrence.

At birth, the tip of the penis is covered with a fold of skin called foreskin. Some parents choose to have the foreskin surgically removed when the baby is born. This procedure is known as circumcision. It is important to know that it is normal if a male child is circumcised and it is normal if he is not.

K E E P I N G   F I T

Examination for Testicular Cancer

Testicular cancer occurs most frequently in males between the ages of 15 and 34. Males should perform regular testicular self-exams for cancer. While shower-ing, feel each testicle using a thumb and forefinger to see if there are hard lumps or notice-able swelling. Be aware of any ache in the groin area. See a doc-tor if any of these signs occur. Self-examination for testicular cancer should be carried out at least once a month for life.

- Impotence, the inability to maintain an erection in order to have intercourse, is a common occurrence. Probably every man has suffered some temporary impotence, especially during periods of extreme stress, tiredness, or illness.
- Sexual potency and functioning do not rely just on the reproductive system but also on the vascular system, brain, nerves, and spinal cord. In addition, the pituitary, thyroid, and adrenal glands play a part in reproductive health.

Problems of the Male Reproductive System

The organs of the male reproductive system can be affected by both functional and structural problems. The effect of sexually transmitted diseases (STDs) on these organs will be discussed in Chapter 27.

Hernia

A hernia occurs when part of an organ pushes through an opening of a membrane or muscle that usually contains the organ. Hernias occur in various parts of the body. A common hernia of the male reproductive system is an inguinal hernia. This is a weak spot in the abdominal wall near the top of the scrotum. Sometimes straining the abdominal muscles can cause a tear in this spot. A part of the intestine can then push through into the scrotum. Sometimes surgery is necessary to correct such a hernia.

Sterility

Sterility is a condition in which a person is unable to reproduce. In a male this can be the result of producing too few sperm, or sperm of poor quality. Temperature changes, exposure to certain chemicals, smoking, contracting mumps as an adult, complications from an STD, or malfunction of the epididymis, vas deferens, Cowper's glands, or the prostate gland can all result in sterility.

Enlarged Prostate Gland

The prostate gland does not usually change in size until after about 50 years of age. It can enlarge for reasons such as infection, or a tumor, or old age. When the gland enlarges, it tends to squeeze the urethra and this affects urination. The treatment is most often a surgical procedure.

Cancer of the Prostate Gland

A cancer is an uncontrolled growth of cells. The prostate gland is often a cancer site in older males. Prostate cancer is the second highest incidence of cancer in males. Only a doctor can diagnose prostate cancer. Early detection is important because prostate cancer can be treated if it is localized in the gland. Radiation therapy and surgical removal of the prostate gland and surrounding tissue are the current treatments.

Cancer of the Testes

Cancer of the testes, or testicular cancer, occurs most frequently in males who are between the ages of 15 and 34. The first sign of testicular cancer is usually a slight enlargement of one of the testes. The male may not experience any pain at all, or he might have a dull ache in the lower abdomen and groin. Hard lumps, or nodules, on the testes may be a sign of this cancer. If discovered early, the condition can be treated effectively. Treatment involves surgery and radiation.

Care of the Male Reproductive System

Caring for the male reproductive system involves cleanliness, protection, and self-examination. Each of these factors plays a key role in maintaining good health.

A daily shower to clean the external organs—the penis and the scrotum—is essential. Avoiding clothing that is too tight and wearing a protector or supporter during strenuous activity will help protect the groin area and the external reproductive organs.

A male who is uncircumcised must practice extra hygiene. It is important that he wash underneath the foreskin daily.

In addition, once a male reaches puberty, he should perform a monthly self-examination of his testes for signs of cancer. Any lumps, thickenings, or change in texture or size of the testes should be reported to a doctor, even though such signs do not always mean there is cancer. If cancer is present, however, early detection usually means successful treatment.

LESSON 1 REVIEW

Reviewing Facts and Vocabulary

1. What is the function of the scrotum?

2. Trace the path that sperm follow from the testes to the urethra.

3. Why is the secretion from Cowper's glands so important?

4. Name two problems that can affect the male reproductive system, and describe them.

Thinking Critically

5. **Analysis.** Classify the organs and glands in the male reproductive system according to function in regard to sperm.
6. **Analysis.** How do Cowper's glands compare with the seminal vesicles?

Applying Health Knowledge

7. Your 11-year-old brother asks you what a "wet dream" is. What would you tell him?

THE FEMALE REPRODUCTIVE SYSTEM

LESSON 2 FOCUS

TERMS TO USE
- Ovaries
- Ovulation (ahv•you•LAY•shun)
- Fallopian tubes
- Fertilization
- Uterus
- Cervix
- Menstrual cycle

CONCEPTS TO LEARN
- Major organs of the female reproductive system are the labia majora, labia minora, the ovaries, Fallopian tubes, uterus, and vagina.

ATTITUDES AND BEHAVIORS TO EVALUATE
- Self-Inventory, page 310.
- Building Decision-Making Skills, page 311.

When a female reaches puberty, hormones released by the pituitary gland stimulate the ovaries to produce the hormones estrogen and progesterone. These hormones are responsible for secondary sex characteristics: breasts develop, hips widen, and pubic and underarm hair appear.

The Function and Structure of the Female Reproductive System

The female reproductive system serves three important functions:
- the production of egg cells, or ova
- the reception of sperm for fertilization to occur
- the nourishment and protection necessary for a fertilized ovum to develop until ready to live outside the female body

Female Reproductive Organs

The external parts of the female reproductive system are known as the vulva, which includes the mons pubis, soft tissue that covers the pubic bone; labia majora, the outer folds of skin that surround the opening of the vagina; and labia minora, the inner folds of skin. Internal reproductive organs include the ovaries, Fallopian tubes, uterus, and vagina.

The Ovaries.   The **ovaries** are female sex glands that house the ova and produce female sex hormones. They are almond-shaped and located on each side of the body in the lower abdominal area. At birth, a female has over 1 million immature ova in her ovaries.

As a female reaches puberty, hormones cause the immature ova to mature. The ovaries begin to release one mature ovum each month. This process is called **ovulation.** Usually one ovary releases a mature ovum one month and the other ovary releases a mature ovum the next month. As endocrine glands, ovaries also produce hormones that are involved in the female reproductive cycle.

The Fallopian Tubes.   When a mature ovum is released from an ovary, it moves into one of a pair of tubes called **Fallopian tubes.** An ovum moves through a Fallopian tube to the uterus. These tiny, muscular tubes lie close to each ovary and have fingerlike projections that, with a waving motion, draw the ovum into the tube. Each tube is about 4 inches (10 cm) long and about $1/3$ inch (0.8 cm) in diameter. Tiny hairlike structures and muscular contractions move the ovum along.

Fertilization can occur if sperm cells are present while the ovum is in the Fallopian tube. One sperm cell unites with the ovum usually in the

The Female Reproductive System

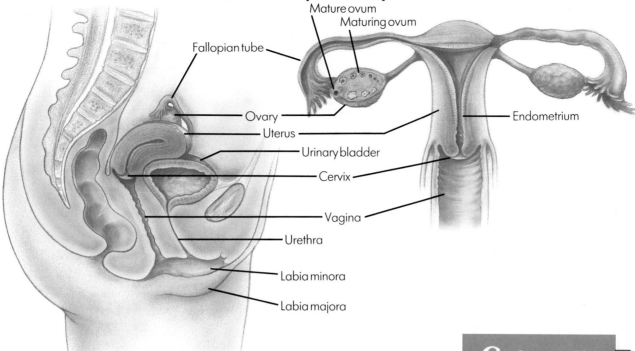

- Fallopian tube
- Mature ovum
- Maturing ovum
- Ovary
- Uterus
- Urinary bladder
- Cervix
- Vagina
- Urethra
- Labia minora
- Labia majora
- Endometrium

upper third of the Fallopian tube. Once fertilization occurs, the female is pregnant, and cell division begins. At the instant of fertilization, a membrane forms around the ovum to prevent any other sperm from penetrating it. The fertilized ovum, or zygote, continues moving through the Fallopian tube to the uterus, where it attaches to the uterine wall and begins to grow and develop.

The Uterus.   The **uterus** is a small, muscular, pear-shaped organ, about the size of a fist. The lining of the uterus has several layers and a rich supply of capillaries.

When an ovary releases an ovum, the hormone estrogen causes the lining of the uterus to thicken in preparation to support a fertilized ovum. If fertilization has taken place, the zygote attaches to the wall of the uterus, where it is nourished for the next nine months of growth.

If fertilization has not occurred, the ovum disintegrates and the thickened lining of the uterus is not needed. As a result of the action of hormones, the lining breaks down and passes through the **cervix,** or neck of the uterus, and the vagina.

The Vagina.   The vagina, also called the birth canal, is a muscular, very elastic tube that is a passageway from the uterus to the outside of the body. It is about 3½ inches (9 cm) long. During intercourse, semen is deposited in the vagina.

Menstruation

The process of shedding the lining of the uterus is called menstruation. The name comes from the Latin word *mensis,* meaning "month."

During menstruation about 2 to 3 fluid ounces (60 to 90 ml) of blood and other tissue leave the body. The menstrual flow usually lasts about 3 to 5 days. After the menstrual period ends, the entire cycle begins again.

Culturally Speaking

Sharing Pregnancy

Distinct rituals are associated with pregnancy and childbirth in many cultures. One interesting practice is the couvade, where the father ritually shares the pregnancy and the pains of childbirth with the mother. In some California Indian groups, the father and mother traditionally avoided certain foods such as salt and meat, ate alone, and limited their activities. Neither would cook or touch tools. Couvade is still practiced in some form by groups in Basque country (Spain), and in the tropical forest cultures of Brazil. Many other cultures also put restrictions on the father-to-be. What ones do you know about?

On average, the menstrual cycle is a 28-day cycle. Ovulation occurs approximately 14 days after Day 1 of the cycle.

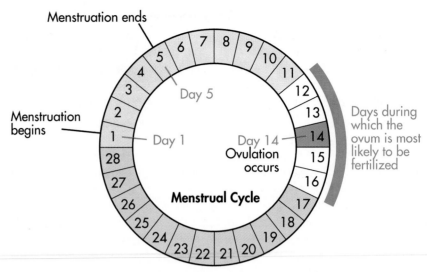

Menstruation ends

Menstruation begins

Day 5

Day 1

Day 14
Ovulation occurs

Menstrual Cycle

Days during which the ovum is most likely to be fertilized

The lining of the uterus thickens again, preparing for the possibility of a fertilized egg. Although there can be great variations, the **menstrual cycle**—the time from the beginning of one menstrual period to the onset of the next—is usually 28 days. The menstrual cycle is regulated by endocrine hormones.

Almost all females begin menstruating between the ages of 10 and 15. The menstrual cycle may be irregular at first. Although hormones control the menstrual cycle, poor nutrition, stress, and illness can influence the cycle.

Problems of the Female Reproductive System

The female reproductive system can be affected both structurally and functionally. The effects of sexually transmitted diseases, STDs, will be discussed in Chapter 27.

Menstrual Cramps

A female may experience abdominal cramps at the beginning of the menstrual period. Menstrual cramps are usually mild, lasting several hours. Light exercise can help relieve cramps. A warm bath or heating pad might also help relax the muscles. However, severe or persistent cramping may be an indication that medical attention is necessary.

Premenstrual Syndrome

Premenstrual syndrome (PMS) refers to a variety of symptoms that some females experience before each menstrual period. Symptoms vary and may be experienced several days to two weeks before the menstrual period. Many females never experience PMS.

The symptoms of PMS include nervous tension, anxiety, irritability, bloating, weight gain, depression, mood swings, and fatigue. The causes of PMS are not completely understood, but it seems to be more common in females in their 30s. Some doctors believe that PMS is related to a hormonal imbalance. Others attribute the cause to a nutritional deficiency.

HELP WANTED

Gynecologist

Sensitivity is an important quality that females look for in their gynecologist. However, integrity and knowledge are equally important. We are seeking a recent medical school grad with these qualities to join our practice. You must have the ability to deal with a female's medical needs. We offer a modern, growing practice and excellent financial rewards.

For more information contact:
American Medical Association
515 N. State Street
Chicago, IL 60610

Most doctors recommend diet and life-style changes as the first treatment of PMS. They also encourage females to find ways to reduce stress. Some PMS sufferers find that reducing their intake of sugar, salt, and caffeine can help alleviate PMS symptoms. An increase in their intake of B vitamins, magnesium, leafy green vegetables, whole grains, and fruit can also help. Finally, a regular exercise program should be followed.

Toxic Shock Syndrome

Toxic shock syndrome (TSS) is a bacterial disease usually found in menstruating females who use tampons. Although the connection between TSS and tampons is unclear, the improper use of tampons increases the risks of developing TSS. Changing tampons regularly every 3 to 4 hours during menstruation is very important to reduce the growth of bacteria already present in the vagina.

The symptoms of TSS are similar to flu symptoms: sudden high fever, vomiting, diarrhea, and dizziness. Any female suffering these symptoms during a menstrual period should seek medical care immediately.

Vaginitis

Vaginitis, or vaginal infection, is a very common condition in females. Nonspecific vaginitis is caused by an excess of normal vaginal secretions and bacteria. This excess can irritate the genital tissue. Symptoms include itching, discharge, and a burning sensation during urination.

Another common vaginal infection is a yeast infection, which is caused by a fungus. The signs of yeast infection are a thick, white discharge and itching in the genital area.

Trichomoniasis often occurs at the end of a menstrual period and is caused by a protozoan, a small microscopic organism. The symptoms include an odorous discharge, genital itching, and occasionally, a burning sensation during urination.

Sterility

Sterility in a female can be the result of a blocked Fallopian tube, the failure of the ovaries to produce ova that can be fertilized, or a sexually transmitted disease that has not been treated.

FINDING HELP

Monthly breast self-examination is an important step in detecting breast cancer. For more information on this subject, contact the following groups:

- American Cancer Society's Reach to Recovery Program 1599 Clifton Road, N.E. Atlanta, GA 30329
- Y-Me National Organization for Breast Cancer Information and Support 18220 Harwood Avenue Homewood, IL 60430

KEEPING FIT

Getting a Routine Pelvic Exam

A pelvic exam is one in which a gynecologist checks a female's pelvic area, first with an instrument called a speculum and then by hand. This is done to check the shape, size, and position of pelvic organs and to check for any tumors or cysts.

The American College of Obstetricians and Gynecologists (ACOG) recommends that young females have pelvic exams by the time they are 18, or earlier if they are sexually active. These exams should occur yearly, even when there are no problems. In addition, females should have pelvic exams if they have menstrual problems, unusual vaginal discharge, or if they are planning to get pregnant.

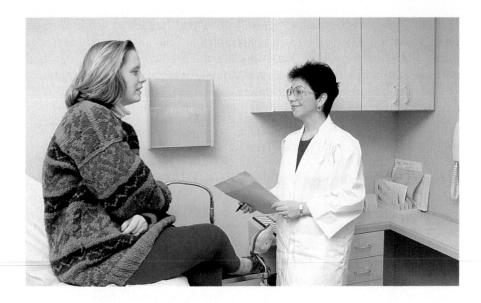

Endometriosis

The endometrium, which is the inner lining of the uterus, sometimes is present abnormally in the abdominal cavity. This condition, endometriosis, usually causes sterility. Treatment involves hormone therapy and surgery.

Breast Cancer

About 1 out of 9 females develop breast cancer at some time in their lives. Most breast lumps are found by the females themselves. About 80 percent of these lumps are benign, which means they are noncancerous. Females with a family history of breast cancer are at a greater risk of developing a cancerous condition.

Ovarian Cysts

An ovarian cyst is a growth on the outside of an ovary. Small, non-cancerous cysts can develop often but usually dissolve on their own. Large cysts may have to be surgically removed.

Cancer of the Cervix, Uterus, and Ovaries

The cervix, uterus, and ovaries are common sites of cancer in females. Cervical cancer is detected through a Pap smear, a test in which samples of cells are taken from the cervix by a doctor and viewed under a microscope. Early detection contributes to successful treatment. Early sexual activity, and a family history of cervical cancer and other factors, is related to an increased incidence of cervical cancer.

Doctors may also sample tissue from the lining of the uterus to check for cancerous cells. Uterine cancer is most common in females between the ages of 60 and 75. However, it can occur at any age. As with cervical cancer, early detection may bring greater success in treatment. The Pap smear is not as accurate in detecting cancer of the uterus as it is for cervical cancer. The American Cancer Society recommends that once a female reaches the age of 18, she begin having a yearly Pap smear.

DID YOU KNOW?

- Multiple births involving four or more babies do not usually occur unless fertility drugs have been used.
- The woman who gave birth to the most children on record gave birth to multiples twenty-seven times. She did this in the 1700s—long before the use of fertility drugs.
- The two heaviest babies on record were born weighing 22 pounds, 8 ounces each. One was born in 1955; the other in 1982.

Frances Hamilton is 44. She is an artist who lives in Boston, Massachusetts, with her artist husband, Peter Thibeault. Together, they not only share an interest in the arts but also a reproductive history that has brought them both pain and joy.

Frances Hamilton says, "I wasn't very interested in having children when I was younger. But then, when I was 35, that changed. It suddenly dawned on me that I really was going to get older. Then I developed a deep interest in becoming a mother."

But becoming a mother was not easy for Hamilton. She had three unsuccessful pregnancies.

But the fourth pregnancy did not fail. It resulted in the birth of Dinah Kate, now 5. "Having gone through the three losses," Hamilton continues, "there wasn't a moment during my pregnancy that I was relaxed. I kept waiting to hear bad news. It wasn't until Dinah was born and in my arms that I could believe she was okay."

Hamilton's fifth and sixth pregnancies again were unsuccessful. But her seventh pregnancy was Anna, her 8-month-old daughter.

For a time, the many losses Hamilton suffered affected her art work. "Because in a mis-carriage a woman bears so much of the responsibility—because it is her body that 'fails'—the losses really affected my self-esteem and my ability to complete projects. The process of creating and bearing a child is not unlike the

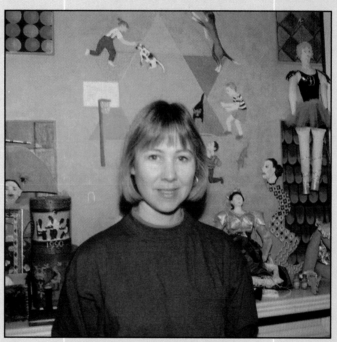

process of creating art. You bring something out of nothing, nurture it, and make it grow. Because of that parallel, in my work, too, I began starting things and losing the thread. I became discouraged very easily in the work.

"I've since made some images about the losses, but I found them so painful that I can't even look at them. I started to focus on images of mothers. I used my own mother and sought magazine images from the '50s, which is when I was growing up. And by identifying with my mother and the mothers of the '50s, I was able to keep working."

These days, Hamilton and Thibeault are very caught up in the lives of their two young daughters. "Every day Peter and I watch them playing together. And when the 5-year-old is making the baby laugh, it just goes through us like music. It's not just their individual presence but their connection with each other that gives us delight. A baby that you've waited for is a source of never-ending pleasure. We're so grateful."

About the experiences she and her husband have gone through in trying to have a family, she concludes, "I think you have to understand that adversity builds a stronger person. When things are difficult, it challenges you to develop your inner resources. In our case, it has made us better parents."

1. How did the repeated loss of her pregnancies affect Hamilton's self-esteem?
2. How did her art struggles parallel those in her reproductive life?
3. What struggles are you facing right now that may be chipping away at your self-esteem? How are they reflected in other areas of your life?

For unknown reasons there has been an increase in the number of cases of ovarian cancer in recent years. There are often no signs of ovarian cancer until late in its development. It is most common in older females, but can affect anyone. Three important ways to detect ovarian cancer include a pelvic examination given by a doctor; a look at a female's family history, since females with a family history of ovarian cancer are at a greater risk of developing the disease; and a blood test called CA 125, which can detect this type of cancer. As with other forms of cancer, the earlier the disease is detected the more successful the treatment can be.

Care of the Female Reproductive System

Cleanliness is an important part of keeping the reproductive system healthy. The vagina is a self-cleansing organ. Once a female goes through puberty, the cells in the lining of the vagina are constantly being shed, causing a slight vaginal discharge. This is normal. Cleanliness is especially important during the menstrual period when menstrual flow may cause a slight odor. Sanitary napkins and tampons should be changed every few hours. Feminine hygiene products such as deodorant sprays and douches should not be necessary and may, in fact, cause irritation to the sensitive tissues around the vagina.

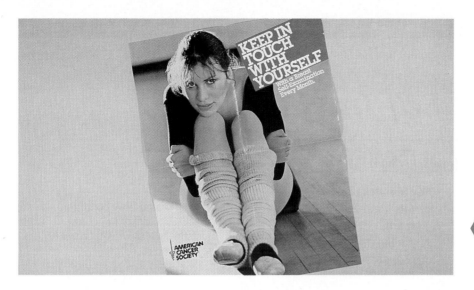

Early detection of breast cancer is still the best preventive health practice. The American Cancer Society recommends the monthly practice of breast self-examination (BSE). The best time to perform it is about one week after the menstrual period—the breasts are then least likely to be tender.

There are three ways to examine the breasts: in the shower, before a mirror, and lying down. Self-examination is most convenient in the shower because hands glide easier over wet skin. Follow this procedure during a bath or shower: With one hand raised over the head and the fingers of the other hand flat, move your hand over every part of each breast. Use the left hand to inspect the right breast and the right hand to inspect the left breast. Pay special attention to the area between the armpit and the breast, checking for any lump, hard knot, or tissue thickening. If you find anything unusual, contact your doctor at once. Only a doctor can make a diagnosis.

Once a female reaches her late 30s, the American Cancer Society recommends that she have a mammogram. This is an X ray of the breasts that detects the presence of abnormal tissue. For more information or to obtain a pamphlet on breast self-examination, contact your local American Cancer Society.

CONFLICT RESOLUTION

Carmina's mother was recently diagnosed with cancer. Her mother's sister Maria is 37 and considered to be at high risk for breast cancer because of family history. However, Maria refuses to get a mammogram. She has all kinds of excuses—she doesn't have time, she doesn't want to be exposed to unnecessary radiation, and she believes the test will hurt. Carmina thinks the real reason is Maria's fear of being diagnosed with cancer.

Help Carmina convince her aunt to get a mammogram.

LESSON 2 REVIEW

Reviewing Facts and Vocabulary

1. What is menstruation?
2. What is PMS?
3. Name two causes of sterility in females.
4. What are two types of vaginal infections?

Thinking Critically

5. **Analysis.** What is the relationship between ovulation, fertilization, and menstruation?

6. **Analysis.** How does the female reproductive system compare with the male reproductive system?

Applying Health Knowledge

7. Make a list of some of the myths you have heard about menstruation. Why do you think there is so much misinformation? Suggest some ways to clear up these types of myths.

Self-Inventory

Care of the Reproductive System

HOW DO YOU RATE?

Number a sheet of paper from 1 through 8. Read each item below, and respond by writing *always*, *sometimes*, or *never* for each item. Total the number of each type of response. Then proceed to the next section.

1. I eat a well-balanced diet.
2. I exercise regularly.
3. I manage the stress in my life.
4. I practice daily health care.
5. I avoid situations that might put me at risk of contracting an STD.
6. I have regular physical check-ups.

For males only:

7. I do a monthly testicular self-exam.
8. I wear a protector or supporter if I am participating in strenuous activity.

For females only:

7. I do a monthly breast self-exam.
8. I avoid the use of feminine hygiene products, such as sprays or douches.

HOW DID YOU SCORE?

Give yourself 3 points for each *always* response, 1 point for each *sometimes* response, and 0 points for each *never* response. Find your total, and read below to see how you scored. Then proceed to the next section.

15 to 24
Excellent. Your health choices show you are taking care of your reproductive system. Keep up the good work!

8 to 14
Good, but there are some things you could do to promote a healthier reproductive system.

Below 8
Look out! You may be taking unnecessary risks that could affect the health of your reproductive system.

WHAT ARE YOUR GOALS?

Complete each statement below.

1. The behavior I would like to change or improve is ____.
2. If this behavior were completely changed, I would look, feel, or act differently in the following ways: ____.
3. The steps involved in making this change are ____.
4. My timetable is ____.
5. People I will ask for support or assistance are ____.
6. The benefits I will receive are ____.
7. My reward at the end of each week will be ____.

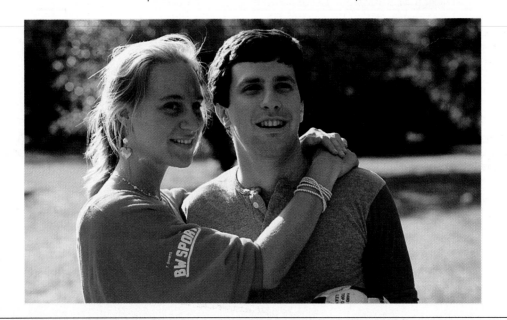

Building Decision-Making Skills

S everal of Shana's girlfriends are at her house for a sleepover to celebrate her 16th birthday. The topic of conversation becomes the girls' sexual experiences. Shana is still a virgin, but it seems that she is in the minority. Her boyfriend, whom she has been dating for several months, has been trying to talk her into "filling in the last piece of the puzzle of their relationship." The idea is admittedly exciting, but she has decided to wait to have sex until marriage. Shana is worried about what to tell the girls. What should she do?

WHAT DO YOU THINK?

1. **Situation.** Why does a decision need to be made?
2. **Choices.** List as many possible ways to handle this situation as you can.
3. **Consequences.** What are the advantages of each possibility?
4. **Consequences.** What are the disadvantages of each possibility?
5. **Situation.** What other decisions will Shana need to make soon?
6. **Situation.** Why should Shana deal with this situation one decision at a time?
7. **Consequences.** What risks are involved in the decision about what to tell her friends?
8. **Consequences.** How might her parents be affected by this decision?
9. **Consequences.** How might Shana's self-esteem be affected?
10. **Consequences.** How might her reputation be affected?
11. **Consequences.** What peer pressure is likely to be used in this situation?
12. **Decision.** What do you think Shana should say to her friends?
13. **Evaluation.** Do you think most teens are truthful when discussing their sexual experiences? Why or why not?

T he guys in the locker room are discussing their sexual exploits and have mentioned several girls Gino has dated as being "easy." The guys have tried to get him to reinforce their comments, but he has never "scored" with any of the girls. In fact he has not had sex with any girl and does not plan to until he is married. How should he handle the pressure from the guys?

WHAT DO YOU THINK?

14. **Choices.** What are Gino's choices?
15. **Consequences.** What are the advantages of each choice?
16. **Consequences.** What are the disadvantages of each choice?
17. **Consequences.** What risks are involved in this decision?
18. **Consequences.** How might Gino's health triangle be affected by this decision?
19. **Consequences.** How might Gino's current girlfriend be affected by this decision?
20. **Consequences.** How might his friends be affected by this decision?
21. **Consequences.** How might his parents be affected by this decision?
22. **Consequences.** How might younger brothers and sisters be affected by this decision?
23. **Decision.** How do you think Gino should handle this situation? Why?

REVIEW

Using Health Terms

On a separate sheet of paper, write the term that best matches each definition given below.

LESSON 1

1. Glands that produce sperm.
2. Tube in which sperm are stored.
3. Sac that protects testes.
4. A disorder of the male reproductive system in which a male is unable to reproduce.
5. A mixture of fluids from glands with sperm; the fluids provide nourishment for sperm and help with their movement.

LESSON 2

6. Cells present in a female ovary from birth.
7. The birth canal.
8. A fertilized ovum.
9. The process in which an ovum is released from the ovaries.
10. The process by which the uterus sheds its lining.
11. The union of a sperm and an ovum.
12. Usual site of fertilization.
13. One possible cause of female sterility characterized by the inner lining of the uterus being present in the abdominal cavity.
14. Site of the development of the ovum if it is fertilized.
15. Lumps that are noncancerous.

Building Academic Skills

LESSON 1 AND LESSON 2

16. **Writing.** The changes one goes through during puberty can be awkward, embarrassing, and difficult. Write a two-page paper describing what it was like for an imaginary friend.

LESSON 2

17. **Reading.** Read Gilda Radner's autobiography, *It's Always Something,* about her struggle with ovarian cancer. Make a list of major events discussed in this book.

Recalling the Facts

LESSON 1

18. What is the function of testosterone?
19. What are the secondary sex characteristics for males?
20. What are the functions of the male reproductive system?
21. What prevents urine and semen from passing through the urethra at the same time?
22. How is acidity neutralized in the urethra thus ensuring that sperm are not killed?
23. Explain what is involved in caring for the male reproductive system.
24. How does the scrotum keep the testes at a temperature that is slightly below normal body temperature?
25. Why is it important for a male to examine his testes regularly? How often should it be done?

LESSON 2

26. What functions does the female reproductive system serve?
27. What causes menstrual cramps in females?
28. What are the secondary sex characteristics for females?
29. What functions do ovaries serve?
30. What are the internal reproductive organs in females?
31. Where does fertilization usually occur?
32. How does a mature ovum travel through the Fallopian tube?
33. What are two suspected causes of PMS?
34. What percentage of females are likely to develop breast cancer?
35. What is the purpose of doing a breast self-examination? How often should it be done? What is the best time to do it and why?
36. How are cervical, uterine, and ovarian cancers detected?
37. What is a Pap smear test?
38. How often should a female get a Pap smear?
39. What is toxic shock syndrome?

REVIEW

Thinking Critically

LESSON 1

40. Analysis. Compare testicular to prostate cancer.

41. Evaluation. When a male is born, a decision needs to be made whether or not to have him circumcised. Research the procedure of this operation and discuss cultural and religious issues regarding circumcision. If you had an infant son, would you choose to have him circumcised? Why or why not?

LESSON 2

42. Synthesis. Ann is 14 years old. She still has not started menstruating, and her breasts have not developed. Some of her friends have started making fun of her. What advice or comfort would you offer to Ann?

43. Synthesis. PMS is still a relatively mysterious ailment. The causes are not yet fully understood. Some medicine companies are producing over-the-counter medications to treat PMS. From what you have learned, how effective do you think the medicines might be? What symptoms do you think the medicines help alleviate?

44. Analysis. Compare the male and female reproductive systems. Highlight similarities and differences.

45. Synthesis. Vaginal infections were once treated with a prescription medicine that is now available over-the-counter. What might the positive aspects of this change be? What might be negative about this?

Making the Connection

LESSON 2

46. Business Education. View ten different television commercials. For each, note the product, the intended customer, the stated message, and the implied message. How many of these commercials used sexual messages? Do you think sexual messages in advertising are appropriate? Explain your reasoning.

Applying Health Knowledge

LESSON 1

47. What would happen if Cowper's glands were not functioning properly?

48. How can a male increase his chances of surviving testicular cancer? Prostate cancer?

49. What do you think might be the result of a male wearing pants that are too tight?

50. Trace the path of sperm through the male reproductive system.

51. Why would it be important for a male to get a medical checkup if he experienced difficulty when urinating?

LESSON 2

52. The ovaries alternately release a mature ovum each month. What might happen if one ovary had to be removed?

53. When a fertilized ovum attaches to the uterine wall, it begins to grow and develop. What happens if the ovum is not fertilized?

54. Why does menstruation take place?

55. When in a female's menstrual cycle is she most likely to become pregnant?

56. Why would it be important for you to be aware of a history of cancer in your family?

57. Sometimes a fertilized ovum fails to move through the Fallopian tube to the uterus. Instead, the zygote continues to grow in the Fallopian tube. Why would it be impossible for this to be a normal pregnancy?

Beyond the Classroom

LESSON 2

58. Parental Involvement. Discuss with your parents feminine health-care ads found on television and in magazines. Discuss what these ads are designed to do. What merits or drawbacks do you and your parents see in them?

59. Community Involvement. Call or write your local American Cancer Society unit for pamphlets describing the correct procedure for breast and testicular self-examination.

CHAPTER

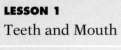

16 PERSONAL HEALTH

LESSON 1
Teeth and Mouth

LESSON 2
Eyes

LESSON 3
Ears

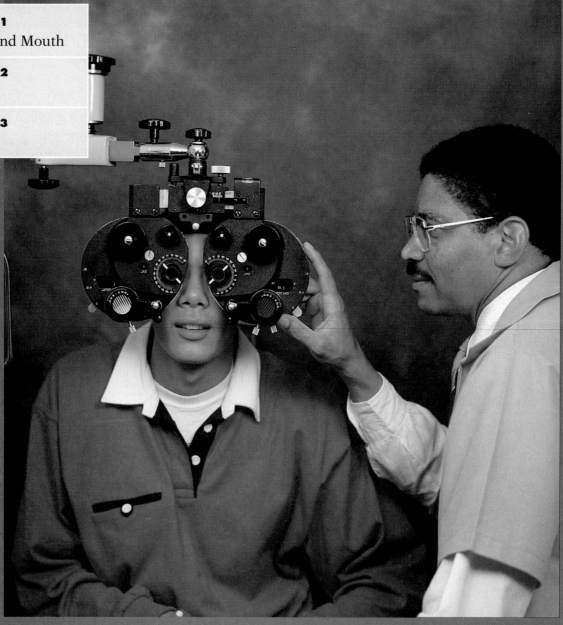

TEETH AND MOUTH

What is the most common noncommunicable disease in the United States? If you guessed tooth decay, you are right. Most Americans have or have had tooth decay. Yet it is one of the most preventable diseases. Before learning more about good oral health, let us first look at the functions and structure of the teeth.

Functions and Structure of the Teeth

Within your mouth, your teeth are the most vital structures and perhaps the single most noticeable contributor to the appearance of your mouth and face. Your teeth not only allow you to chew food, they also form the shape and structure of your mouth.

The Periodontium

The area immediately around the teeth is called the **periodontium.** It is made up of the gums, periodontal ligament, and the jawbone. Together these structures support the teeth.

The Tooth

The tooth itself is divided into three major parts: the root, the neck, and the crown. The crown is the visible part of the tooth.

The **pulp** is the very sensitive, living tissue inside the tooth. The pulp is entirely enclosed by the hard inner walls of the tooth in the root canal. Blood vessels and nerves are also contained in the pulp cavity.

You experience a toothache when the pulp becomes inflamed because of a cavity or disease. Because the inflamed pulp cannot expand within the inflexible walls of the tooth, pressure builds within the tooth and results in pain.

The pulp is surrounded by a material called dentin. The dentin is covered in the root area of the tooth by a substance called cementum. The crown of the tooth is covered with a hard material called enamel.

Enamel is the hardest material in the body. It is the second hardest naturally occurring substance in nature, diamonds being the hardest. However, it is this hard substance, the enamel, that can be the victim of tooth decay.

Problems of the Teeth and Mouth

Good, regular oral health care is necessary for healthy, clean teeth. Oral health care is also an important factor in preventing periodontal disease and other tooth disorders. Let us look at what can happen when teeth and gums are not cared for properly.

LESSON 1 FOCUS

TERMS TO USE

- Periodontium (per•ee•oh•DAHN•tee•uhm)
- Pulp
- Periodontal (per•ee•oh•DAHN•tuhl) disease
- Plaque
- Tartar

CONCEPTS TO LEARN

- Regular oral health care is necessary for healthy, clean teeth.
- Oral health care is an important factor in preventing periodontal disease.

ATTITUDES AND BEHAVIORS TO EVALUATE

- Self-Inventory, page 332.
- Building Decision-Making Skills, page 333.

A tooth is a living structure made up of many parts.

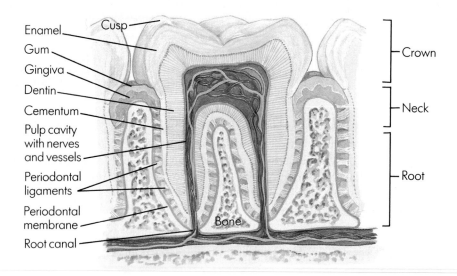

Enamel
Cusp
Gum
Gingiva
Dentin
Cementum
Pulp cavity
with nerves
and vessels
Periodontal
ligaments
Periodontal
membrane
Root canal
Bone

Crown
Neck
Root

Periodontal Disease

Susan has bad breath. Larry's gums often bleed when he brushes his teeth. Michelle's front teeth have begun to spread. All three of these people have periodontal disease—the most common cause of tooth loss.

Periodontal disease is an inflammation of the periodontal structures. It is almost entirely preventable. Periodontal disease is primarily the result of the destructive action of bacteria in your mouth. Bacteria form plaque. **Plaque** is a sticky, colorless film that acts on sugar to form acids that destroy tooth enamel and irritate gums.

Unless plaque is removed once every 24 to 36 hours, it can harden into tartar. **Tartar,** or calculus, as it is sometimes called, is a very hard substance that irritates the underlying bone as well as the surrounding gums of your teeth.

Decay begins as the plaque eats into the enamel and then spreads to the dentin. Your tooth will become more sensitive as the decay reaches the pulp. You will experience a toothache when the decay reaches the pulp and exposes the nerve. If it is not treated, the bacterial infection can spread.

A tooth becomes abscessed when decay progresses to the stage where pus collects in and tissue becomes inflamed around the bone sockets of a tooth. An abscessed or badly decayed tooth in the upper jaw can spread infection into the sinuses.

K E E P I N G   F I T

Knowing the Signs of Gum Disease

Periodontal disease can develop at any age. If you develop any of the following symptoms, see your dentist right away:

- gums that bleed very easily
- chronic bad breath or bad taste in the mouth
- loose or separating permanent teeth
- changes in your bite
- red, swollen, or painful gums sensitive to the touch
- pus between the teeth
- gums that seem to be pulling away from the teeth

Other Tooth and Mouth Disorders

In addition to periodontal disease, several other tooth and mouth disorders can occur. Sometimes they appear as a result of poor oral health, but just as often they develop because of poorly aligned teeth.

Halitosis. Halitosis is bad breath, a condition that can be caused by such factors as decayed teeth, eating certain foods, indigestion, and mouth infections. Mouthwashes and mints may temporarily cover up the odor. However, these breath fresheners do not cure halitosis. Good oral health care can control halitosis. If halitosis is caused by tooth decay or other infections, the only way to cure it is to treat the underlying cause of the problem.

Malocclusion. Malocclusion is a condition in which the teeth of the upper and lower jaws do not align properly. Malocclusion is often hereditary. If the teeth are too large for the jaw to accommodate them, or if a person has an extra tooth, the teeth are pushed out of alignment. Other factors that might cause malocclusion are thumb sucking or tooth loss. Malocclusion can lead to decay and disease and can also affect a person's speech and ability to chew. If malocclusion is severe, a person's appearance and self-esteem can be negatively affected.

Orthodontics is the specialty of dentistry that corrects malocclusion. Orthodontists may recommend the use of braces or other dental appliances to help align the teeth.

Gingivitis. Gingivitis is a disorder in which the gums become red and swollen and bleed easily. The inflammation may be caused by dental plaque, misaligned teeth, or deposits of decaying food. A dentist must determine the cause of the inflammation in order to treat gingivitis.

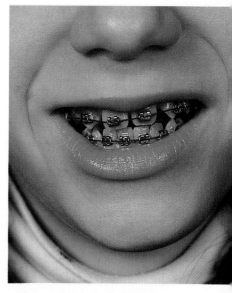

Braces are one orthodontic appliance used to correct misalignment of teeth.

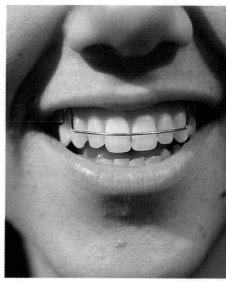

A retainer is another orthodontic appliance used to straighten teeth.

HEALTH UPDATE

LOOKING AT TECHNOLOGY

Lasers: New Light on the Subject

Lasers are now being used in the dentist's office. Dental lasers are being used to vaporize cavities without harming healthy enamel on the patient's teeth. Experimenting with an ophthalmologist's laser, a Michigan dentist found that using a pulsating laser on cavities rather than a continuous beam could zap away cavities without overheating the surrounding gums. In addition to being used for cavities, dental lasers are now also being used to remove and shape gum tissue. This laser use has been found to be as effective as the scalpel usually used in routine gum surgeries. In addition, while 95 percent of people getting scalpel surgery on the gums required some anesthesia, the laser surgery method requires only 20 percent of patients to be anesthetized. The laser, unlike the scalpel, can also get at gum disease in its very earliest stages and in locations that a scalpel may not be able to reach easily.

Periodontitis. If gingivitis is untreated, a more serious form of gum disease, called periodontitis, can develop. This disease results in swollen, tender, and/or bleeding gums. Since bone surrounding the teeth is gradually destroyed, teeth can become loose and may fall out. As with gingivitis, good oral health care, including dental care, prevents this disease.

Care of the Teeth

More than 20 million Americans have already lost most or all of their teeth. This does not have to happen to you. With good care your teeth should last a lifetime. The choice is yours. If you spend 10 to 15 minutes a day cleaning and flossing your teeth, and if you limit foods high in sugar, you will probably be able to keep your teeth your entire life.

Regular brushing after eating and before bedtime is essential. Because a toothbrush often misses hard-to-reach spots, flossing is important. Flossing removes plaque and food particles that are stuck between teeth and between teeth and gums.

Periodontal disease, the most common cause of tooth loss, is almost entirely preventable. By age 15, four out of every five Americans have the beginnings of periodontal disease. In the early stages, the disease can be checked. Checking the progress of the disease requires preventive oral health and periodic visits to a dentist.

Your diet is a major contributor to the presence of plaque on your teeth. Frequent consumption of sugary foods promotes the formation of plaque. If you eat sweets, it is best to brush your teeth as soon as possible. Even if you do not eat sweets you still have to be concerned with plaque removal. Plaque is continually forming. It will form even if you eat nothing at all, so daily plaque removal is essential.

LESSON 1 REVIEW

Reviewing Facts and Vocabulary

1. How can you protect and maintain your teeth?
2. Describe the process of tooth decay.

Thinking Critically

3. **Synthesis.** Develop a message that would be appropriate for people who do not regularly brush or floss their teeth.
4. **Evaluation.** How would you be able to distinguish between a person who practices good oral health and one who doesn't?

Applying Health Knowledge

5. Make a report on the use of fluoride to prevent tooth decay. Is it added to the water in your community? If so, how has the rate of tooth decay changed since the introduction of fluoride?
6. Identify three ads for oral dental health. What do the ads claim? Make up your own ad for oral or dental health. Share it with the class.

EYES

Your eyes have over a million electrical connections and are responsible for about 80 percent of the knowledge you acquire. They can distinguish nearly 8 million differences in color! Of the sense organs, the eyes provide the greatest knowledge of the environment. However, individuals who do not have full use of their sight can and do develop their other senses to a much higher degree.

The Eyes' Built-In Protection

The eyes are situated in orbits protected by the bony sockets of the skull. The general area around the eyes consists of the lacrimal glands, the eyebrows and eyelids, the conjunctiva, and the eyelashes.

The Lacrimal Glands

The **lacrimal gland,** located above each eye, is responsible for producing tears. Tears are made mostly of water and a small amount of salt and mucus. The salt gives the tears an antiseptic effect, which helps them fight pathogens. Tears keep the eyeballs moist and help remove foreign objects from the eyes.

Tears reach the surface of the eye through tiny ducts. Some of the tears evaporate from the eye's surface. Those that do not evaporate are drained into the nasal cavity by two tear ducts located at the inner corner of the eye. These ducts open into larger ducts that run down the nose. When the production of tears increases, the tear ducts are not able to carry away the extra quantity, and tears flow over the lower lid.

Eyebrows, Eyelids, and Eyelashes

Eyebrows are growths of hair that protect the eyes from foreign particles, perspiration, and direct rays of light.

Eyelids are folds of skin that protect the eye by covering its surface. The eyelids are controlled by an automatic reflex action that causes you to blink to protect the eyes. Your eyes are closed a total of about 30 minutes a day because of blinking!

Eyelashes help keep foreign particles out of the eyes. The eyelashes receive a lubricating secretion from oil glands. This oily secretion prevents the eyelids from sticking together.

Conjunctiva

Conjunctiva is a protective mucous membrane attached to the inner surface of the eyelids that continues over the outer surface of the eyeball. Several different conditions, including lack of sleep, can irritate this membrane, causing inflammation.

LESSON 2 FOCUS

TERMS TO USE

- Lacrimal (LAK•ree•mul) gland
- Conjunctiva
- Sclera (SKLER•uh)
- Cornea
- Choroid (KOHR•oid)
- Aqueous humor (A•kwee•uhs HU•mer)
- Vitreous humor (VIT•ree•uhs HU•mer)
- Retina

CONCEPTS TO LEARN

- The parts around the eye provide protection to the eye.
- Your eye adjusts to different intensities of light.
- Many vision problems can be corrected with professional help.

ATTITUDES AND BEHAVIORS TO EVALUATE

- Self-Inventory, page 332.
- Building Decision-Making Skills, page 333.

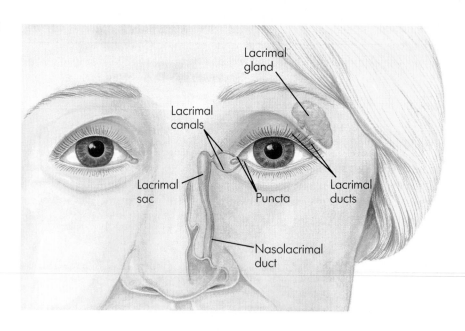

By producing tears, the lacrimal gland helps keep foreign objects out of the eye.

Structure of the Eye

The eyeball is about 1 inch (2.5 cm) in diameter. The eyeball is slightly longer than it is wide. This shape results from the bulge caused by the cornea, known as the window of the eye.

The Eyeball Wall

The wall of the eyeball is made up of three layers: the sclera, the choroid, and the retina.

The Sclera. The **sclera** is a white, tough membrane that helps the eye keep its spherical shape. This is the white part of your eye, and it helps protect the eye's delicate inner structure. In the front part of the eye, the sclera forms the colorless, transparent **cornea,** which is like a round clear dish supplied with many free nerve endings. Thus, the cornea is extremely sensitive to particles that come in contact with its surface.

The Choroid. The middle layer of the eyeball wall, the **choroid,** contains

- the iris, seen from the outside as the color of the eye;
- the suspensory ligaments, which blend with and hold the lens;
- the ciliary muscles, to which suspensory ligaments and the sclera are attached.

The iris is situated at the front of the eye. *Iris,* a Greek word meaning "rainbow," gives the eye its color. The iris is located in front of the lens. The black circle in the center of the iris is the pupil, which actually is a round hole, through which light passes.

Two sets of muscles in the iris change the size of the pupil, thus controlling the amount of light that enters the eye. In dim light one set of muscles, controlled by the sympathetic nervous system, pulls away from the iris, making it larger. This is called dilation.

In bright light the other set of muscles, controlled by the parasympathetic system, makes the pupil smaller. This is called contraction.

Behind the pupil is the lens, held by the suspensory ligaments. These ligaments, in turn, are connected to the ciliary muscles. The lens projects onto the retina an image of what is before it. The lens is curved, and the ciliary muscles help change its shape as the eye focuses on an object.

The cavity between the cornea and the lens is filled with a watery fluid called the **aqueous humor.** The words come from Latin; *aqueous* means "water," and *humor* means "fluid." The aqueous humor is continuously formed and drained off. This helps maintain pressure within the eye. The aqueous humor is a source of nutrients for structures, such as the cornea.

The **vitreous humor,** a thicker fluid, is found behind the lens and keeps the eyeball firm. *Vitreous* means "glasslike."

There are no blood vessels in the sclera, cornea, lens, aqueous humor, or vitreous humor. The choroid, the middle layer, contains the blood vessels that nourish the eyes.

The Retina.   The **retina** makes up the third layer of the eyeball wall. It contains the nerve cells and controls the processes responsible for vision. The retina contains millions of light-sensitive receptors that are classified as either rods or cones. Rods and cones bear names that describe their appearance.

The rods, which are cylindrical, register light and darkness and are used in dim light. They contain a photosensitive chemical called visual purple, which makes it possible to see in dim light. Light breaks down this visual purple so that when you go from a light room to a dark room at first, you cannot see. As the rods re-form the visual purple, you begin to see objects in shades of black, white, and gray. People who do not have enough visual purple experience night blindness. Rods lie toward the edge of the retina. An estimated 125 million rods are in a retina.

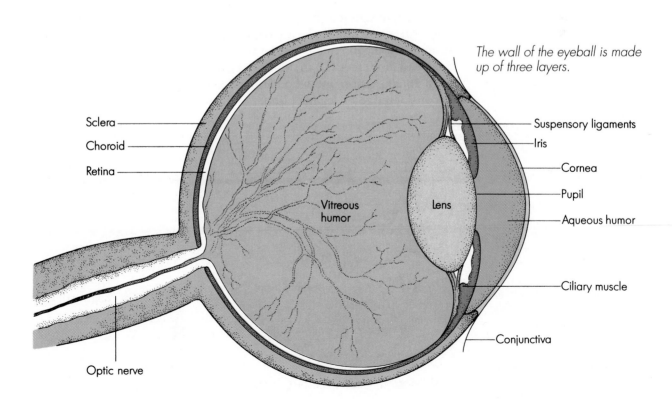

The wall of the eyeball is made up of three layers.

Sclera
Choroid
Retina
Vitreous humor
Lens
Optic nerve
Suspensory ligaments
Iris
Cornea
Pupil
Aqueous humor
Ciliary muscle
Conjunctiva

The cones, which are cone-shaped, are situated with their pointed end nearer the choroid layer. Cones give you vision in bright light and are able to detect differences in color. About 7 million cones are in a retina, concentrated in its back part.

Some people have a deficiency in perceiving colors, which is called color blindness. Almost all color blindness is mild. Color-blind people have trouble seeing shades of red or green. It is rare that a person has complete color blindness—a condition in which the person sees only shades of black, white, and gray.

The Optic Nerve

At the back of the eye is a large nerve cable that connects the eye with the brain. This is known as the optic nerve. At the point where this optic nerve connects with the eye, the nerve spreads and becomes part of the inner surface of the retina.

The point at which the optic nerve enters the eye is called the blind spot. Since there are no cones or rods in this area, vision in this spot is not possible.

Vision

As light rays pass through the cornea and aqueous humor, they are bent and directed through the pupil. The light rays then penetrate the lens, which adjusts to focus the light on the retina. This adjustment is called accommodation. The lens bulges to accommodate near objects and flattens to accommodate faraway objects.

The light-sensitive retina sends impulses along the optic nerve to the occipital lobe of the brain. The brain interprets the light rays as an image.

In normal vision a sharp image is produced. If you stand 20 feet (6 m) from an eye chart and can read the top eight lines, you have 20/20 vision. If you can read at 20 feet (6 m) what a person with normal vision can read at 40 feet (12 m) you have 20/40 vision. A person who has less than 20/200 vision and who cannot see the letter at the top of the chart is considered to be legally blind.

In A-1 the eyeball is too long from front to back, and the image is formed in front of the retina. As a result, distant objects are unclear. In B-1 the eyeball is too short from front to back, and the image is formed behind the retina. In this case, objects that are close are unclear. Corrective lenses in A-2 and B-2 help the image form where it should, on the retina, so objects can be seen clearly.

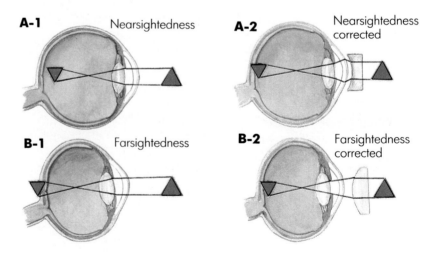

A-1   Nearsightedness

A-2   Nearsightedness corrected

B-1   Farsightedness

B-2   Farsightedness corrected

Overcoming The Odds

Dr. David Hartman is a psychiatrist in private practice in Roanoke, Virginia. He is married and has three children. Dr. Hartman is also blind.

"I lost my sight when I was eight," he says. "I had a congenital eye disease that couldn't be corrected."

When Hartman was 9, he went to a school for the blind, which he attended for about 5 years. He continues, "The school helped me to reorient my thinking and I learned to be treated like everyone else. Even though I lived only 15 minutes from the school, I stayed there from Monday to Friday." Still, despite these separations, Hartman had great family support. "My mom read to me a lot," he says. "My dad figured out creative ways that I could do things. And my sister confronted me with reality."

"In eighth grade, I began public school," he continues. "It was easy for me to adapt to the academics. But the real challenge was to fit in socially. I'd wrestled at the school for the blind from third grade on, so when I wrestled in eighth grade, I was a little better than the other kids. That helped me to be seen by the other students as normal."

Hartman then went on to Gettysburg College where he was active in campus activities, including giving campus tours. With the help of two professors/mentors, Hartman did very well in college and applied to nine medical schools. One by one, eight of the schools rejected him. "At

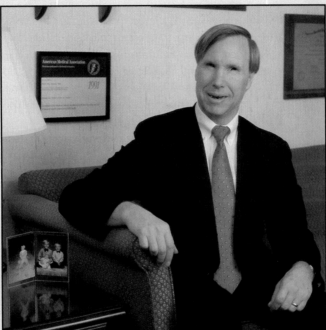

the same time, I was reading The Old Man and the Sea," he says, "and that book helped me more than anything to see that often it's not the goal we are trying to achieve but the process that is most important."

Finally, Hartman was accepted at Temple University School of Medicine. After graduation, he went on to an internship at Temple and then to a psychiatric residency at the University of Pennsylvania. In 1975, a made-for-TV movie called Journey from Darkness about his quest to become a doctor was aired on national TV. Later, he wrote about his life in a book entitled White Coat, White Cane.

Today, Dr. Hartman thinks that his blindness is sometimes an asset. He says, "It allows me to have a different point of view. Some patients say they feel more comfortable because they don't feel I'm peering at them or scrutinizing them." He concludes, "We all have our disabilities. We all have our strengths, too. We need to explore and discover our strengths. We need to recognize that we each have our own uniqueness."

1. Hartman had lots of support along the way—from family, professors, and friends. How can support from caring people motivate someone to achieve goals and develop self-esteem?

2. Hartman says, "We all have our disabilities. We all have our strengths, too." What do you consider your disabilities? Your strengths? How can you accept and/or improve your weaknesses and more fully use and develop your strengths?

Eye Problems

Nearsightedness (myopia) is a condition in which light rays are focused in front of the retina. A person who is nearsighted can see clearly when things are close, but distant objects are blurred. Concave corrective lenses in eyeglasses make the rays focus farther back.

Farsightedness (hyperopia) occurs when the light rays are focused behind the retina. Someone who is farsighted can see distant objects clearly, but things close up are blurred. This condition is corrected by convex lenses in eyeglasses.

Astigmatism occurs when the curvature of the lens is uneven. Light rays focus at different points, causing the image to be blurred. This condition is corrected with specially ground lenses for eyeglasses.

A cataract is a clouding of the lens, which causes blurring or hazy vision and problems with night vision. The clouded lens may be surgically removed and vision restored with corrective glasses. A cataract is the most frequent single cause of blindness among adults.

Crossed eyes (strabismus) might occur when the eye muscles of both eyes do not work together, causing one or both eyes to turn inward or outward. A person with crossed eyes may then see two images because the brain, even though it can interpret the images, cannot fuse the input from each eye.

Amblyopia is a condition of reduced or dim vision in an eye that otherwise appears to be normal. This condition occurs when a child with strabismus favors one eye and the unused eye loses some ability to see. Amblyopia is a major cause of partial vision loss in children. Prevention depends on early diagnosis. Treatment of amblyopia includes wearing corrective lenses, wearing an eye patch on the weaker eye, or possible surgery to correct the eye muscle.

Glaucoma is caused by increased fluid pressure in the eyeball, either because too much aqueous humor is produced or because it drains inadequately. Glaucoma may cause damage to the optic nerve and result in blindness. Glaucoma usually develops slowly and painlessly, and can be diagnosed during an eye examination. If glaucoma is detected early, it can be treated with medication or surgery.

A sty is an eye infection caused by bacteria that lodge in the glands of the eyelids. A physician can prescribe treatment or antibiotic drops for a sty.

Conjunctivitis is an eye infection that affects the sclera and the conjunctiva and causes reddening. It is sometimes called pinkeye when it affects children. A doctor can treat this condition with antibiotics.

Mixed Signals

Raising your eyebrows briefly, "the eyebrow flash," indicates friendliness if you are Balinese, Papuan, Samoan, or American. In Japan, however, it is regarded as an indecent gesture and is avoided. Your culture also influences whether or not to maintain eye contact. Many Americans have learned to make eye contact to show attention, but not to make constant contact, or stare, because it is considered rude. In Japan, eyes are to be lowered as a sign of respect when listening. In Bolivia, constant eye contact is expected.

K E E P I N G   F I T

Preventing Computer Eyestrain

To prevent or decrease the problem of computer eyestrain, remember to
- place your screen so your line of vision is just below eye-level.
- place the screen 20 to 24 inches from your face.
- place the screen away from a window.
- use a glare-filtering cover over the screen.
- look away from the screen, focusing on a distant object, about every 15 minutes.
- remove dust from the screen on a regular basis.
- take breaks.
- adjust the brightness of the letters on the screen so that they are neither too bright nor too faint.

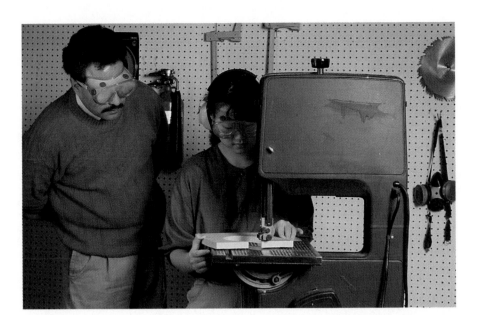

A detached retina is the separation of the retina from underlying tissue. This condition can sometimes be treated and corrected with laser surgery.

Care of the Eyes

Often we take our sight for granted. Yet reports from the National Society to Prevent Blindness indicate that we could do much more to protect and promote healthy eyes. It is important to read and to watch television in a well-lighted room. When viewing television, sit at a comfortable distance from the set. Take breaks from using your eyes for long periods of time by closing your eyes. Avoid rubbing your eyes, and avoid direct sun or bright light. Wear protective goggles or glasses when engaging in an activity or sport that could cause an eye injury. Finally, have regular eye checkups by a trained professional.

LESSON 2 REVIEW

Reviewing Facts and Vocabulary

1. How do lacrimal glands protect the eyes?
2. Describe the main functions of the three layers of the eyeball.
3. How does the eye receive its nourishment?
4. Explain the role of the rods and cones in vision.
5. What is a detached retina?

Thinking Critically

6. **Analysis.** Compare farsightedness and nearsightedness.

7. **Evaluation.** Do you think it is important for school-aged children to have their vision tested on a regular basis? Why or why not?

Applying Health Knowledge

8. Interview someone who is blind or visually impaired, or visit a center for the blind. What special problems do people with visual impairments have? How have their other senses accommodated for their lack of vision?

EARS

TERMS TO USE
- External auditory canal
- Ossicles (AH•si•kuhlz)
- Labyrinth (LAB•uh•rinth)
- Binaural (by•NAWR•uhl) hearing
- Sensory deafness
- Otosclerosis (OHT• oh•skluh•ROH•suhs)
- Tinnitus (TIN•uht•uhs)

CONCEPTS TO LEARN
- Hearing is the result of sound waves moving through the structures of the ear.
- Hearing loss is one of the potential hazards of being around noise.

ATTITUDES AND BEHAVIORS TO EVALUATE
- Self-Inventory, page 332.
- Building Decision-Making Skills, page 333.

Julie, a tenth grader, spends two afternoons a week teaching sign language to children who are deaf. Julie lost her hearing as a young child, but she has not let that slow her down. Julie communicates not only through sign language but also by reading lips.

Julie is among thousands of people who are deaf or hearing impaired. Disorders of the ear may result in a loss of hearing and may affect the sense of balance. Birth defects, injuries, and disease are three causes of hearing loss. Many times the cause is unknown. Before learning how these causes affect hearing, let us learn how the complicated process of hearing takes place.

Structure of the Ear

The ear extends deep into the skull and has three main parts: the outer ear, the middle ear, and the inner ear.

The Outer Ear

The outer ear consists of a fleshy curved part that is attached to each side of the head and is called the auricle. Composed of fatty tissue and cartilage, the cup-shaped auricle collects sound waves and directs them into the ear. Looking directly into the ear, you can see the **external auditory canal.** It is a passageway about 1 inch (2.5 cm) long. The outer part is lined with fine hairs and tiny wax-producing glands. The wax and tiny hairs protect the ear by keeping out foreign substances. The inner two-thirds of the auditory canal is surrounded by the temporal bone, one of the hardest bones in the body. The auditory canal leads to the eardrum, which is a thin sheet of tissue that separates the outer ear from the middle ear.

The Middle Ear

Behind the eardrum are three small bones called the **ossicles,** which are linked together and connect the eardrum with the inner ear:

- The malleus is the first bone. It is attached to the eardrum and is the largest of the three bones.
- The incus is the middle bone. It connects the malleus and the innermost bone, the stapes.
- The stapes is stirrup-shaped and attaches to the inner ear. It is the smallest bone in the body. The ends of the stapes are attached by ligaments to a membrane called the oval window, which leads to the inner ear.

Two other parts of the head connect to the middle ear. Although these parts are not actually a part of the middle ear, they can affect your hearing:

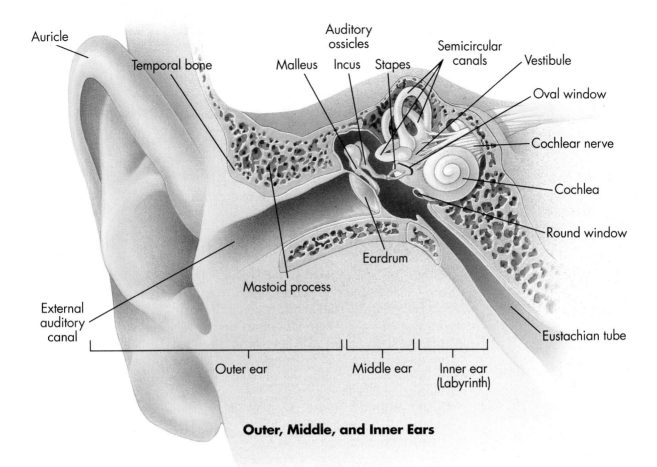

Outer, Middle, and Inner Ears

Auricle

Temporal bone

Auditory ossicles

Malleus *Incus* *Stapes*

Semicircular canals

Vestibule

Oval window

Cochlear nerve

Cochlea

Round window

External auditory canal

Mastoid process

Eardrum

Outer ear *Middle ear* *Inner ear (Labyrinth)*

Eustachian tube

Your ear has three main parts.

- The mastoid process is a series of small air-filled spaces in the bones that lie behind the middle ear. These spaces connect with the middle ear.
- The eustachian tube is about 1½ inches (4 cm) long and connects the nasal cavity in the back of the throat with the middle ear.

Have your ears ever popped as you rode in an elevator? That sensation was your eustachian tube opening to let air pass between your throat and middle ear. The eustachian tube opens when you swallow, blow your nose, or yawn, thus equalizing the pressure on either side of the eardrum. If the eustachian tube did not open, the eardrum would rupture with a sudden change in pressure like the one that occurs when riding in an elevator or an airplane.

The Inner Ear

The inner ear, also called the **labyrinth,** consists of three delicate parts: the vestibule, the semicircular canals, and the cochlea.

The vestibule, which forms the central part of the inner ear, contains the utricle and saccule. These tiny baglike structures are lined with hair cells. These hair cells are specialized sense cells with tiny, hairlike projections. They play an important role in balance.

The semicircular canals consist of three canals set at right angles to one another. Each contains a fluid-filled duct that widens at one end to form a pouch. This pouch contains hair cells attached to nerve fibers. The ducts of the semicircular canals connect with the utricle, which is connected, also by a duct, to the saccule. The three semicircular canals are responsible for your sense of balance.

The cochlea resembles a snail shell. It is made up of three fluid-filled ducts. Within one of these ducts is the basilar membrane, which consists of over 15,000 hair cells. These hair cells make up the organ of Corti, which contains the hearing receptors.

Also in the inner ear is the auditory nerve. Fibers from the auditory nerve extend to each hair cell in the organ of Corti and to the hair cells of the saccule, utricle, and semicircular canals.

The Path of Sound Waves

In order for you to hear, sound waves, which are vibrations in the air caused by anything that moves, must reach the organ of Corti. Sound waves enter the external auditory canal through the auricle, causing the eardrum to vibrate. These vibrations are carried across the middle ear by the malleus, incus, and stapes to the oval window, the opening between the middle and inner ear. Sound vibrations cause the stapes to move like a plunger in and out of the oval window, thus causing fluid in the cochlea to vibrate.

These vibrations travel through the vestibule and along the two strands of tissue coiled up in the cochlea. Hair cells of the organ of Corti, a structure within the cochlear duct, bend, stimulating the nerves attached to them. These nerves send messages through the auditory nerve to the temporal lobe, which is the center of hearing in the brain. It is here that sounds are classified and interpreted.

Binaural Hearing

Binaural hearing is the ability to determine the direction a sound comes from by being able to hear it with both ears. A sound coming from the right is slightly louder in the right ear. It also reaches your

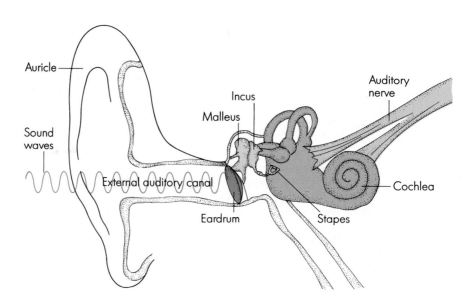

Sounds travel through your ear to be interpreted in your brain.

right ear a fraction of a second sooner than it reaches your left ear. Your brain, picking up on this difference in time and loudness, determines the direction from which the sound comes.

The Sense of Balance

You may not think of balance when you are identifying your senses. How does your body maintain its balance? Your brain receives information from various sense organs about your body's balance. Your eyes and certain pressure-sensitive cells in your arms and legs send messages to your brain about changes in body positions. However, it is the semicircular canals in the ears that provide much of the brain's information about balance.

The Crista

Movement of your head causes the fluid in the semicircular canals to move in a certain direction. At one end of each canal is an organ called a crista. Each crista consists of tiny hairs covered by a dome-shaped, jellylike mass called the cupula. Nerves connect the crista to the brain.

Movements of the head cause fluid to press against a crista, bending the tiny, sensitive hairs. Nerve endings send a message to the brain about these bent hairs. The brain sends a message back, directing the muscles to make the necessary adjustments to maintain balance.

The semicircular canals also enable you to recognize the direction in which your body is moving when you have your eyes closed. The three canals are at right angles to each other. When the head or body moves up or down, forward or backward, or from side to side, the fluid in the canals moves, affecting the delicate hairs in the crista. Again, the nerve endings are stimulated, sending an impulse to the brain.

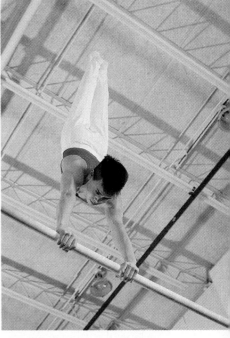

The movement of your head affects the hairs in the crista in the ear to help you maintain balance.

SENSORINEURAL DEAFNESS

Very loud noises that leave your ears ringing can cause permanent damage through accumulative hearing loss. It is usually not noticeable until one reaches the age of 40 or 50.

Sensorineural deafness is hearing loss caused by excessive noise over a long time. Such noise affects the sensitive sensory hair cells in the inner ear. Unfortunately, this type of deafness cannot be corrected. Its cause is all around us—noise. Constant exposure to 90 decibels or above can cause permanent damage to hearing. This type of deafness is gradual. At first, only the high-frequency sounds are lost. Gradually, the nerve cells that transmit lower tones become damaged, and a person cannot hear voices. Whether the sound is rock music or a motorcycle's engine, the damage is caused by the volume of the sound, not the quality.

The prevention of sensory deafness is simple. The first step is to turn down the volume on the stereo, television, radio, or electric guitar to below 65 decibels. (Ordinary conversation is about 60 decibels.) If you work with an object that causes noise of 85 decibels or more—such as a lawn mower, a motorcycle, a vacuum cleaner, factory machinery, trucks, or planes—wear hearing protection.

DID YOU KNOW?

- Rhulin Thomas could not hear when he flew alone across the United States.
- Bonnie Sloan could not hear when she became a psychiatrist.
- Ron Smith could not hear when he bowled a perfect game of 300.
- Walter Wettschreck could not hear when he became Captain of a Civil Air Patrol Squadron.
- Albert Berg could not hear when he coached football at Purdue University.
- Robert Mather could not hear when he passed the bar exam.

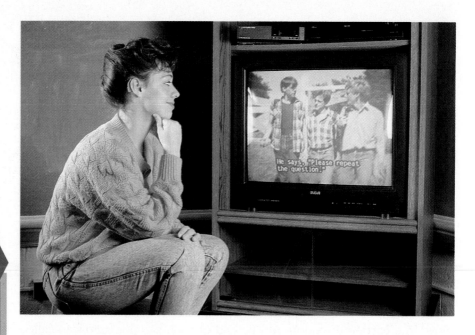

A closed-caption decoder box helps the hearing impaired enjoy television.

Problems of the Ear

Deafness is defined as the loss of the ability to hear, which may be partial or complete. When a hearing problem is associated with the outer or middle ear, it is called conduction deafness. Conduction deafness means that sound waves are prevented from reaching the eardrum or that sound waves are not being transmitted to the cochlea. A buildup of wax or some other form of blockage can prevent sound waves from reaching the eardrum. Middle ear infections or diseases involving the ossicles can result in this type of deafness.

Otosclerosis is a hereditary disease that is a common cause of partial deafness. Otosclerosis occurs when an overgrowth of bone causes the ossicles to lose their ability to move. Thus, sound waves never reach the inner ear. Otosclerosis is usually progressive, meaning that its severity increases with time. Surgical procedures can help people with otosclerosis to regain their hearing.

When hearing loss is associated with the inner ear, this is called sensorineural deafness or nerve deafness. There is damage to the cochlea, auditory nerve, or part of the brain. Nerve deafness can result from continued exposure to high-intensity noise and from tumors.

KEEPING FIT

Communicating With Someone Who Is Hearing Impaired

Follow these guidelines when you are communicating with someone who is hearing impaired:
- Face the person and speak clearly.
- Speak loudly, but do not shout.

- Speak more slowly.
- Don't overly exaggerate your lip movements or facial gestures.
- Don't cover your mouth when you speak.
- Don't chew food or gum.

- Avoid talking from another room or over avoidable background noise, such as running water.
- Don't expect everyone who is hearing impaired to read lips.

Some medicines can damage the hair cells in the cochlea or the auditory nerve, causing a hearing loss. Certain medicines taken by a female during pregnancy can prevent the normal development of the baby's cochlea.

Have you ever experienced a ringing noise in your ears? This common condition is called **tinnitus,** and it can be irritating. Tinnitus can be caused by several conditions, including a buildup of ear wax, fluid in the middle ear, a change in pressure in the inner ear, or an ear infection. Tinnitus itself is not an ear disease. It is usually a symptom of some other problem. Once that problem is identified and corrected, the tinnitus may go away.

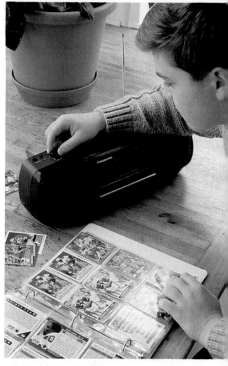

Protecting your ears from loud noise will protect your hearing.

Care of the Ears

The ears are a delicate instrument that must be carefully maintained. It is important to clean them regularly and to protect them against weather, especially the cold.

Cleaning the outer ears should always be done with a cotton swab. Use the soft head of the swab to take out dirt and ear wax, but do not push the swab into the ear. Never use pencils or other sharp items to clean ears.

Sometimes, because of vibrations or a buildup of ear wax, the inside of the ear may feel ticklish. When this happens, gently use your thumb to wiggle the outer ear passage. Do not use swabs or sharp items to stop the tickling.

Cold weather, drafts, and sudden changes of temperature can prepare the way for ear infections. These infections can be very painful. Use ear muffs or a hat that covers the ears in the cold weather to prevent infection in the inner ear and frostbite of the earlobes. If there are bad drafts, you may want to put a piece of cotton in the outer ear passage to stop wind from entering the inner ear.

LESSON 3 REVIEW

Reviewing Facts and Vocabulary

1. What is the function of the auditory canal?
2. How is the ear protected from foreign substances?
3. Describe what makes up the labyrinth of the ear.
4. How should the ears be cleaned?

Thinking Critically

5. **Analysis.** What is the relationship between your sense of hearing and your sense of balance?

6. **Synthesis.** Summarize the kinds of things that one can do to prevent ear problems.

Applying Health Knowledge

7. Make a diagram showing the path of a sound wave from the outside environment to its interpretation in the brain.

Self-Inventory

Your Personal Health

HOW DO YOU RATE?

Number a sheet of paper from 1 through 20. Read each item below, and respond by writing *MT* if the statement describes you all or most of the time, *ST* if the statement describes you some of the time, and *N* if the statement seldom or never applies to you. Total the number of each type of response. Then proceed to the next section.

1. I brush my teeth every day.
2. I brush my teeth more than once a day.
3. I use a soft toothbrush.
4. I brush my tongue when I brush my teeth.
5. I floss my teeth.
6. I floss my teeth every day.
7. I have regular dental check-ups.
8. I am careful not to bump someone who is drinking from a water fountain.
9. I avoid reading in poorly lighted areas.
10. When reading or studying for long periods of time, I rest my eyes periodically by looking at a distant object.
11. I use safety glasses or goggles when involved in activities or sports that could cause an eye injury.
12. I avoid rubbing my eyes.
13. When in bright outdoor light, I wear sunglasses that filter ultraviolet rays.
14. I have my eyes checked by a professional on a regular basis.
15. I wear glasses or contacts when prescribed for me.

16. I clean my ears every day.
17. I protect my ears in very cold temperatures.
18. I avoid extremely loud noise (85 decibels or more).
19. I wear ear protection when I know I will be around loud noises.
20. I am careful to never hit someone in the ears.

HOW DID YOU SCORE?

Give yourself 2 points for each statement that describes you *all* or *most of the time*, 1 point for each statement that describes you *some of the time*, and 0 points for each *seldom* or *never* response. Find your total, and read below to see how you scored. Then proceed to the next section.

36 to 40
Excellent. You are practicing excellent habits.

31 to 35
Good. Although your personal health habits are good, you could improve in some areas.

25 to 30
Fair. Be careful. Your personal habits may be putting some aspects of your total health in danger.

Below 25
Look out! You are not taking a very responsible approach to your own health. More importantly, you may be taking unnecessary health risks.

WHAT ARE YOUR GOALS?

If you received an *excellent* or *good* score, complete the statements in Part A. If your score

was rated *fair* or *look out*, complete Parts A and B.

Part A

1. I plan to learn more about personal health habits for my teeth, eyes, and ears by ____.
2. My timetable for accomplishing this is ____.
3. I plan to share my information with others by ____.

Part B

4. The behavior or attitude toward the health of my teeth, eyes, and ears I would most like to change is ____.
5. The steps involved in making this change are ____.
6. My rewards for making this change will be ____.

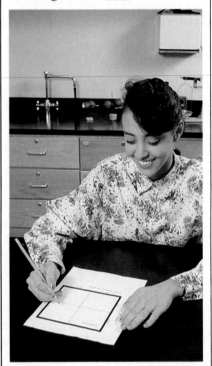

Building Decision-Making Skills

C asey, the class clown, is a great guy with good looks, a super sense of humor, and a very pleasant personality. Unfortunately he also has poor personal health habits that lead to bad breath. He wrote Colleen a clever note asking her out. Colleen likes Casey, but not his breath. She has asked you, a mutual friend, for advice on how to handle the situation. What should Colleen do? Her choices might include:

A. Write a clever note saying she'd love to go, but only if he used toothpaste.

B. Agree to go, but let you or another friend, counselor, or coach talk to him about oral health care.

C. Make up an excuse for not going.

D. Say she is sorry she can't go and honestly explain why.

E. Go with him but wait until she gets to know him better before telling him that his breath is a real turnoff.

WHAT DO YOU THINK?

1. **Choices.** What other options does Colleen have?

2. **Consequences.** What are the pros and cons of each choice?

3. **Consequences.** If Colleen decides to tell Casey he needs to improve his oral health, how may his self-esteem be affected?

4. **Consequences.** If Colleen decides to talk to Casey about this problem, how could she go about it in a caring, thoughtful way?

5. **Decision.** What choice would you recommend to Colleen? Why?

6. **Evaluation.** Have you ever found yourself torn between telling someone something that might be embarrassing or hurtful, but that is offensive to others? Describe the situation, how you handled it, and what you learned from it.

C harmaine is a smart, personable teen and one of Tricia's best friends. Charmaine has long, wavy hair, great eyes, and a clear complexion. She is popular with her classmates, many of whom think she is beautiful. But Charmaine is very self-conscious about her crooked teeth. She would like to have braces, but the cost is quite high. Tricia is finding it harder and harder to be with Charmaine because she keeps calling herself ugly. She's also started refusing to go out with Tricia and her other friends because, although it's untrue, she's convinced that everyone is staring at her crooked teeth. What should Tricia do? Some of her choices might include:

A. Stop including Charmaine in activities until she stops putting herself down.

B. Explain to Charmaine that no one is perfect. Since she has so many other great qualities, she should stop complaining about one little imperfection.

C. Try to support Charmaine by listing her other positive qualities that have nothing to do with physical appearance.

D. Suggest that Charmaine talk with a school counselor who can help her see that looks aren't the only thing in life that's important.

WHAT DO YOU THINK?

7. **Situation.** Why does a decision need to be made?

8. **Choices.** What other choices does Tricia have?

9. **Consequences.** What are the positive and negative aspects of each choice?

10. **Decision.** Which choice do you think is best for Tricia? Explain your answer.

11. **Evaluation.** In our beauty-conscious society, how much do people pay attention to artificial beauty? Name ways people do this. How would you handle a situation in which someone shows favor to another person because he or she is attractive?

REVIEW

Using Health Terms

On a separate sheet of paper, write the term that best matches each definition given below.

LESSON 1

1. The second hardest naturally occurring substance in nature.
2. Hard substance that builds on plaque.
3. Bad breath.
4. The area immediately around the teeth.
5. Swollen and inflamed with pus gathering.
6. Living tissue inside the tooth.
7. Sticky, colorless film that forms on teeth and promotes tooth decay.

LESSON 2

8. Responsible for producing tears.
9. The window of the eye.
10. Photosensitive chemical in rods that enables one to see in dim light.
11. The point where the optic nerve enters the eye.
12. The process in which the pupil of the eye gets larger.
13. A condition in which the eye lens has an uneven curvature.

LESSON 3

14. The ability to determine the direction a sound comes from.
15. A hereditary disease in which an overgrowth of bone causes the ossicles to lose their ability to move.
16. Three small bones that connect the eardrum with the inner ear.
17. The inner ear.
18. Ringing in the ear.

Building Academic Skills

LESSON 1

19. **Writing.** Write a set of directions for third graders describing the best procedures to use when brushing and flossing one's teeth. Make sure your steps are in logical order.

Recalling the Facts

LESSON 1

20. What is the actual physical cause for the pain of a toothache?
21. How can periodontal disease be stopped in its early stages?
22. How can halitosis be cured?
23. What functions do teeth serve?
24. What are the parts of the periodontium and what function do they serve together?
25. What causes periodontal disease?
26. What is good oral hygiene?

LESSON 2

27. What part of the brain is responsible for vision?
28. Name and describe three vision problems that can be corrected.
29. Name and tell the function of the general area around the eyes.
30. What does it mean when someone has 20/20 vision?
31. Why is contraction and dilation of the pupil important?
32. What is the white part of one's eye called and what does it do?
33. Name three things that you can do to protect your eyes.
34. What is behind the pupil and what function does that part serve?
35. What in the retina enables people to see color?
36. How does the lens change and for what purpose does it change?

LESSON 3

37. What is the significance of the semicircular canals?
38. What is binaural hearing?
39. What are some objects that create noises louder than 65 decibels?
40. What is the oval window and what is its significance?
41. What role does the temporal lobe play in the hearing process?
42. What might contribute to ear infections?

Thinking Critically

LESSON 1

43. **Synthesis.** What problems might occur if a person lost all his or her teeth? How might this affect this person's life and/or attitude?

44. **Analysis.** Compare gingivitis and periodontitis.

45. **Synthesis.** Conduct a survey of how many people in your class wear braces. What might these numbers indicate?

LESSON 2

46. **Analysis.** What activities would require protective eyewear? What rule could you give for when to wear protective eyewear?

47. **Evaluation.** Some people overcompensate when they encounter someone with a disability. For example, they may talk louder than normal when speaking to someone who is visually impaired. Why do you suppose people do this? Is it necessary? Support your answer.

LESSON 3

48. **Synthesis.** Why do you suppose the inner ear is also known as the labyrinth?

Making the Connection

LESSON 2

49. **Home Economics.** Research different prices for eyewear. Identify factors that are responsible for price differences.

LESSON 3

50. **Science.** Measure the decibels of sound at a school dance, athletic event, in the cafeteria, or in the parking lot. Compare readings to safety levels. This is also a good way to measure which class can yell the loudest at pep rallies.

51. **Language Arts.** Watch five television commercials. What impact does the auditory part have in selling the product? Is what is seen more or less important in these commercials than what is heard?

Applying Health Knowledge

LESSON 1

52. If your best friend had halitosis, how might you tell him or her?

53. Talk to a person who wears orthodontic braces. Find out how the braces have affected that person's life. How did the person feel before the braces were put on? How does he or she feel now?

54. You may not be aware of how much high-sugar food you ingest in a day. Keep a journal of your daily food intake for one week. Evaluate it. Were the results what you expected? Is there anything in your diet that should be adjusted? Explain.

LESSON 2

55. How might a blind spot affect one's daily life in terms of transportation safety?

LESSON 3

56. An old expression you may have heard is "Never stick anything smaller than your elbow in your ear." What does this mean?

57. Find out about the outer ear ailment known as cauliflower ear. What is it? What causes it? What effect does it have on hearing?

58. Whenever you warn your friends that loud music will damage their hearing, they say it won't happen to them, but if it does they can always get hearing aids. How would you respond? Support your answer.

Beyond the Classroom

LESSON 2

59. **Further Study.** Research the Braille alphabet. Find out all you can about it.

LESSON 3

60. **Further Study.** Take a sign language class or borrow a book on signing from your local library. Practice with a friend. Perhaps you could become proficient enough to volunteer in a community center or a school for the hearing impaired.

CHAPTER
17

FITNESS AND YOUR HEALTH

LESSON 1
The Benefits of Fitness

LESSON 2
Exercise and Physical Fitness

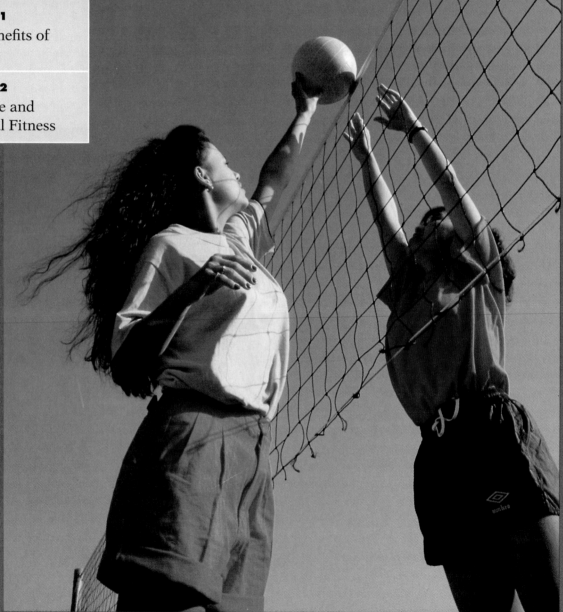

THE BENEFITS OF FITNESS

The word *health* is often associated only with physical fitness, though you know there are other components of health. **Fitness** means "readiness." Fit people are better equipped than nonfit people to handle day-to-day situations.

Your level of fitness includes all aspects of your health and life. It affects your physical, mental, and social health. Your level of fitness affects how you sleep, eat, and learn. If you are fit, you look good, you have energy, and you generally feel good about yourself. Maintaining a high level of fitness is a lifelong challenge.

Fitness in the Past

During the period of growth and frontier settlement in the United States, most people were very active. Fitness and exercise were a part of everyday life. In fact, being fit was necessary for survival. Because people had so much activity during their workday, they looked for ways to make their lives easier.

Soon came the age of labor-saving devices—inventions that ranged from automobiles and dishwashers to electric shavers and hair dryers. Thousands of mechanical and electronic inventions made life so easy for many Americans that they adopted sedentary life-styles. Sedentary living is inactive living, a way of life that is devoid of daily physical activity beyond that required for attending school or going to work.

Medical researchers and scientists have found that a sedentary way of life is not good for one's health. In fact, some consider it to be a health hazard. Muscle strength is lost as a result of an inactive life-style. It has become evident that the lack of regular activity contributes to the risk of cardiovascular diseases.

In addition, immobility negatively affects the respiratory, digestive, and nervous systems. These findings, along with the abundance of new information about disease prevention, have begun to change our attitudes toward fitness.

Fitness Today

The United States experienced a fitness boom during the 1970s that is still growing today. Walking and jogging trails and bicycle paths have been developed in neighborhoods all over the country. At almost any time of day, you can see people of all ages exercising. In fact, millions of Americans make exercise a part of their regular schedule.

Aerobic exercise, dance classes, and weight-training programs have become very popular. More and more people are participating in lifetime sports, such as tennis, swimming, softball, race walking, or jogging. These sports are ones that can be enjoyed and participated in throughout life.

LESSON 1 FOCUS

TERMS TO USE
- Fitness
- Basal metabolism

CONCEPTS TO LEARN
- Exercise improves your physical health.
- Exercise contributes to your social and mental health.

ATTITUDES AND BEHAVIORS TO EVALUATE
- Self-Inventory, page 348.
- Building Decision-Making Skills, page 349.

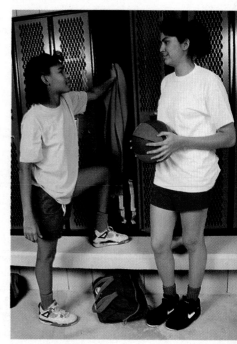

It's important to plan time for exercise.

As you use many labor-saving devices, exercise may become less a part of your routine. For this reason, it is important to plan times for regular exercise or leisure physical activity. In addition, you need to look for opportunities during the day that help build physical activity into your routine.

Exercise and Your Physical Health

Exercise, the primary contributor to good physical fitness, also contributes to mental and social health. Exercise improves the physical part of your health by building a strong body. Exercise can also help reduce the feeling of chronic fatigue, stiffness, and lack of coordination. It can help improve the sense organ functions and motor responses. Sense organ functions refer to your ability to use your senses to their optimal levels.

EXERCISING THROUGHOUT THE DAY

Think about your activity during the day. Whenever possible do you

- stand rather than sit,
- sit up rather than lie down,
- walk rather than ride in a car,
- ride a bike rather than ride in a car,
- use stairs rather than an elevator or an escalator,
- walk around (pace) rather than stand still,
- run or jog rather than walk,
- walk briskly rather than walk slowly,
- use body power rather than a machine?

These behaviors sound simple, but they all add up to an increase in physical activity. Be aware of times throughout your day when you could choose a more active routine.

Exercise for Your Nervous System

Exercise contributes to the functioning of your nervous system by tuning it to a high level, allowing for more skillful body movements. Exercise can improve your reaction time by helping you respond more quickly to stimuli. Your overall mental performance improves too.

K E E P I N G   F I T

Fifteen Great Reasons to Work Out

A regular exercise regimen can bring many benefits to many areas of your life. These include:
- improved cardiovascular health
- better weight control
- improved metabolism
- improved breathing capacity

- improved flexibility
- improved endurance
- improved strength
- improved appearance
- improved self-esteem
- a chance to socialize

- increased mental alertness
- increased ability to handle stress
- less fatigue and more energy
- improved sleep
- a more positive attitude

Overcoming The Odds

Pratima Chaterjee is 17. "Tima," as she is called by her friends, likes to hike and play piano. She has been studying ballet for eight years. Her dream is to dance with a major ballet company. She commutes to the city on weekends to participate in workshops and a performing arts program. With all that she has to do, she sometimes feels very pressured. That's why she says that balance—not just on her toes but in her life—is so important.

Tima says, "This is a very busy time in my life. I work out at the barre every day, and I take dance classes. At school I take Advanced Placement courses. I also have a strong family with lots of time commitments. Sometimes, I feel overwhelmed. That's why I guess I'm grateful for the many perspectives of my grandparents. Because of them I can see different life-styles and pick and choose what will work for me.

"Sometimes it feels as if there's a culture collision in my own living room," she says, laughing. "My American grandmother belongs to a fitness club and a race-walking group. I admire that. She has a great sense of humor, too. However, she eats a lot of high-fat foods. My grandmother from India doesn't exercise at all, but she is a vegetarian, which I admire. I tried the no meat, no eggs, no milk route, but I got weak. I need a lot of good food for the kind of

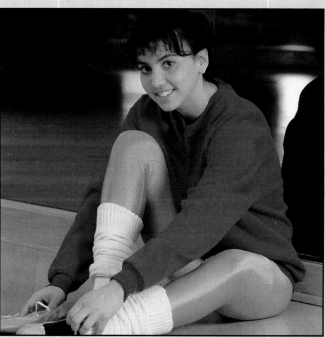

dance training that I do, so now I eat chicken and fish in moderation. My Scottish grandfather has tons of hobbies and knows how to have fun. I'd like to be like that when I'm older; I'd even like to be more like that now. My other grandfather always talks to me about the importance of balance and keeping things in perspective. I try to follow his advice and example, too."

Tima continues, "I don't want to wake up when I'm 40 and realize I have to do radical things all of a sudden just to stay alive because I've abused myself along the way. I want to dance well, but I don't want to starve. I want to be in top shape, but I don't want to ruin my body in the process. I've had too many friends with stress fractures, eating disorders, wrecked knees, and worse—and all in the name of being fit. I want to be a choreographer when I'm older, so I've got to take steps now to make sure my body will work well and work gracefully for a long, long time. I keep hearing my grandfather's words about keeping it all in balance, and I try."

1. Pratima has many examples of different life-styles in her own family. What are the pluses and minuses of having such a variety of life-style models?
2. What are the many kinds of life-styles represented in your extended family? Which do you think are healthiest? Are these the ones you try to follow? Why or why not?
3. Do you ever feel burned out? What do you think causes you to feel this way? What steps can you take to get your life in better balance?

Exercise for Your Respiratory System

With regular exercise, your respiratory system begins to work slower and more efficiently so that you take fewer but deeper breaths. Your lung capacity, the amount of air that you can take in with a single breath, increases. Your body uses oxygen more efficiently as your fitness level improves.

Exercise for Your Cardiovascular System

Regular exercise is a great help to the heart. The heart is a muscle, and like any muscle, the more it is used, the stronger it gets. A strong heart can pump blood more efficiently than a weak one, so more work is done with less effort.

Exercise and Weight Control

One out of every three Americans is overweight. Sedentary living is as much to blame for this situation as is overeating.

Your Metabolism. The absolute minimum amount of energy required to maintain the life processes in your body is called **basal metabolism.** We get our energy from food, and the energy value of food is measured in units of heat called calories. Your body requires a minimum number of calories each day in order to maintain itself. Additional calories must be used, or they will be stored as fat.

Your metabolic rate increases during exercise—during exercise you burn up more calories than when you are at rest. The number of calories you burn depends on the nature of the activity. The benefit of physical activity remains for a short while even after you stop exercising. Your metabolic rate takes some time to return to normal, so during that time you are still burning more calories than before you began exercising.

Your Weight. Much has been written about dieting, weight reduction, obesity, and exercise. There is more information about weight control in Chapter 20. However, the following statements provide an overview.

- If you take in fewer calories than you burn, you lose weight.
- If you take in more calories than you burn, you gain weight.

If you take in more calories than you can use, the excess calories are stored in the body as fat. One pound (0.5 kg) of fat is equal to about 3,500 calories. A person must control calories to control weight.

Exercise is helpful in the prevention of becoming overfat. Overfat is an excessive amount of fat in the body. Being overfat and 20 to 30 percent above recommended weight results in obesity. Both of these conditions have been associated with heart disease and can be a problem among people in all age groups. Vigorous or moderate exercise can help reduce body fat and contribute to weight reduction.

Your Ability to Recuperate. Exercise can help the body's protection against disease by building resistance through improved fitness. A strong, toned body is capable of recuperation, or restoring itself, at a faster rate than a body that is overweight or in poor condition.

Exercise and Your Mental and Social Health

Some people who do sedentary work for long periods of time find that an exercise break refreshes them and leads to more productive work time. Many people have found that after a long day of school or work, exercise gives them an energy boost. They are less fatigued during the evening hours. Feeling better physically has a positive effect on mental and social health.

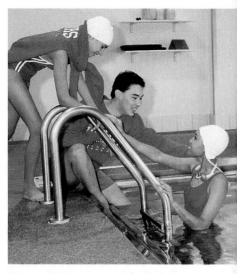

Exercising in organized activities helps you get to know and get along with others.

Mental Benefits

Exercise contributes to mental health in a number of ways:

- Being physically fit gives you a sense of pride and accomplishment for taking care of yourself.
- Getting fit and staying fit contributes to positive self-esteem because you will look better and feel better about yourself.
- Physical fitness helps you deal with strong emotions, stress, and times when you feel down.
- Exercise can be a healthy outlet for tension, anger, or frustration.
- Exercise offers a form of relaxation.

Social Benefits

Some exercise programs can benefit the social side of your health. Through participation in organized exercise activities, you have an opportunity to meet new people. Many people find that exercising with a friend or in a group makes the workout more enjoyable. Working out with someone else can also help motivate a person to continue with an exercise program.

LESSON 1 REVIEW

Reviewing Facts and Vocabulary

1. How does physical fitness relate to health?
2. What are the health implications of a sedentary life-style?
3. What is basal metabolism?
4. What are three ways in which exercise contributes to your physical health?

Thinking Critically

5. **Synthesis.** Suggest ways that people who need regular exercise and are opposed to it can be encouraged to participate.

6. **Evaluation.** Discuss the accuracy of this statement: *He is overweight because he eats too much.*

Applying Health Knowledge

7. Make a list of 10 activities you do almost every day. Next to each, write a statement indicating how a higher level of fitness would help you in each of the activities. Compare your list of statements with those of other class members.

EXERCISE AND PHYSICAL FITNESS

LESSON 2 FOCUS

TERMS TO USE

- Physical fitness
- Body composition
- Flexibility
- Muscular strength
- Muscular endurance
- Cardiorespiratory endurance
- Anaerobic exercise
- Aerobic exercise

CONCEPTS TO LEARN

- Physical fitness includes many components.
- There are benefits to both anaerobic and aerobic exercise.
- Weight training contributes to muscular strength and endurance.

ATTITUDES AND BEHAVIORS TO EVALUATE

- Self-Inventory, page 348.
- Building Decision-Making Skills, page 349.

Pattyann is the school's star soccer player. She moves up and down the field with speed and grace. Pattyann can outmaneuver almost any other player. Yet she cannot touch her toes or reach her hands to the ground.

Karen has competed on the balance beam since she was 8 years old. Last year she won the city title for her event. Yet when Karen is late for the bus, she gets completely out of breath after running half a block.

Jerry runs 4 miles every day. He also runs in races all over the state. Yet Jerry cannot do 25 sit-ups or push-ups.

Would it surprise you to know that the physical fitness program of each of these students is lacking?

Basic Components of Physical Fitness

Physical fitness can be defined as the ability to carry out daily tasks easily and have enough reserve energy to respond to unexpected demands. Physical fitness includes these components:

- **Body composition** refers to the percent of fat, lean muscle, bone, connective tissue, water, and so forth in the body. The term *percent body fat* refers to the amount of fat in the body in relation to total body weight.
- **Flexibility** is the ability to move a body part through a full range of motion.
- **Muscular strength** is the ability to exert force against resistance.
- **Muscular endurance** is the ability of muscles to keep working over a period of time without causing fatigue.
- **Cardiorespiratory endurance** is the ability of the heart, lungs, and blood vessels to send fuel and oxygen to the body's tissues during long periods of vigorous activity.

Measuring Body Composition

Appearance is probably one of the biggest reasons people exercise and watch what they eat. A combination of diet and physical activity is essential for weight control. One way to improve physical fitness is to control the percentage of body fat to total body weight. Two ways to determine percent body fat include underwater weighing and skinfold measurements done with calipers.

Using calipers is easy and inexpensive. Underneath your skin is a layer of fat. By having the thickness of skinfolds in specific areas of your body measured with calipers, a percentage of body fat can be determined. There is a high relationship between the measure of this fat and the fat inside your body. The measurements taken are compared to those on a chart for an estimated percent body fat.

Exercising is an effective way to control body fat. Exercise that is aerobic, continued for a fairly long period of time, and done regularly is most effective for losing body fat. The key is to expend as many calories as possible during each regular exercise period.

Measuring Flexibility

Flexibility is specific to each moving joint. For this reason, it is difficult to measure total body flexibility. However, the following test will give you a general measure of your level of fitness in this area. You should remember two important points when taking this flexibility test. First, do some light stretching to warm up your muscles. This will help prevent injury from too vigorous a movement. Second, avoid quick, jerking movements. Your reach should be gradual and slow.

Now follow these directions to measure your flexibility.

- Sit on the floor with your legs straight in front of you with your shoes off. Your heels should touch a piece of tape on the floor and be about 5 inches (13 cm) apart.
- Place a yardstick or meter stick between your legs so that it rests on the floor with the 36-inch (or 1 meter) end pointing away from your body. The 15-inch (38 cm) mark on the stick is to be even with your heels. (It is best to tape the measuring stick in place so that it does not move.)
- Slowly reach with both hands as far forward as possible and hold this position. Practice three times and measure the fourth.
- The score is the most distant point the fingertips reach on the measuring stick.

BODY FLEXIBILITY

Scoring		Rating
Male	**Female**	
22 inches (56 cm) or more	23 inches (58 cm) or more	Excellent
17–21 inches (43–53 cm)	20–22 inches (51–56 cm)	Good
13–16 inches (33–41 cm)	17–19 inches (43–48 cm)	Average
9–12 inches (23–30 cm)	14–16 inches (36–41 cm)	Fair
8 inches (20 cm) or less	13 inches (33 cm) or less	Poor

Measuring Upper Body Strength and Endurance

Pull-ups can measure upper body strength and endurance. Follow these directions:

- Hang from a horizontal bar with your palms facing away from your body. Arms and legs should be fully extended.
- Raise your body, keeping your legs still, until your chin clears the bar.
- Lower your body to the starting position. Repeat as many times as you can with no time limit.

CONFLICT RESOLUTION

Ana and Luis are having an argument about whose exercise program is better. Ana works out on a weight machine for an hour after school each day and does calisthenics at home on weekends. She always works up a sweat, so she feels she must be giving her heart a good workout. Luis walks three miles every day and goes swimming or cross-country skiing just about every weekend. Luis assumes that if his heart is healthy, he's physically fit. Ana and Luis have asked you to help them resolve their disagreement.

Assess their programs, suggest improvements, and explain the merits of both anaerobic and aerobic exercise.

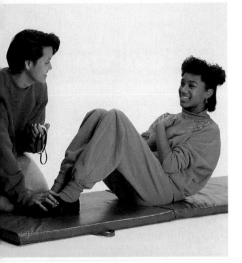

UPPER BODY STRENGTH AND ENDURANCE

Scoring (number of pull-ups)		Rating
Males	**Females**	
ages 13-14	ages 13-14	Excellent
7-10 times	2 times	
ages 15-16	ages 15-16	Excellent
11 times	2 times	
ages 13-14	ages 13-14	Good
5-6 times	1 time	
ages 15-16	ages 15-16	Good
9-10 times	1 time	

Doing modified sit-ups tests abdominal muscular strength and endurance.

Abdominal Strength and Endurance. Test your abdominal strength and endurance with a one-minute modified sit-up test. You will need a stopwatch and a partner.

■ Start by lying on your back with your knees slightly bent. Your partner should hold your ankles for support. Your heels should be 1 to 1½ feet from your buttocks.
■ With your arms crossed on your chest, do as many modified sit-ups as you can in one minute. Your elbows should touch your thighs each time.
■ Return to full starting position with your back to the floor in between each sit-up.
■ Be sure you do not hold your breath during the test. Breathe freely.
■ Your partner should keep the time and your sit-up count.

ABDOMINAL STRENGTH AND ENDURANCE

Scoring (number of sit-ups in 1 minute)		
Male	**Female**	**Rating**
40 or more	30 or more	Excellent
33–39	24–29	Good
29–32	18–23	Average
21–28	11–17	Fair
Less than 21	Less than 11	Poor

K E E P I N G   F I T

Exercise Programs

Dr. Kenneth Cooper, the "father of aerobics," recommends that 14- to 18-year-olds try some of these regular exercise programs to increase their levels of fitness:
■ walking 3 miles, 4 times per week, in less than 45 minutes

for girls and less than 43 minutes for boys;
■ swimming 1,000 yards, 4 times a week, in less than 25 minutes for girls and less than 24 minutes for boys;
■ running or jogging 3 miles, 4

times a week, in less than 27 minutes for girls and 24 minutes for boys;
■ cycling 8 miles in less than 40 minutes for girls and less than 32 minutes for boys.

Measuring Cardiorespiratory Endurance

One way to measure cardiorespiratory endurance is the 1-mile (1.6 km) run/walk. On a measured course, cover the distances as fast as you can. If you need to walk some of the distance, walk as fast as you can.

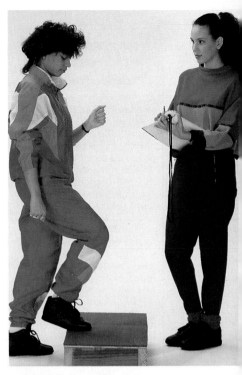

A step test measures your cardiorespiratory fitness.

CARDIORESPIRATORY ENDURANCE

Scoring		Rating
Male	**Female**	
Under 7 minutes	Under 8 minutes	Excellent
7:01–7:30	8:01–8:30	Good
7:31–8:00	8:31–9:00	Average
8:01–8:30	9:01–9:30	Fair
8:31–9:00	9:31–10:00	Low
9:01 or longer	10:01 or longer	Poor

This 3-minute step test also will measure your cardiorespiratory fitness:

- Using a sturdy bench about 8 inches (20 cm) high, step up and down every 2 seconds for 3 minutes.
- Fully extend each leg as you step. Step up with your right foot, then your left. Step down with your right foot first. Stepping should be continuous.
- Step at the rate of 24 steps per minute for 3 minutes.
- After 30 seconds, count your pulse for 1 minute.
- Find your pulse either on your wrist or on the side of your neck. This count gives you your pulse recovery rate, which is the rate at which your heart beats following activity.

PULSE RECOVERY RATE

Scoring (number of heartbeats)	Rating
70–80	Excellent
81–105	Good
106–119	Average
120–130	Fair
131 or more	Poor

Types of Exercise

Sensible exercise is good for you. The more muscles and joints you use, the greater the health gain. Exercise is generally one of two types, anaerobic or aerobic.

Anaerobic exercise is intense physical activity in which the body's supply of oxygen to produce energy does not meet the demand. Running a 100-meter dash is an anaerobic activity. **Aerobic exercise** is vigorous activity that uses continuous oxygen. This activity usually needs to last at least 20 minutes. During this time heart rate increases and oxygen is transported to the muscles to be used as energy to do more work. Running for a couple of miles is an example of an aerobic exercise.

DID YOU KNOW?

- The Centers for Disease Control and Prevention reported in January 1992 that fewer than 40 percent of high school students get enough vigorous exercise each week.
- The average 14- to 17-year-old American is now 5 to 7 pounds heavier than in 1980.
- Many health clubs, once centered only on exercise, have expanded their offering to include seminars in nutrition, stress management, smoking cessation, weight loss, and even attitude-enhancement and self-esteem.

Anaerobic Exercise

Anaerobic exercises improve muscular strength, muscular endurance, and flexibility. Anaerobic exercises may not raise your general level of fitness because they do not require the body to increase its use of oxygen. Weight training is considered an anaerobic exercise.

WEIGHT TRAINING

Weight-training programs are designed to build muscular strength and endurance. Weight training is a good way to tone muscles. However, you may not lose weight. Muscle tissue weighs more than fat tissue.

There are three types of weight-training programs:

- Isometric. This type of exercise involves muscular strength with little or no movement of the body part. With this type of exercise, you use muscle tension to build strength. Putting the palms of your hands together in front of you and pushing is an example of an isometric exercise. Pushing against a wall is another example.
- Isotonic. This type of exercise involves muscular contraction with movement. You develop muscular strength and flexibility with repeated movements using weights. Push-ups, pull-ups, and modified sit-ups are isotonic exercises. Lifting weights also is isotonic exercise.
- Isokinetic. This type of exercise involves muscular strength and endurance, and flexibility. With this type of exercise, resistance is moved through an entire range of motion, such as pushing or pulling against a hydraulic lever of certain exercise equipment.

During exercise muscle fibers become thicker and are able to do more work. Eventually, repeating the same amount of exercise causes muscles

HEALTH UPDATE

LOOKING AT TECHNOLOGY

Biomechanics: Sports on a Screen

Training for athletic performance and fitness is no longer just limited to the playing field. Advanced technology is now being used to measure and analyze athletes' motions and body functions. This science, called *biomechanics*, involves using computers to measure those forces that act both within and upon the athlete's body. Computers also monitor such things as breathing, heart rate, muscular contractions, pressure changes, and calories consumed. Using high-speed film or videotapes of athletes performing, it can provide mathematical analysis of both the athlete's motion and his or her energy consumption. Using such high-tech statistics can help athletes in training develop specific ways to perform at their best levels of athletic achievement, minimize fatigue, and avoid injuries.

In addition to helping athletes, biomechanics is now also being used to help people with various skeletal or muscular diseases, conditions, or injuries.

to reach a limit. For muscles to keep getting stronger, it is necessary that you gradually increase how often, how hard, or how long you use a particular muscle group.

Conditioning programs are reversible. A person in good physical condition can lose much strength and endurance in just two or three weeks of inactivity.

Aerobic Exercise

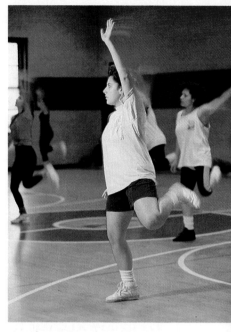

Brisk walking, jogging, swimming, dancing, cycling, and any other nonstop vigorous exercises are aerobic activities. During aerobic exercise the body has a greater demand for oxygen to provide the muscles with the energy they need to carry out the activity. This kind of exercise increases the lungs' capacity to hold air.

Aerobic exercises are rhythmic and sustained and use the large muscle groups, particularly those in the hips and legs.

Aerobic exercise causes the arteries to enlarge and increases the dilation of capillaries that take blood to the muscles. Blood flow increases to the skeletal muscles.

As these large muscles contract, they press against the blood vessels, sending increased amounts of blood to the heart. The heart becomes a stronger and more efficient pump, so it beats slower during exercising and at rest. The slower the heart rate the longer the heart can rest between beats.

Aerobic exercise is important in maintaining and improving one's fitness level.

Exercises that improve the condition of the heart and lungs have three essential characteristics:

- They must be brisk. They should raise the heart rate and breathing rate.
- They must be continuous. They should be done for 20 to 30 minutes without stopping.
- They must be regular. They should be repeated at least three times a week to maintain one's fitness level.

LESSON 2 REVIEW

Reviewing Facts and Vocabulary

1. Define the term *physical fitness.*
2. What two important points should you remember before taking a body flexibility test?
3. Define the term *pulse recovery rate.*

Thinking Critically

4. **Analysis.** Compare muscular strength to muscular endurance.
5. **Evaluation.** Discuss the accuracy of this statement: *Aerobic exercise is better for you than anaerobic exercise.*

Applying Health Knowledge

6. Interview a person who exercises regularly. What motivates that person to exercise? What benefits does he or she receive? Then interview one who does not exercise regularly. What conclusions can you draw?
7. Write an advertisement to promote physical fitness. Include at least five selling points.
8. Find advertisements in magazines or newspapers for equipment that claims to increase physical fitness and well-being. Discuss the claims in class. Evaluate the accuracy of the advertisements.

Self-Inventory

Figuring Out Your Fitness

HOW DO YOU RATE?

Number a sheet of paper from 1 through 30. Read each item below, and respond by writing *yes* or *no* for each item. Total the number of *yes* and *no* responses. Then proceed to the next section.

1. I exercise because I enjoy it.
2. I am more active than I am sedentary.
3. I do at least 20 minutes of aerobic exercise at least three times a week.
4. I keep an activity log or journal of my daily exercise workouts.
5. I use the stairs instead of escalators or elevators whenever possible.
6. I do not use tobacco.
7. I do not use alcohol or illegal drugs.
8. I regularly participate in lifetime sports, such as tennis, swimming, and softball.
9. I walk or ride a bike when possible, rather than take a car.
10. I take in about the same number of calories that I burn.
11. I often use exercise to deal with tension, anger, or frustration.
12. I keep within 5 pounds (2 kg) of my ideal weight.
13. I seldom feel tired or run-down.
14. I get at least 8 hours of sleep each night.
15. I plan regular times for exercise.

16. I stand rather than sit whenever possible.
17. I make daily, personal decisions to be fit.
18. I avoid consuming high-fat foods and snacks.
19. I usually follow through with my exercise plans.
20. I tend to eat nutritious meals and snacks.
21. I usually warm up before starting an exercise session.
22. I usually cool down after an exercise session.
23. Stretching is a part of my warm-up.
24. Stretching is a part of my cool down.
25. I enjoy a variety of physical activities.
26. I feel better after I exercise.
27. I motivate myself to exercise regularly.
28. I vary my exercise activities.
29. I encourage my friends to exercise.
30. I encourage family members to exercise.

HOW DID YOU SCORE?

Give yourself 1 point for every *yes* answer. Read below to see how you scored. Then proceed to the next section.

21 to 30
Excellent. Fitness is a part of your daily life. Keep up the good work.

11 to 20
Good. Your fitness behavior is positive, but limited in scope. Ask your family and friends to

support and encourage you in making fitness a part of each day.

5 to 10
Fair. You need to increase your activity level in order to get more benefits.

Below 5
Poor. You're missing out on a lot of fun that comes with exercise. Get off the couch and move your body! No one else can do it for you.

WHAT ARE YOUR GOALS?

If you received an *excellent* or *good* score, complete the statements in Part A. If your score was *fair* or *poor*, complete the statements in Parts A and B.

Part A

1. I plan to learn more about fitness and health by ____.
2. My timetable for accomplishing this is ____.
3. I plan to share my information with others by ____.

Part B

4. The behavior or attitude toward fitness that I would most like to change is ____.
5. The steps involved in making this change are ____.
6. My rewards for making this change will be ____.
7. My timetable for making this change is ____.
8. The people or groups I will ask for help are ____.

Building Decision-Making Skills

A ndrew is quite overweight and is constantly making fun of his physique and his lack of activity. Kevin believes that Andrew really would like to do something about his problem, but that he doesn't know how to go about it. Kevin works out regularly and would like to invite Andrew to join him, but he doesn't know if he should.

WHAT DO YOU THINK?

1. **Situation.** What might be holding Andrew back from regular workouts and becoming fit? Is it possible that there are health issues that Kevin doesn't know about?

2. **Situation.** What decision does Kevin need to make?

3. **Choices.** Assuming he decides to ask Andrew, what are some possible approaches Kevin could use?

4. **Consequences.** What are the advantages and disadvantages of each approach?

5. **Consequences.** How might Kevin's asking Andrew to work out affect Andrew's self-esteem? How might it affect Kevin's self-esteem?

6. **Consequences.** What's the worst thing that might happen if Kevin asks Andrew to join him in a workout? What's the best thing that might happen? What would probably happen? Do you think the risks are worth it?

7. **Decision.** What do you think Kevin should do? How should he go about it?

8. **Evaluation.** Have you ever been in a situation where you wanted to help someone but didn't because you were afraid of what others would think? How did you handle the situation? How would you handle it now?

B yron's father is very athletic. He pushed Byron into a lot of sports when Byron was young and today Byron is really turned off by any mention of sports. He knows it's important to be active but he also knows that sports are not for him. What should Byron do?

WHAT DO YOU THINK?

9. **Situation.** What reasons might Byron have for being turned off by sports?

10. **Choices.** If sports are out, what other choices does Byron have?

11. **Consequences.** What are the advantages of each choice?

12. **Consequences.** What are the disadvantages of each choice?

13. **Consequences.** Who will be affected by Byron's decision?

14. **Consequences.** How might Byron's self-esteem be affected by this decision?

15. **Consequences.** What risks are involved in this decision?

16. **Consequences.** How might Byron's health triangle be affected by this decision?

17. **Decision.** What should Byron do? Explain your answer.

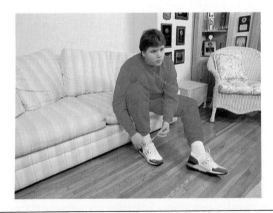

REVIEW

Using Health Terms

On a separate sheet of paper, write the term that best matches each definition given below.

LESSON 1

1. An excessive amount of fat in the body, often associated with heart disease.
2. The minimum amount of energy required to maintain the life processes in your body.

LESSON 2

3. The amount of fat in the body in relation to total body weight.
4. Intense physical activity lasting a few seconds to a few minutes.
5. Continuous vigorous activity lasting at least 20 minutes, during which the heart rate increases.
6. A type of weight-training exercise that involves muscular contraction but little or no movement of the body part stressed.
7. A type of exercise that involves repeated movements using weights.

Building Academic Skills

LESSON 1

8. **Reading.** Use the context clues below to define the term *sedentary*:
   As a receptionist, Claudia sits at a desk for eight hours a day answering the telephone. She has a sedentary job.
9. **Math.** One pound of fat is equal to about 3,500 calories. How many calories must be eliminated from the diet each day in order to lose 2 pounds in a 1-week period?

LESSON 2

10. **Reading.** Which of the following statements is the best summary of Lesson 2?
    a. Physical fitness is the ability to carry out daily tasks easily and to respond to unexpected demands.
    b. Sensible exercise is good for you.
    c. Physical fitness can be achieved through weight control and a variety of exercises.

Recalling the Facts

LESSON 1

11. What aspects of your overall health does fitness affect?
12. What body systems are negatively affected by immobility?
13. Is it better for your respiratory system to work slow or fast?
14. Is it better for your lung capacity to be high or low?
15. What makes a muscle grow stronger?
16. How is the energy value of food measured?
17. What happens to calories your body takes in but does not use?
18. If you take in more calories than you burn, do you lose or gain weight?
19. How many calories equal one pound of fat?

LESSON 2

20. Explain how calipers measure percent body fat.
21. Describe one way to measure cardiorespiratory endurance.
22. Why do anaerobic exercises generally not raise a person's level of fitness?
23. What are the benefits of including weight training in an exercise program?
24. Which kind of weight training would you use to build muscular strength with little or no body movement?
25. Which kind of weight training would you use to increase muscular strength and endurance, and flexibility?
26. Which weighs more, muscle tissue or fat tissue?
27. What kind of weight training builds muscular strength and flexibility with repeated movements using weights?
28. What are three requirements for exercises to improve the condition of the heart and lungs?
29. Give three examples of aerobic exercises.
30. Is weight training an aerobic or an anaerobic exercise?
31. What benefits can a person gain from anaerobic exercise?

REVIEW

Thinking Critically

LESSON 1

32. Analysis. What advantage does a totally fit person have over an unfit person on a day-to-day basis?

33. Synthesis. What are two possible social benefits of an exercise program? Explain your answer.

LESSON 2

34. Synthesis. Participating in an aerobics class three times a week will contribute to cardiovascular fitness. Some people cannot afford this, or do not want to exercise in front of a group. What would accomplish the same goal and be more private—as well as less expensive?

35. Evaluation. The following students participated in the school's annual assessment of upper body strength and endurance. Rate each student's performance based on the information provided in your text. All students were age 13 or 14.
  a. Jerry Ono: 7-10
  b. Sheila Gordon: 2
  c. Sam Miller: 5-6
  d. Shirley Obetz: 1

36. Evaluation. During a 1-mile run/walk cardiorespiratory endurance test, what would be the rating for each of the following persons?
  a. Frank Deerwater: 9 minutes
  b. Juanita Gonzalez: 8 minutes, 15 seconds
  c. Jake Karpels: 7 minutes, 2 seconds
  d. Shelley Jones: 8 minutes, 12 seconds

37. Synthesis. What factors should you consider in selecting exercises for your total fitness program?

Making the Connection

LESSON 1

38. Art. Design a poster with a slogan that illustrates the benefits of being physically fit. Display the posters throughout your school.

Applying Health Knowledge

LESSON 1

39. For each pair described below, which individuals are choosing the more physically fit way of living?
  a. Dave and Donna both work for Fidelity Insurance, which is located on the third floor of the Grover Building. Dave always takes the elevator to the third floor; Donna always uses the stairs.
  b. The Jacksons and the Smiths live next door to each other. Their lawns are identical in size. The Jacksons use a hand mower to keep their lawn trim; the Smiths use a riding mower.

LESSON 2

40. Label each type of exercise described below as *isometric, isotonic,* or *isokinetic.*
  a. using a rowing machine
  b. doing push-ups
  c. pushing against a wall

Beyond the Classroom

LESSON 1

41. Community Involvement. Interview five working adults. Ask each what kind of exercise they get on their jobs and what kinds of exercise they get outside their jobs.

LESSON 2

42. Community Involvement. Call or visit a health spa, physical fitness center, or your local YMCA or YWCA. Find out what kinds of fitness exercises they recommend for teenagers. Discover what types of equipment and facilities they have. Also find out what other services they provide. Report to your class on the services and equipment offered and the fees charged.

43. Parental Involvement. Talk to your parents and siblings about a family exercise program. Work together to set up a regular plan of family fitness and exercise.

LESSON 1
Beginning an
Exercise Program

LESSON 2
Avoiding Injury

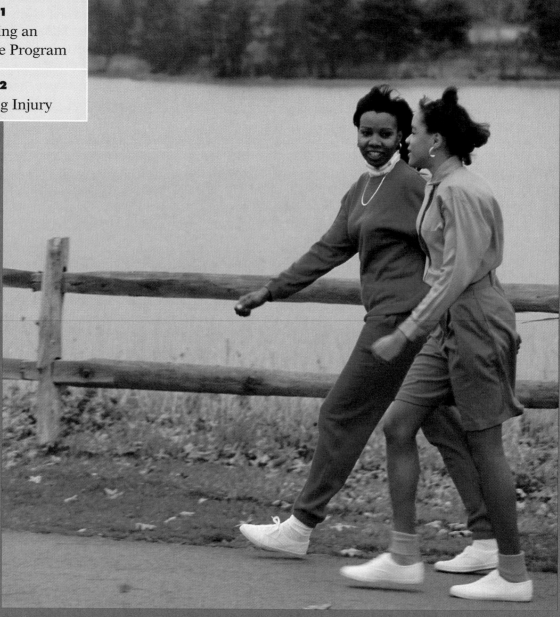

BEGINNING AN EXERCISE PROGRAM

In the previous chapter you learned what exercise does for the body and how exercise influences your level of fitness. You also had an opportunity to determine your level of physical fitness. Now you are ready to plan an exercise program to improve or maintain your fitness level. To design an exercise program for yourself, you need to consider what you hope to accomplish and what you enjoy doing.

Setting Your Goals

If your goal is to strengthen muscles, you will probably choose an anaerobic exercise program, such as lifting weights or using a strength-training machine.

If your goal is to improve your endurance, you will probably develop a program of aerobic exercise, such as walking, jogging, cycling, or swimming. It could be that you have a combination of these goals in mind.

Finding the Right Exercise

Choose exercises that are appropriate for the location in which you live. The available facilities and weather are important considerations. You also need to consider any physical problems or limitations you may have. Seek medical advice, especially if you have not been exercising at all or if you have any health problems.

As you consider what exercise to do, it is important to pick something you enjoy. It is unlikely that you will continue an exercise activity if you do not enjoy it or cannot do it very well. In addition, consider exercise that you already do during a day. You may walk briskly to and from classes, so you might want to pick an exercise that does not involve walking.

By developing a regular plan of exercise, you prepare yourself for dealing more effectively with the problems and challenges of daily living. You will look and feel better. As you begin to improve your level of fitness, you may actually find you have more energy each day.

By developing these exercise habits now, you will find that they can become part of your life as an adult. You will continue to enjoy activities that others are not able to enjoy because you have chosen to take care of yourself. More than likely, you will live longer because people who take care of their bodies are less likely to develop poor health and disease.

When and Where to Exercise

It is best to find a regular time during the day to exercise so that exercise becomes a part of your routine. Try not to exercise after eating.

LESSON 1 FOCUS

TERMS TO USE
- Warming up
- Target heart rate
- Cooling down
- Resting heart rate

CONCEPTS TO LEARN
- To be successful, a personal exercise program must meet the needs of the individual.
- Regular exercise is a major part of a healthy life-style.
- Specific, realistic, attainable goals are essential to any personal exercise program.
- Every exercise session should include a warm-up, a workout, and a cool down.

ATTITUDES AND BEHAVIORS TO EVALUATE
- Self-Inventory, page 366.
- Building Decision-Making Skills, page 367.

Carla runs on her school's cross-country team and thinks she has a really good coach. The team recently placed in a regional meet and qualified to run in the state meet. To get more practice time in, the coach has extended the workout part of the practice the last couple of weeks. Consequently, some team members have skipped the usual cool down. Some say they cool down as they catch rides to go home. Carla thinks a cool down is important after the workout.

What should Carla say to her teammates about this?

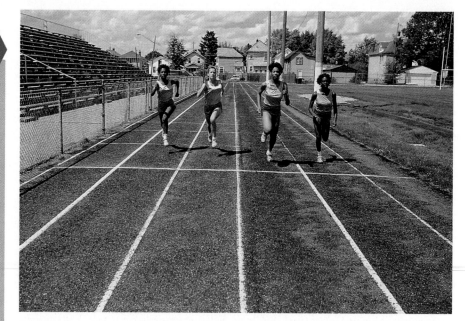

By joining a team or a league, you set up situations that will encourage you to participate in activities you want to do more often.

During exercise more blood is diverted to the skeletal muscles, depriving the stomach of oxygen, affecting the rate of digestion. Exercising on a full stomach can result in stomach cramps or nausea.

Consider safety in choosing when and where to exercise. If your program takes you outside at night, wear reflective clothing and practice good safety habits. Consider working out with a partner, and avoid unlighted streets, dark alleys, and remote areas.

COMMON MYTHS ABOUT EXERCISE

A myth is a belief or opinion based on false reasoning. There are many myths about fitness and exercise. Here are a few, with explanations of why they are false:

■ Myth 1: Exercise makes you tired. As you get in better shape, you will find that exercising gives you more energy than you had before. Regular exercise can actually reduce stress and fatigue.

■ Myth 2: Exercise takes too much time. Regular exercise does not have to take more than 25 to 40 minutes, three times a week.

■ Myth 3: All exercise gives you the same benefits. All physical activities can give you enjoyment, but only frequent, continuous activity helps the heart and lungs, and burns off fat and calories.

■ Myth 4: Exercise is expensive. Some of the most beneficial exercises are very inexpensive, such as walking or jogging. Swimming is another excellent activity that is reasonably priced.

■ Myth 5: Exercise means playing a sport. While team sports are exercise, individual activities such as walking, running, biking, or swimming are excellent forms of exercise, too.

■ Myth 6: You have to be athletic to exercise. Most aerobic activities, such as those mentioned above, do not require any special athletic abilities. In fact, many people who find school sports difficult have discovered that these other activities are easy to do and are enjoyable.

Components of an Exercise Session

There are three components of an exercise session. They include

- the warm-up,
- the workout,
- the cool down.

The Warm-Up

Warming up is engaging in activity that prepares the muscles for the work that is to come. The first step in warming up is to stretch the large muscles. Stretches should be slow and smooth, not jerky. Stretching helps increase the elasticity of muscles and tendons. Stretching can prevent injury to the muscles and tissue surrounding the joints.

The second stage of the warm-up is to perform the activity slowly for about 5 minutes. So if you are going to jog 2 miles, you might walk briskly for about 5 minutes before you begin to jog. If you are going to bike 10 miles, you might ride at an easy pace for the first 5 minutes, then pick up the pace.

Warming up allows your pulse rate to increase gradually. A sudden increase in the pulse rate puts unnecessary strain on the heart and the blood vessels.

The Workout

This is the component of your exercise program in which you are actually performing the exercise at its highest intensity. The intensity depends on your current fitness level. Choose an activity that continually uses the large muscle groups. Biking, walking, swimming, and running are good examples. You should work hard, but not overdo it. Studies have shown that doubling the amount of exercise does not double its effectiveness. Overdoing exercise can cause sleeplessness or chronically sore muscles.

Frequency.   To begin both anaerobic and aerobic programs, you should schedule workouts three times a week, with no less than one day and no more than two days between sessions.

Many people enjoy their aerobic exercise routine so much that they do it more often than three times a week. There is no real harm in doing aerobic exercise five times a week once one is physically fit.

Exercising more than three times a week for six months should help get you physically fit. You then must maintain your program at least three times a week to maintain your fitness level.

Intensity.   It is very important not to overdo exercise. You must start slowly and build endurance. In weight training, start with a lighter weight and build to the heavier ones. In aerobic programs, work toward your target heart rate. Your **target heart rate** is 70 to 85 percent of your maximum heart rate. The target rate provides a range for exertion.

To find your target heart rate, first estimate your maximum heart rate by subtracting your age from 220. For example, if you are 15 years old, subtract 15 from 220 to get 205. Your maximum heart rate would be 205 beats per minute. Your target heart rate would be between 70 and

High Altitude Exercise

Exercising at high altitudes (above 10,000 feet) poses special problems to people who usually live and exercise at lower altitudes. Because air at high altitudes is at a lower pressure, breathing rate is affected. Non-natives who exercise at high altitudes become tired easily, and may have difficulty breathing. Because of this, professional athletes who compete in cities of high altitude may travel there early so that team members can adjust to the different air pressure.

People in the Andes mountains of Peru and the Himalayas of Tibet live at high altitudes all the time. As a result, they have developed larger lungs, and produce more red blood cells than people living at sea level. This allows them to take in more air in a breath and to carry oxygen more effectively to the tissues that need them.

85 percent of 205, or between 144 and 174 beats per minute. You should never exercise to your maximum heart rate. Exercise at a level to stay within the range of your target heart rate.

You can learn to take your heart rate, but a general rule of thumb is that if you cannot talk while you are exercising, you are probably doing too much.

Duration. In weight training, do the exercises slowly, taking at least 2 seconds each time you lower a weight. Rest for 1 or 2 minutes between sets, and do a variety of exercises to strengthen your muscles in the full range of motion. A set consists of 10 to 14 repetitions.

The time spent doing aerobic exercises should be built up gradually. The goal in aerobics is to spend 20 to 30 minutes in your target heart rate.

The Cool Down

Just as your body needs to be readied for increased activity, it needs to be returned gradually to a less active state. During exercise an increased amount of blood is pumped to the heart with the help of contractions of large leg muscles that push against the veins. If the leg muscles relax suddenly, pooling may result. The blood will collect in your extremities instead of getting back to the heart. The heart is still pumping hard, but less blood is returning to it. Pooling can cause lightheadedness, even fainting.

When you are **cooling down,** you gradually decrease activity. Your muscles continue to assist in returning the blood to the heart until your pulse rate slows. During cool down, the metabolic processes can gradually return to resting levels.

The best way to cool down is simply to slow down activity. Slower activity should be done for about 5 minutes, followed by 5 minutes of stretching. You have cooled down adequately when your heart rate is within 20 to 30 beats of your regular heart rate.

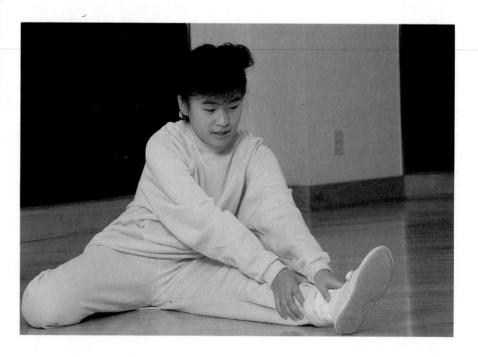

Always warm up and cool down when you exercise.

THE VALUE OF VARIOUS ACTIVITIES FOR THE HEART AND LUNGS

Column A

High level of conditioning

Bicycling
Cross-country skiing
Uphill hiking
Ice hockey
Jogging
Jumping rope
Rowing
Running in place
Soccer
Stationary cycling
Swimming

Column B

Moderate level of conditioning

Basketball
Calisthenics
Field hockey
Handball
Racquetball
Squash
Tennis (singles)
Walking

Column C

Low level of conditioning

Baseball
Bowling
Downhill skiing
Football
Golf (on foot or by cart)
Softball
Volleyball

Column A
These exercises are naturally very vigorous. They need to be done for at least 20 minutes, three times a week. They maintain fitness and contribute to weight control.

Column B
These activities are moderately vigorous, but they can be excellent conditioners if done briskly for at least 30 minutes, three times a week. When done briskly, they offer benefits similar to those activities in column A.

Column C
These activities, though they may be vigorous, are usually not sustained long enough to provide conditioning benefits. They can improve coordination, flexibility, and muscle tone. However, they must be combined with activities in column A or B to improve total fitness.

Checking Your Progress

In planning your fitness program, you need to include an evaluation to see how well you are doing. You need to take time to think about your program. Do you feel better? Can you lift more weight and for a longer period of time? Are you walking farther in a shorter amount of time? The questions you ask yourself depend on the program you developed and the goals you set.

Many people like to keep a journal to track their progress. If you decide to do this, begin the journal the day you begin your exercise program, or as close to it as you can. In the journal list your goals and some information about yourself, such as weight, measurements, how you feel, how well you sleep, how long you sleep, and how energetic you feel. Keep track of the frequency, intensity, and duration of your workouts.

At the end of 6 weeks, check the same information about yourself that you checked when you started the journal. Compare the figures. Do not be discouraged if the change is not dramatic: it often takes 12 weeks to see any change. Check yourself every 6 weeks and compare your most recent figures with your initial figures. You will be living proof that exercise works!

HEALTH UPDATE

LOOKING AT TECHNOLOGY

Magnetic Resonance Imaging

In the past, when people were injured while exercising or playing sports, diagnosing the injury was often guesswork. Now, with magnetic resonance imaging, or MRI, experts can evaluate neck, knee, shoulder, and other injuries in a painless way using a strong magnetic field. For example, they can tell how severely a ligament is torn and easily determine if an operation will be necessary. An MRI even allows physicians to see through both organs and bones.

How does MRI work? The patient lies on a table inside a giant magnet, and its magnetic field works on the patient's body. Instead of using X rays or contrast dyes, as many diagnostic tests do, the MRI uses radio waves and magnetism to make images. A computer analyzes the pattern of magnetic energy. It takes into account the length and strength of radio signals and makes the pattern into a picture. The radiologist then interprets the picture and can more clearly diagnose the problem. In addition to getting a three-dimensional image of inside the body, the physician can also get a two-dimensional "slice" of any body part and have that image displayed on a screen.

Your Resting Heart Rate

Your **resting heart rate** is found by taking your pulse at intervals when you are not active—perhaps while you are reading a good book. If you measure your pulse several times, the average is your resting heart rate. Your resting heart rate indicates your level of fitness. A person of average fitness has a resting heart rate between 72 and 84 beats a minute. After only 4 weeks of an exercise program, that rate can decrease by 5 to 10 beats a minute. A resting heart rate below 72 beats a minute indicates a good fitness level. A young athlete at the top of his or her form may have a resting rate as low as 40 beats a minute.

K E E P I N G   F I T

Exercising: Some Basic Principles

In *The Family Fitness Handbook*, authors Bob Glover and Jack Shepherd present these basic fitness principles:
- Exercise should be progressive. Never increase your exercise by more than 10 percent from one week to the next.
- Exercise with regularity.
- Use specific exercises to achieve specific fitness benefits.
- Vary the exercises you do.
- Make the exercises adaptable to your body and level of fitness, as well as to your schedule, fitness goals, environment, weather, and the seasons.
- Try to be patient. Fitness takes time.
- Exercise in moderation.

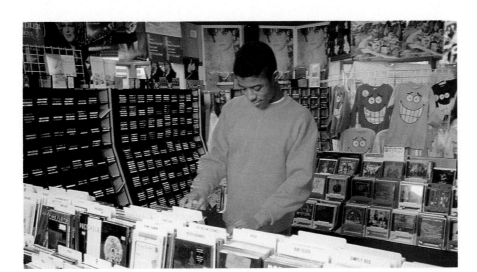

Your Body Measurements

Many people begin an exercise program to lose weight and to improve muscle tone. If you are exercising and not eating any more calories than you need, you will lose weight and improve muscle tone.

It is possible to lose fat without losing weight, so do not be discouraged if the scale is not moving very much when you write your 6-week measurements in your journal. Muscle tissue is heavier than fat tissue. If you are building muscle, the scale may even go up a bit. That does not matter; getting rid of the fat and becoming fit is what matters. When you take your measurements, you will probably see a change there. Use a standard measuring tape and measure your waist, upper arm, upper leg, and hips. Record and date your measurements.

LESSON 1 REVIEW

Reviewing Facts and Vocabulary

1. What should you consider in selecting exercises for your fitness program?
2. Why should you exercise on an empty stomach?
3. Why is a warm-up an important part of your workout?
4. How does the warm-up contribute to physical fitness? How should warm-up exercises be done?
5. What is cooling down?

Thinking Critically

6. **Analysis.** What is the difference between aerobic and anaerobic exercise?

7. **Evaluation.** Are there any justifications for engaging in physical activity that is not aerobic?
8. **Analysis.** How is your resting heart rate an indicator of your fitness level?

Applying Health Knowledge

9. Keep a record of your pulse rate during different physical activities. Which activity makes your heart work the hardest? Compare your pulse rate record with your classmates' records.
10. Some people start an exercise program only to give it up, claiming that exercise is boring or too hard or that they just do not have time. What suggestions can you give to help them stay with their exercise programs?

Avoiding Injury

LESSON 2 FOCUS

TERMS TO USE
- Sprain
- Bruise
- Strain
- Tendinitis (ten•duh•NYT•uhs)
- Hernias
- Frostbite

CONCEPTS TO LEARN
- There is always a risk of injury during exercise.
- Most injuries or conditions can often be prevented by taking adequate precautions, including a good warm-up and the use of good equipment and proper technique.

ATTITUDES AND BEHAVIORS TO EVALUATE
- Self-Inventory, page 366.
- Building Decision-Making Skills, page 367.

With any movement activity, there is always a risk of accident or injury. There are many ways to prevent the more common injuries associated with exercise. The risk of injury during exercise increases when a person is not in good physical condition or has not sufficiently warmed up. To attempt activities beyond your level of ability also increases the risk of injury.

Injuries most often occur when the body is not prepared for the demands placed on it. Even when people are in good physical condition there is risk of injury based solely on the nature of the activity.

The most common injuries that occur from exercise are to the muscular and skeletal systems. This is because movement is fundamental to muscle and joint activity, as well as to exercise. Injury to these areas is likely when you exercise too long or too hard.

Injuries to the Skeletal System

Sprains and dislocations are the most common injuries of the skeletal system. They involve joints and result from too much stress being placed on a joint. If you experience a sudden blow or twist or stretch, the tissues that join the bones can strain, pull, or tear.

Have you ever stepped off a curb in the wrong way and twisted your ankle? Sprains can occur as easily as that! A **sprain** is an injury to tissues surrounding a joint. Ligaments may be stretched and torn. A sprain may be accompanied by severe pain, swelling, and difficulty in moving.

If you suffer a sprain, apply cold packs or ice to the sprained area. Elevate the area, if possible, to help control swelling. Also, apply an elastic wrap to the area. Wrapping and cold exposure cause the blood vessels to become narrower, lessening the internal bleeding. Elevating the injured area increases the flow of blood in the veins that lead away from the injury.

Stress on a joint can result in torn cartilage when the strong connective tissue has been pulled out from the bone. Surgery is usually required for this injury. Because it can be difficult to distinguish a sprain from a dislocation or a fracture, a health professional should check more serious sprains.

A dislocation is also a serious injury. A dislocation occurs when the end of a bone is pushed out of its joint. The ligaments holding the bones are severely stretched and may even be torn. Dislocations are usually quite painful. The joint must be set back into its normal position and held there while the surrounding tissue heals.

Never attempt to replace a dislocation yourself. Joints are surrounded by many tiny blood vessels and nerves. You risk further damage to them if you do not know what you are doing. Keep the injured area very still, apply cold packs or ice, and seek medical attention right away.

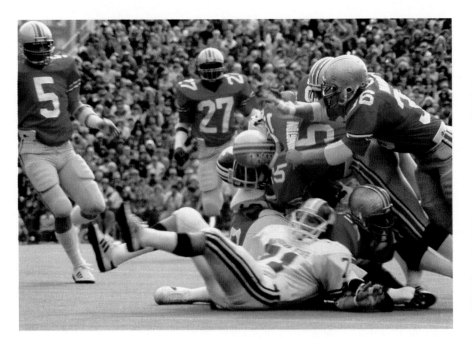

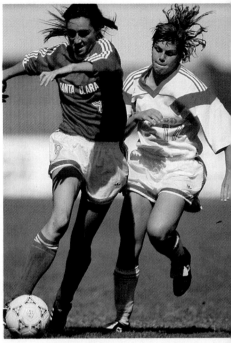

Injuries to the skeletal system can occur during many activities.

Injuries to the Muscular System

Some of the most common injuries to muscles are bruises, strains, tendinitis, pulled and torn muscles, muscle cramps, and hernias.

A **bruise** is an injury to tissue under the skin. Bruises usually result from a blow to the muscle. Discoloration results when the capillaries break and ooze blood. If cold packs are applied immediately, swelling and discoloration will be reduced.

A muscle **strain** results when muscles are overworked. Have you ever participated in a strenuous activity you were not used to and then been sore the next day? You experienced muscle strain. Resting the muscles and applying ice for the first 24 hours are the best ways to treat muscle strains. You can prevent some strains by warming up properly and gradually building up your level of exertion. In other words, avoid going all out your first day of exercise.

Tendinitis occurs when a tendon—the connective tissue of the muscles and bones—is stretched or torn. The injured area becomes inflamed. A common example of tendinitis is tennis elbow. To treat tendinitis, first rest the injured area to decrease the inflammation, and then use prescribed medicines or physical therapy to help cure the injury.

A pulled or torn muscle can cause severe pain and require you to cease your activity. In a pulled or torn muscle, the large muscle is separated or torn from its point of attachment. This injury can damage the blood vessels that supply nourishment to that muscle. Immediate medical care may be necessary. Cold packs should be put on the muscle area right away.

As with other muscle injuries, lack of warm-up and overexertion of an unprepared muscle are the major causes of a pulled or torn muscle.

Muscle cramps occur when a muscle contracts tightly and will not relax. Cramps usually happen as the result of an irritation within the muscle. When a muscle cramp occurs, all fibers contract at the same time. This may be caused by temporary lack of food or oxygen to the muscle. Sometimes cramping occurs as a result of a person's losing

DID YOU KNOW?

- You can put unnecessary strain on your muscles if the heels of your athletic shoes wear down too far.
- Runners should not run in walking shoes because they do not have enough cushioning. Walkers should not walk in running shoes because they do not have much heel and the Achilles tendon is not supported.

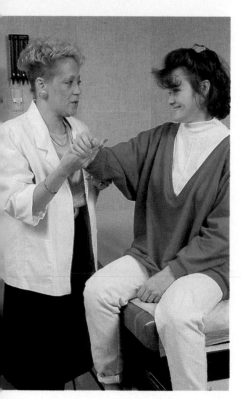

This physical therapist is helping this teen regain the mobility in her arm.

large amounts of salt and water through perspiration. Tired, overworked muscles sometimes cramp.

Massaging the muscle area firmly can help a cramp. Continuing to work the muscle lightly can help relieve the cramp. Heat can also help. You can help prevent cramps by warming up properly and by drinking enough fluids before and during exercise.

Cramps are dangerous if they occur while swimming. You could drown before you are able to relieve a severe cramp. The most important point to remember is to remain calm. Your body will float if you do not panic. It is best to take a deep breath, curl over, and massage the muscle. Although cramps are painful, they do not involve injury.

Hernias, or ruptures, are weak areas in the muscle supporting various organs. This usually occurs in the abdominal area. Part of an organ such as the intestine may push through this weak area. Hernias can be caused by a lack of warm-up exercises or by picking up heavy objects improperly. Surgery is usually necessary to correct a hernia.

Weather-Related Risks

Certain health problems can occur in hot and cold weather. The major ones are heat cramps, heat exhaustion, heatstroke, and frostbite.

Heat cramps can occur when a person loses a large amount of water and electrolytes—for example, body salt—through perspiration. Massaging and drinking small amounts of salt water every 15 to 20 minutes will usually relieve the condition.

Heat exhaustion usually results from exercise or overexertion in a hot, humid atmosphere. The body becomes overheated with the loss of a large amount of water and electrolytes. The skin becomes pale and moist. A person may also experience dizziness, headache, shortness of breath, and nausea. The person should be moved to a cool place and kept lying down, with the feet raised.

You can prevent heat exhaustion by drinking plenty of fluids before and during exercise. Activities on hot, humid days should be restricted, especially if you are not accustomed to the weather.

Heatstroke is a more serious condition. Heatstroke usually follows prolonged exposure to direct sun, dehydration, and profuse sweating. It may also be caused by obesity or the inability of the body to adapt to a weather situation. The body loses its ability to rid itself of the heat that has built up. The body retains the heat, the person does not perspire,

K E E P I N G   F I T

Training

Here are some steps to follow before participating in any sport.
- Make sure you first get in good condition.
- Work to improve cardiopulmonary function, endurance, flexibility, and strength.

- Forget the no-pain-no-gain approach. Train slowly and progressively.
- Eat a variety of complex carbohydrates.
- Drink lots of liquids.

- Get regular, uninterrupted sleep.
- Wear proper equipment. Make sure it fits.
- If it is too stressful or too painful, stop.

and body temperature can get as high as 108 degrees. The person may collapse suddenly, have a rapid pulse, twitching muscles, and difficulty breathing. The skin will be dry and hot, and blood will rush to the head and face.

If you are present when someone experiences heatstroke, call for help right away. Heatstroke is a life-threatening situation. Serious organ damage can result from such a high body temperature. Move the person to a cool place, loosen the clothing, and spray or sponge the person with cold water. Monitor the person's breathing. It may be necessary to administer artificial respiration.

When there is prolonged exposure of a body part to a freezing or near-freezing temperature, **frostbite** occurs. In this situation, the exposed tissue freezes. The normal activity of the cells is stopped. When circulation of the blood stops, cells begin to die.

Frostbite occurs most often to the chin, cheeks, nose, ears, fingers, and toes. Dressing warmly, covering all exposed skin—especially the head, face, fingers, and toes—and avoiding fatigue and excessive exposure to cold while exercising helps prevent frostbite.

If frostbite does occur, apply blankets to warm the body. The frostbitten body part should never be rubbed or exposed to intense heat. This causes further damage. The body must be gradually warmed. If frostbite is severe, the person should be kept quiet and watched for signs of shock or difficult breathing. Because of tissue damage, medical care should be sought.

STEROIDS: TOO BIG A RISK

Weight lifters and shot-putters began using anabolic steroids more than 35 years ago to improve performance. Unfortunately, anabolic steroids are now used in junior and senior high schools around the United States.

Anabolic steroids are chemicals similar to the male hormone testosterone. They are taken by athletes and bodybuilders to increase muscle mass without increasing fat while doing weight training.

Many young people have not been warned of the dangerous physical and psychological effects of using these drugs. Some people think the drugs are only training aids. The short-term gain from anabolic steroids seems to motivate some people to use these drugs regardless of their long-term health risks.

The negative consequences of taking these drugs are enormous. Consider the health risks involved:
- increased risk of cancer and heart disease
- sterility
- skin problems
- unusual weight gain or loss
- sexual dysfunction
- suicidal or depressive tendencies

Consider also the following facts:
- Illegal distribution of steroids is a felony.
- Possession without a prescription is illegal.
- Athletes who test positive for steroids risk their careers.
- Purchasing "street steroids" adds risks because you do not know what you are getting.

Even when steroids do increase muscle mass, the effects are short-term. The conclusion: steroids mean trouble.

Applying heat can help relieve a cramp.

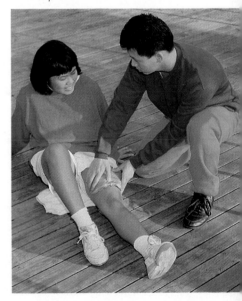

Overcoming The Odds

Missy Meharg is 28. She has an advanced degree in psychophysiology of sports. She is a master field hockey player and head coach at the University of Maryland. She knows a lot about winning and physical fitness. But she also knows a lot about losing and injuries.

In college, she played both lacrosse and field hockey and was voted Most Valuable Player in both. Soon, however, she began to channel most of her athletic energies toward field hockey, an Olympic sport. As a member of the U.S. National Team, her new goal was to compete in the Pan American Games or an Olympic event, but she was cut from the team and became a first alternate in 1988. Not one to give up, Meharg tried out again for the U.S. National Team in 1989, made it, and went on tour in Russia and other countries. Two years later, again a member of the National Team, she competed in the Pan American Games and the Olympic Qualifying Tournament. Unfortunately, the team did not qualify for the Olympics in Barcelona in 1992, but Meharg is upbeat about the loss. "It's okay because I really did what I wanted to do, and I tried my best."

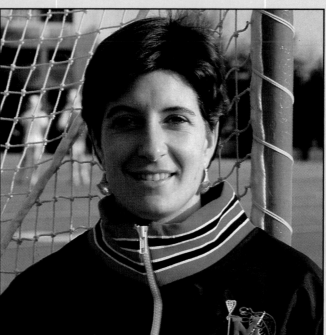

In her athletic career, Meharg has had three major injuries. The first was a really bad ankle injury in which she stretched the ligaments. So was the second. The last injury, however, was the most serious. She had just gotten a new pair of in-line skates and was using them as a form of aerobic training. "I was going down a hill a little fast, thinking I was a little better than I was, and I was not being safety conscious. I was flying. The next thing I knew, my feet were straight above my head. I came down backwards on both wrists. I broke my scaphoid bone in half in my left wrist. It's the slowest healing bone in your body." Meharg then had a difficult choice to make: have a long arm cast for three months and not be able to play, or have an operation in which a screw would be put into the bone to keep it together. She opted for the latter. She was back playing — more cautiously —just one month later. She continues, "Ever since, I don't take the risks I used to."

What advice does Meharg give young athletes? "Know your limitations. Most athletic injuries are acquired because of lack of knowledge or lack of preparation. Every time I go out to play anything now I always do a small run—8 to 10 minutes to warm up, then a full stretch to take care of all the major muscle masses, and then I start the activity slowly and work up to 100 percent. I do the cool down the same way." She concludes, "When I was younger, I didn't realize how important total fitness was. I do now. I'd say that overall health is so dependent on your overall fitness level. I know that decision making and being mentally stable are closely related to being healthy and physically fit."

1. What advice does Meharg give about avoiding injury when exercising?
2. How does your level of fitness affect your mental and social health?

Dressing Properly and Choosing the Proper Equipment

Sports and exercise equipment are big business. Clothing, shoes, apparatus, and food supplements are all part of a multi-million dollar industry. How much money you spend on dress and equipment for an activity depends on you. It depends on your motives. Some people want to wear the highest-priced clothing, have the most expensive athletic shoes, or use some name-brand sports equipment endorsed by a major sports performer. These choices may have nothing to do with safety, comfort, or performance during your activity—factors that other people consider to be most important. Here are some tips for making wise buying decisions:

- Clothing should be comfortable and loose around the joints. Cotton or other porous materials are best because they absorb perspiration and allow air through.
- Footwear should have a cushioned heel, good arch support, and ample toe room.
- If you are starting a new sport, rent or borrow the equipment to see how you like the sport before spending a lot of money on equipment.

Avoiding Risk and Injury During Exercise

What can you think of that would help you avoid being injured during exercise? Think back to your own experiences during exercise or to the experiences of others you know who have been injured.

Why do people get hurt? As you begin your own exercise program, think carefully about safety and caring for your body. If you think of your body as a valuable resource, one that needs care and attention, then you will see that prevention is the best way to avoid injuries.

LESSON 2 REVIEW

Reviewing Facts and Vocabulary

1. Describe five injuries that can occur during exercise.
2. Name two injuries to the muscles and to the joints that may occur when the body is not in condition or when there is not sufficient warm-up.
3. What is tendinitis?

Thinking Critically

4. **Analysis.** Compare heatstroke and heat exhaustion.
5. **Analysis.** What is the difference between a sprain and a strain?

Applying Health Knowledge

6. Compile a list of at least 10 sports and recreational activities adults engage in as part of an exercise program. Evaluate the risk of injury in each.
7. Research the cost of dress and equipment for a particular exercise program. Make two detailed lists: one of what is necessary for the program; the other of what might be used in the program. Use newspapers, catalogs, and other means to compare prices. Show how little could be spent and how much could be spent for the exercise program chosen.

Self-Inventory

Aerobic Alternatives

HOW DO YOU RATE?

Number a sheet of paper from 1 through 12. Read each item below, and respond by writing *MT* for any activity you do more than three times a week. Write *TT* for any activity you do two or three times a week and *OW* for any activity you do once a week.

1. I walk continuously 20 minutes or more.
2. I walk continuously 20 minutes or more using hand weights.
3. I jog or run continuously 20 minutes or more.
4. I swim continuously 20 minutes or more.
5. I ride a bike continuously 20 minutes or more.
6. I dance continuously 20 minutes or more.
7. I roller-skate or use rollerblades continuously 20 minutes or more.
8. I play basketball continuously 20 minutes or more.
9. I play volleyball continuously 20 minutes or more.
10. I play tennis or badminton continuously 20 minutes or more.
11. I play football or soccer continuously 20 minutes or more.
12. I play softball or baseball continuously 20 minutes or more.

HOW DID YOU SCORE?

Give yourself 5 points for every *MT* response, 3 points for every *TT* response, and 1 point for every *OW* response. Find your total, and read below to see how you scored. Then proceed to the next section.

15 and above
Excellent. You are to be commended for promoting your health. Keep up the good work.

5 to 14
Good. It's great you are active. More activity will increase your fitness and health.

Below 5
Needs Improvement. Join in the fun and fitness. Feel good about yourself. Try some of the activities listed above. You are sure to find one you will enjoy.

WHAT ARE YOUR GOALS?

If you received an *excellent* or *good* score, complete the statements in Part A. If your score *needs improvement*, complete Parts A and B.

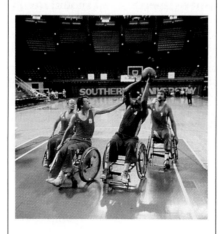

Part A

1. I plan to learn more about different types of aerobic exercise by ____.
2. My timetable for accomplishing this is ____.
3. I plan to share my information with others by ____.

Part B

4. The behavior or attitude toward aerobic exercise that I would most like to change is ____.
5. The steps involved in making this change are ____.
6. My rewards for making this change will be ____.
7. My timetable for making this change is ____.
8. The people or groups I will ask for help are ____.

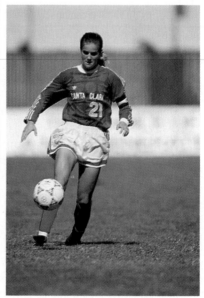

Building Decision-Making Skills

Dan and his friend, Tony, have always shared a commitment to good health and fitness. Their fitness program includes eating nutritious foods, working out together, and avoiding alcohol and other drugs. The boys' workout program is varied. Some days they jog or cycle; other days they lift weights and do calisthenics. Recently Tony has had to cut back on his workout time with Dan in order to study for final exams. Dan has noticed that sometimes Tony stays up all night studying. He seems to have unpredictable mood swings, and he's been seen in the company of some of the school's known drug users. Dan suspects that Tony is using steroids, but he doesn't know for sure. He wants to confront his friend, but if he is wrong, he could ruin a great friendship. What should Dan do?

A. Look for more evidence before confronting Tony. Then talk with him about his concern.

B. Forget it and do nothing. Final exams will be over in a few weeks and things will probably be back to normal.

C. Tell Tony's parents of his suspicions and let them handle it.

D. Stop being friends with Tony since he no longer seems to share a commitment to good health and fitness.

WHAT DO YOU THINK?

1. **Choices.** What other choices does Dan have?
2. **Consequences.** What are the advantages of each choice?
3. **Consequences.** What are the disadvantages of each choice?
4. **Decision.** What do you think Dan should do?
5. **Evaluation.** Have you ever been in a situation where a friend appeared to be losing his or her energy and health? How did you handle the situation? Would you do the same thing now? Explain your answer.

Dana loves her part-time job at a local restaurant. She likes the people she works with and all the things she's been able to do with the money she's earned. The only bad part about the job is that she's gaining weight and feeling sluggish, probably because of her love for the restaurant's famous double fudge sundaes and because she has quit running track in order to work more hours. What should Dana do?

A. Reduce her hours and rejoin the track team.

B. Control the number of sundaes she eats.

C. Get into some other kind of exercise program.

D. Get a different job—one that doesn't tempt her with food.

WHAT DO YOU THINK?

6. **Choices.** What other choices does Dana have?
7. **Consequences.** What are the advantages and disadvantages of each choice?
8. **Decision.** Which choice should Dana make?
9. **Evaluation.** Why might it be important for teens to have a job and be part of a school activity?
10. **Evaluation.** Staying active can be one of the most difficult things to do. How does one overcome this difficulty?

REVIEW

Using Health Terms

On a separate sheet of paper, write the term that best matches each definition given below.

LESSON 1

1. Type of activity that targets specific muscle groups, usually to strengthen them.
2. The optimum heart rate one should sustain during exercise.
3. How often something is done.
4. Type of exercise designed to improve one's endurance.
5. How long something is done.

LESSON 2

6. Occurs when a muscle contracts tightly and will not relax.
7. Chemicals used to increase muscle mass without increasing fat.
8. Weak area in a muscle through which part of another organ, such as the intestines, may push out.
9. Injury to tissue under the skin, resulting from a blow to the muscle.
10. Frozen tissue as a result of prolonged exposure to extreme cold.

Building Academic Skills

LESSON 1

11. **Reading.** Many people believe that exercise will help them live longer, healthier, happier lives. There are those who disagree, however. Read *The Exercise Myth* by Henry A. Solomon, M.D. Decide what the author's point of view is and what his purpose for writing is. Then decide if you think his point is valid or not. Support your opinion in writing.

LESSON 2

12. **Writing.** Many fiction writers research background to make their accounts more realistic. Using accurate facts, write a short fiction story in which the main character has chosen to use anabolic steroids.

Recalling the Facts

LESSON 1

13. What can happen as a result of pooling?
14. How does a person's resting heart rate indicate his or her level of fitness?
15. Give examples of anaerobic exercises and aerobic exercises.
16. Why should a person not exercise too soon after eating?
17. What three components should every exercise program consist of?
18. How is warming up beneficial to a person's pulse rate?
19. If someone does not know his or her target heart rate, what is a good rule of thumb to follow?
20. Why might a person weigh more instead of less after starting to exercise?
21. Give two examples of activities that promote a high level of conditioning, two that are moderate level, and two that are low level.
22. What is the purpose of an exercise journal and what might be included in it?
23. How often should someone check his or her improvement due to exercise?
24. What should an exercise program do?
25. How long will it likely take for a person to become physically fit?

LESSON 2

26. What are three factors that increase the risk of injury?
27. What should be done for a dislocation?
28. What causes and prevents muscle cramps?
29. What can be done to relieve a muscle cramp?
30. What is tennis elbow and how should it be treated?
31. What are two things one should never do to treat frostbite?
32. Which two body systems are most likely to be injured during exercise?
33. Why does a bruise become discolored?
34. What are the two most common injuries to the skeletal system?

REVIEW

Thinking Critically

35. Synthesis. Explain the phrase "No pain, no gain," and tell why it is not true.

36. Synthesis. Outline an exercise program for yourself. Include alternative activities if poor weather should interfere with your program.

37. Evaluation. Interest in exercise is a fairly recent trend. Do you think it will continue? Support your answer.

38. Analysis. What types of safety equipment would be needed for the following activities? Explain.

a. bicycling	**e.** playing basketball
b. skateboarding	**f.** playing soccer
c. running at night	**g.** playing football
d. playing softball	**h.** playing ice hockey

39. Analysis. For each of the following situations, tell what injury the victim has suffered and how you would help him or her.

a. Mr. Smythe had been working in his garden for 3 hours in the hot sun. Suddenly, he fell to the ground. He was not perspiring, and he felt very hot. His pulse was racing, breathing was difficult, and his face was very red.

b. After jogging 5 miles in 96-degree heat, Jenny felt she could not go on. She was perspiring a lot. She became pale, dizzy, nauseated, and had trouble breathing.

Making the Connection

40. Language Arts. Prepare a short talk about physical fitness for an elementary school class. Present and define these components of physical fitness—flexibility, muscular strength, muscular endurance, and cardiorespiratory endurance. Demonstrate at least one fitness test that could be used to assess each component.

Applying Health Knowledge

41. What exercise limitations might be posed by weather in the area where you live?

42. Give examples of physical limitations someone your age might have.

43. Which of the following schedules would be better for exercise? Explain why.
a. Monday, Tuesday, Wednesday
b. Monday, Friday, Sunday
c. Monday, Wednesday, Saturday

44. Plan a warm-up for an activity you enjoy.

45. What is a good cool-down activity for jogging?

46. For treatment of a sprain, why should heat not be applied to the injured area?

47. According to Peter Francis, Ph.D., and Lorna Francis, Ph.D., authors of *If It Hurts, Don't Do It*, 40 percent of America's adult population does not exercise at all. Discuss why you think that is. What do you think you could say or do to convince these people to start exercising?

Beyond the Classroom

48. Community Involvement. Research aerobic programs available in your community. Contact the instructor of each program to find out what type of warm-up, workout, and cool down is practiced. Publish your information in a directory or an article in the school newspaper.

49. Parental Involvement. Sometimes exercising with someone provides needed support and motivation. With a parent, develop an exercise program with activities appropriate and convenient for everyone in your family. Do your exercises together.

50. Further Study. Find out all you can about sports medicine and what types of careers this field might lead to.

CHAPTER

19

MAKING RESPONSIBLE FOOD CHOICES

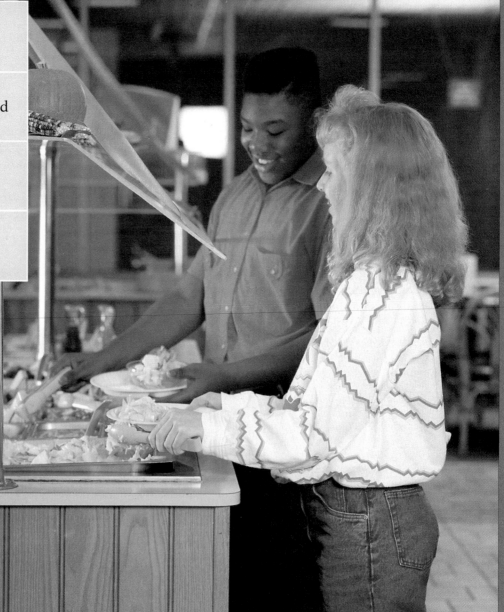

YOUR NEED FOR FOOD

In one way or another, food affects almost everything you do. It affects how you look, feel, and act. It affects how you grow. It even affects your abilities—how well you function each day. Conversely, how you look, feel, and act influences what you eat.

Food has an impact on life because it supplies nutrients. **Nutrients** are substances in food that the body needs to function properly such as in growing, in repairing itself, and in having a supply of energy.

Nutrition is both a pure science and a social science. As a pure science it looks at how the body uses nutrients. As a social science it looks at the relationship between food and human behavior and the environment, or how and why people eat.

Why Do You Eat?

Have you ever wondered why you eat and why you make certain food choices? The reasons may be more complex than you realize. Your choices about food are linked to your physical needs, your environment, and your emotions.

Your Physical Health

The most basic reason for eating is physical. Eating is a matter of survival, as well as growth, energy, and fitness.

Food, along with air and water, is one of life's basic needs. When you go without food for a long time, you feel hungry. This is your body's signal that it needs more food. After you eat, the feelings of hunger disappear. You have satisfied your physical need for food.

Eating the right amounts and kinds of food gives energy and stamina for active life-styles. A nutritious diet provides for growth and maintenance of a healthy body and helps keep you mentally alert.

If good food choices aid health and performance, then what you eat affects everyday living. In addition, six out of ten leading causes of death in the United States are linked in some way to food. Eating well not only reduces health risks, it also adds to the quality and the length of your life.

Your Environment

Your food choices are linked to many factors. Your cultural heritage, your family and social relationships, media messages, and life-style all influence the foods you like and choose.

Culture. What foods do you associate with picnics, baseball games, county fairs, holidays, and birthday parties? Your food choices reflect

---

LESSON 1 FOCUS

TERMS TO USE
- Nutrients (NOO•tree•uhnts)
- Nutrition

CONCEPTS TO LEARN
- Your body depends on you to provide nutrients that it needs to function.
- Food choices are linked to cultural heritage, family and social relationships, media messages, and life-style.
- At every stage of life, good nutrition is essential for health.

ATTITUDES AND BEHAVIORS TO EVALUATE
- Self-Inventory, page 398.
- Building Decision-Making Skills, page 399.

the culture you live in, as well as your ethnic background and perhaps your religious beliefs. Teenagers have a culture of their own, too. What food practices seem to be part of teen culture?

Family and Friends. Children pattern their food habits after their role models, perhaps parents or older brothers and sisters. What you ate as a child, what you learned to like and dislike, and when you ate meals were all influenced by your family. These influences affect your food decisions and preferences now—and they will continue to influence you throughout your life.

As you have grown older, friends have influenced your food choices. Perhaps you tried new foods at their homes or tasted different foods at parties. Because eating can be a social experience, food is the focus of many gatherings. Many people use food as gifts. A gift of food may show someone you care.

Advertising. Food ads are everywhere—on television, in magazines, and on billboards. Food ads are created to make you aware of certain foods and, perhaps, of their benefits. Most importantly, they shape food decisions. Think of food ads you see and hear on television. Which foods have you bought or tried as a result of an ad?

Many people believe everything they read in newspapers and see and hear on television and radio. Yet, an ad may tell just part of the truth. For example, an ad may state that a food is low in fat without mentioning that it is high in calories. Advertisers spend millions of dollars on powerful persuasion techniques. Ads may try to persuade you that status, sex appeal, weight loss, or a terrific appearance will be yours if you buy the product.

To make informed food choices, you need to know about food and health. You need to listen and judge advertising messages carefully. That way, you—not advertisers—control what foods you buy and eat.

Time and Money. Cost, convenience, taste, nutrition, and food safety are the factors that influence food shopping most, according to consumer studies.

With today's busy life-styles, people rely more on foods they can cook and eat quickly, such as convenience foods and microwave meals. To stay healthy, choose nutritious foods that you can prepare and eat within the time you have available. Skipping meals is not the answer.

Cost also affects food choices. How has cost affected food decisions you have made?

K E E P I N G   F I T

Your Family's Cooking Heritage

Many families have family recipes or foods that they serve only on special occasions. Sometimes these food choices stem from particular tastes of the individuals within that family. But often, specific ingredients, recipes, serving styles, or food lore hold valuable family history. A family's food choices often have strong ties to the culture of one's ancestors or relatives. Learning to grow, prepare, and cook these foods can become a hands-on way of learning about your cultural heritage. It can also be an effective way to preserve and pass on your family's history.

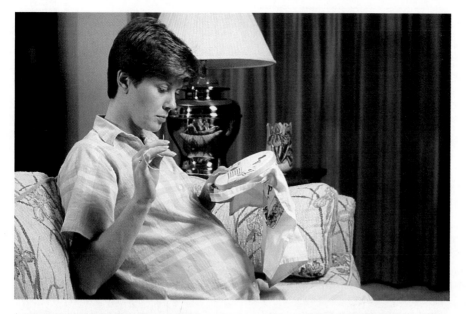
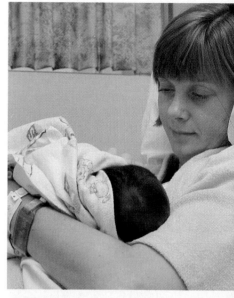
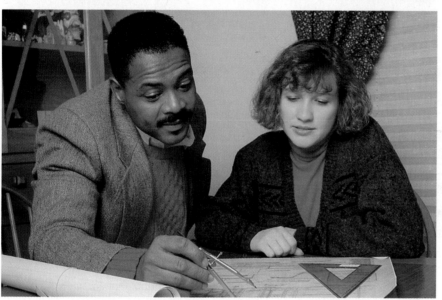
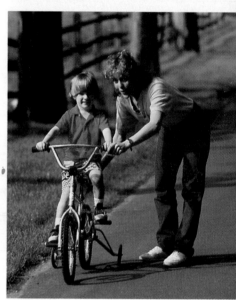

Nutritional needs are different at various stages of life. Which of these individuals probably need more calories than other individuals of the same age?

Your Emotions

Think about some of your eating habits. Have you ever headed to the refrigerator just because you had nothing else to do? Do you tend to eat more—or less—when you feel stressed, frustrated, or depressed? Do you tend to eat when you are watching an exciting game? What do you eat when you feel really good or when you want to celebrate? What foods do you think are just plain fun to eat?

Eating is closely tied to emotions. Eating to relieve tension or boredom can result in overeating. However, if you lose your appetite when you are upset or bored, you may miss out on getting essential nutrients. By understanding how eating relates to emotions, you can make more healthful food choices.

Overcoming The Odds

"My name is Ray Winnemucca. I'm 16 years old. I've always been pretty healthy. My parents have always talked about respecting and nourishing our bodies. We've always had a garden. We don't buy much junk food. So when I started having a problem, food was the last thing anybody suspected."

The problem Ray is talking about is celiac sprue disease. It is a chronic disease caused by the body's inability to tolerate gluten, a protein found in wheat, rye, barley, and oats. It causes the body to have a hard time absorbing essential nutrients and digesting food properly. "I started having these awful stomach cramps. I was losing weight and feeling really tired all the time. My stomach was bloated. Our doctor gave me antibiotics in case I had an intestinal infection. Then my bones started to hurt. I even seemed to stop growing, and that's when they took me to the medical center for all kinds of tests. For the first time, I was scared. I started to think all kinds of awful things. I even thought I might be dying.

"Then they diagnosed celiac sprue disease. They told me I'd just have to eat a gluten-free

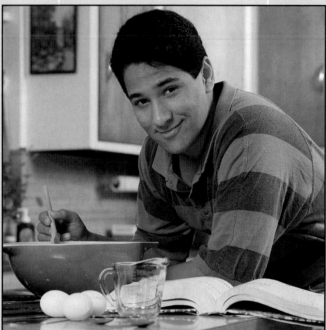

diet, which sounded like no big deal. What I didn't realize at the time was that many foods I eat come from these grains. Many thickeners, additives, and emulsifiers used in processed foods are on my 'No' list, so chocolate milk, many salad dressings, canned soups, and even ice cream are out.

"For a while I was really depressed and then I got angry. I felt bad about myself because I had to say no to foods my friends could eat. It was hard. Eventually, I got sick of feeling depressed and got motivated to learn all I could about food. Now, my friends ask me to cook for them sometimes because I'm really creative about it. My energy is back, and my size is normal for my age. Still, I wish I didn't have this problem. I'll be on this special diet for the rest of my life. So I have to make the best of it.

"Right now, I'm working on a gluten-free cookbook with recipes like gluten-free pizza for people my age that have celiac sprue disease. I feel good that out of this I'm learning new skills and reaching out."

1. How did Ray's health problem affect his self-esteem?
2. When faced with a health concern, what are some ways a person can, as Ray has, "make the best of it"?
3. How can learning new skills and reaching out help a person cope with dietary, health, or other problems?

Nutrition Throughout Your Life

At every stage in life, good nutrition is essential for health. Even before you were born, then as an infant and a child, and now as a teen, nutrients in food have provided you with substances you needed to grow and develop. At each age you have needed the same nutrients. As you have grown and developed, however, you have needed them in increasing amounts.

Adults of all ages continue to need the same nutrients, though in slightly smaller amounts. As people become less active and as metabolic rate declines with age, caloric needs go down. However, the need for the right nutrients in the right amounts is still important. No matter what age a person is, choosing foods wisely is a major key to health.

Nutrition and Adolescence

Next to the first years of your life, adolescence is the period of the fastest and most growth you will experience. Adolescence is also a time when your life-style is probably a very active one. Good nutrition is important to both your growth and the energy you need to maintain an active life-style.

Many teenagers, however, skip meals or substitute high-fat or sugary foods for more nutritious choices. Why do you think this is true?

As you read about nutrition and its effect on your body and health, evaluate your own eating habits. Identify food choices you can control, changes you might need to make, and food choices that could affect your total health and level of performance. Then plan to promote your health by making wise food choices.

Culturally Speaking

Foods on the World's Table

As you learn about other cultures, you may also increase your knowledge about food and learn to like various foods or new ways to prepare foods. Consider these international food facts:

- In Israel, salad may be served for breakfast.
- Arab foods often include heavily spiced lamb and chicken mixed with rice.
- The national drink in Iran is tea.
- On holidays in India, sweetened milk is served.
- In Vietnam, fish is often served in the form of a sauce called nuoc mam. Buffalo is sometimes a main dish.

LESSON 1 REVIEW

Reviewing Facts and Vocabulary

1. Define the terms *nutrients* and *nutrition*.
2. Describe factors that influence food choices, and give five examples.
3. Why is good nutrition so important during adolescence?
4. Describe how your nutritional needs will change between your teen years and adult years.

Thinking Critically

5. **Analysis.** How have your culture and family influenced your food habits?

6. **Analysis.** Compare your food habits with those of a friend. What might account for the differences?
7. **Synthesis.** Describe how emotions can affect food choices. Give two examples.

Applying Health Knowledge

8. Evaluate five food advertisements on radio or television. Discuss the approach each one uses to influence your food choices.
9. Read the newspaper for a week. Find five stories that show how the world around you influences food choices. Summarize your findings in writing.

YOUR BODY'S NEED FOR NUTRIENTS

LESSON 2 FOCUS

TERMS TO USE
- Carbohydrates
- Lipids (LIP•uhds)
- Saturated (SACH•uh•RAYT•uhd)
- Cholesterol (kuh•LEHS•tuh•rohl)
- Proteins
- Amino (a•MEE•noh) acids
- Recommended Dietary Allowances (RDA)

CONCEPTS TO LEARN
- Nutrients nourish the body in three ways.
- Nutrients can be grouped into six main categories.
- Carbohydrates are the most important source of energy.
- Proteins are a vital part of every body cell.
- Water is the body's most essential nutrient.

ATTITUDES AND BEHAVIORS TO EVALUATE
- Self-Inventory, page 398.
- Building Decision-Making Skills, page 399.

Nutrients in food perform life-sustaining functions in the body. During digestion, food is broken down into simpler forms of nutrients that are released and absorbed. Through the blood, nutrients are taken to body cells where nourishment takes place.

Nutrients nourish the body in three main ways. They provide energy; build, repair, and maintain body tissues; and regulate body processes.

Scientists have identified more than 40 different nutrients for good health. These nutrients can be grouped into six main categories: carbohydrates, fats, proteins, vitamins, minerals, and water. Each has a unique function in the normal growth and functioning of the body. As you will see, no one food provides all the nutrients your body needs.

Carbohydrates

For most body functions, **carbohydrates** are the body's preferred source of energy, or calories. There are several forms of carbohydrates, including sugars, starches, and fiber.

Many people think of sugar only as table sugar. However, sugars really are the simplest form of carbohydrate. They include fructose in fruit, lactose in milk, maltose in grain, and sucrose in table sugar.

Complex carbohydrates, such as starches, have a more complicated chemical structure. Digestion breaks them down into glucose, a simple sugar, which is absorbed in the blood.

Roles of Carbohydrates

Carbohydrates, found mainly in plant sources of food, are your body's most important sources of energy, or calories. Health experts recommend that 55 to 65 percent of your calories come from carbohydrates, mainly complex carbohydrates.

Eating enough carbohydrates allows protein to be used for building and repairing the body. When protein is used for energy, it cannot be used for other purposes.

Contrary to popular belief, carbohydrate-rich foods are not necessarily fattening. Ounce for ounce, carbohydrates have the same number of calories as proteins do, and fewer calories than fat.

Sources of Carbohydrates

Good sources of complex carbohydrates include vegetables and legumes (especially peas, beans, and potatoes), pasta, seeds, and nuts. Sugars, or simple carbohydrates, are present naturally in many foods, including fruits, some vegetables, and milk. Table sugar, syrups, and molasses are examples of processed sugars. Processed sugars are added to many foods, including sweet desserts, candies, and soft drinks.

Fiber

Dietary fiber is another form of complex carbohydrate, but it is not a nutrient in the true sense. Fiber is the tough, stringy part of vegetables, fruits, and grains. Because it cannot be digested, fiber serves other functions. It helps move waste through your digestive system and helps prevent constipation, appendicitis, and other intestinal problems. Eating enough fiber throughout your life may help protect you from some cancers and heart disease and can help you control diabetes. Just how fiber is involved is not yet clear, though some types of fiber are known to lower blood cholesterol and control blood sugar.

If you are watching your weight, fiber has other benefits. Fiber-rich foods are bulky, so they offer a feeling of fullness. They tend to be lower in fat and calories, and they may take longer to chew.

Most Americans may benefit from eating more high-fiber foods. To increase the amount of fiber in your diet, eat vegetables and fruits, especially those with edible skins and seeds; and whole-grain products, including whole wheat breads and pasta, whole rye bread, bran, brown rice, oatmeal, corn tortillas, and popcorn.

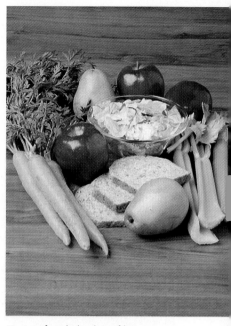

Eating foods high in fiber is one way to care for your digestive system.

Fats

With all the talk about fat these days, some people wonder why they really need it. The nutrient fat has several important functions in health.

Fat is known by the scientific name *lipid.* **Lipids** are fatty substances that do not dissolve in water.

Fats are composed of the same three elements as carbohydrates—carbon, hydrogen, and oxygen. The chemical makeup of fats determines their type: saturated, or polyunsaturated. Fats are made up of fatty acids attached to a glycerol molecule. Each fatty acid is a long chain of carbon, hydrogen, and oxygen. A fatty acid is **saturated** when the carbon chain holds all the hydrogen it can. Polyunsaturated fatty acids have two or more missing hydrogen atoms on the carbon chain.

There are about 30 different fatty acids. Fats are neither totally saturated nor totally unsaturated. Instead, they are a mixture.

Animal fats and some vegetable oils (palm, palm kernel, and coconut) have a high proportion of saturated fats. Fats in beef, pork, egg yolks,

---

KEEPING FIT

Calculating Your Ideal Fat Intake

- According to Sushma Palmer, a nutritional biochemist, you can quickly become a fat calculator. To determine your daily fat allowance, she offers the following formula to calculate your ideal fat-gram number. Take your ideal weight and cut it in half. For someone whose ideal weight is 120 pounds, that would be 60 grams of daily fat, or 2.1 ounces.
- Sushma Palmer also says that only one-third of your daily allowance of fats should come from saturated fats. To calculate your recommended amount of daily saturated fats, she advises that you take your daily fat allowance (calculated above) and divide that by 3.

DID YOU KNOW?

- Too much saturated fat, as well as total fat, in the diet puts an individual at risk of heart disease.
- To reduce the amount of saturated fat in your diet, substitute nonmeat sources of protein for meat occasionally, substitute margarine for butter and skim milk or low-fat milk for whole milk, and substitute vegetable (unsaturated) oils for solid (saturated) fats.
- To reduce total fat intake, substitute poultry and fish for beef, lamb, and pork frequently; use less margarine, butter, and oils; avoid fried foods and rich, creamy sauces; substitute low-fat and skim milk for whole milk; eat fewer pies, pastries, and cakes; and reduce the amount of ice cream, whipped cream, and cookies you eat.

and dairy foods are higher in saturated fats than fats in chicken and fish. Fats high in saturated fatty acids are usually solid or semisolid at room temperature.

Most vegetable fats, including soybean, corn, cottonseed, and olive oils, have a higher proportion of unsaturated fatty acids. Fats high in unsaturated fatty acids are liquids, or oils, at room temperature.

Processing can change the characteristics of fats. By adding missing hydrogen to fatty acids, hydrogenation makes fats more saturated and firmer in texture. For example, margarine is hydrogenated vegetable oil. As a general rule, firmer fats are more saturated.

Roles of Fats

Fats are an important source of calories. Ounce for ounce, fats provide more than twice the energy of carbohydrates or proteins. For good health, fats should supply no more than 30 percent of your daily calorie intake.

Fats carry fat-soluble vitamins A, D, E, and K into your blood. Without fats, our bodies could not use these nutrients.

Fats provide essential fatty acids. The body cannot make linoleic acid, a fatty acid essential for growth and healthy skin. It must come from your diet. Dietary fats offer other benefits, too. Fats add flavor, and they help satisfy hunger because they take longer to digest than carbohydrates and proteins do.

Body fat, or adipose tissue, is a form of stored energy. It accumulates when people consume excess calories from any source—carbohydrates, fats, or proteins. Your body needs some body fat. It surrounds and cushions your vital organs, protecting them from injury. The fat layer under your skin insulates your body from heat and cold.

Sources of Fats

Almost every food has some fat—at least in very small amounts. Some have much more fat than others.

Visible fats—butter, margarine, vegetable oil, and the fat layer on meat and poultry—account for about 40 percent of the fat in our diets. Many fats also are hidden in foods, for example, fat marbled in meat. Chocolate, seeds, nuts, egg yolks, ice cream, cheese, cream soups, croissants, and doughnuts all have hidden fats. Some food preparation methods—frying and cooking with sauces—add fats to food, too.

Cholesterol

Cholesterol is a fatlike substance. In many ways cholesterol resembles fat, but its structure is quite different. Because the human liver can make the cholesterol it needs, cholesterol is not considered a nutrient.

Cholesterol is an essential part of each cell membrane in the human body. The body uses cholesterol to produce certain hormones, vitamin D (in the presence of sunlight), and the protective sheath around nerve fibers. The liver uses cholesterol to make bile acids that aid in digestion.

The terms *dietary cholesterol* and *serum cholesterol* often are confused. Dietary cholesterol comes from food. Serum, or blood, cholesterol circulates in your blood.

Dietary cholesterol is present only in foods of animal origin—meat, poultry, fish, eggs, and dairy products. Egg yolks and organ meats are especially high in cholesterol. Fruits, vegetables, grains, legumes, and other foods from plant sources are, by nature, cholesterol-free.

In some people, the body makes too much cholesterol. High blood cholesterol is a major risk factor for heart and other circulatory diseases. Consuming too much cholesterol may contribute to elevated serum cholesterol; limiting cholesterol intake may reduce the risk.

Proteins

Proteins are a vital part of every body cell. Muscle, bone, connective tissue, teeth, skin, blood, and vital organs all contain protein. The term *protein* comes from the Greek *proteins,* meaning "of prime importance." The name fits because without protein, life could not exist.

Proteins actually are made of chains of building blocks called **amino acids.** Just as letters of the alphabet are arranged to make different words, amino acids are arranged in countless ways to make different body proteins.

Your body can make all but 9 of the 20 different amino acids. These 9 are called essential amino acids, because they must come from foods you eat. The rest your body can make if you eat enough protein-rich foods.

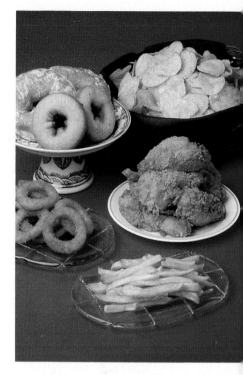

These foods are all high in fat. They have been fried.

Roles of Proteins

Your body uses proteins mainly for building and maintaining all body tissues. During periods of growth—infancy, childhood, adolescence, and pregnancy—amino acids build new body tissues. Throughout life new proteins form constantly to replace damaged or worn-out body cells.

Proteins in enzymes, hormones, and antibodies also help regulate many body processes. Enzymes are substances that control the rate of thousands of biochemical reactions in your body cells. Hormones regulate reactions. Antibodies help identify and destroy bacteria and viruses that cause disease in the body.

If you do not get enough calories from carbohydrates and fats, proteins from food provide the necessary energy. However, proteins are a less efficient energy source than carbohydrates and fats. When proteins are used for energy, they are not available for building and repairing body tissue. Proteins should supply only 10 to 15 percent of the calories in your diet.

K E E P I N G   F I T

Pumping Iron—Nutritionally

Many teens consume amounts of iron that are below the RDA, or Recommended Dietary Allowance. Females who menstruate are particularly likely to be low in iron. Yet during the teen years, when growth is rapid, high iron levels are needed for increasing blood volume and muscle mass. Iron is needed for the hemoglobin in your blood, which carries oxygen throughout your body. Without it, you may feel tired and have little endurance when playing sports.

To make sure you get enough iron, eat foods that contain high levels of it. These include liver, clams, beef, black beans, chick peas, raw spinach, pumpkin seeds, shrimp, and navy beans.

Sources of Proteins

Animal sources of foods, such as fish, meat, poultry, eggs, milk, cheese, and yogurt, contain all the essential amino acids. For this reason they are called complete protein sources.

Legumes, seeds, and nuts are the best source of plant proteins. However, no single plant protein has all essential amino acids in adequate amounts. For this reason they are called incomplete protein foods.

Plant proteins can be combined with either animal proteins or certain other plant foods to make complete protein foods. Following are some of these combinations:

- legumes + seeds or nuts (peanuts with mixed nuts)
- legumes + grains (beans and rice, peanut butter on bread, tortilla and refried beans, tofu-vegetable stir fry over noodles)
- any plant protein + dairy products or eggs (macaroni and cheese, rice pudding)

WATER-SOLUBLE VITAMINS

Vitamin	Role in Body	Food Source
C (ascorbic acid)	Protects against infection; helps with formation of connective tissue; helps wounds heal; maintains elasticity and strength of blood vessels.	Citrus fruits, tomatoes, cabbage, broccoli, potatoes, peppers
B_1 (thiamine)	Changes glucose into energy or fat; helps prevent nervous irritability; necessary for good appetite.	Whole-grain or enriched cereals, liver, yeast, nuts, legumes, wheat germ
B_2 (riboflavin)	Transports hydrogen; is essential in the metabolism of carbohydrates, fats, and proteins; helps keep skin in healthy condition.	Liver, green leafy vegetables, milk, cheese, eggs, fish, whole-grain or enriched cereals
Niacin	Hydrogen transport; important to maintenance of all body tissues; energy production; needed by body to utilize carbohydrates, to synthesize human fat, and for tissue respiration.	Yeast, liver, wheat germ, kidney, eggs, fish
B_6	Essential to amino-acid and carbohydrate metabolism.	Yeast, wheat bran and germ, liver, kidneys, meat, whole grains, fish, vegetables
Pantothenic acid	Functions in the breakdown and synthesis of carbohydrates, fats, and proteins; necessary for synthesis of some of the adrenal hormones.	Liver, kidney, milk, yeast, wheat germ, whole-grain cereals and breads, green vegetables
Folacin (folic acid)	Necessary for the production of RNA and DNA and normal red blood cells.	Liver, nuts, green vegetables, orange juice
B_{12} (cyano-cobalamin)	Necessary for production of red blood cells and normal growth.	Meat, liver, eggs, milk

Vitamins

Vitamins are known as micronutrients because they are needed in small amounts. Vitamins help regulate many vital body processes. They work with enzymes by triggering specific chemical reactions that allow the digestion, absorption, metabolism, and use of other nutrients.

Contrary to popular belief, vitamins do not supply calories. Some, however, do speed up reactions that produce energy in body cells.

Vitamins are classified into two groups: water-soluble vitamins and fat-soluble vitamins. Their solubility determines certain characteristics: how they are absorbed and carried in the blood, whether they are stored in the body, and what may happen during food preparation.

Water-Soluble Vitamins

Vitamins B complex and C are water-soluble vitamins, meaning they dissolve in water. For this reason they pass easily into the blood in the process of digestion. However, water-soluble vitamins are not stored to any extent in the body tissue. Instead, any excess is excreted in urine. Since there are no reserves, your diet needs an adequate supply of foods that contain water-soluble vitamins every day.

Foods need to be cooked carefully so that water-soluble vitamins are not destroyed by heat or lost through steam or in cooking water. To retain water-soluble vitamins in fruits and vegetables, follow these tips:

- Cook fruits and vegetables quickly.
- Steam them, or use only small amounts of cooking water.
- Cover food during cooking.
- Use leftover liquid in soups and stews.

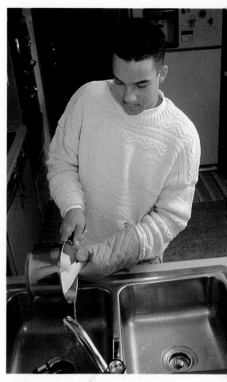

If the liquid from these potatoes is thrown away, many vitamins will be lost. It would be much better to cook vegetables in a small amount of water and use the liquid that is left in a soup or sauce.

FAT-SOLUBLE VITAMINS

Vitamin	Role in Body	Food Source
A	Maintenance of epithelial tissue; strengthens tooth enamel and favors utilization of calcium and phosphorus in bone formation; growth of body cells; keeps eyes moist.	Milk and other dairy products, green vegetables, carrots, animal liver
D	Promotes absorption and utilization of calcium and phosphorus; essential for normal bone and tooth development.	Fish oils, beef, butter, eggs, milk; produced in the skin upon exposure to ultraviolet rays in sunlight
E	May relate to oxidation and longevity; may be a protection against red blood cell destruction.	Widely distributed in foods; yellow vegetable oils, and wheat germ
K	Essential for blood clotting; assists in regulating blood calcium level.	Spinach, eggs, liver, cabbage, tomatoes; produced by intestinal bacteria

Fat-Soluble Vitamins

Vitamins A, D, E, and K are fat-soluble vitamins, meaning they are absorbed and transported by fat. The body stores fat-soluble vitamins in fatty tissue. Excess buildup of these vitamins can have a dangerous toxic effect. People who take nutrient supplements with very large doses of fat-soluble vitamins are especially vulnerable to the toxic effects.

Minerals

Minerals are inorganic substances that the body cannot manufacture. Like vitamins, they are micronutrients and act as catalysts, regulating many vital body processes. Despite the small amounts our bodies need, each mineral has its own unique function in health.

ELECTROLYTES

Sodium, chlorine, and potassium are important minerals in the body. They are present in relatively large amounts when compared to many other minerals. They are unique among nutrients because they become electrically charged when in solution as they are in the body fluids. Because of their electrical charges they are called electrolytes.

Sodium and chlorine combine to form table salt. Potassium is found in most foods, particularly bananas, oranges, prunes, and meats. Electrolytes also are found in water and other liquids.

These and other electrolytes must be present in the body and must be present in certain concentrations. Electrolyte balance requires that the intake of water and electrolytes is equal to the amounts of water and electrolytes eliminated from the body in perspiration, feces, and urine.

Water

Water is your body's most essential nutrient. Only oxygen is more important to life. Flesh feels solid, but the human body actually is about two-thirds water.

Water is a regulator and is vital to every body function. Mainly through the plasma in your blood, water carries nutrients to and transports waste from your cells. Water lubricates your joints and mucous membranes. It enables you to swallow and digest foods, absorb nutrients, and eliminate wastes. Through perspiration, water helps your body cool down and prevents the buildup of internal heat.

Most people use about 10 cups (2.4 l) of water a day. If they sweat a lot from fever, hot weather, or strenuous exercise, they use more. Some water can be replaced by drinking fluids (juice, milk, water)—about 6 to 8 cups (1.4 to 1.9 l) daily.

Food also supplies water. On average, fruits, vegetables, and milk products contain about 75 percent water; poultry and meat, 50 to 60 percent; and grain products, between 5 and 35 percent.

Mineral	Primary Function	Food Source
Calcium	Building material of bones and teeth (about 99 percent of body calcium is in your skeleton); regulation of body functions: heart muscle contraction, blood clotting.	Dairy products, leafy vegetables, apricots
Phosphorus	Combines with calcium to give rigidity to bones and teeth; essential in cell metabolism; helps to maintain proper acid-base balance of blood (calcium and phosphorus are the most abundant minerals in the body).	Peas, beans, milk, liver, meat, cottage cheese, broccoli, whole grains
Iron	Part of the red blood cell's oxygen and carbon dioxide transport system; necessary for cellular respiration; important for use of energy in cells and for resistance to infection.	Liver, meat, shellfish, peanuts, dried fruits, eggs
Iodine	Essential component of the thyroid hormone, thyroxine, which controls the rate of cell oxidation; helps maintain proper water balance.	Iodized salt, seafood
Manganese	Enzyme activator for carbohydrate, protein, and fat metabolism; also important in growth of cartilage and bone tissue.	Wheat germ, nuts, bran, green leafy vegetables, cereal grains
Copper	An essential ingredient in several respiratory enzymes; needed for development of young red blood cells.	Kidney, liver, beans, Brazil nuts, whole meal flour, lentils, parsley
Zinc	The function is unknown, although it is a component of many enzyme systems and is an essential component of the pancreatic hormone insulin.	Shellfish, meat, milk, eggs
Cobalt	An essential part of Vitamin B_{12}.	Sources of Vitamin B_{12}, such as meats, milk, and milk products
Fluorine	Essential to normal tooth and bone development and maintenance; excesses are undesirable.	Drinking water in some areas
Molybdenum	Essential for enzymes that make uric acid.	Legumes, meat products, some cereal grains
Sodium	Regulates the fluid and acid-base balance in the body.	Table salt, milk, meat, fish, poultry, egg whites
Chloride	Associated with sodium and its functions; a part of the gastric juice, hydrochloric acid; the chloride ion also functions in the starch-splitting system of saliva.	Same as sodium
Potassium	Part of the system that controls the acid-base and liquid balances; thought to be an important enzyme activator in the use of amino acids.	Readily available in most foods
Magnesium	Enzyme activator related to carbohydrate metabolism.	Readily available in most foods
Sulfur	Component of the hormone insulin and the sulfur amino acids; builds hair, nails, skin.	Nuts, dried fruits, barley and oatmeal, eggs, beans, cheese, and brown sugar

Nutrients: How Much Do You Need?

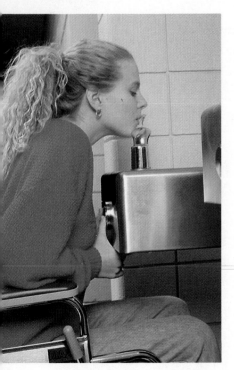

Without water, our bodies could not survive.

No matter what age, everyone needs the same nutrients. The only significant difference is the amount needed. However, at your age, without the nutrients needed for growth and development, your body will not reach its full potential.

Age and sex are two factors that determine how many nutrients you need. Teenagers, who are growing rapidly, have the highest nutrient need. Compared to females, males tend to be bigger, and their body composition is different, so they usually need more nutrients. For females, pregnancy and lactation or nursing require extra calories and nutrients to support the needs of both mother and baby.

Recommended Dietary Allowances

How much of each nutrient does your body need every day? The Food and Nutrition Board of the National Research Council, the National Academy of Sciences, has developed nutrient guidelines for people in the United States. The recommendations are listed by age and sex, and for females during pregnancy and lactation. The amounts recommended are considered to be adequate to maintain health for everyone, from infancy through adulthood.

The **Recommended Dietary Allowances (RDA)** suggest the amounts of 19 essential nutrients that most people need daily to stay healthy. The RDA also include guidelines for calories and estimated intake for vitamins and minerals. Your own nutritional and caloric needs may be slightly more or slightly less.

Every few years scientists update the Recommended Dietary Allowances. Each new edition reflects the latest research on nutrition and health. RDA were first published in 1943.

LESSON 2 REVIEW

Reviewing Facts and Vocabulary

1. Name the six classes of nutrients.
2. What three nutrients provide energy?
3. Describe the importance of dietary fiber, and list three sources.
4. Name three functions of fats.
5. What is cholesterol? What does it do?
6. What is protein? What does it do?

Thinking Critically

7. **Analysis.** Compare fat- and water-soluble vitamins.

8. **Evaluation.** Why do you think water is considered a nutrient?

Applying Health Knowledge

9. Is a bean burrito a complete or incomplete protein food? Explain your answer.

CHOOSING A HEALTHY DIET

W hat should you eat to stay healthy, to grow, and to have the energy you need? Along with exercise, eating a varied, moderate, and balanced diet is an important strategy for fitness. Your **diet** is everything you eat and drink.

Many Americans feel bombarded with information linking food, nutrition, and health. Food selection guides, such as the Dietary Guidelines and Daily Food Guide, help you choose a healthy diet that is right for you.

Dietary Guidelines for Americans

To help you sift through thousands of foods on store shelves and restaurant menus, the U.S. Department of Agriculture has published nutritional advice on how to eat to stay healthy. The Dietary Guidelines are meant for healthy Americans aged 2 years and over. Following the Dietary Guidelines will decrease your risk of diet-related problems now and in the future.

Eat a Variety of Foods

Your body needs about 40 nutrients. However, no one food has all the nutrients—in adequate amounts—that you need for growth, energy, and health. By eating a variety of foods daily, your body can get the many nutrients it needs. The **Daily Food Guide** offers an easy way to choose a varied, balanced, and moderate diet. Just eat adequate amounts from the following five food groups daily:

- bread, cereal, rice, and pasta
- fruit
- vegetable
- meat, poultry, fish, dry beans, eggs, and nuts
- milk, yogurt, and cheese

Combination foods, such as pizza or burritos, contain ingredients from more than one food group and supply the same nutrients as the foods they contain.

Foods in a particular food group supply similar amounts of key nutrients. However, the nutrient value of foods within a group differs, so eating a variety within each food group is important, too.

How many servings from each food group do you need? That depends on your age, sex, physical condition, body size, and activity level. Most people need at least the minimum servings daily. Teenage boys and active men usually need the most. Young children may need fewer servings. Except for additional iron and calcium needed by females, eating the recommended number of servings should supply all the nutrients most people need.

LESSON 3 FOCUS

TERMS TO USE
- Diet
- Daily Food Guide
- Empty-calorie foods

CONCEPTS TO LEARN
- Your diet is everything you eat and drink.
- You should eat adequate amounts from the five food groups daily.
- A varied, moderate, and balanced diet is the basis of a healthy eating pattern.
- Applying principles of good nutrition is important when eating out.

ATTITUDES AND BEHAVIORS TO EVALUATE
- Self-Inventory, page 398.
- Building Decision-Making Skills, page 399.

The Food Guide Pyramid focuses on fat because most American diets are too high in fat. Note that some fat and sugar symbols are shown in all the food groups. This is to remind you that even foods that are naturally low in fat may be prepared in ways that add to their fat or sugar content.

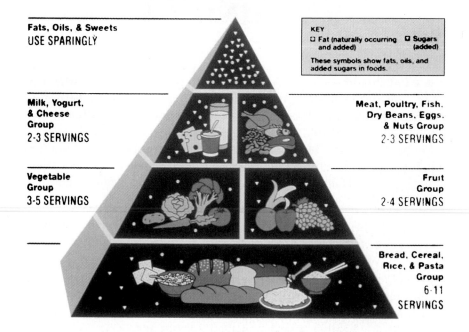

Food Guide Pyramid
A Guide to Daily Food Choices

Fats, Oils, & Sweets
USE SPARINGLY

KEY
□ Fat (naturally occurring ▽ Sugars
and added)   (added)
These symbols show fats, oils, and
added sugars in foods.

**Milk, Yogurt,
& Cheese
Group
2-3 SERVINGS**

**Meat, Poultry, Fish.
Dry Beans, Eggs.
& Nuts Group
2-3 SERVINGS**

**Vegetable
Group
3-5 SERVINGS**

**Fruit
Group
2-4 SERVINGS**

**Bread, Cereal,
Rice, & Pasta
Group
6-11
SERVINGS**

Food Groups

Bread, Cereal, Rice, and Pasta.   Enriched and whole-grain products are good sources of complex carbohydrates, iron, and B vitamins. Whole-grain foods are also good fiber sources. You need 6 to 11 servings daily.

Fruits.   Fruit and fruit juices (as long as the juice is 100 percent juice) can be good sources of vitamins A and C and carbohydrates. Some fruits provide more vitamins than others, so eat a variety. Fruits with edible skins are good fiber sources, if you eat the skin. You need 2 to 4 servings of fruit daily.

Vegetables.   Many vegetables and vegetable juices are good sources of vitamins A or C. Starchy vegetables, such as potatoes and squash, also supply complex carbohydrates—starch and fiber. Each day eat at least 3 to 5 servings. Eat dark green leafy vegetables several times a week.

Meat, Poultry, Fish, Dry Beans, Eggs, and Nuts.   Eggs, dry beans, nuts, and seeds are alternates. These foods along with meat, poultry, and fish are good sources of protein, iron, and B vitamins. At least 2 to 3 servings equal the recommended 5 to 7 ounces (142 to 198 g) daily.

Milk, Yogurt, and Cheese.   These foods are good sources of protein, calcium, and riboflavin, a B vitamin. You need at least 2 to 3 servings daily.

Fats, Oils, and Sweets.   Some foods do not belong in the five food groups: for example, cakes, cookies, doughnuts, soft drinks, candy, jam, salad dressing, chips, condiments, gravy, mayonnaise, margarine, butter, coffee, and tea. Many provide carbohydrates (mainly sugars) or fats, but few other nutrients, so they are often called **empty-calorie foods.**

Fatty and sugary foods provide taste and interest to meals and snacks. Because they supply mainly calories but few nutrients, health experts recommend using these foods sparingly.

Maintain Healthy Weight

According to nutrition experts, being too fat or too thin increases the chance of health problems. In the next chapter, you will learn more about managing weight. The following principles apply to everyone—whether the goal is to lose, gain, or maintain weight:

- Controlling body fat is more important to health than controlling body weight.
- Smart eating and regular exercise are the best ways to keep a healthful weight.
- No matter what their source, all calories add up the same way.
- Watching your diet and exercising is more important than watching the scale.

Choose a Diet Low in Fat, Saturated Fat, and Cholesterol

Too much fat in your diet is not healthy; neither is too much fat on the body. Diets high in fat, saturated fat, and cholesterol increase the risk of heart disease. A buildup of cholesterol and fat on arterial walls can lead to heart attacks. For some people, eating less fat, especially saturated fat, and cholesterol lessens the problem. High-fat diets are linked to obesity and some cancers.

Most Americans eat too much fat. Even after cutting back, many people still get 37 percent of their calories from fat. Health experts recommend getting 30 percent or less, including less than 10 percent from saturated fats.

Controlling dietary cholesterol can control blood cholesterol. That is why many experts recommend limiting cholesterol intake to 300 milligrams per day. Cutting back on fat, especially saturated fat, has an even greater effect on controlling blood cholesterol.

Controlling Fat in Foods.   Follow these tips to help control the fat and cholesterol in your diet:

- Cut off the fat you see on meat. Remove skin from chicken and turkey; there is a fat layer under the skin.

KEEPING FIT

Smart Snacking

- Snack mostly on foods from the five food groups. Limit fats and sweets!
- Plan your snacks when you can. Carry fresh fruit, such as grapes or a pear, instead of candy or chips.

- Help keep nutritious snacks on hand, such as plain popcorn, fruit, yogurt, fresh vegetables, cheese, and whole-grain crackers.

- Snack early, well before mealtime so that you do not spoil your appetite.
- Choose a substantial snack, if it must replace a meal.

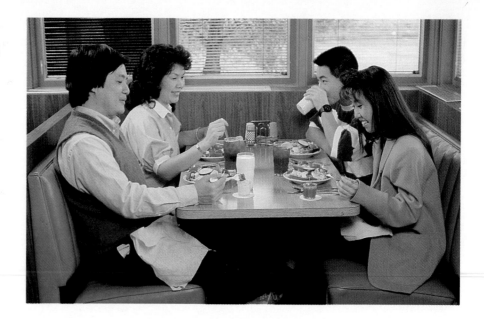

Asking for your salad dressing on the side is one way to control and reduce the quantity you use.

- Eat lean meat, fish, and poultry.
- Choose lower-fat milk, cheese, and yogurt.
- Eat less salad dressing. Spread only a little margarine, butter, or mayonnaise on bread. Use less gravy or sour cream on potatoes.
- Cut down on fried foods. Eat roasted, baked, broiled, or grilled meat, poultry, or fish instead.
- Eat vegetables that are steamed, boiled, or baked, rather than fried. (Limit the amount of french fries and fried onion rings in your diet.)
- Eat plenty of vegetables, fruits, and whole-grain foods.

Choose a Diet With Plenty of Vegetables, Fruits, and Grain Products

Why do vegetables, fruits, and grain products get special attention? They are excellent sources of complex carbohydrates and fiber, and are usually low in fats. Unlike many sugary foods, they provide essential vitamins and minerals. These foods are good choices and are low in calories.

From the viewpoint of disease prevention, a diet high in fiber and complex carbohydrates, yet low in fat, is advised. It seems to decrease the risk for heart disease, obesity, and some cancers. The National Cancer Institute recommends 20 to 35 milligrams of fiber a day. The average American eats only 10 to 15 milligrams daily.

To cut back on fat and reach the goal of 55 to 65 percent of calories from carbohydrates, eat plenty of vegetables, fruits, and grain products. Because they also are low in calories, these foods can help you control weight, too.

Use Sugars Only in Moderation

Sugars are carbohydrates; they taste good. Why limit them? On average, Americans eat a lot of sugar, up to 120 pounds (54 kg) yearly. Some sugars are present naturally in food, but much sugar is added during processing. Added sugars provide energy, but no other nutrients.

Most people can eat moderate amounts of sugar unless they must limit caloric intake. However, there are health cautions for eating too much, too often.

Carbohydrates—sugars and starches—contribute to tooth decay if they are eaten frequently and if they stick to teeth. Sipping a soda for an hour causes more harm than drinking it all at once.

Between-meal sweet snacks can damage teeth more than sweets eaten with a meal. Other foods in the meal help neutralize damaging acids that result from carbohydrates. After eating sweets, brush your teeth to remove food debris.

Control your sweet tooth for other reasons. Too much added sugar may mean too many calories, which can lead to obesity. When sweet desserts, sugary snacks, and sodas replace nutritious foods, you may miss out on essential nutrients. Sodas will not replace the calcium you would get in milk.

Controlling Sugars in Foods.   To control the added sugar in your food choices follow these tips:

- Cut back on foods with added sugars, such as soda, candy, cakes, and fruits canned in syrup. A 12-ounce (355-ml) regular soda has 9 to 12 teaspoons (45 to 60 ml) of sugar.
- Read food labels. Choose foods with less added sugar.

Use Salt and Sodium Only in Moderation

What is the salt-sodium connection? Salt is made from two essential nutrients, sodium and chloride. Both help maintain the body's fluid balance. In so doing, sodium helps transport nutrients into your cells and helps wastes move out. It helps maintain your normal blood pressure and nerve function.

Sodium comes from many foods. About 10 percent of the sodium we eat is naturally present in food. Celery, for example, is high in sodium. Salt is added to preserve and flavor food; 75 percent of the sodium we eat comes from processed foods. The rest comes from the salt shaker.

Most people consume more salt and sodium than they need. For some, a high-sodium diet increases the risk of hypertension.

Most Americans consume too much salt. Think about other options before you add salt to your food.

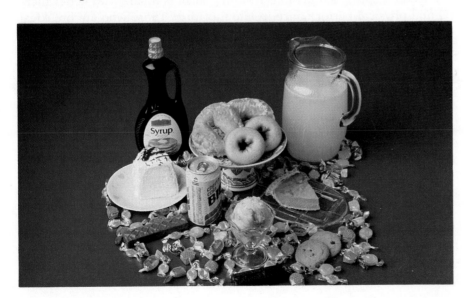

These foods are all high in sugar. Eat them sparingly for good health.

Controlling Sodium in Foods. Follow these tips to help control sodium and salt:

- Taste foods before you salt. If you must add salt, shake once, not twice.
- Limit salty snack foods, such as chips, crackers, pretzels, and nuts.
- Season foods with herbs and spices, and use less salt in cooking.
- Read food labels for sodium content. Buy lower-sodium foods when you can.
- Use catsup, mustard, other condiments, and foods in salt solutions (such as pickles) sparingly.

Healthful Eating Patterns

A varied, moderate, and balanced diet forms the foundation of a healthful eating pattern. Whether you eat three meals a day, or four, five, or six minimeals instead, follow Dietary Guidelines and the Daily Food Guide, and avoid overeating.

Meals and snacks that represent all five food groups provide nutrients you need. Variety is important within each meal because nutrients in one food affect how your body uses nutrients in another.

When planning menus, remember that there are no good or bad foods. Any food that supplies calories and nutrients can be part of a nutritious diet. Nutrition guidelines apply to all your food choices for a day or more, not for just a single meal or food. You can enjoy a soft drink or fries occasionally, as long as your total diet is healthy.

Meals

A healthy meal includes variety from the food groups. Calories and nutrient intake are also spread throughout the day.

Breakfast. Breakfast may be your most important meal. After 10 to 12 hours without food, your body needs to be refueled. According to breakfast studies, eating a nutritious morning meal is linked with better mental and physical performance in late morning. Those who ate breakfast also reacted faster and experienced less muscle fatigue than those who skipped breakfast.

Breakfast can include any foods you enjoy—pizza, a peanut butter sandwich, a salad. Just make it nutritious. To get enough vitamin C during the day, choose citrus juice or fruit for breakfast. Choose fiber-rich, whole-grain breads and cereals. Breakfast is also a good time to get one calcium-rich serving of milk, cheese, or yogurt.

Lunch and Dinner. Eating other nutritious meals is important for health and energy. Typically, Americans eat a midday and an evening meal. Other cultural groups may follow a different pattern.

For most lunches and dinners, plan around a high-protein main dish. Then balance your meal with foods from the other food groups. Add side dishes, such as salads, fruit, vegetables, pasta, rice, or bread; a beverage; and perhaps a dessert. Each meal should provide about one-third of your daily needs for nutrients and calories.

Snacking

Many teenagers need snacks. Nutritional and caloric needs are at their highest level because adolescents are active and growing. It is important to choose snack foods that are high in nutrients, and not just high in calories.

Carefully chosen, snacks provide essential nutrients, but they should never replace meals. Snacks offer a chance to get nutrients you may miss at mealtime. For example, if you did not drink vitamin C-rich juice for breakfast, an orange or tangerine can be a great snack. Make milk a snack, too.

HEALTH UPDATE

LOOKING AT THE ISSUES

How Much Meat Should We Eat?

Because a high-fat diet has been linked to many diseases and other health problems, many Americans are listening and cutting their consumption of animal foods. Some people, however, claim that people should not only eat less animal food, they should eat none at all.

Analyzing Different Viewpoints

ONE VIEW. Many people who eat meat say they enjoy it, and as long as they eat it in moderation and cook it in healthful ways, there is no problem.

A SECOND VIEW. Some nutritionists claim that meat provides amino acids, the building blocks of protein, as well as important vitamins and minerals. They also point out that strict vegetarians may suffer ill health effects from deficiencies in minerals such as calcium, and vitamins such as B_{12}.

A THIRD VIEW. Some people choose to be vegetarians for health reasons. They cite studies linking animal products with heart disease, high cholesterol, and some cancers. In addition, they point out that meat eaters are more likely than vegetarians to ingest agricultural chemicals.

A FOURTH VIEW. Other people choose not to eat meat on moral grounds. They believe that animal life should not be sacrificed for human beings. They talk about the unnecessary pain, abuse, and slaughter of animals raised for human consumption.

A FIFTH VIEW. Still others refuse to eat meat because they claim the process of raising animals for food uses up resources that should instead be used to feed hungry humans. They point to the destruction of forests for grazing land and the huge amounts of water needed for cattle raising.

Exploring Your Views

1. If you are a meat and dairy consumer, what steps can you take to make sure you are not getting too much of your food from animal sources? If you are a vegetarian, what steps can you take to make sure you are getting enough protein, minerals, and vitamins?

Eating Out

On average, people eat 30 percent of their calories and more than 20 percent of their meals away from home. Fast-food restaurants serve 40 percent of those meals. You need to apply principles of good nutrition to restaurant, cafeteria, vending machine, and fast-food eating.

Most restaurants offer enough variety for nutritional choices. To eat fewer calories, you might skip the appetizer, order a small portion (a cup instead of a bowl of soup), ask for salad dressing or butter on the side, split dessert with a friend, or order fruit rather than a sweet dessert.

Fast Foods. Fast foods are convenient, relatively low-cost, predictable, and quick. Carefully chosen, fast-food meals supply many essential nutrients. However, they tend to be high in calories, fat, and sodium.

Today, with more salad bars, vegetables, yogurt, and low-fat, low-sodium menu items, you can make healthy fast-food choices. Many restaurants provide free nutritional information on menu items, too. Consider these tips for healthy fast-food choices:

- Order the regular sandwich instead of the double or deluxe size.
- Enjoy salad bars. Go heavy on fresh fruits and vegetables, but light on creamed salads and dressings. One ladle often holds 2 tablespoons (30 ml) of dressing, which can be 150 calories.
- At potato and pasta bars, avoid overloading sauces, sour cream, and butter.
- Avoid breaded chicken and fish sandwiches. Order lean meats and grilled chicken and fish instead.
- Skip high-fat, high-sugar desserts.
- Choose milk instead of a soft drink for added nutrients.
- When fixing your sandwich, load up on lettuce, tomato, and onion.
- Skip the french fries or fried onion rings, especially if you order a fried poultry or fish sandwich. At the very least, order a small serving with no salt.

LESSON 3 REVIEW

Reviewing Facts and Vocabulary

1. Name the five food groups and the recommended range of servings for each.
2. What are four weight-control principles that apply to everyone?
3. Why should you limit the added sugar in your diet?
4. Why are people urged to control sodium and salt in their diets?

Thinking Critically

5. **Analysis.** What are some possible results of an unhealthy eating pattern?

6. **Evaluation.** What foods in your diet are empty-calorie foods? How often do you eat them?
7. **Evaluation.** What foods in your diet may be high in sodium or salt?

Applying Health Knowledge

8. Record your meals and snacks for a day. Evaluate them using the Daily Food Guide and Dietary Guidelines. Make recommendations for any improvements.
9. Go to a fast-food restaurant. Plan a nutritious, fat-controlled meal from the menu.

BEING A WISE FOOD CONSUMER

Now that you know the basics about nutrition, how can you be a wise consumer and make healthy food choices? Information on food labels, on supermarket shelves, and on restaurant menus can help you know what you are buying and eating.

Food Labeling

Food labels say more about food than you may realize. By knowing how to use them, you can be a smart consumer. All labels on processed foods must state the following information:

- name of the food, including the variety, style, packing medium, and special dietary properties
- net amount in weight or volume
- name and address of the manufacturer, packer, or distributor

In addition, labels must carry information about ingredients and nutrient and caloric content. Some labels also give nutritional or health claims and preparation instructions.

The Food and Drug Administration (FDA) and U.S. Department of Agriculture (USDA) regulate food labeling. Because labels have become confusing, Congress recently passed a law requiring the food industry to create straightforward, standardized labels for most foods. In 1993 the FDA released its new guidelines, which went into effect the following year.

Nutrition Labels

Nutrition labels indicate the nutritional and caloric content of foods. This information helps you find good sources of nutrients, compare nutrients and calories in various brands, and choose foods for special diets.

Under the new FDA guidelines, all foods require nutrition labels with the exception of the following:

- food served in restaurants
- plain coffee and tea
- some spices and other foods that contain no nutrients
- fresh meat, poultry, and fish; and fresh fruits and vegetables
- food produced by very small companies or offered in very small packages

What nutritional information goes on a food label?
- serving size
- servings per container
- calories per serving and calories per serving from fat
- grams of total fat, saturated fat, cholesterol, sodium, carbohydrates, dietary fiber, sugars, and protein per serving
- percentage of the recommended Daily Value (DV) the product supplies of the above nutrients plus some important minerals and vitamins

LESSON 4 FOCUS

TERMS TO USE
- Food additives
- Enriched
- Fortification (fawrt•uh•fuh•KAY•shuhn)
- Unit pricing

CONCEPTS TO LEARN
- Knowing how to use food labels can make you a smart consumer.
- Governmental and private agencies exist to protect the consumer in various ways.
- The federal government maintains an ongoing program of enacting new regulations and providing important information to consumers.
- Unit pricing allows you to compare food prices.

ATTITUDES AND BEHAVIORS TO EVALUATE
- Self-Inventory, page 398.
- Building Decision-Making Skills, page 399.

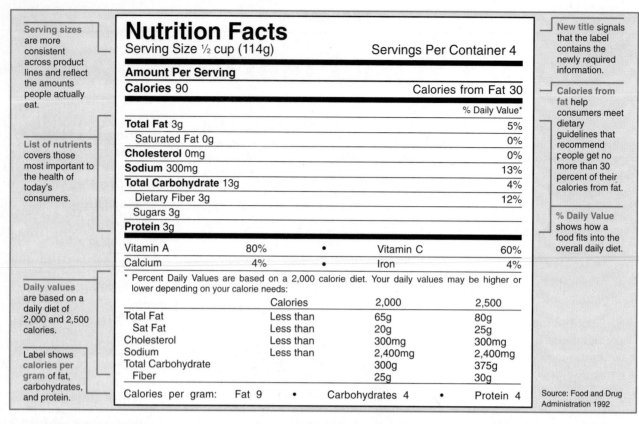

Nutrition Facts

Serving Size ½ cup (114g)   Servings Per Container 4

Amount Per Serving

Calories 90   Calories from Fat 30

	% Daily Value*
Total Fat 3g	5%
Saturated Fat 0g	0%
Cholesterol 0mg	0%
Sodium 300mg	13%
Total Carbohydrate 13g	4%
Dietary Fiber 3g	12%
Sugars 3g	
Protein 3g	

Vitamin A	80%	Vitamin C	60%
Calcium	4%	Iron	4%

* Percent Daily Values are based on a 2,000 calorie diet. Your daily values may be higher or lower depending on your calorie needs:

	Calories	2,000	2,500
Total Fat	Less than	65g	80g
Sat Fat	Less than	20g	25g
Cholesterol	Less than	300mg	300mg
Sodium	Less than	2,400mg	2,400mg
Total Carbohydrate		300g	375g
Fiber		25g	30g

Calories per gram: Fat 9 • Carbohydrates 4 • Protein 4

As this sample shows, the new food label will provide easy-to-use nutrition information.

The new guidelines require that labels on beverages containing fruit juice specify the percentage of fruit juice they contain.

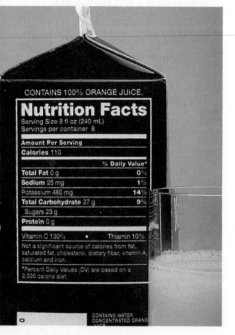

In addition to this information, the new labels contain guidelines on the amount of nutrients people need in their daily diets. For example, the FDA recommends 25 grams of dietary fiber and a maximum of 65 grams of fat each day for an average woman or child, slightly more for an adult man. The DV is the reference value for labeling food. Individual nutrient needs vary depending on age, sex, size, health, and activity level.

Some nutrient labels have two lists. If a food is eaten with another food, for example, cereal with milk, nutritional information is given for the product alone and with the other food.

Regulations now permit labels of certain foods to claim *possible* benefit in combatting a disease or condition. For example, labels on products that are high in calcium can claim to be a possible help in preventing osteoporosis. Labels on foods high in fiber, low in fat, or high in vitamins A and C can claim they "may help" to prevent cancer.

Ingredient Listing

Almost all food labels must have an ingredient list. The only exceptions are foods with one ingredient, such as some peanut butters and canned fruits and vegetables.

Labels list ingredients by weight, in descending order. The ingredient in greatest amount is first. Food labels with several similar ingredients are confusing. For example, when three sweeteners—corn syrup, sugar, and honey—are used, instead of just sugar, each is listed separately and lower on the list.

Food Additives. Additives must be listed on food labels. **Food additives** are substances added to food intentionally to produce a desired effect. They are used to:

- add nutrients,
- lengthen storage life,
- give flavor or color,
- maintain texture,
- control food's acidity,
- help age foods, such as cheese.

Foods are enriched or fortified to improve nutrient value. In **enriched** foods, nutrients lost in processing are added back. Breads, pastas, and rice made of refined grains are enriched with B vitamins and iron. **Fortification** adds nutrients not naturally present. Because vitamin D helps deposit calcium in bones, milk is fortified with vitamin D.

The FDA and USDA regulate most foods that cross state lines. This includes foods with additives. If food manufacturers want to use regulated additives in their products, they must prove to the appropriate government agency that the additives are safe in the amounts used.

Some additives, such as sugar and salt, are termed *generally recognized as safe (GRAS)*. Because they have been used safely for years, these 700 or so additives can be used without permission. The GRAS list is constantly reviewed.

To avoid eating too much of any one additive, health experts recommend eating a variety of foods. People with allergies to certain additives must check food labels.

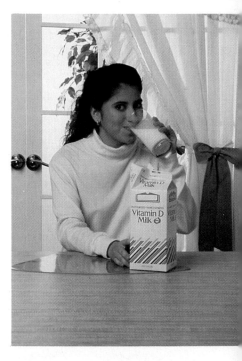

Milk is fortified with vitamin D.

MAKING SENSE OF LABEL TERMS

Terms such as *low-fat*, *low-calorie*, *low-cholesterol*, and *low-sodium* must now refer to foods that can be eaten frequently without a person exceeding dietary guidelines for the substance. For example, a low-fat food must contain 3 grams or less of fat per serving and a low-calorie food must contain 40 calories or less per serving. Low-calorie *meals*, such as frozen dinners, may contain no more than 120 calories.

- **Light:** This term now means that calories in an item have been reduced by at least a third, or the fat or sodium by at least a half.
- **Less and more:** A food must contain 25 percent less of a nutrient or of calories than a comparable food and 10 percent more than the regular food to be able to use these terms.
- **-free:** A product can contain no amount, or only a negligible amount, of the substance, such as fat, cholesterol, sodium, sugars, or calories.
- **High:** This term may be used if the food supplies 20 percent or more of the Daily Value of a particular nutrient in a serving. A good source must supply 10 to 19 percent of the nutrient.
- **Fresh:** Only foods that are raw, unprocessed, contain no preservatives, and have never been frozen or heated can be labeled fresh.
- **Natural:** This term is defined for meat and poultry only. According to the USDA, it means the food is minimally processed with no artificial or synthetic ingredients.

The FDA is also considering a definition for the term *healthy* based on a food's fat, cholesterol, and sodium content.

Sugar and Fat Substitutes. The food industry has responded to many consumer concerns about nutrition. In many cases, the industry has been very creative in substituting ingredients that lower either the calorie count or the fat content.

CONFLICT RESOLUTION

In 1986, California voters approved a toxic right-to-know law. Other states are considering similar legislation. Such laws require warning labels on foods and other products that contain chemicals known to cause cancer or birth defects. Consumer groups that support the legislation believe this law would eliminate the use of dangerous chemicals. Opponents, largely from business and industry, argue that the law would cost billions of dollars, lead to a loss of jobs and an increase in the number of lawsuits.

Explain how you would vote on a toxic right-to-know bill.

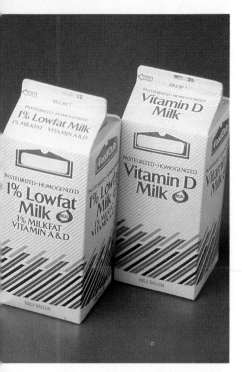

These containers of milk cannot be sold after the date shown on the labels.

Fructose, natural fruit sugar, is used as a caloric substitute. Because it is sweeter than table sugar, less is needed, so it supplies fewer calories.

Two noncaloric sweeteners are used in the United States—saccharin and aspartame. They are commonly added to soft drinks and frozen desserts, or you can buy them in powdered form. These sweeteners are considered safe when used in moderation.

With the public's recent concern about fat, the food industry has developed several types of fat substitutes. They have the potential for widespread use in processed foods, fried foods, and home cooking as a way to reduce fat intake.

Open-Dating

Many food products are open dated with a system that consumers can easily interpret. Look for these dates on labels:

- expiration date—last date you should use or consume the product
- freshness date—last date a food is thought to be fresh
- pack date—packaging date
- sell date—last date product (for example, milk) should be sold (although you can store it past this date).

Shelf Labeling

Shelf labeling helps consumers get the most nutrition for their food dollar. Unit pricing and, to a lesser extent, nutritional shelf labels are posted under food products. Many stores also display printed information about fresh products.

Unit Pricing

Unit pricing allows you to compare food prices. It shows the cost per unit of different-size packages. Suppose an 8-ounce can of Jiffy Beans cost 88¢; the unit price per ounce is 11¢. A 12-ounce can of the same brand costs $1.04, which is 8.7¢ per ounce. Instead of calculating these amounts, you can look at unit price labels on the shelf. Unit pricing also helps you compare different brands.

There is a caution. Before you buy the larger size, which may cost less per unit, decide whether you can use the extra amount.

K E E P I N G   F I T

Preservative and Additive Alert

Some people have severe allergic reactions to some of the nearly 3,000 additives and preservatives in foods.

When you know you are allergic to a certain substance, learn its alternate names. For example, sulfites may be listed on labels as sodium sulfite, sodium bisulfite, sulfur dioxide, potassium metabisulfite, or sodium metabisulfite.

Otherwise, when you read labels, you may miss the fact that the very thing you are allergic to is in the food you are about to consume.

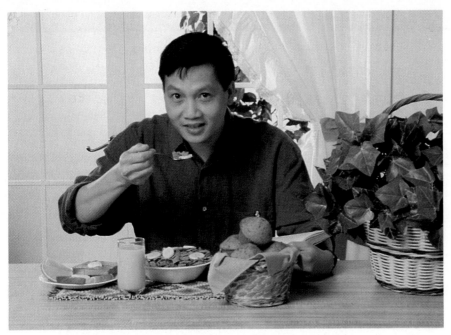

Good nutrition during adolescence is a vital link to total health.

Nutritional Shelf Labels

More and more stores have nutritional information on grocery shelves, next to the unit price. These labels might describe fat, sodium, or caloric content. Currently, no standard format exists for nutritional shelf labels. If your supermarket has them, ask the customer service staff how to use them.

LESSON 4 REVIEW

Reviewing Facts and Vocabulary

1. List the information required on a nutritional information label.
2. What do the terms *enriched* and *fortified* mean?
3. Describe the way ingredients are listed on food labels.
4. What are four reasons food additives are used in food?
5. What do *open dating* and *unit pricing* mean?

Thinking Critically

6. **Analysis.** How can food labels help you make smart food choices?
7. **Analysis.** Compare two similar food products using the information on their labels.

8. **Evaluation.** What information could you use to find hot dogs that had less fat and less sodium than the standard?

Applying Health Knowledge

9. Create a food label for a food of your choice. Include all the required information, including a nutritional information label. Support any nutrient claim with specific nutritional information.
10. Visit the grocery store, and compare the cost of several foods using unit pricing: two brands of the same size product and two sizes of the same product. Which would you buy? Why?

Self-Inventory

Making Healthy Food Choices

HOW DO YOU RATE?

Number a sheet of paper from 1 through 25. Read each item below and respond by writing *almost always, sometimes, seldom,* or *never* for each item. Then proceed to the next section.

1. I eat foods from several food groups at each meal.
2. Each day I eat at least six servings from the breads, cereals, grains, and pasta group.
3. Each day I eat at least three servings from the vegetable group.
4. Each day I eat at least three servings from the fruit group.
5. Each day I eat at least two servings from the meat, poultry, fish, and alternates group.
6. Each day I eat at least two servings from the milk, yogurt, and cheese group.
7. I eat fried foods, such as french fries and fried onion rings sparingly.
8. I avoid high-fat desserts and baked foods.
9. I eat gravies and rich sauces sparingly.
10. I cut all visible fat off meat and remove the skin from chicken.
11. I reach for fresh fruit instead of a sweet dessert or snack.
12. I buy fruit packed in water or juice rather than heavy syrup.

13. I eat whole-grain breads and cereals instead of highly refined grains.
14. I eat whole fruit with the skin or peel.
15. I taste food before salting it.
16. I avoid eating too many salty snack foods.
17. I avoid alcoholic beverages.
18. I eat a nutritious breakfast.
19. I drink milk or juice at meals rather than soft drinks.
20. I snack mostly on foods from the five food groups, rather than on empty-calorie foods.
21. If I snack, I do so well before mealtime.
22. At potato and pasta bars, I avoid overloading on sauces, sour cream, and butter.
23. At salad bars I go heavy on fresh fruits and vegetables and light on creamed salads and desserts.
24. I use information on a nutrient label and the ingredient list of a food label when I shop for food.
25. I compare prices using the unit price label when I shop for groceries.

HOW DID YOU SCORE?

Give yourself 2 points for every *almost always* response; 1 point for every *sometimes* response; and 0 points for each *seldom* or *never* response. Find your total, and read ahead to see how you scored. Then proceed to the next section.

38 to 50
Excellent. Your food choices show that you are taking good care of your health.

13 to 37
Good. You may understand that good nutrition is important to your health, but you need to make wiser food decisions.

0 to 12
Needs Improvement. Your food choices may be putting your body at risk.

WHAT ARE YOUR GOALS?

If you scored between 38 and 50, complete the statements in Part A. If your score was under 38, complete Parts A and B.

Part A

1. I plan to learn more about making wise food decisions in these ways: ____.
2. My timetable for completing this is ____.
3. I plan to share food and nutritional information with others by ____.

Part B

4. The food behavior I would like to change or improve is ____.
5. The steps involved in making this change are ____.
6. My timetable for making this change is ____.
7. The people or groups I will ask for support or assistance are ____.
8. My rewards for making this change are ____.

Building Decision-Making Skills

L eon works at the newest restaurant in town, which is doing a thriving business. He really likes his job and the people that work there, and he definitely needs the money. However, he has discovered that other employees engage in unsanitary practices while they are at work. The manager, a family friend who hired him, is aware of what is happening but has not spoken to the other employees. In fact, the one time Leon tried to speak with the manager about the problem she told him she would take care of it. That was two weeks ago. Nothing has changed. What should Leon do?

WHAT DO YOU THINK?

1. **Situation.** Why does a decision need to be made?
2. **Choices.** What possible choices might Leon have?
3. **Consequences.** What are the advantages and disadvantages of each choice?
4. **Consequences.** How will the other employees and the manager probably feel about each choice?
5. **Consequences.** What risks are involved for Leon in this decision?
6. **Decision.** What do you think Leon should do? Explain your reasoning.
7. **Evaluation.** Have you ever been in a similar situation? If so, how did you handle it? What did you learn from the experience?

D enise feels very strongly about eating wisely. She has made a commitment to avoid fat, refined sugar, salt, and red meat. However, she is in a social situation with friends who are going to a fast-food restaurant. What should she do?

WHAT DO YOU THINK?

8. **Choices.** What choices does Denise have?
9. **Consequences.** What are the advantages and disadvantages of each choice?
10. **Decision.** What do you think Denise should do?
11. **Evaluation.** Have you found yourself in a dilemma such as this? Describe the situation, how you handled it, and what you learned.

K ari's high school has a student body that includes many different cultures and ethnic groups. The cafeteria manager does a great job and has won considerable praise for the quality of the food. Although Kari likes the food, a group of friends have decided that the cafeteria does not serve enough ethnic foods. As part of a cultural awareness week, Kari's friends have made it a project to try to get the manager to add more ethnic foods to the menu. The manager was offended by their suggestion and refuses to consider it. Kari's friends are organizing a boycott of the cafeteria and have asked for her support. Students are not permitted off campus during lunch, and Kari hates to carry her lunch. Should Kari join the boycott?

WHAT DO YOU THINK?

12. **Consequences.** What are the advantages and disadvantages of joining the boycott?
13. **Consequences.** What are the advantages and disadvantages of not joining the boycott?
14. **Decision.** Which choice do you think is best for Kari?
15. **Evaluation.** Have you ever found yourself in a similar situation? Describe the situation, how you handled it, and what you learned.

Using Health Terms

On a separate sheet of paper, write the term that best matches each definition given below.

LESSON 1

1. Substances in food that the body needs to function properly.
2. Study of how the body uses food.

LESSON 2

3. Starches, sugars, and fiber.
4. Building blocks of protein.
5. Fatlike substance found only in animal sources of food.
6. Body fat.
7. Vitamins A, D, E, and K.

LESSON 3

8. Guideline for helping people choose a varied, balanced, and moderate diet.
9. Everything you eat and drink.
10. Foods that provide calories but few essential nutrients.
11. Must accompany smart eating for weight control.
12. Food substances linked to tooth decay.
13. A nutrient found in salt, which is often linked with high blood pressure.

LESSON 4

14. A governmental agency that is responsible for food labels.
15. Substances added for a specific effect.
16. Consumer aid for judging foods' freshness.
17. Information on a food label that tells the specific contents of the product.

Building Academic Skills

LESSON 1

18. **Writing.** Write a food autobiography describing food habits unique to you.

LESSON 2

19. **Reading.** Read a magazine or newspaper article about a current nutritional issue. Summarize the article in writing.

Recalling the Facts

LESSON 1

20. Where do food preferences come from?
21. How does your environment affect your food choices?
22. Give two examples of how eating is tied to emotions.
23. What are the two fastest growth periods in your life?

LESSON 2

24. Refute the claim that carbohydrates are fattening.
25. What is the simplest form of carbohydrate?
26. Why are some amino acids known as essential amino acids?
27. What is the nondigestible part of some foods that helps move waste through the digestive tract?
28. What is the RDA?

LESSON 3

29. What is the purpose of the Dietary Guidelines for Americans?
30. Why should you eat a variety of foods from each of the five food groups?
31. What are the key nutrients supplied by each of the five food groups?
32. Why do fats and sweets not belong in any of the five food groups?
33. What are the benefits of controlling the fat and cholesterol in a person's diet?
34. List three ways you might reduce the fat in your diet. Which would be most effective for you? Why?
35. What are some benefits of controlling the amount of sugar in your diet?
36. Explain ways you could lower the amount of fat in food you order in a restaurant.

LESSON 4

37. What useful information can you find on food labels?
38. What is required on a nutritional information label?
39. What is the GRAS list?
40. How are ingredients listed on food labels?

REVIEW

Thinking Critically

LESSON 1

41. Synthesis. Identify a holiday, and describe the food customs that usually surround the celebration.

42. Evaluation. Is it right or wrong for parents to reward or punish their child with food?

43. Analysis. How might a limited budget influence your food choices?

44. Evaluation. How do boredom, stress, frustration, and happiness affect eating habits? Give examples.

LESSON 2

45. Evaluation. What is the primary source of calories in your diet?

46. Synthesis. What would you expect of a product labeled *hydrogenated corn oil?*

47. Synthesis. Create an accurate and persuasive advertisement for a nutritious food.

LESSON 3

48. Evaluation. Compare your eating habits with those of a friend. Which of you makes more healthful choices?

49. Synthesis. Create a nutritious daily menu plan for someone who typically eats six minimeals during the day.

50. Synthesis. Suppose your friend skips breakfast because she does not like traditional breakfast foods. What advice might you offer?

51. Evaluation. What standards would you apply to decide if a snack is healthy?

Making the Connection

LESSON 1

52. Home Economics. Compare the fat content in ½ pound of various types of ground beef (regular, chuck, round) by breaking the ground beef apart and browning it with no additional fat. Remove the meat from the frying pan, pour the fat into a measuring cup, and measure. What conclusions can you draw from this experiment?

Applying Health Knowledge

LESSON 1

53. Discuss the pros and cons of food advertising on children's television.

LESSON 2

54. How might a vegetarian who eats no meat, poultry, or fish get all of the nutrients he or she needs?

55. Suppose your friend said, "Milk is only for children." How would you refute this?

LESSON 3

56. The typical fast-food meal (burger, fries, and shake) has over 800 calories. How could you lower this meal's caloric and fat content?

57. Suppose a family member has high blood pressure. How could you help control the sodium in his or her diet?

58. As a teenager, you probably enjoy snacks. What might you do to keep snacks from promoting tooth decay?

LESSON 4

59. You are buying a breakfast cereal. One has 100 percent of the Daily Value for all nutrients listed. The other has 25 percent of B vitamins, 15 percent of iron, and small amounts of other nutrients. Which would you buy? On what basis do you decide to buy a cereal? What factors do not enter into your decision?

60. If you had the opportunity, what information would you include on food labels?

Beyond the Classroom

LESSON 1

61. Parental Involvement. Ask your parents what criteria they use when shopping for food.

LESSON 4

62. Further Study. Research the recent food labeling debate, and report on its current status.

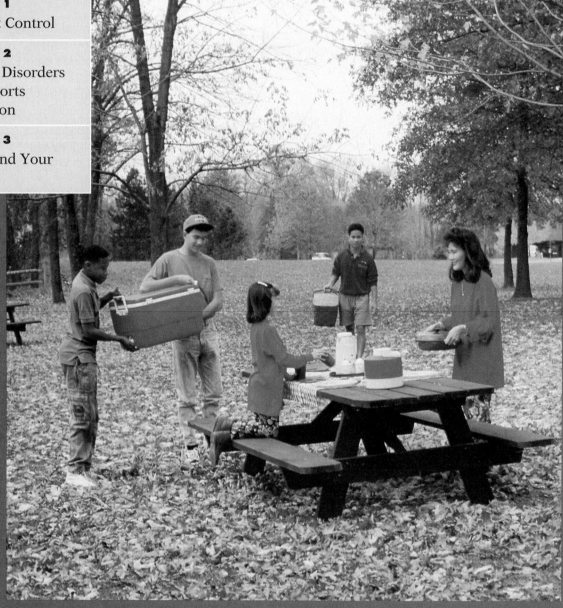

WEIGHT CONTROL

To be truly fit, you need to maintain a healthy weight—now and throughout your lifetime. Your own healthy weight probably will not be the same as the weight of a high-fashion model or that of your best friend. You can use some general guidelines, however, to judge your weight and to keep it within a healthy range.

Calorie Basics

To understand weight management, you need to understand calories—what they are, where they come from, and how they affect body weight. When people hear the word *calories,* they often think of fattening foods. **Calories,** or more correctly, kilocalories, are simply a unit to measure energy. Calories are a measure of the energy in food and the energy your body burns. Calories are not nutrients.

Calories: Their Source

Some foods have more calories than others. The specific number depends on the amount of carbohydrate, fat, and protein in the food—as well as the portion size. The way a food is prepared or cooked also affects the calorie count.

In the previous chapter you learned about three nutrients that supply energy, or calories. Carbohydrate, the main source, and protein each supply four calories per gram. Fat supplies more than twice as much—nine calories per gram. For this reason, even small amounts of fat in a food significantly increase its calorie content.

The look and taste of many foods often provide clues to their calorie content. High-fat foods may be sweet and gooey, crisp and greasy, or oily. Low-fat foods may be watery, crisp (but not greasy), or bulky (high-fiber). Can you give examples of both types of foods?

Calories to Burn

Calories in foods provide your body's fuel. Your body uses calories 24 hours a day, even while you are asleep. You need a "full tank" to provide the fuel for basic metabolism, or all life-sustaining body processes, and all of your physical and mental activities.

How many calories do you need? Several factors play a role, such as rate of growth, body size, sex, age, and metabolic rate. For example, some people have a higher metabolic rate than others so they need more calories. Children and teens need more calories than adults because they are still growing. Taller and bigger people need more than shorter and smaller people. A person's activity level also plays a major role. Active people need more calories than sedentary people do in order to remain active.

LESSON 1 FOCUS

TERMS TO USE
- Calories
- Overweight
- Obesity (oh•BEE•suh•tee)
- Underweight
- Undernutrition
- Nutrient-dense
- Weight cycling

CONCEPTS TO LEARN
- Both obesity and being underweight are health risks.
- Exercise is an important part of weight management.
- Fad diets and gimmicks do not result in permanent weight loss.

ATTITUDES AND BEHAVIORS TO EVALUATE
- Self-Inventory, page 420.
- Building Decision-Making Skills, page 421.

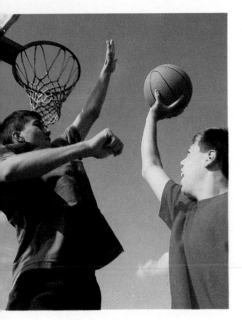

Being active is a necessary factor in balancing the energy equation.

Balancing the Energy Equation

Keeping a healthy weight is an issue of energy balance. Simply stated, calories consumed must equal calories burned. You gain or lose weight by tipping the balance. By taking in fewer calories than you expend, you lose body weight. When you take in more calories than you expend, you gain. Your body banks the extra calories as body fat.

Each pound (0.5 kg) of body fat equals about 3,500 calories. To lose 1 pound (0.5 kg) a week, which is a realistic, healthy goal, you need to consume 500 fewer calories than normal each day. Here is the calculation: 500 calories per day × 7 days = 3,500 calories = 1 pound (0.5 kg) of body fat. What will happen if you also burn 250 extra calories a day through exercise?

Weight Problems: Risky Business

Being too heavy or too thin increases the risk of developing health problems later on. In the meantime, weight problems can certainly affect the quality of life.

Body Fat versus Body Weight

Although we use the terms *overweight* and *obesity* interchangeably, these conditions are not the same. **Overweight** means weighing more than 10 percent over the standard weight for height; **obesity** means excess body fat, or adipose tissue. Usually obesity and overweight go together.

From a health standpoint, being overweight or being obese is risky. However, in certain situations, being overweight might not be a risk. A football player or bodybuilder may be overweight because of excess muscle but not have excess fat. Body composition, rather than weight, is a better measure of fitness.

Obesity: A Hazard to Health

Obesity is a common health risk in the United States. Excess body fat strains the body frame and increases the work load of the heart and the lungs. Obese people have a higher risk of health problems, including hypertension, diabetes, high blood cholesterol, atherosclerosis, and some cancers. Also, obese people are often inactive, which increases the health risks even more.

Adolescent obesity is increasing. Besides the health risks later in life, excess body fat during adolescence may affect self-esteem and social health. Unfortunately, many teens who are overweight or obese as adolescents continue to be so through adulthood.

Why do people gain too much weight? There are two main reasons:

- sedentary life-style
- poor food habits

Interestingly, studies show that many obese people actually eat less than normal-weight people who exercise more.

Obesity may be more complex, however. Heredity may play a role, but the exact relationship is unclear. Some scientists believe that obese

DID YOU KNOW?

- Regular exercise is one effective way to lose weight. These activities, performed by a 110-pound woman for just 10 minutes, can burn the following numbers of calories:

dancing	26
tennis	55
walking	41
sitting quietly	11
climbing hills	61
playing piano	20
running	97
swimming	78

people have more fat cells, which may get smaller but never go away. Other researchers are exploring the set point theory. This theory says that each person has a biological set point for weight and body fat. The body works to maintain that point by lowering metabolic rate when caloric intake goes down. Then it is hard to lose weight and keep it off.

Underweight: A Health Risk

Being thin does not mean being fit. With so much attention on obesity, we sometimes forget the health risks related to **underweight,** or being 10 percent or more below normal weight. Being too thin means a person has little body fat as an energy reserve, and perhaps less of the protective nutrients the body stores. This condition makes it harder for an overly thin person to fight off infection and increases the risk of health problems when surgery is needed.

Underweight people may be undernourished, too. **Undernutrition** is not consuming enough essential nutrients or calories for normal body functions. Among other health risks, underweight people have a greater chance for iron-deficiency anemia and osteoporosis.

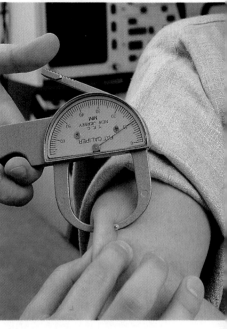

There are expensive and inexpensive versions of calipers. All of them measure percentage of body fat.

Managing Body Weight

How many people do you know who have gone on a diet? How many lost weight only to regain it shortly afterward? Why? Perhaps they did not follow realistic weight-control strategies.

Determining a Healthy Weight

Height and weight charts are often used to determine a person's proper weight. However, the range of weights listed on these charts can vary a great deal when accounting for different size body frames. For example, two people who are the same height can have very different weights. A large-boned person will weigh more than a small-boned person of the same height.

Measuring a person's body composition is a more accurate way to determine a healthy weight. By measuring the thickness of skinfolds in three specific areas of the body with calipers, percent body fat can be determined when compared on a chart. For males 15 years and older, measurements can be taken at the chest, abdomen, and thigh. For females 15 years and older, measurements can be taken at the triceps,

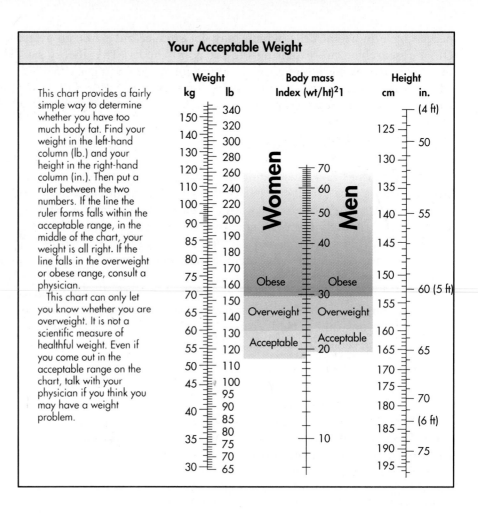

Your Acceptable Weight

This chart provides a fairly simple way to determine whether you have too much body fat. Find your weight in the left-hand column (lb.) and your height in the right-hand column (in.). Then put a ruler between the two numbers. If the line the ruler forms falls within the acceptable range, in the middle of the chart, your weight is all right. If the line falls in the overweight or obese range, consult a physician.

This chart can only let you know whether you are overweight. It is not a scientific measure of healthful weight. Even if you come out in the acceptable range on the chart, talk with your physician if you think you may have a weight problem.

Weight		Body mass	Height	
kg	lb	Index (wt/ht)^{2}1	cm	in.

Weight kg/lb scale: 150–340, 140–320, 130–300, 120–280, 110–260, 100–240, 90–220, 85–200, 80–190, 75–170, 70–160, 65–150, 60–140, 55–130, 50–120, 45–110, 40–100/95/90/85, 35–80/75/70, 30–65

Body mass index: Women / Men; 70, 60, 50, 40, Obese 30, Overweight, Acceptable 20, 10

Height cm/in: 125–(4 ft), 130–50, 135, 140–55, 145, 150–60 (5 ft), 155, 160–65, 165, 170, 175, 180–70, 185–(6 ft), 190–75, 195

thigh, and over the top of the hip. A desirable percent body fat is about 11 to 18 percent for males and 16 to 23 percent for females. A person with an excess of body fat is considered obese.

Knowing the amount of body fat you have is important for weight control. Equally important is the location of body fat. Excess abdominal fat increases the chance of heart disease and diabetes more than excess fat elsewhere, such as on the hips and thighs.

The chart shown above provides an indicator for acceptable weight. This chart uses a body mass index.

Starting a Weight Control Plan

The true meaning of the word *diet* is everything a person eats and drinks, not a restrictive eating plan. People who manage their weight well never need a restrictive eating plan. Instead, they eat and exercise to maintain a healthy weight throughout life.

These steps can get you started in a smart weight control plan:

- Target your weight. Based on your body frame, choose a target weight that is within a healthy range, and not too thin. Ask your doctor what range is healthy for you.
- Set smart goals. Losing or gaining ½ to 1 pound (0.2 to 0.5 kg) a week is realistic, attainable, and safe.
- Make a personal plan, preferably one that includes both a nutritious diet and regular exercise. Consider your own food preferences and

DID YOU KNOW?

- Researchers from the United States and Sweden, looking over data from 247 sets of identical twins and 426 sets of fraternal twins, discovered that, whether or not the twins are raised apart, they are likely to end up with similar weights. They are also much more likely to have weights similar to natural parents rather than adoptive ones. This and other new research indicates that one's weight may have more to do with one's genes than previously thought.

406 CHAPTER 20 AVOIDING PROBLEMS WITH FOODS

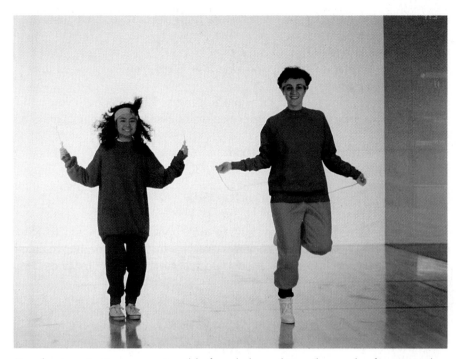

Regular exercise in some enjoyable form helps achieve the goals of any weight-control program.

life-style. Choose an exercise you will enjoy doing. It is easier to follow a plan that you create yourself.
- Put your goal and plan in writing.
- Stick to your plan. To help, keep a diary of what you eat and when, so that you become more aware of your food habits. Eat a variety of foods with at least the minimum number of servings from the Daily Food Guide. Avoid meal skipping; eat three or more meals a day.
- Think positively. If you slip up occasionally, that is okay. Focus on your progress, and get back on track.
- Evaluate your progress, but avoid weighing yourself every day. Instead, weigh yourself once a week at the same time of day.
- Recognize that plateaus are normal. Plateaus are a period of time when your weight does not change.

Smart Weight-Loss Strategies

The best weight-loss strategies are easily summed up as follows:

- Eat fewer calories (and make them nutrient dense). **Nutrient-dense** foods are those high in nutrients relative to their caloric content.
- Burn more calories through exercise.
- Better yet, do both.

This advice is the same no matter how much you need to lose—5, 15, even 50 pounds (2.3, 6.9, even 22.7 kg).

These strategies can help your weight-loss plan work for you:

- As a teen, eat at least 1,400 calories daily. Otherwise, you may miss out on essential nutrients.
- Eat mainly low-calorie foods from the five food groups, including fruits and vegetables.

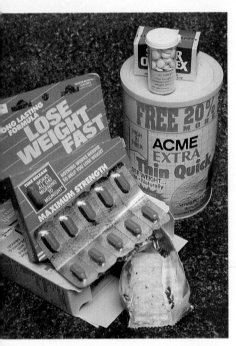

There is no safe way to take weight off quickly, no matter what claims and promises the ads make.

- Eat foods you like. If your favorites are high in calories, have just a tiny portion from time to time.
- Make meals last. Take small bites.
- If you are tempted to snack, do something else, even if you need to leave the house.
- Avoid shopping for food when you are hungry. This will help you avoid the temptation to buy empty-calorie desserts and snacks on impulse.
- Avoid rewarding yourself with food.

Smart Weight-Gain Strategies

Some people want to gain weight to look better; others want to gain for sports. Smart weight gain includes exercise and a diet higher in calories. Without exercise, extra food calories turn mainly to body fat. Consider these tips:

- Increase caloric intake, especially with foods high in complex carbohydrates, such as bread, pasta, rice, potatoes, beans, and vegetables.
- Eat more frequently. Take second helpings.
- Eat nutritious snacks, but space them two to three hours before meals to avoid spoiling your appetite.

Exercise and Weight Management

People can lose body fat just by dieting, but increased physical activity helps them reach their target weight faster, easier and, over the long run, more effectively. Whether you need to lose, gain, or maintain weight, you should exercise. Consider the following benefits of regular exercise:

- It burns calories, which promotes loss of body fat.
- It tones and builds muscles to give a firm, lean body shape. Without exercise, the weight lost may be lean tissue as well as body fat.
- It helps promote a normal appetite response, which helps anyone trying to gain, lose, or maintain weight.
- It helps relieve the stress that leads to overeating or undereating.
- It helps increase metabolic rate, so the body burns more calories even while resting. It takes more calories to maintain muscle tissue than body fat. Exercise may help lower your set point.
- It increases self-esteem, which helps keep your plan on track.

To build muscles and spend calories, you really need to work your muscles on a regular basis. Even adding exercise to your daily routine, such as using stairs instead of an elevator or walking instead of driving, helps. To set up a realistic, yet effective exercise program, refer to Chapter 18.

Popular Diets and Gimmicks

Perhaps no area of health receives more attention—or is more lucrative—than weight control. People want to take off the pounds quickly even though it took months, even years, to put them on. That is why

LOOKING AT TECHNOLOGY

The Calorimeter

The calorimeter is a high-tech room that measures human energy. It monitors the number of calories a body takes in and gives off. On the outside, the calorimeter looks like a square space capsule. It has a control panel filled with mysterious dials. It also has an observation window and a special slot where food trays can be passed through to the interior. Inside, it is a small room equipped with a TV, bed, toilet, and sink plus enough room to do certain kinds of exercise. The purposes of the calorimeter, nicknamed "The Box," are to try to determine why and how some people become overweight and to understand how efficiently a particular body utilizes and produces energy.

How does "The Box" operate? A test subject enters the 9×12-foot metal box for a 24-hour period. The entire time the person is inside the enclosed environment, 80,000 energy sensors in the walls of "The Box" register how much heat the subject's body takes in and gives off. Also measured are the oxygen and carbon dioxide involved in the subject's breathing.

The calorimeter has already been used to dismiss the common myth that most people who get fat do so because of faulty or slow metabolisms. It will also be used to disprove other misconceptions about dieting, obesity, and the effectiveness of various diets.

---

fad weight-loss diets and gimmicks are so common. Fad diets are approaches to weight control that are very popular for a short time. Diet gimmicks are deceptive approaches that are costly, unsafe, and ineffective. You can find both in books, magazines, and newspapers. Health food stores, drugstores, and grocery stores provide products that promise weight loss in a few, short steps.

Dieting the Wrong Way

Many popular diets are extreme and hard to stick to. Many promise quick results without offering adequate nutrition. Some are dangerous; others are costly. Most do not result in long-term weight loss.

Quick weight-loss regimens may seem to work at first. However, the initial weight lost is usually water, not body fat.

Weight cycling, or the cycle of losing, regaining, losing, and regaining, is the result of following one weight-loss regimen after another. This is also called seesaw or yo-yo dieting.

Weight cycling may be more unhealthy than weighing a bit extra. The reason? Lean body tissue lost with body fat is replaced by more body fat. Because body fat burns fewer calories than muscle does, the person continues to require fewer and fewer calories to maintain weight. Weight loss gets harder and harder.

Culturally Speaking

Ice Cream Anyone?

Sometimes problems with food are genetically caused. Infants have an enzyme (lactase) that allows them to digest milk sugar (lactose). People from cultures with histories of dairy farming also are more likely to be able to digest milk sugar. For example, only 2 percent of Danish adults are lactose intolerant (cannot digest milk sugar).

Most adults worldwide, however, lose this ability. The Thai or Pima Indians, with no dairy farming heritage, have 98 percent lactose intolerance. If these adults eat milk products, they experience diarrhea and other problems.

BEWARE

Many people look for quick, effortless weight reduction. Consumers need to be aware that many such diets or products may be not only ineffective but also unsafe. Beware of any diet or product that

- consists of only one food;
- promises quick results;
- supplies too few calories (below 1,200 calories a day) for energy and health;
- requires a weight-loss aid, such as a vitamin pill, a body wrap, a liquid shake, or an appetite suppressant;
- promises spot reducing—an unrealistic claim because weight loss occurs all over;
- does not teach a person how to make changes for permanent weight loss.

Other Risky Weight-Loss Strategies

Three other weight-loss approaches—fasting, liquid protein diets, and diet pills—are not worth the risks.

Fasting. Avoiding food, or fasting, is dangerous even for a short time. For health, growth, and energy, you need a fresh supply of nutrients daily. For example, without protein, the body uses its own muscle tissue for energy.

Liquid Protein Diets. High-protein, low-carbohydrate diets can have such serious side effects that the FDA requires a warning label on these products. Using them as the only source of nutrients can result in serious health problems, even death.

Diet Pills. The side effects of diet pills can be very serious. Some cause drowsiness; others may produce anxiety. In addition, diet pills may be addictive. Most important, they do not result in permanent weight loss.

LESSON 1 REVIEW

Reviewing Facts and Vocabulary

1. Name three health risks related to being obese and being underweight.
2. What is a skinfold test? How is it used?
3. What is the set point theory?

Thinking Critically

4. **Analysis.** Compare being obese to being overweight.
5. **Synthesis.** How would you explain energy balance?

6. **Synthesis.** Suppose you want to lose 1 pound (0.5 kg) per week for the next five weeks. How would you change the calories you eat and the calories you burn in exercise to reach that goal?

Applying Health Knowledge

7. Find a magazine article about a current weight-loss or weight-gain plan. Evaluate it using principles of good nutrition and health. Discuss whether the program could allow permanent weight change.

EATING DISORDERS AND SPORTS NUTRITION

Fitness-minded people usually care about their diets. They choose what they eat to maximize their overall performance. Sometimes people take a wrong turn on the road to good nutrition, however. They may have misconceptions about the role of food in their lives. Others, obsessed by their body weight, may fall victim to eating disorders.

Eating Disorders—Serious Health Risks

Today's society is obsessed with being thin. The average high-fashion female model is about 5 feet 8 inches (1.7 m) tall and weighs less than 110 pounds (50 kg). Does this model represent an accurate picture of a healthy, typical female figure? In truth, no, but many people compare themselves to these models.

An obsession with thinness, along with psychological pressures and perhaps genetic factors, can lead to two eating disorders: anorexia nervosa and bulimia. Thousands of people in the United States, mainly females, suffer from these disorders.

Anorexia Nervosa

Anorexia nervosa involves the irrational fear of becoming obese and results in severe weight loss from self-induced starvation. Many adolescents who develop anorexia were not above a normal weight to begin with. This disorder often starts as ordinary dieting. *Anorexia* means "without appetite"; *nervosa* means "of nervous origin."

Anorexia nervosa is a psychological disorder with emotional and physical consequences. It relates directly to an individual's self-concept and coping abilities. Being thin becomes an obsession. Outside pressures, high expectations, the need to achieve, and the need to be popular help lead to this disorder.

What are the signs of anorexia? Each person with anorexia is different, but these behaviors and emotions are typical: a very low caloric intake, a great interest in food, an obsession with exercising, emotional problems, a distorted body image (feeling fat even though underweight), and a denial of an eating problem.

A person with anorexia has physical symptoms related to malnutrition and starvation: extreme weight loss, constipation, hormonal changes, heart damage, impaired immune function, decreased heart rates, and in females, no menstrual cycle. In severe cases, anorexia can result in death.

Most people with anorexia are females, in their teens or twenties. However, this eating disorder is not unknown among males. All cases of anorexia require professional medical help.

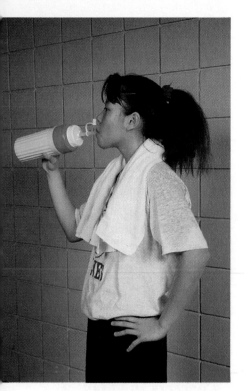

Taking care of your body's fluid requirements helps you perform at your best.

CONFLICT RESOLUTION

Her friends think Tracey has it all: she's a good student and very popular. However, Tracey is unhappy. She thinks she's overweight. Tracey's parents worry that she's getting too thin. Because they nag her to eat more, Tracey lies about how much food she eats away from home. As her weight drops, she feels more and more in control, but she still sees a chubby image in the mirror. Only the low numbers on the bathroom scale make her feel good.

How can Tracey be helped to resolve her unhappiness with herself?

Bulimia

Bulimia is another very serious eating disorder involving cycles of overeating and some form of purging, or clearing of the digestive tract. Often the person with bulimia follows a very restrictive diet, only to binge in response to hunger. To binge is to eat a large amount of food in a short time. This eating behavior is followed by self-induced vomiting or purging through laxative abuse. Often after a binge, a person may try to follow a severely restrictive diet in order to restore a sense of control and avoid the possibility of weight gain.

The desire to become thin, more attractive, and more physically perfect can be overwhelming until vomiting or purging becomes a daily routine. Associated with this behavior may be the misguided notion that once the perfect figure is attained, everything in life will be fine. Bulimics are often secretive, but they know they have a problem.

Bingeing, purging, or fasting should never be viewed as a smart way to control weight. Bulimia can lead to serious health problems, even death. Vomiting and diarrhea lead to dehydration, kidney damage, and irregular heartbeat. Chronic vomiting erodes tooth enamel, causes tooth decay, and damages tissue of the stomach, esophagus, and mouth. Because laxative abuse interferes with digestion and absorption, nutrient deficiencies may occur. Laxative abuse can also lead to serious damage of blood composition.

Anorexia and bulimia are not diseases; they are symptoms of other problems. Both are psychological in nature. People suffering from these disorders need medical help and qualified counseling immediately. Recovery is a long process, but early diagnosis and care improve the chance of recovery.

If you believe a friend has symptoms of anorexia or bulimia, advise your school nurse, or, in a caring way, encourage your friend to get help. Do not try to counsel your friend yourself.

Food for Sports

Are you a serious athlete? Do you engage in pick-up basketball or tennis? Do you swim for fun and relaxation? No matter what type of athlete you are, good nutrition can help you do your best. Smart food choices can help you reach your top physical performance as you train.

The Training Diet

No one food or nutrient builds muscle or increases speed. The best training diet is balanced, moderate, and varied. Athletic training does not significantly alter the body's requirements for protein, vitamins, or minerals. The main difference is the increased need for calories, or food energy. Nutrient-dense foods are the best sources.

Physical activity requires an increase in fluids, especially during hot weather, to prevent dehydration and heatstroke. Drink several cups of fluid two hours, and then 15 minutes, ahead of a heavy workout. During exercise drink a half cup of fluid every 15 minutes. Afterwards drink two cups of fluid for every pound of body weight lost through sweat. Water is an athlete's best source of fluid.

Making Weight

In some sports maintaining a certain body weight is important. For example, wrestlers compete in a specific weight class. In contact sports, a little extra body weight may offer some advantages. Athletes are wise to meet their weight requirements in a healthful way.

Trying to compete in a weight class that is below your healthy weight can be dangerous. Fasting, crash dieting, or trying to sweat off extra weight before weigh-in can cause dehydration and can compromise performance. Over time these practices may result in loss of muscle mass, too. If you do need to lose weight, follow the sensible plan—1/2 to 1 pound (0.2 to 0.5 kg) a week—described earlier in this chapter.

Athletes who train to gain weight need to follow a healthy diet and to exercise to build muscle mass. Extra calories should come mainly from nutrient-dense foods. Slow, steady weight gain, no more than 2 pounds (0.9 kg) a week, is best. Using hormones, such as steroids, to increase muscle mass is not healthy. They may stunt growth and damage the body's reproductive system.

Pre-Competition Meal

Many athletes ask, "What should I eat before competing, and how far ahead of the event?" Eating three to four hours before an event allows the stomach to empty, yet keeps the athlete free from hunger pangs while competing.

Before competing, choose a meal high in carbohydrates and low in fat and protein. Fats and proteins stay in the digestive tract too long. Good sources of carbohydrates are pasta, rice, breads, vegetables, and fruits. Drinking plenty of fluids before a workout is important, too.

Carbohydrates are stored in the body in the form of **glycogen.** Athletes who participate in endurance sports, such as cross-country running or long-distance bicycling, may benefit by **carbohydrate loading,** or storing extra glycogen in the muscle before strenuous exercise. Several days ahead, the athlete eats a high-carbohydrate diet to store plenty of muscle glycogen. Practice is light for two days before competition, too, so stored glycogen is not depleted.

Carbohydrate loading is not recommended for teenage athletes who are still growing. A balanced diet supplies enough glycogen for most sports as long as the diet includes a wide variety of foods and the recommended 55 to 65 percent from carbohydrates.

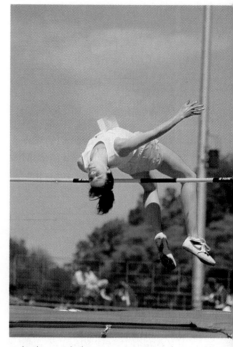

A balanced diet is an essential ingredient in achieving peak athletic performance.

K E E P I N G   F I T

Muscle Up and Trim Down

New research indicates that exercises that help you to build muscle mass, such as working out with weights or even just doing abdominal crunches, can help you lose weight. Why? Because such exercises get your "calorie-burning engines" working extra hard. The larger the muscle mass you are working, the greater the number of calories you will burn. So don't just rely on aerobic exercise to trim down or maintain your weight. Add strength training to your workout regimen.

Overcoming The Odds

Janelle is 17. She is an A student and a fine gymnast. She is also a bulimic. She begins, "I have an eating disorder that will stay with me for the rest of my life. But now that I'm getting help, I know I can deal with it.

"All my life I've always had this older sister with this great figure. My mom was heavier when she was a kid, but she's really thin now and into exercise, so I had these women in my life who were living examples of what I wasn't: Thin. I felt like I could never measure up. But my real problem didn't take hold until I was about 13."

The "real problem" Janelle talks about is bulimia. Janelle continues. "It all started innocently. I went on a diet and lost some weight. So I figured I could reward myself and get away with it. I love ice cream. I crave it. So I started to buy pints on my own after school, scarf them down, then force myself to throw up. Then I started bingeing on other things like cakes and cookies and chips. I'd usually do it when I knew no one was at home, but when they were, I found ways

around it. It was all this massive shameful cover-up.

"By the time I was 15 I was doing this a lot. I was afraid of going out of control. I felt like there was this deep empty black hole inside me and

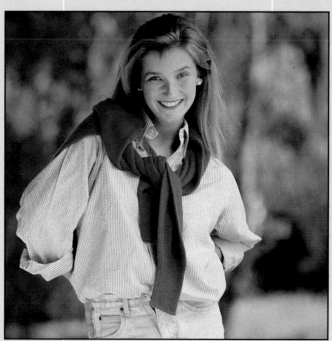

nothing could fill it up— except food. I got scared that my dentist would figure out what I was doing, so that's when I started using laxatives. In a while that got out of control, too. Finally, I started to look kind of bad. My energy level was down. Then, at a gymnastics meet, I just passed out. That was the beginning of the next stage."

The "next stage" to which Janelle refers was getting help. She was taken to her doctor for a full medical evaluation. "I was dehydrated. My electrolytes were way out of whack. So they got me physically straightened out, and then they started on my head," she laughs.

"I had individual therapy for a while. I've started to be able to look at myself for who I am, not for what I weigh or how well I compete. It isn't easy. It's a lifelong challenge, I know. But there are pluses. My family communicates better. I do, too. There's hope. That's not to say that the problem has gone away. It hasn't. But I realize that I don't have to be so perfect, that maybe I'm okay as I am."

1. What were some of the characteristic bulimic behaviors and feelings that Janelle exhibited? What caused her to get into recovery?
2. How do you feel about your body? Your weight? How is your self-esteem tied to your body image, your weight, and the comments others make about the way you look?

SPORTS NUTRITION QUESTIONS

Do vitamin pills give extra energy? Because vitamins do not supply calories, extra amounts will not give extra energy. Although B vitamins help release energy from carbohydrates, fats, and proteins, athletes usually get enough in the extra foods they eat. No so-called energy-giving aids really work; these include bee pollen, wheat germ oil, and others.

Will extra protein or amino acid supplements build extra muscle? The only way to build muscle mass and strength is through exercise. The body does not store protein. Extra protein is expended as energy or stored as body fat.

Does eating a candy bar or honey before a workout provide quick energy? Energy for physical activity comes from foods you ate several days, not an hour or so, before a workout.

Will drinking tea, colas, or coffee before a workout improve performance? All three beverages contain the stimulant caffeine. A good warm-up gets you moving just as well. Caffeine can cause headaches, stomach upset, nervousness, irritability, and diarrhea. Caffeine has a diuretic, or urine-producing, effect, so it also increases the chance of dehydration.

Will sucking on ice before a workout prevent dehydration? Ice does not provide much fluid. To avoid dehydration and heatstroke, athletes need to drink enough fluid before, during, and after a workout.

Do athletes need salt tablets? A normal diet has enough sodium to replace losses through sweat. Salt tablets may worsen the problem of dehydration.

FINDING HELP

Overeaters Anonymous is a group of men and women who support one another in their attempts to deal with food addictions. The OA program is modeled on Alcoholics Anonymous. There are therefore no dues or fees. What is said at the meetings and who attends them remains anonymous, and members' last names are not used. People who join OA generally get special friends, called sponsors, who help to guide them through their recovery.

For more information about the OA program in your area, look in your phone book under Overeaters Anonymous.

For some athletes, eating special foods before competition offers a psychological lift. As long as those foods are part of a healthy diet, enjoy them!

Contrary to popular belief, having a steak dinner before competing has no physical benefits. In fact, a high-fat, high-protein meal will not digest as fast as one high in carbohydrates.

LESSON 2 REVIEW

Reviewing Facts and Vocabulary

1. What is anorexia nervosa? What is bulimia?
2. Write three health risks related to anorexia and to bulimia.
3. What is carbohydrate loading?
4. What characterizes the best training diet for athletes?

Thinking Critically

5. **Synthesis.** Why do you think that most people with anorexia are females in their teens or twenties?

6. **Synthesis.** If you had a friend who might have an eating disorder, how would you help?
7. **Synthesis.** What would you say to a friend who decided to double protein intake to build muscles?

Applying Health Knowledge

8. Using library resources, write a research report on eating disorders. Consider reading about a celebrity who struggled with the problem, such as performer Karen Carpenter, who died from the complications of anorexia. Share your findings with the class.

FOOD AND YOUR SAFETY

LESSON 3 FOCUS

TERMS TO USE
- Foodborne illness
- Cross-contamination
- Nutrient supplements
- Megadoses (MEHG•uh•doh•sehz)
- Food allergy
- Allergens (AL•uhr•juhns)

CONCEPTS TO LEARN
- Foodborne illness is caused by bacteria.
- Getting nutrients from a balanced, varied diet, rather than from supplements, is the safest, healthiest approach.
- Food allergies can come from food additives as well as various kinds of food.

ATTITUDES AND BEHAVIORS TO EVALUATE
- Self-Inventory, page 420.
- Building Decision-Making Skills, page 421.

How can you be sure the food you eat is safe? Are nutrient supplements necessary if you eat a balanced diet? How common are food allergies? Food is at the center of many issues related to health.

Food Safety

Food safety has been described as one of the major health issues of the 1990s. Foodborne illness is on the rise. The increased use of pesticides and additives has more and more people asking about their impact on health and on the environment.

Foodborne Illness

Reports suggest that millions of Americans experience foodborne illness every year. **Foodborne illness,** or food poisoning, comes from eating food contaminated by bacteria. Many times these bacteria cannot be seen, smelled, or tasted. Protecting yourself from foodborne illness comes from knowing the causes and ways to keep food safe.

Foodborne illnesses related to food spoilage are commonly caused by four types of bacteria: *Salmonella, Staphylococcus aureus, Clostridium perfringens,* and *Clostridium botulinum.* Parasites and intestinal viruses can cause other food-related diseases.

You may not realize when you have foodborne illness because many of the symptoms are similar to flu symptoms. Nausea, vomiting, diarrhea, fever, and body aches are common symptoms of foodborne illness. People often get over these symptoms in a few days. However, for those who are elderly, very young, ill, or malnourished, foodborne illness is very risky. One form of foodborne illness, botulism, is especially dangerous because it can be fatal. It comes from food contaminated in a canned or vacuum-packed container. If you come down with foodborne illness, rest, drink plenty of fluids, and, if the symptoms continue, call a doctor.

Health Foods

Is there really such a thing as health food? Not really; no food has special abilities to promote health. Whether you are active or sedentary, nothing beats a balanced, varied diet for good health.

The term *health food* has no legal definition. The Food and Drug Administration has called the health food business a racket and one of the most widespread forms of deception in the United States. Yet many people perceive that these higher-priced foods offer extra benefits. Foods or ingredients commonly sold as health foods include brewer's yeast, lecithin, honey, and alkaline salts. Some out-of-the-ordinary vegetables and grains may also be available in health food stores.

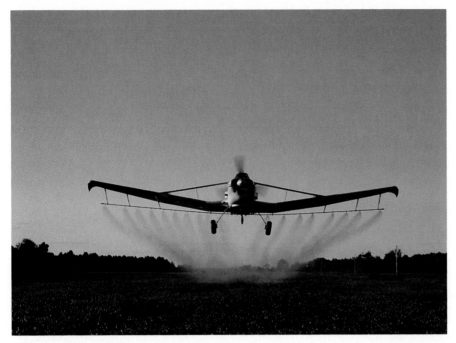

Many people are beginning to examine and question the impact that various pesticides may have on health.

Some health foods are referred to as organic foods. Actually, all foods are organic. However, some foods are organically grown, which means they are grown without pesticides or synthetic fertilizers. Production of organically grown foods is not monitored in most states, so you have no way of knowing whether the claims are true unless you actually see how the plants were grown.

KEEPING IT SAFE!

Bacteria need three conditions for growth: nutrients, moisture, and warmth. Bacteria in food multiplies rapidly between 40° and 140°F (4.4° and 60°C). At these temperatures, bacteria double in number in 30 minutes.

Keep food safe by selecting and handling it with care. Follow these guidelines:

■ Do not buy or eat food from damaged packaging. Check all packaging for cracks, leaks, bulging lids, or popped safety buttons.
■ Store and prepare foods according to package instructions.
■ Keep hot foods hot. Bacteria is destroyed when food reaches an internal temperature of 160°F (71.2°C). Be especially careful with a microwave oven because cooking is uneven; that is why you need to rotate foods.
■ Keep cold foods cold. Below 40°F (4.4°C), bacteria grow more slowly.
■ Keep all foods and food preparation surfaces clean. Wash hands, work surfaces, and utensils with hot, soapy water to keep bacteria away.
■ Avoid **cross-contamination,** or spreading bacteria from one food to another. Wash work surfaces, utensils, and hands after handling raw foods.
■ Refrigerate leftovers so that they do not stay at room temperature longer than two hours. Do not thaw food on the counter!
■ Throw away suspicious foods without tasting them.

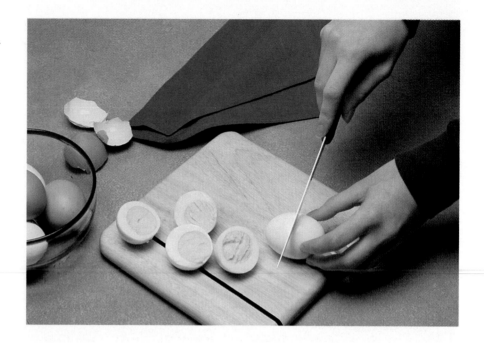

If you use a wooden cutting board, be sure it has no cracks. Bacteria can get trapped in the cracks, multiply, and contaminate other foods.

Nutrient Supplements

Nutrient supplements are pills, powders, and liquids—not foods—that contain nutrients. If you believe everything you hear or read, you might think that vitamin pills or protein supplements are the cure-all for just about any pain or disease. For some people nutrient supplements in safe amounts make health sense. Unfortunately, people also misuse them.

Under some health conditions or during certain stages of life, people can benefit from nutrient supplements. Following are some of these situations:

- Pregnant and nursing women have somewhat increased nutrient needs.
- Some illnesses affect appetite or nutrient absorption.
- Women may need extra iron to replace iron lost through menstruation.
- Menopausal women may need extra calcium to protect against osteoporosis.
- Elderly adults need a supplement if they do not eat adequately.
- Some medications may interfere with nutrient absorption.

K E E P I N G   F I T

Nutrient Supplements

The annual sales of nutrient supplements has more than doubled during the last decade. But the use of supplements is often unnecessary, costly, and sometimes unsafe. It often keeps people from getting the medical attention they need.

- Supplements won't improve athletic performance. The extra food athletes eat provides the added vitamins they need.
- No evidence proves that vitamin B_6 supplements relieve menstrual cramps. In fact, large doses may cause nerve damage.
- Emotional stress doesn't require extra vitamins. So-called "stress" vitamins aren't needed, but rest and recreation are.

What dose of nutrient supplements is safe? Very large amounts, or **megadoses,** are an unnecessary cost and are potentially dangerous. Excess amounts of fat-soluble vitamins A, D, E, and K, for example, stay in the body and become toxic. Excess amounts of vitamin C, a water-soluble vitamin, are excreted, putting a heavy strain on the kidneys. A safe dosage of vitamins is near or less than the RDA levels. The supplement's label gives the dosage.

Fiber supplements are also on the market. However, the benefits of a higher-fiber diet come from high-fiber food, not fiber alone. The excess fiber from supplements may increase the risk of intestinal problems and decrease the absorption of some nutrients.

Getting vitamins, minerals, and other nutrients from a balanced diet, rather than from supplements, is the healthiest, safest approach.

Food Allergies

An *allergy* is the body's reaction to a toxin. With a true **food allergy,** the body's immune system overreacts to substances in some foods. These substances, called **allergens,** are usually proteins. The immune system responds to them as it would to pathogens, or foreign invaders. The body produces antibodies for defense.

Some people with food allergies show no symptoms. Others may experience one or more reactions: rash, hives, or itchiness on the skin; vomiting, diarrhea, or abdominal pain; or hay fever-like symptoms in the respiratory tract.

Most food allergies come from nuts, eggs, milk, wheat, and soy. Fish, shellfish, chicken, and tomatoes may cause problems, too. Sulfites, or food additives that help preserve food, cause allergic reactions in some people. To identify an allergy, doctors ask patients to cut out certain foods one at a time from their diet or to keep a food diary. They also test for antibodies.

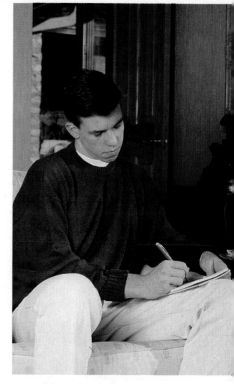

A well kept food diary can provide invaluable information in tracking down an allergy.

LESSON 3 REVIEW

Reviewing Facts and Vocabulary

1. Define the term *foodborne illness.*
2. What are the common symptoms of foodborne illness?
3. List five ways to protect your food supply from bacterial growth.
4. Give three examples of situations in which nutrient supplements might be beneficial.

Thinking Critically

5. **Analysis.** Explain why some people may be more vulnerable to foodborne illness than others.

6. **Synthesis.** Describe how a doctor might find out if you are allergic to peanut butter.

Applying Health Knowledge

7. Plan a picnic meal, keeping in mind the principles of food safety. List what you could do to prevent foodborne illness. Report to the class.

Self-Inventory

How Do You Manage Your Weight?

HOW DO YOU RATE?

Number a sheet of paper from 1 through 20. Read each item below and respond by writing *yes* or *no* for each item. Then proceed to the next section.

1. Would you consider exercise to be as important as diet if you needed to lose weight?
2. Do you think that very slim models have the "perfect" body?
3. Would you eat all you could at all-you-can-eat places to get your money's worth?
4. If you had a weight problem, would you be satisfied to lose or gain one pound per week?
5. Do you think that your weight as a teenager will have any effect at all on your health 30 to 40 years from now?
6. Have you ever bought a book or magazine because it had a quick weight-loss or weight-gain scheme you might try?
7. Would you be willing to set 30 minutes aside 3 times a week to work out?
8. Do you think that being obese can effect the quality of your life?
9. Do you consciously try to eat a variety of nutritious foods, even when you are trying to lose or gain weight?
10. Would you ever eat just for something to do when you were bored or stressed?
11. Would you use stairs rather than an elevator if you had a choice?
12. If you had a choice, would you go grocery shopping on an empty stomach?
13. Do you reward yourself with food?
14. Do food advertisements on TV lure you to the refrigerator or kitchen cabinet?
15. Have you ever fasted or gone on a quick weight-loss or weight-gain diet?
16. Do you eat even when you are not hungry?
17. Do you keep snack foods around you?
18. Do you think you must give up high-calorie favorites to lose weight?
19. Would you be willing to put your fork down between bites to make meals last?
20. Are you willing to change your eating habits for your lifetime, if necessary, in order to control your weight?

HOW DID YOU SCORE?

Give yourself 1 point for each *yes* answer to these items: 1, 4, 5, 7, 8, 9, 11, 19, 20. Give yourself 1 point for each *no* answer to these items: 2, 3, 6, 10, 12, 13, 14, 15, 16, 17, 18. Add the total, and see how you scored. Then proceed to the next section.

15 to 20
Excellent. Your attitudes and behaviors toward weight management can help keep you at a healthy weight.

10 to 14
Good. Many of your attitudes and behaviors are positive, but you could benefit from a few changes.

5 to 9
Fair. You need to examine your attitudes and behaviors carefully to maintain your healthy weight.

0 to 4
Needs Improvement. You need to rethink your attitudes and behaviors toward food before your weight is out of control!

WHAT ARE YOUR GOALS?

If you scored *excellent* or *good*, complete Part A. If your score was *fair* or *needs improvement*, complete Parts A and B.

Part A

1. I plan to learn more about controlling my weight by ____.
2. My timetable for accomplishing this is ____.
3. I plan to share what I learn with others by ____.

Part B

4. The weight management attitude or behavior I would most like to change is ____.
5. The steps involved in making this change are ____.
6. To be successful, my support must come from ____.
7. I will be successful if ____.
8. If I slip along the way, I will ____.
9. My rewards for making this change are ____.

Building Decision-Making Skills

R amad's girlfriend, Felicia, has lost 20 pounds in the last couple of months. He really likes her new, 110-pound, trim look. However, he is concerned because she still thinks she is fat. She has become very irritable and seems obsessed with exercising. She has promised that she won't continue to lose weight. What should Ramad do?

WHAT DO YOU THINK?

1. **Situation.** Why does Ramad need to make a decision?

2. **Choices.** What possible choices might Ramad make?

3. **Consequences.** What are the benefits of each choice?

4. **Consequences.** What are the costs of each choice?

5. **Consequences.** What health risks are present here? Explain your answer.

6. **Consequences.** How will Ramad feel about each choice?

7. **Consequences.** How will Felicia feel about each choice?

8. **Consequences.** How will Ramad's health triangle be affected by each choice?

9. **Decision.** Which choice do you think is best for Ramad?

10. **Evaluation.** Have you ever found yourself in a situation in which you were faced with a decision that might jeopardize a relationship? Describe the situation, how you handled it, and what you learned from it.

L ing's boyfriend, Chris, is the star of the school's varsity wrestling team and a top prospect for a college scholarship. It is now wrestling season, and she has very mixed emotions. She loves the excitement of the sport and of being the star's girlfriend, but she hates the fact that he goes from the 185 pounds he weighed during football season to 157 for wrestling. To do this, he goes through all kinds of diets, exercises, and various other tricks to lose weight. In the meantime he becomes sullen and sometimes mean. He's counting on the scholarship to go to college. His parents and coach believe that he will be only an average wrestler if he competes at a higher weight class. Ling has spoken to Chris about her concerns. He says he has the situation under control, but he doesn't. What should Ling do?

WHAT DO YOU THINK?

11. **Situation.** How should Ling deal with her conflicting feelings (her pride and her concern for his health)?

12. **Situation.** How should Ling deal with people that reinforce the situation by complimenting Chris?

13. **Choices.** What possible choices might Ling make?

14. **Consequences.** What are the benefits of each choice Ling might make?

15. **Consequences.** What are the risks of each choice Ling might make?

16. **Consequences.** Does Chris's athletic success and college scholarship justify the risk to his health?

17. **Consequences.** How will Chris probably feel about each choice?

18. **Consequences.** How will Chris's parents probably feel about the choices Ling might make?

19. **Consequences.** How will Chris's coach probably feel about Ling's choices?

20. **Consequences.** How will Ling's health triangle be affected by each choice?

21. **Decision.** Which choice do you think Ling should make and how should she implement it?

22. **Evaluation.** Have you ever found yourself in a similar situation? Describe the situation, how you handled it, and what you learned.

Using Health Terms

On a separate sheet of paper, write the term that best matches each definition given below.

LESSON 1

1. Excess body fat.
2. Device used to measure body fat.
3. Weighing more than 10 percent over a standard weight for height.
4. Term used to describe foods high in nutrients compared with their caloric content.
5. Unit of energy.
6. Equals 3,500 calories.
7. Ten percent or more below normal weight.
8. Deceptive approaches to dieting that are costly, unsafe, and ineffective.

LESSON 2

9. Disorder characterized by an irrational fear of becoming obese.
10. Eating large amounts of foods in a short time, followed by self-induced vomiting.
11. Eating large amounts of starches on days leading up to athletic competition.
12. Best fluid replacement for sports.

LESSON 3

13. Comes with eating food contaminated by bacteria.
14. Pills, powders, and liquids that contain nutrients.
15. When the body's immune system overreacts to food substances.

Building Academic Skills

LESSON 1

16. **Math.** Suppose you need to lose 10 pounds (4.5 kg). Currently, you eat 3,000 calories daily. To lose this weight in 15 weeks, calculate how many calories you should eat and expend in extra daily exercise.

LESSON 3

17. **Math.** Bacteria double in number every 30 minutes. Determine how many bacteria are produced from one bacterium in 24 hours.

Recalling the Facts

LESSON 1

18. Why is obesity considered a health risk?
19. What are the characteristics of a high-caloric food?
20. What health problems do obese adolescents face?
21. Explain why a person might be obese but not overweight.
22. What do you learn from a skinfold test?
23. What is the main reason people gain weight?
24. What health risks are associated with being underweight?
25. How does exercise promote healthy weight?
26. List the steps in smart weight control.
27. Why does yo-yo dieting make permanent weight loss difficult?
28. What are five clues to an unsound weight-loss diet or product?

LESSON 2

29. What are four signs of anorexia nervosa?
30. What are the behavioral differences between bulimia and anorexia?
31. What is the best high-performance diet for sports?
32. Why is fasting an unhealthy way to make weight for sports competition?
33. Why is carbohydrate loading not recommended for teenage athletes?
34. How much fluid should a person drink to replace 2 pounds (0.9 kg) of weight lost through perspiration?
35. Can vitamin pills give a person extra energy? Why or why not?

LESSON 3

36. What conditions promote the growth of bacteria in food?
37. Who is especially vulnerable to foodborne illness?
38. What illness is associated with bulging canned foods? What is the risk?
39. Why can vitamin pills taken in large doses be unhealthy?

REVIEW

Thinking Critically

LESSON 1

40. Synthesis. Besides overeating, what personal habits could lead to the problem of obesity?

41. Evaluation. Why do you think many people fail in their attempts to lose weight?

42. Analysis. From what you know about the characteristics of high-caloric and low-caloric foods, make a list of snacks for each category.

43. Analysis. Why are teenagers urged to eat at least 1,400 calories a day in a weight-loss eating plan?

44. Analysis. Compare dieting the right way with dieting the wrong way.

LESSON 2

45. Synthesis. Discuss how the pressures faced by today's teenagers might lead to eating disorders.

46. Synthesis. How should you respond to someone who says, "Athletes need more protein than other people do"?

LESSON 3

47. Analysis. Why do food service establishments post signs for employees that say, "Wash hands before returning to work"?

48. Synthesis. Describe how you might decrease the risk of foodborne illness if you gave an afternoon barbecue party.

49. Evaluation. Explain how you would judge a food labeled "health food."

Making the Connection

LESSON 1

50. Social Studies. In many parts of the world starvation is the result of poverty, drought, political upheaval, poor transportation, insect infestation, and overpopulation. Choose an area of the world where people are starving, and research the causes, the public health consequences, and the aid provided to the victims.

Applying Health Knowledge

LESSON 1

51. Make an advertisement for a weight-loss program that follows the two basic principles of healthy weight loss.

52. Conduct a survey in your school to find out how teenagers lose, gain, or maintain their weight. Evaluate the responses based on good nutrition.

53. Study one weight-loss plan that is available to the public today. What questions would you ask yourself in determining whether this plan would or would not be a healthy approach to weight control?

LESSON 2

54. Suppose you have a friend who wants to put on a little weight for contact sports. What would you advise? Explain your response.

LESSON 3

55. Present a lesson for preschool or kindergarten children on the importance of washing hands before handling food.

Beyond the Classroom

LESSON 1

56. Community Involvement. Investigate three weight-loss programs available in your community. Judge them based on sound nutritional principles and their ability to sustain long-term weight loss. You might ask a local dietitian for advice.

LESSON 2

57. Community Involvement. Locate reliable services in your community for people with anorexia or bulimia. Learn about their programs, and report to the class.

LESSON 3

58. Further Study. Interview your school's food service director to learn the health department rules for maintaining food safety. Report to the class.

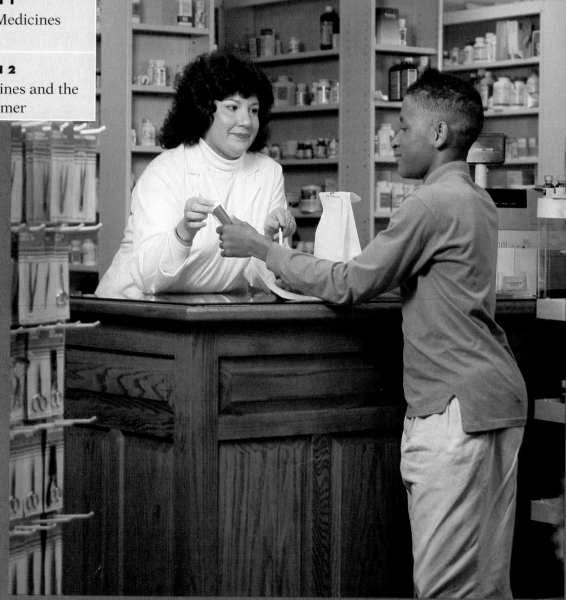

CHAPTER

21

UNDERSTANDING MEDICINES

LESSON 1
How Medicines Help

LESSON 2
Medicines and the Consumer

How Medicines Help

Years ago some people were crippled from polio. Others with tuberculosis spent time in sanitariums, isolated from family and friends. Thousands suffering from smallpox died. Since 1900 many medical discoveries and the development of more effective medicines have provided better treatment and prevention of medical problems. A **medicine** is a substance that, when taken into or applied to the body, helps prevent or cure some disease, injury, or medical problem.

At one time medicines also were called drugs. The term *drug* referred to any substance that, when taken into the body, caused a change in physiological or psychological activity. The term *drug* included medicines—both prescribed and over-the-counter (OTC), legal substances such as caffeine, and illegal substances such as marijuana, cocaine, and heroin. The term *drug* is now used primarily to refer to dangerous and illegal substances. Alcohol and tobacco, which are legal for adults but not for children and teenagers, are also considered to be drugs. Medicines sold on the street for purposes other than those intended by the manufacturer become dangerous drugs. Chapter 24 focuses on these drugs.

Classification of Medicines

Medicines are generally grouped according to their effect on the body. Some of the most widely used kinds of medicines

- prevent disease,
- fight pathogens,
- relieve pain,
- help the heart and regulate blood pressure.

Medicines That Prevent Disease

Your immunization schedule shows a record of what shots or vaccines you were given as an infant, child, and teen. You received these to help prevent you from contracting certain diseases. A **vaccine** contains weakened or dead pathogens of a particular disease. These weakened or dead pathogens stimulate your body to produce specific antibodies against these pathogens. Once these antibodies are produced, they give your body long-lasting protection against these specific pathogens should they enter your body in the future.

Antivenins are blood fluids that contain antibodies and act more quickly than vaccines. Antivenins are produced in animals, such as horses, sheep, or rabbits, in response to an infection or vaccination. The antivenin can then be used to help protect someone against certain diseases or poisonous bites or stings.

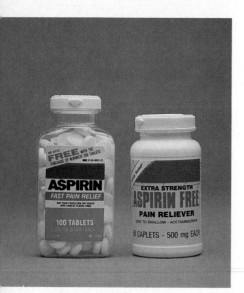

Aspirin and its substitute acetaminophen are medicines that relieve pain.

The American Academy of Pediatrics (AAP) and the Advisory Committee on Immunization Practices (ACIP) issue recommendations for childhood vaccinations.

Medicines That Fight Pathogens

Sulfa medicines were the first disease-fighting medicines discovered. Today sulfa medicines are used to fight urinary tract infections and to treat malaria.

Antibiotics are medicines that kill or reduce harmful bacteria in the body. Antibiotics are made from bacteria, fungi, and some plants. The most commonly used antibiotics are penicillin and tetracycline.

Penicillin is an antibiotic that kills a wide variety of bacteria. It is the most effective and well-known antibiotic. When penicillin was first used, it was known as the wonder medicine because it was so effective in killing bacteria causing strep throat and pneumonia.

Tetracycline is a group of antibiotics used to treat infections and fight many microorganisms. Widespread use of tetracycline has resulted in some microorganisms becoming resistant to the effects of this antibiotic.

Medicines That Relieve Pain

Analgesics are medicines that relieve pain without loss of consciousness. Some can be bought without a prescription. Aspirin is by far the most widely used nonprescription analgesic medicine in the United States. Some 20 billion tablets are sold annually. Aspirin contains a chemical, acetylsalicylic acid, that helps relieve pain and reduce fever. Aspirin is used for headaches, toothaches, and muscular pain. Aspirin is one of the most effective anti-inflammatory medicines; that is why it is so effective with arthritis. Because of aspirin's wide and common use, many people do not realize that aspirin can be dangerous. Even small amounts can irritate the stomach, especially an empty one. Aspirin can interfere with blood clotting, and large doses can cause dizziness and ringing in the ears. Children who take aspirin are at risk of developing Reye's syndrome. Because this is a potentially life-threatening illness of the brain and liver, aspirin should not be given to children when illness with fever is present and undiagnosed.

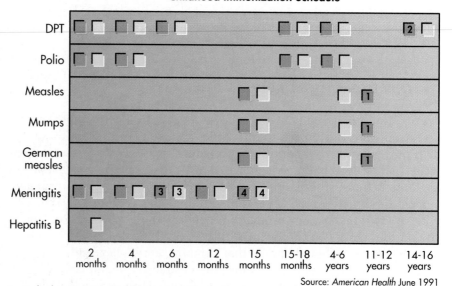

Childhood Immunization Schedule

Source: *American Health* June 1991

1 Earlier booster recommended in the event of local outbreaks.
2 Only for diphtheria and tetanus, not pertussis.
3 Shot may not be required, depending on the vaccine used.
4 May be given at 12 months, depending on the vaccine used.

■ = AAP   □ = ACIP

Some people who are sensitive to aspirin take acetaminophen, an aspirin substitute. It does not contain acetylsalicylic acid and does not cause most of the side effects of aspirin.

Codeine and morphine are much more powerful medicines than aspirin. They are narcotics—medicines that relieve pain and cause sleep by slowing down the brain and central nervous system. Narcotics are used for some types of cancer, pain resulting from severe injury, or for postoperative care. Codeine is often found in cough syrups and analgesics. Only a doctor can prescribe narcotics because they can cause both physiological and psychological dependence.

Medicines That Help the Heart and Regulate Blood Pressure

There are five main kinds of cardiovascular medicines:
- Beta blockers block the action of nerves that constrict blood vessels. This helps slow heartbeat and lower blood pressure.
- Diuretics increase urine production to reduce the amount of water and sodium in a person's body. Removing water from blood vessels helps reduce blood fluid volume. This is particularly important after heart failure.
- Vasodilators dilate the veins and arteries to increase the area for blood and oxygen flow. When there is a decreased blood supply in the arteries because of a spasm, blood clot, or a buildup of cholesterol, vasodilators are very useful.
- Antiarrhythmics are medicines given to help cases of arrythmia—any disturbance in the rhythm of the heart.
- Clot-dissolving medicines work to lower high blood pressure and to prevent blood clots.

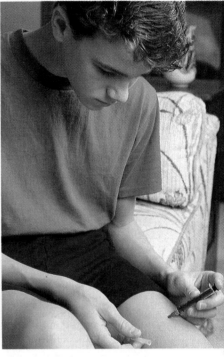

When a diabetic takes insulin intramuscularly, the insulin goes immediately to the bloodstream.

Medicines in the Body

The effect of a medicine in the body depends on the type and amount of medicine a person takes and the method by which the person takes it. If the person swallows a medicine, it goes into the stomach, much like food. Sometimes the instructions on medicine labels will state that the medicine should be taken at mealtime. This allows absorption of the medicine with the least irritation to the gastrointestinal tract. Medicines usually dissolve in the stomach or small intestine. From there they are absorbed into the bloodstream and carried to the liver.

K E E P I N G   F I T

Read Medicine Labels Carefully

Many over-the-counter medicines contain some alcohol. This can be dangerous for alcoholics in recovery who do not want to relapse, or return to alcohol use. It can also be dangerous to others, including young children or people who are about to drive.

Before taking any medicine, read the ingredient label carefully. If a medicine contains alcohol, do not take it if you have to drive or operate machinery. Consult with your doctor to see if there are any alcohol-free alternatives. If there are not, beware. Let someone else drive you where you have to go while you are on the medication.

When a medicine is taken intravenously, in the veins, or intramuscularly, in the muscles, by injection, the effects are much more immediate because the medicine goes directly into the bloodstream and then to the liver. A medicine that is inhaled must pass through the lungs before being absorbed into the bloodstream. A medicine that is sniffed must pass through the mucous membranes before being absorbed.

The Body's Reaction to Medicines

Each person's body chemistry is different. This means medicines will have different effects on different people. Some people experience side effects, or reactions, to certain medicines. They may even be allergic to a medicine. Several factors, including age, weight, and the use of other medicines, influence the effects of medicines. When you have questions about medicines, ask your doctor and pharmacist for accurate information.

HEALTH UPDATE

LOOKING AT THE ISSUES

Generic Versus Brand-Name Medicines

Though some people buy brand-name medicines at some times and generic drugs at others, there are people who feel strongly about choosing one or the other.

Analyzing Different Viewpoints

ONE VIEW. Some people are dedicated to using generic medicines. They cite the fact that they can cost from 30 to 80 percent less than the brand-name versions. In addition, brand-name and generic medicines not only contain the same chemical components, they are also often made by the same companies. Additionally, since generic medicines are so much less expensive than their often better-known alternatives, many people think they are essential in the treatment of the nation's elderly and poor, who otherwise might be even less likely to have necessary medications made available to them.

A SECOND VIEW. Recent reports that not all generic medicines are safe and that there are some abuses in the industry have kept some people from using them. Some critics of generic medicines call for the FDA to have stricter regulations for generic medicines. Other people buying brand names feel more secure dealing with established pharmaceutical companies. Still others claim that with certain medicines, such as thyroid medications, brand names offer greater control of dosages than generic versions.

Exploring Your Views

1. What are the advantages and disadvantages of using generic medicines?
2. The next time you might need a prescription, will you specify that you want a generic medicine or brand-name medicine or simply leave the decision up to your physician and/or pharmacist? Why?

Medicine Interaction

Based on extensive scientific research, scientists can predict side effects that might be expected. These reactions, however, can be quite different when two or more medicines are present in the body at the same time. It is difficult to predict medicine interaction.

When medicines work together in a positive way, an **additive interaction** occurs. For example, both an anti-inflammatory and a muscle relaxant may be prescribed to treat someone with joint pain. A **synergistic effect** is the interaction of two or more medicines that results in a greater effect than when the medicines are taken independently. It occurs when one medicine increases the strength of the other. For example, the analgesic effect of a painkiller increases when cough medicine with codeine is taken at the same time. An **antagonistic interaction** occurs when the effect of a medicine is canceled or reduced when taken with other medicine. For example, someone who receives an organ transplant will take antirejection medicines. If this person is diabetic and takes insulin, the effectiveness of the insulin may be decreased.

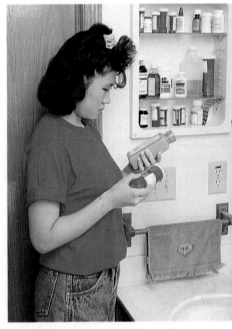

Because of unknown effects, medicines should not be mixed without the advice of a doctor or pharmacist.

Problems Using Medicines

Sometimes people develop dependence on a particular medicine. In psychological dependence, a person believes he or she needs a medicine to feel good or to provide some form of an escape from reality. The medicine may be used to relax, sleep, or feel energetic. Soon the user is unable to relax, sleep, or feel energetic without the medicine.

Physiological dependence is a chemical need for a medicine. Physiological dependence is determined when a person experiences tolerance and withdrawal. **Tolerance** means the body becomes used to the effect of the medicine. The body then requires larger doses of the medicine to produce the same effect. **Withdrawal** occurs when the person stops taking a medicine to which he or she is physiologically dependent. Withdrawal symptoms include nervousness, insomnia, severe nausea, headaches, vomiting, chills, and cramps. These symptoms gradually ease or disappear after a period of time off the medicine. Withdrawal from certain medicines may require medical attention.

LESSON 1 REVIEW

Reviewing Facts and Vocabulary

1. Define the term *antibiotic* and list what antibiotics are made of.
2. Describe when withdrawal occurs and give examples of symptoms.

Thinking Critically

3. **Analysis.** Explain the difference between medicines and drugs.

4. **Analysis.** Compare psychological and physiological dependence. Give specific examples of each.

Applying Health Knowledge

5. Research the major health threats today and compare them to the leading killers 100 years ago. What are the differences? How can you account for the differences?

LESSON 2

MEDICINES AND THE CONSUMER

Throughout history in the United States, there have been medicines that did people little or no good. Because some of these medicines were actually harmful, the federal government set up a system for protection of the consumer.

Two forces regulate the use of medicines and drugs: the Food and Drug Administration (FDA) and increasing consumer awareness of what is available on the market.

Governmental Control

A consumer receives accurate information about the effectiveness and labeling of medicines from the FDA. In the United States all medicines must meet specific FDA standards before being approved and made available to the public.

The FDA requires a manufacturer of medicines to supply information about the chemical composition, the intended use, the effects, and the possible side effects of a medicine. Medicines are usually tested on animals first and then with different experimental groups of people. Since the FDA requires information about the long-term effects of a medicine, it takes about five years for a manufacturer of a medicine to meet all FDA requirements. The FDA decides which medicines require a doctor's prescription and which can be sold as OTC medicines. OTC medicines are safe to use without a doctor's supervision.

The FDA also controls all of the advertising of prescription medicines. These advertisements are generally found in medical journals and magazines because doctors make the decisions about particular prescription medicines to use. Laws also govern the advertising of OTC medicines. These advertisements cannot imply results that the medicines cannot provide.

When the FDA approves a medicine, it is saying that the medicine is safe when used as directed. FDA approval also means a medicine is effective in treating the illness or condition for which it was prescribed.

The FDA assists the consumer in using medicine properly by requiring companies to put certain information on all medicine labels. OTC medicine labels include more information than prescription medicines because they are self-prescribed and self-administered.

The FDA has many controls, but there are still risks and responsibilities when using medicines. **Medicine misuse** is using a medicine in a way that is not intended. Examples of medicine misuse include
- giving your prescription medicine to someone else,
- taking too much or too little of a medicine,
- taking someone else's medicine,
- discontinuing use of a medicine without informing one's doctor,
- taking medicine for a longer period of time than was prescribed,
- mixing medicines.

THE CONTROLLED SUBSTANCES ACT

The purpose of the Controlled Substances Act was to set guidelines for the distributors of medicines and to prevent improper use of medicines. As a result, medicines for use in the United States were categorized into five schedules based on their potential for improper use.

	Use of Medicine
Schedule I	Research only No current accepted medical use in United States Risk involved in use
Schedule II	Obtain with written prescription No refills Severe restrictions on medical use Improper use may lead to psychological or physiological dependence
Schedule III	Obtain with written or oral prescription Refill up to five times in six months Has accepted medical use Improper use may lead to high psychological or low physiological dependence
Schedule IV	Written or oral prescription Refill up to five times in six months Has accepted medical use Improper use may lead to limited psychological or physiological dependence
Schedule V	OTC or prescription limited to doctor's order Has accepted medical use in treatment Improper use may lead to limited psychological or physiological dependence

CONFLICT RESOLUTION

It seems to Maryann that there's a new and improved allergy medicine on the market almost every year for her sister's hay fever. However, for her own rare, congenital eye disease, which is slowly depriving her of her sight, there's virtually no research being done. Maryann and her parents think that if more people were aware of her disease and others like it, more pressure could be given to companies to search for a treatment or cure.

Can you think of ways Maryann and her family could increase public awareness of her disease?

Over-the-Counter Medicines

OTC medicines include a wide variety of medicines you can buy without a doctor's prescription. These medicines can be purchased in pharmacies and other stores that sell medicines. They are not as strong as prescription medicines. However, any OTC medicine has the potential of being harmful if it is not used as directed.

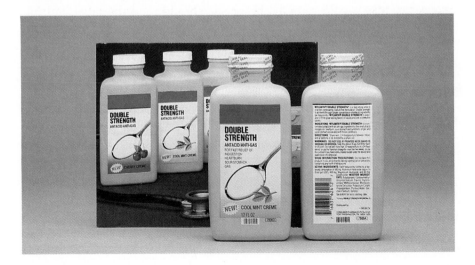

The FDA governs the advertising and labeling of OTC medicines.

OTC Medicines for Colds

Your nose is dripping, your eyes are watering, your head aches—you have a cold and want relief. You can find shelves of nonprescription cold remedies. There are hundreds of them, and people spend millions of dollars a year trying to cure their colds. The fact is, although cold remedies may relieve your symptoms, only time will cure a cold.

A virus in the respiratory system causes colds. When this pathogen invades your body, special cells release a substance called **histamine.** This natural body substance causes the blood vessels in the respiratory tract to dilate. It also causes tissues to swell, which accounts for a stuffed-up nose and a seepage of fluid into surrounding spaces. This causes a runny nose and watery eyes.

When taken orally, cold remedies containing antihistamines block the effects of the histamine. They can reduce swelling and a runny nose for up to 12 hours. They also can reduce sneezing and watery eyes. Antihistamines in decongestants relieve sinus congestion.

A person using an antihistamine should check the label closely. One side effect of most antihistamines is drowsiness. In addition, cold remedies containing antihistamines often contain a variety of other chemicals.

OTHER CHEMICALS IN COLD REMEDIES

Some or all of the following chemicals are often included in cold remedies:
- caffeine, a stimulant to counteract the drowsiness
- aspirin or acetaminophen, medicine to lower fever and relieve aching and inflammation
- codeine to suppress a cough
- antacids to counteract the burning quality of aspirin and nauseating effect of antihistamine

All of this information points to the fact that just because a product is sold over the counter does not mean that the consumer should not take precautions or consider side effects or possible dangers. If a person chooses to take a cold remedy, he or she should read the label and follow the directions for use.

K E E P I N G   F I T

Ask the Right Questions About Prescribed Medicines

Ask your doctor and pharmacist these questions before taking a prescription medicine:
- Why is the medicine being prescribed?
- Was the dosage tailored to your body's needs?

- Is this dosage the lowest possible level to be effective?
- What are the benefits and side effects of this medicine?
- Are there printed instructions?
- Is this medicine compatible with other medicine you take?

- When, how often, and how long should the medicine be taken?
- Is there a less expensive, yet still effective, generic medicine?
- Are there any storage requirements?
- Are there any food restrictions?

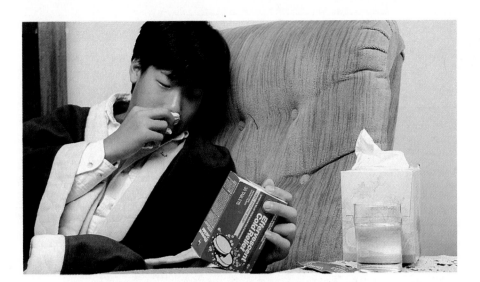

Prescription Medicines

Prescription medicines require more controls because of their strength and potential harm. A prescription is a doctor's written order to a pharmacist to give a certain medicine to a patient. Only a physician can order them, and only a licensed pharmacist can sell prescription medicines.

Cautions about Medicines

Certain precautions should be taken with all medicines. Keep in mind the following guidelines for safe use of medicines.

- Keep medicines out of the reach of children. If anyone, particularly a child, takes a large dose, get medical help immediately.
- Do not use medicines for extended periods of time without medical supervision. If symptoms persist or unexpected symptoms develop, see your physician right away.
- Read the label on the container carefully. It will tell you how much medicine to take and when and how to take it.
- Do not take any medicine that contains aspirin if you are allergic to aspirin or have ulcers or a bleeding problem.
- Seek medical help immediately if you experience any bleeding or vomiting of blood after taking aspirin.

DID YOU KNOW?

- The average number of new approved medicines available to the consumer per year in the United States is about 25.
- Of every 5 medicines trying to be approved, only 1 makes it.
- In the U.S. there are over 1,000 pharmaceutical companies.
- The states that produce the most pharmaceuticals are New Jersey, New York, and Pennsylvania.

K E E P I N G   F I T

Avoiding Quacks

Medical quackery can result in a waste of money. Even more serious, it can result in injury, illness, or death. Be on the lookout for the following:

- "secret formula"
- "miracle cure"
- "overnight results"
- "limited offer"
- endorsements by stars
- availability only through mail order
- foreign medicine not usually available in the U.S.
- passionate testimonials of those supposedly "cured"
- hard-sell approaches

Overcoming The Odds

Lorenzo Odone is 13. As a small child, he spoke three languages and traveled to 16 different countries. These days, Lorenzo is an opera fan, loves to have the classics read to him, and still understands three languages. His mother, Michaela Odone, speaks with pride of her son's accomplishments. Unfortunately, Lorenzo can no longer speak. He is hearing impaired, and he cannot walk. His father, Augusto Odone, explains. "Our son was struck by a little-known, very rare disease. The medical establishment told us that he was going to die, and that he had about two years." Lorenzo's parents began a passionate search for a cure for the disease. They succeeded, inventing a treatment that saved his life.

The rare genetic disease that Lorenzo has is called ALD, which weakens, paralyzes, and kills young boys.

Refusing to accept the doctors' death sentence for their son, the Odones began doing extensive medical research. "We talked to everyone," Lorenzo's father says. "The world is large. There are other towns, other countries. We called everywhere." The next step was to get these experts from around the world together to brainstorm about the disease and its treatments. "We

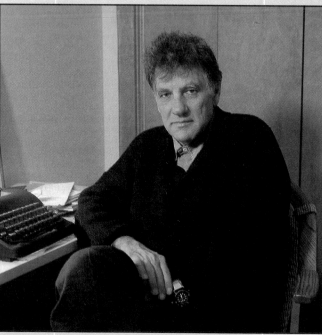

organized the first international symposium on the disease," he continues. "This gave us ideas, and after gathering information, our next step was action."

Based on others' research and their own research and ideas, Augusto Odone eventually hypothesized that a combination of oleic acid and erucic acid might be the answer. He tested the oil on members of his wife's family, who are carriers of the disease. The experiment worked. "Then I immediately gave it to Lorenzo," he says. "In three weeks, his blood was normalized."

The treatment was not a cure, however. It did not reverse the symptoms already under way, but it stopped them in their tracks and kept Lorenzo from dying. The Odones have named the edible oil mixture "Lorenzo's Oil" in honor of their son, and it has now been patented. Still an experimental medicine in this country, the FDA has given permission for a U.S. doctor to prescribe the oil to patients with the disease. In addition, its use has been adopted in other nations, including the Imperial Institute of Neurology in Japan and a major children's hospital in London, England. So far, 30 boys with ALD have taken Lorenzo's Oil. All remain symptom-free.

Mrs. Odone advises young people to become responsible health consumers, to ask tough and thorough questions about their conditions and their treatment. "Don't run out and make your own medicine," she advises. "But do develop a very critical sense about what is being done to you."

1. How is the way you deal with doctors or experts in other areas of your life related to your level of self-esteem?
2. For what reasons do you think people sometimes accept the opinions of the experts as the final word without questioning them?

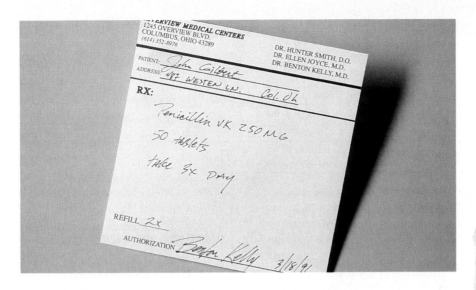

HELP WANTED

Pharmaceutical Sales Representative

If science is your love, but sales is your game, maybe your career should be selling our products to doctors and hospitals. We need people who can sell in a highly competitive environment, but who have the scientific background to understand our products and the professional qualities to relate to our sophisticated clientele. High ethical standards, intelligence, an assertive attitude, and the ability to communicate are musts. You will likely have extensive college training in business as well as the sciences, especially chemistry. Experience in a medical field is a plus.

The Pharmacist

A **pharmacist** is a person concerned with the preparation, distribution, and sale of medicines. A pharmacist is trained in medical therapy and therefore knows what a medicine is supposed to do and what adverse effects can occur. Pharmacists keep a profile of all medicines someone takes. The pharmacist can then monitor potential medicine interaction or medicine misuse. A pharmacist can fill your prescription, inform you of any side effects or precautions to take when using the medicine, and indicate the directions for taking the medicine.

Your pharmacist can provide the following information about prescriptions:

- the name and dosage of the medicine
- how and when it is to be taken
- possible side effects
- whether a prescription can be refilled
- whether an available generic medicine can be substituted
- what the shelf life of a medicine is—how long it can be kept before it becomes ineffective or dangerous
- how to store the medicine
- whether two or more medicines can be taken together safely.

LESSON 2 REVIEW

Reviewing Facts and Vocabulary

1. What is the role of the FDA?
2. Define the term *histamine* and tell when it is released.

Thinking Critically

3. **Analysis.** Compare medicines with brand names with generic medicines.

4. **Synthesis.** Suggest possible reasons why a physician, not a pharmacist, is licensed to write prescriptions.

Applying Health Knowledge

5. Interview a pharmacist to determine what questions consumers most often ask about their medicines. Draw conclusions about how active consumers are in their own health care.

Self-Inventory

Using Medicines Carefully

HOW DO YOU RATE?

Number a sheet of paper from 1 through 15. Read each item below, and respond by writing *MT* if the statement describes you most of the time, *ST* if the statement describes you some of the time, and *N* if the statement never applies to you.

1. I try at least one healthful way to relieve physical discomfort before taking an OTC medicine.
2. I use OTC medicines only when necessary.
3. I use only one kind of medicine at a time, unless otherwise instructed by my physician.
4. If I am not sure about a medicine, I ask my parent, physician, or pharmacist.
5. I ask my physician for information about a medicine that is being prescribed for me.
6. I read all the enclosed information and follow the directions carefully when taking medicines.
7. I never take someone else's prescription medicines.
8. I take prescription medicine only according to my doctor's advice.
9. I check the expiration date on all medicines before taking them and properly dispose of those that are out of date.
10. I check all OTC medicines to see that the tamper-proof seal has not been broken.
11. I keep all medicines away from younger children.
12. I keep myself informed about types of medicines, the effects on the body, and their proper use.
13. I alert my parents or physician immediately if side effects occur when taking medicines.
14. I do not take OTC medicines for an extended period of time without my doctor's knowledge.
15. I compare the ingredients and prices on generic and brand-name medicines.

HOW DID YOU SCORE?

Give yourself 2 points for each statement that describes you *most of the time*, 1 point for each statement that describes you *some of the time*, and 0 points for each *never* response. Find your total, and read below to see how you scored. Then proceed to the next section.

23 to 30
Excellent. Keep it up. Your behavior and knowledge concerning medicines is healthful.

15 to 22
Good. You exercise some caution when taking medicines, but could improve your knowledge of medicines.

7 to 14
Fair. While you are acting carefully in some ways, you are omitting some important precautions that would protect you and others.

Below 7
Poor. You could be taking some unnecessary and dangerous risks with medicines.

WHAT ARE YOUR GOALS?

If you received an *excellent* or *good* score, complete the statements in Part A. If your score was rated *fair* or *poor*, complete Parts A and B.

Part A

1. I plan to learn more about medicines by ____.
2. My timetable for accomplishing this is ____.
3. I plan to share my information about medicine with others by ____.

Part B

4. The behavior I would most like to change is ____.
5. The steps involved in making this change are ____.
6. My timetable for accomplishing this is ____.
7. The people or groups I will ask for support and assistance are ____.
8. My rewards for making this change will be ____.

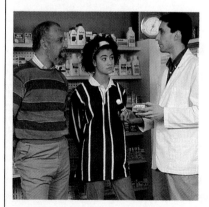

Building Decision-Making Skills

*H*eather has suffered from severe allergies for which her allergist has prescribed regular injections and a nasal spray that has a steroid ingredient that violates the school's athletic policy. Heather was a good athlete long before taking the medication, and this particular medicine does not have a performance-enhancing element. What should Heather do? Some of her choices are:

A. Find a different therapy or medication that does not violate the policy.
B. Ask for an exception to the policy, pointing out the fact that it is prescribed by a doctor for a legitimate medical situation and not for performance-enhancing purposes.
C. Challenge the system in court.
D. Use the medication and try not to get caught.

WHAT DO YOU THINK?

1. **Choices.** What other options does Heather have?
2. **Consequences.** What are the probable consequences of each of the choices given?
3. **Decision.** Which strategy do you think Heather should choose? Explain your answer.
4. **Evaluation.** How will Heather know whether or not her decision was a good one?
5. **Evaluation.** Have you ever been affected—positively or negatively—by a bureaucratic policy that seemed very arbitrary and wrong to you? What did you do about it? Describe the situation, how it turned out, and what you would do differently the next time.

*L*ucia's twin, Alicia, has missed school again, complaining of a migraine headache. Lucia realizes Alicia has headaches but doesn't think they have ever been diagnosed as migraines. Alicia treats herself by taking over-the-counter medicine in excessive doses and going to bed. It seems to Lucia that these headaches occur at very convenient times, such as before school tests and unpleasant social situations. Lucia finds this especially irritating because her parents won't allow the girls to miss school for just any reason. Her sister is getting around the rule by being dishonest. How should Lucia handle this situation?

WHAT DO YOU THINK?

6. **Situation.** Is this a problem with which Lucia should concern herself?
7. **Choices.** If so, what are the possible solutions Lucia has for handling the situation with her sister?
8. **Consequences.** What are the advantages and disadvantages of each solution?
9. **Decision.** Which solution should Lucia choose?
10. **Evaluation.** How do you think Lucia will know whether or not her decision was a good one?

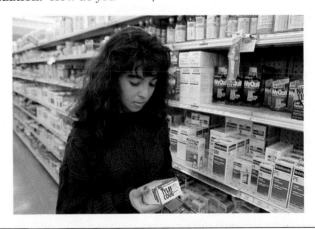

REVIEW

Using Health Terms

On a separate sheet of paper, write the term that best matches each definition given below.

LESSON 1

1. Blood fluids that contain antibodies and act more quickly than vaccines.
2. Medicines that relieve pain and cause sleep by slowing down the brain and central nervous system.
3. Interaction in which two or more medicines react with greater potency than each would when taken independently.
4. Antibiotic once known as the "wonder medicine."
5. Condition in which one's body becomes used to the effect of a medicine.
6. Antibiotic used in place of penicillin.
7. The most commonly used nonprescription analgesic medicine in the United States.

LESSON 2

8. Substance released in one's body when a cold virus invades the respiratory system.
9. A person trained in the preparation, distribution, and sale of medicines.
10. Using a medicine in a way that is not intended.

Building Academic Skills

LESSON 2

11. **Writing.** Using animals to test products is a controversial issue. However, some people believe that using animals to test medicines is necessary. Take a stand and write an editorial for your school or local newspaper.
12. **Reading.** Occasionally, an FDA approved substance becomes the subject of controversy. In recent years, red dye number 5 was one such substance. Research this substance or a current controversy involving the FDA. (News magazines are a good source.) Decide what position the news magazine has taken. Cite supporting facts and details.

Recalling the Facts

LESSON 1

13. What is the active ingredient in aspirin? What is aspirin used for?
14. What factors affect how one's body will interact with medicine?
15. How has the meaning of the term *drug* changed over the years?
16. What are the most widely used medicines used for?
17. Name and describe three types of medicine interactions.
18. Define psychological dependence.
19. Define physiological dependence.
20. Where and why are antivenins produced?
21. When does withdrawal take place?
22. What are the symptoms of withdrawal?
23. What is a vaccine?
24. How does a vaccine work?
25. Name four ways in which medicine can be taken into the body.

LESSON 2

26. How do OTC medicines differ from prescription medicines?
27. How long does it usually take for a medicine to be approved by the FDA?
28. What information must a manufacturer of medicines provide to the FDA?
29. What controls does the FDA place on the advertising of OTC medicines?
30. List four ways in which medicine might be misused.
31. Medicines are categorized into five schedules. How did this come about?
32. What are common chemicals found in OTC cold medicines?
33. Tell why generic medicines are just as good as those with brand names.
34. List five things a pharmacist can tell a person about a prescription.
35. What does FDA approval of a medicine mean?
36. What information is always given on OTC medicine labels?
37. What do cold medicines actually do?

REVIEW

Thinking Critically

LESSON 1

38. Analysis. How would you answer a person who said that vaccines are dangerous substances because they contain pathogens?

LESSON 2

39. Evaluation. Do you think it is better to have a government agency or a privately owned company regulating approval of medicines? Support your answer.

40. Analysis. In later stages of development, experimental medicines are often tested on groups of people. Where do you think these groups of people come from? What would be the ramifications of being in this experimental group?

41. Evaluation. Sometimes insurance companies will not pay for a prescription if a generic equivalent was available but not dispensed. Do you feel this is justified? Support your answer.

42. Evaluation. What is the role of the Food and Drug Administration in monitoring medicines? Do you think this role should be altered in any way? Explain your answer.

Making the Connection

LESSON 1

43. Math. Study a newspaper or a magazine. Determine the percentage of ads for medicines. Display this information in a pie graph.

44. Home Economics. Conduct a home safety check by determining if all medicines at home are safely stored and outdated medicines are properly discarded. Summarize your findings and recommendations in writing.

45. Language Arts. In writing, describe one of the dilemmas teens may face in regard to OTC medicines. Then provide three different solutions to the dilemma.

Applying Health Knowledge

LESSON 1

46. If you had strep throat, the doctor might give you a choice between taking medicine orally or receiving an injection. Which would you choose and why?

47. Give an example of medicines that are taken into the body in each of the four ways described in this chapter.

48. You are watching your 3-year-old sister, and she develops a sudden fever. In the medicine cabinet, you find acetaminophen but the directions on the label only give dosage amounts for children six and older. Should this medicine be given to your sister? Why or why not?

LESSON 2

49. What are some appropriate questions to ask the doctor before he or she writes a prescription?

50. Select an advertisement of a medicine that is used to alleviate pain. Analyze the claims and benefits of the medication and determine the accuracy of the ad. Note ways the ad influences a person's decision to buy the medicine.

51. Look through a magazine and count the number of advertisements for OTC medications. What conclusions can you draw about the public's attitude toward taking medicines to relieve pain? Pick an ad and rewrite it, giving suggestions for relieving a health problem without medicine.

Beyond the Classroom

LESSON 1

52. Further Study. Some people still oppose mass vaccinations and reject these procedures as a requirement for admission to public schools. Is this the right of each family, or is it the responsibility of the school to protect the students? Defend your answer.

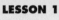

CHAPTER

22

TOBACCO

LESSON 1
Problems for the
Tobacco User

LESSON 2
Choosing Not to
Smoke

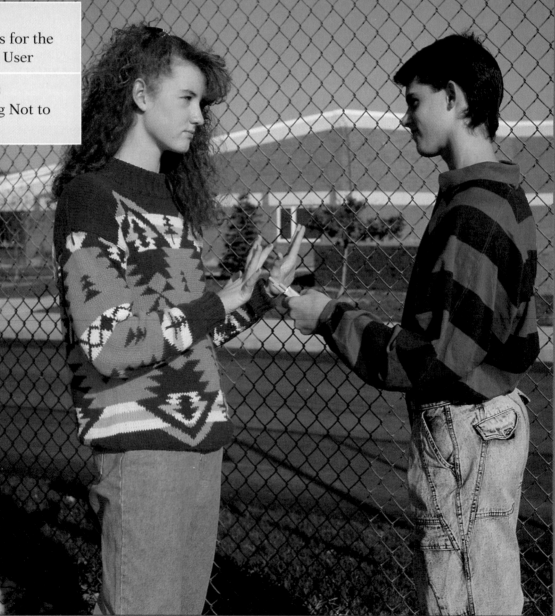

PROBLEMS FOR THE TOBACCO USER

When it comes to using tobacco, there is good news and bad news. The good news is that more and more people are becoming aware of the dangers of tobacco and are giving up the use of tobacco products. Consider these facts:

- At least 30 million Americans have quit smoking.
- An estimated 65 percent of doctors, 61 percent of dentists, and 55 percent of pharmacists who once smoked have now quit.
- In 1965, 40 percent of American adults smoked, while in 1990 that figure dropped to 29 percent.
- During the past 25 years almost half of the adults who once smoked have now given up the use of tobacco.

In short, emphasis on quitting smoking or never starting to smoke increases every day.

The bad news is that there are still some 50 million Americans who do smoke, despite the fact that most of them know of the dangers—from allergies, cancer, and heart and lung disease, to early death. According to the World Health Organization, in developed countries ". . . the control of cigarette smoking could do more to improve health and prolong life . . . than any single action in the whole field of preventive medicine." Yet too many people are still lighting up.

Why Young People Smoke

Every day in the United States 3,000 teens start smoking. Even though the media and schools keep sending out the message that tobacco use is hazardous to one's health, teens are smoking, chewing, and dipping tobacco in large numbers. Consider these facts:

- Teenage females are smoking more than ever before. The number of teenage females who smoke has doubled over the past 20 years.
- It is estimated that about 15 percent of 12- to 17-year-olds use cigarettes.
- In national samples of high school seniors, 13 percent of males and 12 percent of females describe themselves as daily smokers.
- One-quarter of high school seniors who smoke had their first cigarette by sixth grade, one-half by eighth grade.
- Over the last 20 years, the age at which teens start to smoke has continued to fall.
- According to the Centers for Disease Control and Prevention, an agency of the United States Public Health Service, each year an estimated 1 billion packs of cigarettes are sold to people younger than 18—even though it is against the law in many states.

According to U.S. Surgeon General Antonia Novello, "If current smoking rates were to continue in the United States . . . . 5 million children now living in this country would die of smoking-related diseases."

LESSON 1 FOCUS

TERMS TO USE
- Nicotine
- Stimulant
- Tar
- Carcinogens
- Carbon monoxide
- Leukoplakia

CONCEPTS TO LEARN
- Tobacco use is a major cause of illness and death.
- Being in the company of smokers is risky behavior.

ATTITUDES AND BEHAVIORS TO EVALUATE
- Self-Inventory, page 454.
- Building Decision-Making Skills, page 455.

Several recent studies have found that passive smoke, the smoke inhaled by nonsmokers, is dangerous. As a result, efforts to discourage cigarette smoking are increasing.

Some people who continue to smoke complain of being treated as social outcasts. For this reason, some experts suggest a kinder attitude toward smokers. They argue that nicotine addiction is a medical problem, and smokers need treatment, not isolation.

What additional efforts can be used to discourage cigarette smoking and not have smokers feel like social outcasts?

So why do teens ever start to smoke? One major reason some teens smoke is that they feel insecure in social situations. Before they begin smoking, some teens believe that puffing on a cigarette will somehow remove their fears or insecurities, something a cigarette simply cannot do.

Teens may smoke because of peer pressure. Or they may smoke because advertising on billboards and in magazines has made them associate a particular brand with the attractive models pictured.

Teens may smoke because they think the bad effects of smoking on health occur only after many years of smoking. They may not realize that health risks begin from the moment the cigarette smoke from that first cigarette enters the body.

Perhaps the greatest reason young people smoke is that they believe that they can drop the habit at any time. They do not realize that for many smokers, smoking is no habit; it is an addiction that is difficult to shake. Still, some teens realize that people sometimes get addicted to cigarettes, yet feel certain that they are the exception and can stop at any time.

In a large survey of teens who smoke, half claimed they either definitely or probably would not be smoking after five years. They viewed it as a passing habit. The problem is that after five years of smoking, many of these same teens found that they had an addiction to cigarettes. Addiction includes physiological or psychological dependence. Many adult smokers who began smoking as teens are still at it because they are addicted.

Cigarettes

With each puff of a cigarette, a smoker comes in contact with more than 4,000 chemicals, and at least 43 of these are known to cause cancer. But the chemicals in tobacco can cause other ailments as well. Tobacco contains **nicotine,** the addictive drug in cigarettes. People smoke to reduce the craving for nicotine, which is a poisonous stimulant. A **stimulant** is a drug that increases the action of the central nervous system, the heart, and other organs. Nicotine raises blood pressure and increases heart rate.

The flavor of a cigarette is due mostly to the tar in tobacco. **Tar** is a thick, sticky, dark fluid produced when tobacco burns. Several substances in tar are known **carcinogens,** cancer-causing substances. Tar penetrates the smoker's airways and lungs. Combined with the drying

K E E P I N G   F I T

The Benefits of Being a Nonsmoker

Nonsmoking means
- being able to take a deep breath,
- tasting food and having the full sense of smell,
- having good endurance during physical activity,
- using money for other things,

- preventing bad breath and having a clean mouth,
- unstained teeth and fingers,
- having hair and clothes that smell fresh,
- being free from addiction to nicotine,

- reducing the risks of heart disease, cancer, and leading respiratory diseases,
- taking pride that you are part of a growing, health-conscious no-smoking movement.

effect of cigarette smoke, tar paralyzes or destroys cilia, the waving hair-like projections that work to keep the respiratory tract clear.

Carbon monoxide is a colorless, odorless, poisonous gas in cigarette smoke that passes through the lungs into the blood. This is the same gas in automobile fumes that, if inhaled, could prove fatal. It unites with the hemoglobin in red blood cells, preventing them from carrying the oxygen needed for energy to the body's cells.

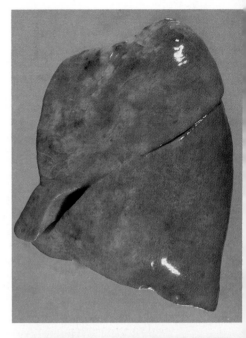

Pipes and Cigars

Like smoking cigarettes, smoking pipes and cigars also presents major health risks. Pipe and cigar smokers usually inhale less smoke, yet they are more likely to develop cancers of the lip, mouth, and throat because more tar and other chemicals are generated by pipes and cigars. If the pipe or cigar smoker makes it a habit to inhale the smoke, his or her chances of lung cancer also increase.

Specialty Cigarettes

Specialty cigarettes are those prepared with tobacco and other ingredients. They are often made with strong tobacco and contain spices that make them taste and smell sweet. However, the effects they can have on the body of the user are anything but sweet. Experts say that specialty cigarettes actually contain more cancer-causing tars than standard cigarettes.

The most common specialty cigarette is the clove cigarette, which contains about 60 percent tobacco and 40 percent cloves. Most of these cigarettes are imported from Indonesia and have been used in the United States since the 1970s. Young people started smoking them in the early 1980s. Use of these cigarettes has dropped sharply in recent years for several reasons. There have been complaints of lung problems and possible deaths as a result of smoking clove cigarettes. The ingredient that produces the aroma of cloves anesthetizes the back of the throat and allows deeper inhalation.

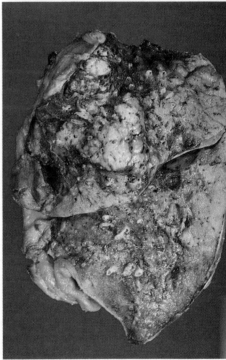

Top: Normal lung.
Bottom: Cancerous lung.

Smokeless Tobacco

Use of smokeless tobacco has increased, especially among teenagers. Many people believe that using smokeless tobacco is safer than smoking it. These users claim it is safer because they are not taking in smoke or putting smoke into the air. In addition, advertisements using famous people to promote smokeless tobacco have contributed to an increase in its use, especially among teenagers. The picture of a cowboy or an athlete using smokeless tobacco gives the impression that chewing and dipping contribute to one's masculinity. They do not. Instead, they contribute to one's ill health. The fact that many teens who use smokeless tobacco started chewing tobacco or dipping snuff when they were between the ages of 13 and 15 means that they can develop serious health problems early in life. Some of those health problems include mouth sores that can turn into cancer of the lip, mouth, or throat; damage to teeth and gums; and damage to the digestive system.

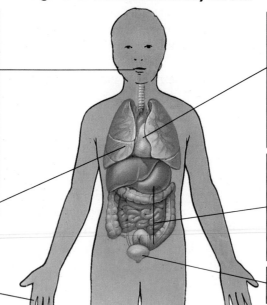

Mouth. Just one cigarette causes "cigarette breath" and dulls the taste buds. The hot smoke is harmful to the mouth and throat tissues. Cigarette smoking plays a major role in causing cancer of the oral cavity and larynx.

Teeth. Tar stains the teeth, causing brown spots.

Bronchioles. As smoke is drawn into the respiratory tract, harmful gases and particles settle into the surrounding membranes (bronchioles). One point of great concentration is where the bronchus divides into left and right bronchi. This is also where most lung cancer begins.

Lungs. Efficiency decreases.

Fingers. Cigarettes cause yellow stains on fingers.

Cardiovascular system. Nicotine causes blood vessels to constrict, forcing the heart to pump faster and increase blood pressure. Smokers have a higher death rate from strokes. Smoking is also a risk factor in the development of cardiovascular disease, affecting the circulation in the arms, hands, feet, and legs.

Gastrointestinal tract. Cigarette smoking appears to be connected to increased illness and a higher death rate from peptic ulcers. Cigarette smoking reduces the effectiveness of standard ulcer treatment and slows the rate of ulcer healing.

Bladder. Smokers have a greater risk of bladder cancer than nonsmokers.

Dangers of Smoking

Every day in the United States at least 1,000 people die from diseases caused from smoking. Cigarette smoking is responsible for well over 400,000 deaths in the United States each year.

Smoking and the Respiratory System

Cigarette smoking is a major factor associated with the two principal diseases that make up chronic obstructive pulmonary disease (COPD). These are chronic bronchitis and pulmonary emphysema, which are 10 times more likely to occur among smokers than among people who do not smoke.

Chronic bronchitis is a condition in which the bronchi are irritated. As cilia become useless, tar from cigarette smoke builds up, which results in chronic coughing and excessive mucous secretion of the bronchial tree.

Pulmonary emphysema involves the destruction of the tiny air sacs in the lungs through which oxygen is absorbed into the body. As the walls between the sacs are destroyed, they lose their elasticity, becoming larger and thus providing less total surface from which oxygen can be absorbed. More breaths are required, and instead of using 5 percent of one's energy in breathing, a person with advanced emphysema uses up to 80 percent of personal energy just to breathe.

Lung cancer, directly linked to cigarette smoking, is the leading cause of cancer deaths among males. With the increase in female smokers, lung cancer is becoming a more significant cause of cancer death among females, too.

Lung cancer begins as the bronchi are irritated by cigarette smoke. Cilia are destroyed and extra mucus cannot be expelled. The smoker develops a cough. Cancerous cells can grow in these conditions, block the bronchi, and move to the lungs. In advanced stages, cancerous cells can travel to other organs through the lymphatic system.

DID YOU KNOW?

According to *Prevention's Giant Book of Health Facts:*

- About 75 percent of deaths from lung cancer among women are caused by smoking.
- On average, a cigarette smoker is 10 to 15 times more likely to get lung cancer than a nonsmoker.
- Someone who smokes 2 or more packs of cigarettes a day is 20 to 25 times more likely to die from lung cancer.
- A male smoker who is between 30 and 40 years old can expect to lose about 8 years of his life because of smoking.

Overcoming The Odds

Todd and Ramon have been friends since junior high. They live in the same apartment building. They're on the same basketball team. They like to hang out together. Todd and Ramon have also been smoking together since eighth grade—at least until recently.

Not long ago Todd's dad was diagnosed with lung cancer. He was a two-pack-a-day smoker and thought nothing of it. Ramon's grandmother, a chain smoker, has emphysema. She can barely make it up the stairs. Both boys have seen firsthand what smoking can do to a person.

Then Todd's dad told him he was really sorry he'd ever set such a bad example for him by smoking all those years, and he begged Todd to stop smoking so he wouldn't end up like him—losing weight and gasping all the time—because of cigarettes. Todd decided to take action.

"I asked Ramon if he'd give up smoking, too," Todd says. "Ramon said he'd try but he didn't know for sure if he could do it. He said his grandmother had been trying to quit for 20 years, but he'd give it a shot.

"We worked out a system for helping each other," says Ramon. "We made a pact. We decided we'd call each other or just drop in at least three times a day—unannounced—to make sure the other guy wasn't cheating. My sister said we should write up a contract

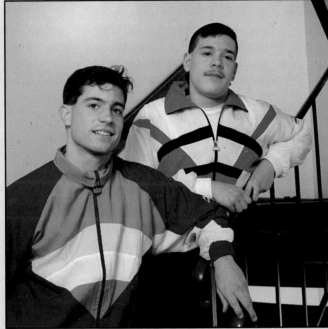

and sign it, but we told her we didn't need one—that we took each other's word for it."

Todd and Ramon started running in the park every day after school instead of hanging out with the other smokers. They cut down on the number of cigarettes gradually, and on the day of the last cigarettes, they chucked their ashtrays in the dumpster in a little ceremony. "We promised if we made it through the first week, we'd buy each other a new tape," says Todd, "and if we made it through the month,

we'd buy each other tickets to the play-offs. That took away some of the pain."

The first few days Todd says he felt like he would jump out of his skin. Ramon described it as feeling like his fingers were plugged into a socket.

Todd chewed packs and packs of gum. Ramon bit down on what seemed like hundreds of lollipop sticks but then, they actually started to feel better—calmer, less strung out than before.

It's been over four months now for Ramon. Todd, after one slip, is back on track, helping out his dad, and staying away from the cigarettes. He's running better than ever now, beating everybody's times, and his coach is talking about helping him apply for an athletic scholarship. "What I started out doing for my dad," he says, "I'm now doing for myself."

1. What factors motivated Todd and Ramon to try to stop smoking?
2. What strategies did they use for stopping? Do you think these methods will work over time? Why or why not?
3. How do you think this experience has affected their self-esteem? Their friendship?

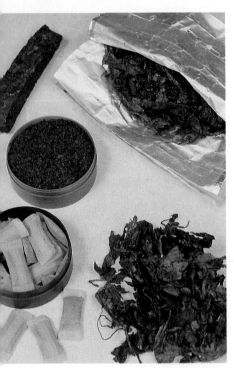

Smokeless tobacco can present some serious health problems.

Smoking and the Circulatory System

You already know that nicotine makes the heart work harder and speeds up the pulse. Smoking constricts blood vessels, which cuts down on the circulation, or blood flow, to the limbs. This can result in a tingling feeling in a smoker's hands and feet. Nicotine contributes to plaque buildup in blood vessels. The formation of these fatty deposits in the arteries increases the chance of arteriosclerosis, or hardening of the arteries, and gradually clogs the blood vessels to the heart. This condition increases the risk of heart attack.

Cigarette smoking also damages the heart. The risk of sudden death from heart disease is three times greater for smokers than nonsmokers. This risk increases for those who smoke more than a pack a day.

Smoking raises blood pressure and leads to increased risk of stroke. If a smoker has high blood pressure and high cholesterol, the risks of coronary heart disease are even greater. Experts estimate that if all Americans stopped smoking, deaths from heart diseases could be cut by almost a third, saving more than 20,000 lives a year.

The Dangers of Smokeless Tobacco

Although smoke does not get into the lungs, smokeless tobacco presents other health problems, some of which can be serious, even life-threatening.

The nicotine in smokeless tobacco is as addictive as the nicotine in cigarettes. Once a person starts chewing and dipping, it can become very difficult to stop.

KEEPING FIT

Sixteen Good Reasons Not to Light Up

- lung cancer
- bad breath
- throat cancer
- yellow teeth
- stained fingers
- premature wrinkling of the skin
- birth defects
- irritated eyes
- increased heart rate
- increased blood pressure
- emphysema
- increased bronchitis
- sinus problems
- increased cholesterol, even as a teen
- lower life expectancy
- often being treated as a social outcast

SMOKING, APPEARANCE, AND SOCIAL HEALTH

Smoking not only can harm a person's insides, it can damage a smoker's outsides, too. In fact, cigarette smoking may be hazardous to a person's looks.

How? For one thing, it can yellow the smoker's teeth and stain the fingernails and fingers that hold cigarettes. In addition, according to a new study at the University of Utah, smoking can triple the average person's likelihood of getting wrinkled skin early. Heavy smokers studied were 5 times more likely to develop premature wrinkles than nonsmokers. According to the study, people who smoke and sunbathe have even greater wrinkling risks. They are 12 times more likely to develop wrinkles earlier in life than nonsmokers.

Smoking also causes bad breath, a smoke odor on clothes and in hair—as well as in a car, house, or workplace. All of this can have a negative impact on one's social health.

People who use smokeless tobacco have more saliva. Although the chewers usually spit out the saliva, they do swallow some without realizing it. This introduces tar and other chemicals into the digestive and urinary systems. Tobacco juices also contain chemicals that may delay healing of wounds.

Tobacco and its by-products are extremely irritating to the sensitive tissues in the mouth. Irritation from direct contact with tobacco juices is responsible for **leukoplakia,** thickened, white, leathery-appearing spots on the inside of a smokeless tobacco user's mouth. These areas can develop into cancer of the mouth.

Smokeless tobacco users also tend to show greater tooth wear than nonusers. The gums tend to be pushed away from the teeth where the tobacco is held. The roots of the teeth become exposed and more susceptible to decay. Dip and snuff products may cause people to lose their teeth while they are still young. Users of smokeless tobacco also develop bad breath and discolored teeth. Tobacco products decrease the user's ability to smell and taste, especially salty and sweet foods.

LESSON 1 REVIEW

Reviewing Facts and Vocabulary

1. Give three reasons some teens smoke.
2. Write a paragraph identifying some of the dangers of smoking, using the words *nicotine, carcinogens,* and *carbon monoxide.*

Thinking Critically

3. **Evaluation.** Do you think a doctor has the right to refuse to treat a person for a disease related to smoking if the individual refuses to quit smoking? Why or why not?

4. **Synthesis.** What would be the health risks to someone who smokes cigarettes *and* uses smokeless tobacco?

Applying Health Knowledge

5. Design a label that could be put on cigarette packs to alert the potential smoker to the many hazards of smoking.
6. Write a public service announcement for your school on the dangers of using any form of tobacco.

CHOOSING NOT TO SMOKE

LESSON 2 FOCUS

TERMS TO USE

- Passive smoke
- Mainstream smoke
- Sidestream smoke

CONCEPTS TO LEARN

- There are many successful approaches to stopping smoking.
- Smokers must recognize their personal desire to quit and believe they are in control.

ATTITUDES AND BEHAVIORS TO EVALUATE

- Self-Inventory, page 454.
- Building Decision-Making Skills, page 455.

Increasingly, people who smoke cigarettes, pipes, and cigars are frowned upon by nonsmokers. They may be asked to move or to leave places where smoking is prohibited. More likely, individuals bothered by their smoke may simply cast them dirty looks or get up and move. In short, smoking can make a person feel like an outsider with strangers and friends—sometimes even in the smoker's own home.

In addition, many people object to the smell of smoke on hair or clothes. Even people who have already extinguished a cigarette, cigar, or pipe may experience disapproving looks from people who find the odor their tobacco has left behind offensive.

There is increasing concern and interest in the United States and around the world that the nonsmoker is being affected by the smoke of those using cigarettes, pipes, and cigars. In a recent report by the Environmental Protection Agency (EPA), it was estimated that being exposed to others' smoke kills 53,000 nonsmokers in the United States every year. In fact, passive cigarette smoke has recently been classified as a cause of cancer in its own right, and it is now considered the nation's third-leading preventable cause of death.

Environmental Tobacco Smoke

Each year the evidence grows that people who breathe someone else's cigarette smoke can receive the same unhealthy effects as the person who smokes. **Passive smoke** is cigarette, cigar, or pipe smoke inhaled by nonsmokers. It is also smoke that remains in a closed environment after the smoker is through smoking. Passive smoke includes **mainstream smoke,** what a smoker blows off, as well as **sidestream smoke,** what comes from burning tobacco.

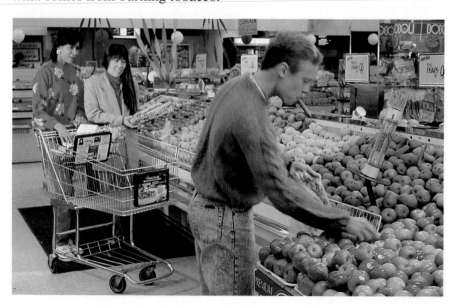

Passive smoke is cigarette, cigar, or pipe smoke inhaled by nonsmokers. Passive smoke is offensive to nonsmokers.

Passive smoke contains large amounts of the same harmful ingredients as the smoke inhaled into a smoker's lungs. However, mainstream smoke may contain less nicotine and tar than sidestream smoke. This may be because sidestream smoke is hotter than mainstream smoke and has not been filtered through the cigarette.

A smoke-filled room may have levels of carbon monoxide and other pollutants as high as those that occur during an air pollution emergency. A nonsmoker could inhale enough nicotine and carbon monoxide in an hour to have the same effect as having smoked a whole cigarette.

Passive smoke causes eye irritation, headaches, and coughing. It causes more frequent ear infections, asthma attacks, and other respiratory problems, and aggravates existing heart and lung diseases, including lung cancer. Lengthy exposure to these conditions can result in the same kinds of health problems that the smoker may experience. Consider these facts:

■ New studies indicate that passive smoke not only makes existing heart disease worse; it can actually cause it.
■ Nonsmokers who live with smokers have a higher risk of dying from heart disease than do nonsmokers.
■ An estimated 37,000 people die annually from heart disease directly caused by passive smoke.
■ At least 3,700 people die annually from lung cancer and 12,000 from other forms of cancer because of exposure to others' smoke.

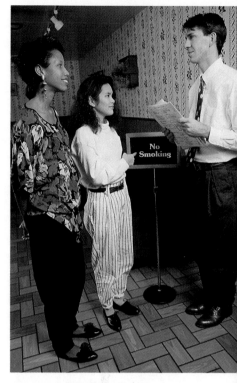

Most restaurants provide non-smoking sections.

Smoking During and After Pregnancy

Cigarette smoking during pregnancy is associated with small fetal growth, an increased chance of spontaneous abortion and prenatal death, increased stillbirths, and a low birth weight, as well as growth and developmental problems during early childhood. Babies born to mothers who smoked during pregnancy may be adversely affected in intellectual development and behavioral characteristics.

Nicotine constricts the blood vessels of the fetus in the mother's uterus as carbon monoxide reduces the oxygen level in the mother's and fetus's blood. Smoking is especially harmful during the second half of pregnancy. After the baby is born, nicotine can be transferred during breast-feeding.

Most people would not give a child a cigarette, but people who smoke around children are doing the same damage to these youngsters that they would if they were helping them light up.

K E E P I N G F I T

Getting Smoke-Free: Some Things that Help

If you want to give up cigarettes, consider these steps:
■ Decide once and for all that you want to quit.
■ Make a list of what smoking is costing you, in terms of money, health, appearance, and social acceptance.
■ Set a target date for quitting and stick to it.
■ Cut down on the number of cigarettes gradually.
■ Begin an exercise program.
■ Plan some fun to fill your time.
■ Ask a friend to quit with you. Offer one another daily—or even hourly—support.
■ Plan a healthy way to reward yourself when you have achieved a smoke-free status.

A federal study of 47,000 households shows that children of cigarette smokers are nearly twice as likely to be in poor or fair health as the children of nonsmokers. Among their ailments, they have more bronchitis and other respiratory problems. They have poorer lung function and a higher incidence of wheezing.

In addition, children of parents who smoke have twice the chance of developing lung cancer as children of nonsmokers.

Rights of the Nonsmoker

Despite the growing awareness of the dangers of passive smoke, nearly half of all smokers light up without asking those around them if they mind. According to a recent medical report, even though at least 80 percent of nonsmokers report that they are bothered by passive smoke, only about 4 percent actually ask smokers to stop. Because of the dangers of passive smoke, that fact has to change. You can help change it.

You have a right to express that you prefer that people not smoke around you. By doing so, you protect the air you breathe and the air of those around you. If you are allergic to smoke or the smell of it makes you sick, it is particularly important that you learn to speak up and let people know.

If you are out in a restaurant, ask for the nonsmoking section or at least ask to be seated away from smokers. If you are a member of some group or club, ask that no smoking be allowed during meetings or at least that the smokers sit near ventilated areas or windows.

It is considerate of smokers to ask others in an enclosed area if they mind their smoking. It is also important that smokers avoid smoking in very small or poorly ventilated areas, or in the presence of small children or people with allergy, lung, or heart problems. In fact, smokers should take responsibility to smoke elsewhere whenever nonsmokers are around. When they do not, nonsmokers also should take responsibility for their own health by asking smokers to extinguish their cigarettes or by moving to a smoke-free space.

Kicking the Habit

More and more people are taking responsibility for their health by giving up the use of tobacco. Giving up tobacco can be tough, but there are many ways to stop and many places that offer support and help with the process.

A person who wants to quit using tobacco should be reminded that he or she will probably go through a period of withdrawal. As you remember, withdrawal occurs when something on which a person is physiologically dependent is no longer used. During this period the person might feel nervous, moody, or have difficulty sleeping. These symptoms of withdrawal do not last long.

Some people may use a series of filters over a period of weeks to stop smoking. Each filter reduces the tar and nicotine levels so that withdrawal is gradual. Other people get a prescription from their doctors for gum that contains nicotine. The aim is to gradually cut down on the amount and frequency of gum use until they are eventually nicotine-free. A nicotine patch that is prescribed can also be used. This patch, placed on the body, gives off decreasing amounts of nicotine. The

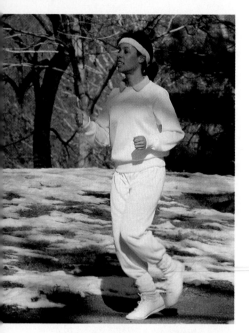

Concentrating on an exercise program, such as running, is one way to overcome the urge to smoke.

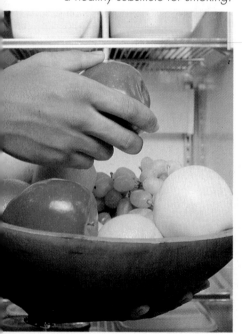

Snacking on nutritious foods is a healthy substitute for smoking.

smoker can give up cigarettes while withdrawing gradually from the nicotine. Many people combine several of these approaches and techniques to get and stay tobacco-free. In addition, there is a variety of support groups for people to join when they want to stop smoking and need group support to do so.

Tips for Quitting

Those who want to quit smoking might take these steps:

- Identify the times when they usually reach for a cigarette out of habit.
- Change their daily routine so that they avoid situations that trigger smoking.
- Avoid people who smoke and situations that are conducive to smoking during the first few weeks.
- Make a list of the reasons they want to quit smoking, post it around the house, and read it when they feel like smoking.
- Chew sugarless gum, suck on sugarless candy, or munch on carrot sticks or other healthy snacks when they feel a desire for cigarettes.
- Drink plenty of water to flush out toxins.
- Avoid alcohol, coffee, tea, and colas for a while because these substances often stimulate the craving for tobacco.
- Exercise frequently.
- Think in terms of quitting for a few minutes, then an hour, and then a day, saying things to themselves like, "I choose not to smoke during this hour," or "I have to do this only one day at a time."
- Take deep breaths to aid relaxation when the craving to smoke gets strong.
- Brush their teeth often to remove tobacco residue.
- Stop buying cigarettes by the carton; buy them by the pack instead.
- Set a final target date for being tobacco-free and stick with it.
- Make a ceremony out of smoking the last cigarette, and declare their intentions to family and friends.
- Get rid of smoking reminders, such as ashtrays, matches, and lighters.
- Plan rewards for themselves each time they resist lighting up.
- Become aware of improvements in how they feel, in their senses of smell and taste, and in how they look.
- Get positive reinforcement and support from nonsmoking friends.
- If they relapse, or go back to smoking, know that they are not failures and that they can try to quit again.
- Think about all of the benefits of being smoke-free.

Culturally Speaking

Toward a Smoke-free World

- In Canada, very high taxes on cigarettes now put the price of a carton of cigarettes at about $40.
- Because of these high taxes on cigarettes, the number of smokers in Canada continues to fall.
- Thailand has a ban on all cigarette advertising. Because of this, tobacco use is less common than in most Western countries.
- Singapore is holding a campaign to make itself a nation of nonsmokers.
- The French National Assembly called for a halt to all tobacco advertising by 1993.
- By 1990, all print advertising for tobacco products was outlawed in Australia.

K E E P I N G   F I T

More Ways to Give Up Smoking

- Surround yourself with people who support your decision and who, themselves, don't smoke.
- Decide how many cigarettes you will smoke that day. Stick to that plan.
- Find a substitute to put in your mouth such as sugar-free gum.
- Don't buy cartons of cigarettes.
- Ask nonsmoking friends what it's like for them to breathe your smoke.
- Try to stay smoke-free one day at a time.
- Have your teeth cleaned.
- If you do smoke again, don't give up. Many people have relapses. Start again on the smoke-free trail. It's worth it.

HEALTH UPDATE

LOOKING AT THE ISSUES

The Debate Over the Sale of Tobacco to Minors

Today in the United States, 45 states and the District of Columbia have laws that outlaw the sale of tobacco to people younger than 18. Now there is a move by many groups to get laws passed to raise the age to 21.

Analyzing Different Viewpoints

ONE VIEW. Some people are opposed to such laws. They think that it is unfair to single out teens when 18-year-olds can perform other adult responsibilities, such as enlist in the military.

A SECOND VIEW. Other people claim that these laws could not be properly enforced. They claim that despite statewide bans on tobacco sales for minors, it is still very easy for most teen smokers to buy cigarettes and other tobacco products.

A THIRD VIEW. Still others think that it is necessary to protect the health of the youth throughout the country by passing and enforcing policies that prohibit the sale of tobacco products to minors.

A FOURTH VIEW. Some anti-tobacco activists think that laws alone are not enough. They believe that there should be stiff penalties for stores and store owners that allow the sale of tobacco products to minors. They also recommend that towns and cities issue tobacco-selling licenses that require store owners to sign statements that indicate they know that the sale of tobacco to minors is against the law. People who hold this view advocate that tobacco-selling licenses should then be taken away from those who do not comply with the law.

Exploring Your Views

1. Which of these views seems most reasonable and fair to you? Which seems most likely to protect the health of young people?
2. Do you think tobacco sales should be banned for those younger than 18? Why or why not?
3. Should the buying age for tobacco products be raised to 21? Why or why not?
4. Should this age policy be decided by each state or should there be a uniform nationwide policy? Explain your reasoning.

Weight Gain: A Common Concern

A common concern of smokers is the risk of weight gain if they try to quit. The following information has been reported about people who have faced up to their habit or addiction and quit smoking:

- One-third gain weight because they substitute eating for smoking.
- One-third lose weight because they start a fitness program at the same time they stop smoking. They fill their need for smoking by eating carrot sticks or other low-calorie snacks.
- One-third of those who quit find their weight remains the same.

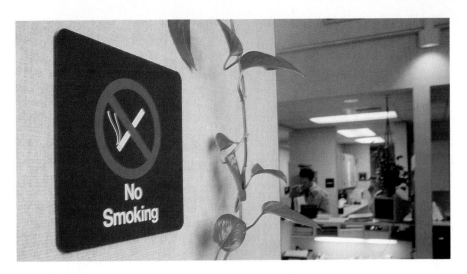

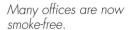
Many offices are now smoke-free.

A Smoke-Free Society

Increasingly, the American public is working toward becoming smoke-free. As people realize that the decision to smoke can affect not only their own health but also the health of loved ones, the drive to become a smoke-free society increases.

There are now whole towns that are banding together to restrict smoking. Tobacco licenses are being revoked by stores and store chains that sell cigarettes to minors. Vending machines are being moved out of unsupervised areas. Many cities are passing laws that restrict smoking in public places, such as in restaurants, civic buildings, business offices, even lobbies. Airplanes now prohibit smoking on commercial flights. Hotels have whole floors for nonsmokers. Laws are being proposed to ban smoking in all enclosed public spaces, and increasingly, the law is on the side of the nonsmoker.

These days smoking is less common in private social settings, too. Meetings of all kinds are now often designated as smoke-free. Even people giving parties no longer put out ashtrays; instead, they ask smoking guests to smoke outside. With continued commitment to health, the remaining bad news about tobacco use can be turned into good news about nonuse as Americans aim toward a smoke-free 2000.

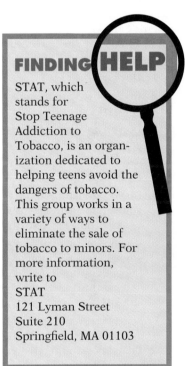

FINDING HELP

STAT, which stands for Stop Teenage Addiction to Tobacco, is an organization dedicated to helping teens avoid the dangers of tobacco. This group works in a variety of ways to eliminate the sale of tobacco to minors. For more information, write to
STAT
121 Lyman Street
Suite 210
Springfield, MA 01103

LESSON 2 REVIEW

Reviewing Facts and Vocabulary

1. What is passive smoke?
2. What are some of the effects of passive smoke on the health of a nonsmoker?

Thinking Critically

3. **Evaluation.** Why do you think people sometimes do not stand up for their rights as nonsmokers?

4. **Synthesis.** In what ways do you predict American society will move toward becoming smoke-free?

Applying Health Knowledge

5. Make a booklet listing the programs and other resources available in your area to teens who want to get tobacco-free.

Self-Inventory

Are You Passive About Passive Smoke?

HOW DO YOU RATE?

Number a sheet of paper from 1 through 15. Read each item below and respond by writing *yes* or *no* for each item. Total the number of *yes* responses for items 1 through 5, 6 through 13, and 14 and 15. Then proceed to the next section.

1. Do you smoke?
2. Do you live with a smoker or smokers?
3. Do you have good friends who smoke?
4. Are you often exposed to other people's smoke?
5. Do you sometimes find yourself in enclosed spaces, where people are smoking?
6. When around people who smoke, do you let them know that you do not like to smell or breathe their smoke?
7. Have you ever given smokers disapproving looks to let them know indirectly that you are bothered by their smoke?
8. Have you ever made negative comments about someone's smoking to others but not directly to the smokers themselves?
9. Have you ever asked people who smoke to extinguish their cigarettes, cigars, or pipes?
10. Have you ever asked smokers to move so that you would not have to breathe their smoke?
11. If a smoker does not stop smoking or move, have you ever moved to a smoke-free space?
12. If you are in a car and someone is smoking, do you roll down the windows?
13. Instead of asking smokers to stop exposing you to their smoke, do you move away from them instead?
14. Are you ever passive about passive smoke, choosing to say and do nothing?
15. Are you afraid that if you speak up and ask a smoker to stop smoking or to move, that the person will laugh at you, get mad at you, or think you are not cool?

HOW DID YOU SCORE?

If you said *yes* to any of the first five questions, you may be at great risk from exposure to smoke.

Now look at your answers for questions 6 through 13. If you said *yes* to none of these, you are in the "passive zone" and need to stand up for your rights as a nonsmoker. If you said *yes* to one or two of these questions, you may be in the passive zone but are at least beginning to stand up for your right to breathe. If you said *yes* to three or four of these questions, you are heading for the "active zone," beginning to stand up for your health and your right to breathe. If you said *yes* to five or more questions, you are in the active zone, where people know they have a right to protect their health from others' smoke.

If you said *yes* to questions 14 and 15, it is very important that you learn to become assertive in standing up for your rights. Now proceed to the next section.

WHAT ARE YOUR GOALS?

If you are in or near the passive zone when it comes to standing up for your rights around smokers, complete Part A. If you are completely in the active zone, complete Part B.

Part A

1. I plan to take a first step in standing up for myself when I am exposed to someone else's smoke by ____.
2. The last time I was exposed to someone else's smoke and did not stand up for my rights, I was passive because ____.
3. I will take the following steps to become less passive and more active about avoiding passive smoke: ____.
4. The benefits will be ____.

Part B

5. I protect myself from exposure to passive smoke in the following ways: ____.
6. I will help others who are afraid or embarrassed to speak up for themselves on the issue of passive smoke by ____.
7. I will continue to give this person support for his or her rights as a nonsmoker by ____.
8. The benefits I will receive from sharing this information will be ____.

Building Decision-Making Skills

Karl is a popular student leader. A group of students in his school, including some of his friends, are lobbying the administration for a smoking area for students. Karl himself doesn't smoke, and he hates the smell of cigarette smoke, but his friends want his support for the idea that having such an area will reduce smoking in the bathrooms. This would eliminate a serious passive smoke problem for nonsmokers. Karl is concerned that, if he endorses the plan, he will be called a "grit," the label attached to the smoking group in the school.

WHAT DO YOU THINK?

1. **Situation.** What decision needs to be made?

2. **Situation.** What issues does Karl have to address in order to make this decision?

3. **Choices.** What possible choices does Karl have?

4. **Consequences.** What are the probable consequences of each choice?

5. **Consequences.** How will others be affected by this decision?

6. **Consequences.** How will Karl's health triangle be affected by this decision?

7. **Consequences.** How might the school board and the school administrators be affected?

8. **Decision.** What should Karl do?

Darlene's boyfriend smokes. She dislikes the fact that his clothes smell, his breath smells, and he spends so much money on cigarettes. She worries about the health risks to both of them, but she is afraid that he'll break up with her if she tries to get him to quit. What should Darlene do?

WHAT DO YOU THINK?

9. **Choices.** List three possible methods of dealing with this problem.

10. **Consequences.** What would be the probable outcome for each?

11. **Consequences.** How might Darlene address the problem and still be sensitive to her boyfriend's feelings?

12. **Situation.** Where might Darlene find help in addressing this problem?

13. **Decision.** What do you think Darlene should do? Why?

14. **Evaluation.** Have you ever faced a similar situation? If so, describe it and tell how you handled it. Would you handle a similar situation differently now? Explain your answer.

15. **Evaluation.** Every nonsmoker has experienced a situation where they have felt that their space was invaded by smoke. If you are a nonsmoker, are there certain situations that bother you? How do you handle these situations? Would you rather do it differently?

16. **Evaluation.** If you are a smoker, how do you feel about nonsmokers' rights? Have you ever been asked not to smoke? What have you done? How will you handle these situations in the future?

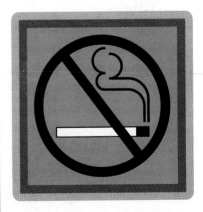

REVIEW

Using Health Terms

On a separate sheet of paper, write the term that best matches each definition given below.

LESSON 1

1. A physiological or psychological dependence.
2. An addictive drug found in cigarettes.
3. The type of drug that increases the action of the central nervous system, the heart, and other organs.
4. A thick, sticky, dark fluid produced by burning tobacco.
5. Cancer-causing substances.
6. A colorless, odorless, poisonous gas found in cigarette smoke.
7. Thickened, white, leathery-appearing spots on the inside of the mouth of a smokeless tobacco user.

LESSON 2

8. A condition characterized by nervousness, moodiness, and difficulty in sleeping, caused by giving up a substance on which a person is physiologically dependent.

Building Academic Skills

LESSON 1

9. **Reading.** Below are three statements describing effects. Write *nicotine, tar,* or *carbon monoxide* as the cause of each effect.

   a. paralyzes or destroys the cilia that help keep the respiratory tract clear
   b. unites with the body's hemoglobins, preventing them from carrying oxygen to the body's cells
   c. increases the action of the central nervous system, raises blood pressure, and increases heart rate

LESSON 2

10. **Writing.** Write a letter to a 14-year-old who has just begun to smoke. Use your best persuasive arguments to convince this person to stop smoking.

Recalling the Facts

LESSON 1

11. Label each statement below *true* or *false.*

    a. Among high school seniors, more males than females smoke.
    b. Between 1965 and 1990, the number of adult Americans who smoked dropped by 11 percent.
    c. More than half of all doctors, dentists, and pharmacists who once smoked have quit smoking.
    d. During the last 20 years, teens who begin to smoke have been doing so at younger and younger ages.

12. According to the Centers for Disease Control and Prevention, about how many packs of cigarettes are sold each year to persons under the age of 18?
13. Who is Antonia Novello?
14. List four reasons some teens start to smoke.
15. What kinds of cancers are more likely to occur in pipe and cigar smokers than in cigarette smokers?
16. What are specialty cigarettes?
17. Are specialty cigarettes generally more or less harmful than standard cigarettes? Why?

LESSON 2

18. Why do many nonsmokers object to living, working, and socializing with smokers?
19. How serious is the threat of cancer from passive cigarette smoke?
20. What is the difference between mainstream smoke and sidestream smoke?
21. List five risks that have been associated with smoking during pregnancy.
22. Is smoking more harmful during the first or second half of pregnancy?
23. List three tips for quitting smoking.
24. What have studies shown about weight change in people who quit smoking?
25. List three places where smoking used to be allowed but is no longer permitted.
26. How does gum that contains nicotine help someone quit smoking?

REVIEW

Thinking Critically

LESSON 1

27. Evaluation. How effective are the warning labels on cigarettes in influencing people not to smoke?

28. Synthesis. Suggest ways that cigarette smoking is a problem for an entire society.

29. Analysis. Compare the amount of energy used for breathing by a person with advanced pulmonary emphysema and the amount used by a healthy person.

30. Analysis. Comment on this statement, "Smoking is the single, most preventable cause of death in the world."

31. Analysis. How addictive is the nicotine in smokeless tobacco compared to the nicotine in cigarettes?

LESSON 2

32. Analysis. How does the risk of developing lung cancer compare for children of smokers and children of nonsmokers?

33. Synthesis. Develop a list of protective measures that a nonsmoker can put into place to live in a smoke-free environment.

34. Evaluation. Three of your best friends have started to smoke. You have several choices. You can stop seeing these people. You can start smoking yourself, or you can try to convince your friends to quit. How will you decide what to do?

35. Evaluation. America is striving for a smoke-free society by the year 2000. What do you think about this goal?

Making the Connection

LESSON 2

36. Social Studies. Research the influence of tobacco production and sales on the United States economy. Something to consider: How would a ban on cigarette smoking affect tobacco growers and tobacco manufacturers? If cigarette smoking were banned, how would this affect the health of United States consumers?

Applying Health Knowledge

LESSON 1

37. You've noticed that some of the other members of the high school baseball team have begun chewing tobacco. They say professional players do it, and they are not hurting their lungs. What could you tell them about the effects of chewing tobacco?

LESSON 2

38. Which of the following would be good advice to give a person who wishes to quit smoking? Write *yes* for each one that should help. Write *no* for those that probably won't help. Give reasons for your answers.

   a. Eliminate foods and beverages that stimulate the craving for tobacco, such as alcohol and beverages that contain caffeine.

   b. Keep your intention to quit smoking a secret from friends and relatives.

   c. Stay away from other people who have quit smoking.

   d. Spend some time with people who still smoke to build up your resistance.

   e. Eat healthy snacks when you feel a desire to put a cigarette in your mouth.

   f. Drink lots of water to flush toxins from smoking out of your system.

   g. Brush your teeth often so your mouth will feel clean.

   h. Start an exercise program.

Beyond the Classroom

LESSON 1

39. Community Involvement. Interview 10 people who smoke or used to smoke. Choose people from different age groups. Prepare a list of questions to ask them about their smoking habit. Draw conclusions about your findings.

40. Parental Involvement. Ask your parents about changes in the smoking policies at work. Report your findings to the class.

CHAPTER

23

ALCOHOL

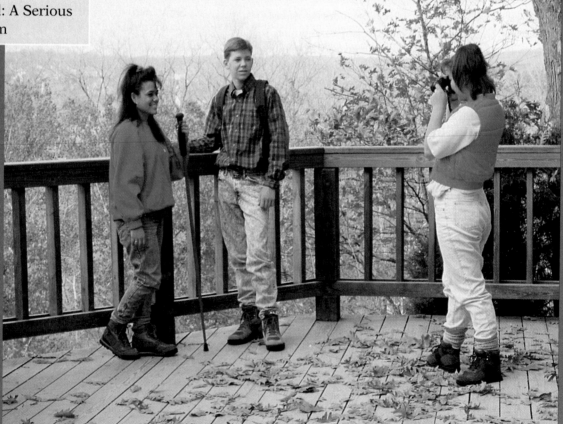

ALCOHOL: A PHYSICAL PROBLEM

E thyl alcohol, also known as ethanol, is the type of alcohol found in alcoholic beverages, such as beer, wine, and liquor. It can be made synthetically, or it can be produced naturally by fermentation of fruits, vegetables, or grains. Fermentation is the chemical process that produces alcohol through the action of yeast on sugars.

The source of the sugar varies from drink to drink. In beer, malted barley is the sugar source; in wine, it is berries or grapes; in whiskey, it is malted grains, such as rye or corn. Potatoes are the source of sugar for vodka; molasses, the source for rum.

All alcoholic drinks are only partly alcohol. The rest is water, flavoring, and minerals. Beer is 4 to 6 percent alcohol; wine, 12 to 20 percent; and liquor, 40 to 50 percent. Yet there is the same amount of alcohol in 12 ounces (355 ml) of beer, 5 ounces (148 ml) of wine, and 1 1/2 ounces (44 ml) of liquor.

Alcohol provides little of the taste but all of the intoxicating effect in alcoholic beverages. Because alcohol contains calories, it is a food substance. However, it is of little or no nutritional value. The term *empty calories* is often used with such food substances. Because of its effects on the body, alcohol is considered a drug.

How Does Alcohol Work in the Body?

When someone has a drink, the alcohol follows the same path that food does as it travels through the digestive system. About 20 percent of the alcohol passes directly into the blood from the stomach. So within minutes after a person takes a drink, some alcohol is circulated throughout the body. The majority of the alcohol passes into the small intestine, where it is absorbed into the blood.

Some of the effects of alcohol are short-term, or immediate. Others are not seen for some time, perhaps even years. These are called long-term effects.

Immediate Effects

Alcohol affects several parts of the body immediately. Several factors are involved, such as the amount of alcohol consumed, the size of the person, and whether or not there is food in the person's stomach.

Brain. Alcohol reaches the brain almost as soon as it is consumed. It depresses the activity of the brain, slowing the work of the nervous system. Thought processes are disorganized, and memory and concentration are dulled.

Liver. The liver, in a process called oxidation, changes alcohol to water, carbon dioxide, and energy. The liver can oxidize only about 1/2 ounce (15 ml) of alcohol an hour. There is no way to speed up this pro-

---

LESSON 1 FOCUS

TERMS TO USE
- Fatty liver
- Cirrhosis (suh•ROH•suhs)
- Multiplier effect

CONCEPTS TO LEARN
- Alcohol affects many parts of the body.
- Regular use of alcohol can result in tolerance and dependence.

ATTITUDES AND BEHAVIORS TO EVALUATE
- Self-Inventory, page 474.
- Building Decision-Making Skills, page 475.

■ *Blitzed* and *bombed* are two words still used to mean "drunk." But just as the state of drunkenness isn't funny, neither is the derivation of these words. They were first introduced during the Blitzkrieg, or German bombings of London during World War II—deadly pursuits, just as drunkenness can be.

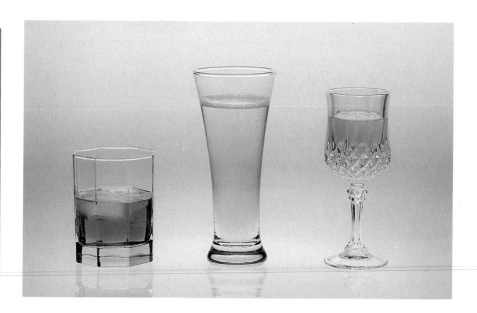

1½ oz of 80 proof liquor is equal to 12 oz of beer or to 5 oz of wine. "Proof" is an indicator of the concentration of alcohol in a beverage. The higher the proof, the greater the intoxicating powers of the alcoholic beverage.

cess. Until the liver has time to oxidize all the alcohol, the alcohol keeps circulating through all body parts.

Blood Vessels. The blood carries the alcohol to all parts of the body, including the heart, liver, and brain. When alcohol enters the blood, it causes the blood vessels to dilate or widen. The result is an increased flow of blood, especially to the skin. This makes the skin feel flush and warm. However, it is an artificial warmth. The increase of blood flow near the surface of the skin causes the body to lose heat by radiation—body temperature actually decreases. Alcohol causes an increase in heart rate and an increase in blood pressure.

Kidneys. Alcohol affects the kidneys by causing them to produce more urine. (This is done indirectly. Alcohol affects the pituitary gland, which, in turn, acts on the kidneys.) This is one reason a person feels dehydrated the day after heavy drinking.

Stomach. Because the alcohol molecule is very small and water soluble, it does not have to be digested. It can be immediately absorbed into the blood from the stomach. Having food in the stomach slows the

K E E P I N G   F I T

Alcohol and Tobacco: A Smoking Gun

The harmful physical effects of alcohol are well-known. So are those of tobacco. But combining alcohol and tobacco can cause added health risks. Overconsumption of alcohol and cigarettes has recently been linked to increased risks for various kinds of cancer, including cancer of the larynx, esophagus, and mouth.

absorption process. Even so, food will not keep a person from getting drunk if he or she drinks too much. Alcohol increases the flow of gastric juices from the stomach lining. Larger amounts of alcohol cause a larger flow of these high-acid juices, irritating the stomach lining. Repeated irritation can cause an open sore called an ulcer.

Long-Term Effects

There are several long-term effects of alcohol use.

Tolerance. Regular use of alcohol may result in tolerance, making it necessary to drink more and more in order to produce the same effects. As tolerance develops, a person may drink an increasing amount without appearing to be intoxicated. The person may continue to function reasonably well until some severe physical damage results or until he or she is hospitalized for some other reason. Then the individual will experience withdrawal, symptoms that occur when the person stops drinking alcohol. These symptoms range from jumpiness, sleeplessness, sweating, and poor appetite to tremors, convulsions, and hallucinations.

Dependence. Some people become physiologically dependent on alcohol. The body develops a chemical need for alcohol. Physiological dependence is marked by tolerance and withdrawal. The symptoms of withdrawal are so unpleasant, a person tends to drink more alcohol in order to avoid the symptoms. As a result, the level of tolerance increases.

Liver Problems. Alcohol interferes with the liver's ability to break down fats. As fats build up in the liver, a condition known as a **fatty liver** develops. This increased amount of fat prevents the normal work of the

Alcohol in the Body

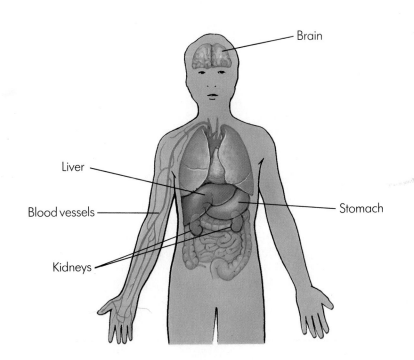

Brain

Liver

Blood vessels

Kidneys

Stomach

Alcohol affects various parts of the body.

- Alcohol is used by more Americans than any other drug. It is estimated that at least 1 in 20 Americans is addicted to alcohol.
- On average, alcohol shortens the life of an alcoholic by 10 to 12 years.
- One recent study of juveniles in jail indicated that 40 percent of them had been under the influence of illegal drugs and 33 percent had been under the influence of alcohol when they committed crimes.

liver cells. It also interferes with the growth of new liver cells. As a result, old liver cells are not replaced as quickly as they normally would be. The excess fat in the liver blocks the flow of blood in the liver cells, resulting in reduced oxygen, and eventually, cell death. This condition has been found in both moderate and heavy drinkers. It can be reversed when drinking stops.

Heavy alcohol use destroys liver tissue, which is then replaced with useless scar tissue. This condition is called **cirrhosis** of the liver. *Cirrhosis* means "scarring." There is no blood flow in the scarred area because there are no blood vessels, so the work of the liver is greatly reduced by cirrhosis. The symptoms of cirrhosis are high blood pressure, hemorrhages, abdominal swelling, tendencies toward infection, and a jaundiced appearance. Jaundice can be recognized by a yellowing of the skin or eyes.

Brain Damage. Long-term, excessive use of alcohol invariably leads to major brain damage. People have been hospitalized in mental institutions for severe brain damage caused by excessive alcohol use. Even moderate drinking can destroy brain cells. There can be a loss of intellectual abilities, such as remembering and problem solving. These losses can be enough to interfere with everyday functions.

Mixing Alcohol with Other Drugs

The interaction that occurs when a person takes alcohol with other drugs or medicines is called the **multiplier effect.** Alcohol is a depressant drug. When a person takes another depressant, such as a tranquilizer, with alcohol, the effects can be drastic. Impairment of both mental and physical abilities result. Many accidental deaths result from combining alcohol with other drugs or medicines. Some multiplier effects are not always predictable.

Both over-the-counter medicines like aspirin and prescription medicines can alter the way that alcohol affects the body. Medicines that might cause reactions with alcohol have warnings on their labels. The labels warn about drinking any alcoholic beverages while using the medicine.

LESSON 1 REVIEW

Reviewing Facts and Vocabulary

1. Name the major parts of the body that alcohol affects and tell how it affects them.
2. Explain what is meant by the *multiplier effect.*

Thinking Critically

3. **Analysis.** Compare the short- and long-term effects of drinking alcohol.

Applying Health Knowledge

4. Find two different magazine or newspaper advertisements for alcoholic beverages. How do they compare? What do they not tell you?
5. Consider the impact of labeling every alcohol container with the word *drug.* How do you think this would affect alcohol use or attitudes toward alcohol?

ALCOHOL: A MENTAL AND SOCIAL PROBLEM

In 1991 the average American drank 23 percent less hard liquor, 14 percent less wine, and 7 percent less beer than in 1980. What do these statistics have to do with you? At this stage of your life, you will undoubtedly be faced with increased pressure to use alcohol. You can learn about all the problems associated with drinking and the effect of alcohol on the body. However, what really matters are the decisions you make in regard to alcohol. Those decisions can mean the difference between life and death.

Why Young People Drink

The reasons that teenagers give for drinking often are not very different from the reasons that adults give:

- to escape pressures or problems
- to feel better; to get over being sad or lonely
- to relax
- to gain more self-confidence
- to get away with something that they are not supposed to do
- to fit in

Friends are often an important influence on a teenager's choice to drink. There is pressure to drink, and it can be very difficult to say no, especially when you want to be accepted as part of the group.

The family is another major influence on teenage drinking behavior. The example the family sets regarding drinking has much to do with the

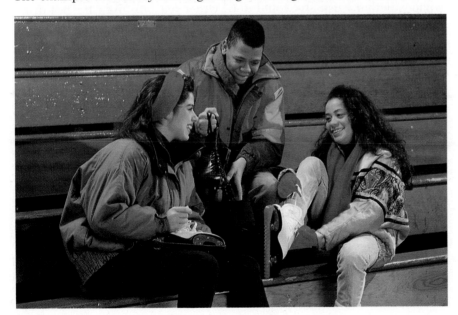

There are many ways to have a good time without alcohol.

A Nonalcoholic Drink, Please. . .

Evidence shows that early in human history, fermentation of sugar-containing mashes (crushed grains) was discovered, and alcoholic beverages became a part of many cultures. Drinking establishments are mentioned in the oldest known code of laws, the Hammurabi of Babylonia, from 1770 B.C. Choosing not to drink alcohol probably has almost as long a history. There are accounts of several attempts made by the Chinese to prohibit alcohol consumption, but all met with incomplete success. Religious prohibitions have been more successful. Buddhists in India have avoided alcohol since the 6th century B.C., as do the members of the Hindu Brahmin caste. The Qu´ran, written in the 7th century, prohibits drinking of alcohol for all faithful followers of Islam.

teenager's attitudes and behavior toward alcohol. If the teenager sees the parents use alcohol when they have problems, or when they want to socialize or celebrate, chances are the teenager will do the same.

Everyone has the need to belong, to feel loved, and to be important. You can go about meeting those needs in many ways. Drinking does not have to be one of them.

THE HIGH COST OF DRINKING

According to the Alcohol, Drug Abuse, and Mental Health Administration, alcoholism and problem drinking cost the economy over $136 billion in 1990 in lost work, accidents, health-care costs and treatments, research, education, and criminal justice costs. In addition, alcohol is

- a major factor in the four leading causes of accidental death in the United States (motor vehicle crashes, falls, drownings, fires and burns).
- a significant factor in 20 to 35 percent of all suicides.
- a factor in family violence, including spousal and child abuse.
- a major reason for marital separation and divorce.

Other facts about drinking are these:

- **Alcohol-impaired driving,** or driving under the influence of alcohol, is the leading cause of death among teenagers.
- The earlier one begins to use alcohol, the greater the chances of using other drugs later in life.
- Each day 11 teenagers are killed and over 350 are injured in alcohol-related car crashes.

Why Young People Choose Not to Drink

So much attention is focused on the reasons for teenage drinking that the nondrinking teenage group is often slighted. Why do millions of young people choose not to drink?

The most common reason given for not drinking is: "I do not need it." Perhaps the person is really saying, "I do not have to drink to be popular," or "I do not need to drink to be accepted, to have fun, or to act in some way that I usually would not." Other reasons given for not drinking include the following:

- It makes me sick.
- I hate the taste.
- It is fattening.

KEEPING FIT

What to Do If a Friend Who's Been Drinking Wants to Drive

- Don't let the person drive.
- Encourage him or her to ride home with a nondrinker.
- Walk the person home.
- Take away the person's car keys.

- Give the person bus, subway, or cab fare.
- Call a safe-rides service.
- Call the person's parents.
- Ask the host's family to let the person spend the night.

Do whatever you can to keep the person from getting behind the wheel. You could be saving your friend's or someone else's life.

- It costs too much.
- It leads to other problems.
- I do not want to lose control.
- I want to enjoy what is going on around me.
- It is harmful to my health.
- My parents are opposed to it.
- I would be breaking training rules.
- In most states, it is illegal for teenagers to buy or possess alcohol.

Negative Social Consequences of Drinking

Bad things can happen as a result of even one drinking episode. The negative consequences can affect not only the drinker but also the drinker's family and friends, as well as anybody else with whom the drinker comes in contact.

Whether drinking is a cause or a symptom, problem drinkers have difficulties with family, friends, school, and police. This situation becomes circular, meaning that if you had some problems at home in the first place, and then started drinking, the drinking would probably lead to more family problems.

Alcohol and Advertising

It is not very difficult to picture what is in a television beer commercial and why such commercials are so popular. Many, if not all, include the following:

- young people who are handsome, attractive, fit, and healthy-looking
- a partylike atmosphere with upbeat music
- an otherwise healthy environment, often in the beauty of the outdoors
- problem-free drinking
- a verbal message that really does not say anything about the product

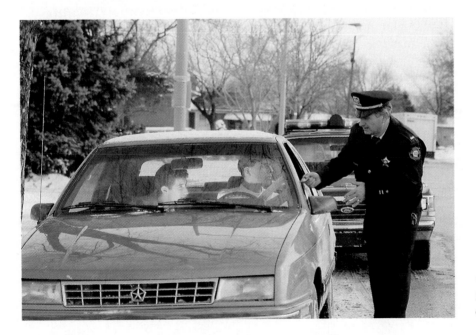

What penalties would these teens suffer for drinking and driving in your state?

Overcoming The Odds

My name is Colleen O'Conner. I want the people who read this book to know that there are teens out there who are popular, who do just fine in school and with friends, and who don't drink. I also want them to know that nothing grizzly out there got me to make the decision. It was more like a whole number of messages that added up over time that made me decide that I wasn't going to drink. And I don't. Sure, you hear in the news that ten or eleven million teens drink beer and other booze. But you don't hear enough about the other half—millions and millions like me who don't. So it's my turn, and I'm taking it.

"I saw what happened to my older brother when he became a teen. One time when he was about 15 he went to this 'All you can drink' party for three bucks. He came home crawling. And he swore he'd never do it again. Barry—that's my brother—had at least one friend who had a DUI, lost his license, had to go for special classes, the works. Then there are all those awful stories about drinking and driving and people losing legs and dying. When they brought a wrecked car to be displayed on the front lawn of our

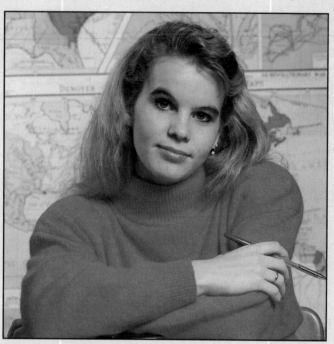

school, I just stood there and stared. It really cut through me.

"In health class we had an alcohol and drug education program. It really hit home that you could mess up your life and the lives of others in a big way if you let the drinking take over. And I guess I just decided one day that I wanted to be in more control than that, that I wanted to be healthy, live a long time, not ruin my life or anybody else's. I guess I 'got it' that nobody sets out to get addicted, but lots of people get that way anyway.

"After that, there was this growing level of disgust in me. Like, why are these people at

the parties I go to doing this to themselves? Seems like it's the only way they know how to fit in or have fun. And I've seen and heard enough about people throwing up or passing out or ending up with people they didn't want to be with or having to drink to get up the courage to do what they don't want to do anyway, and it's . . . well, really sad, I think. And I don't want any of it. Besides that, more and more of my friends are choosing not to drink, so that makes it easier.

"I used to be afraid of being singled out, but now I kind of like it. I let the negative comments roll. But it feels real good when someone knows they can always rely on me to drive because I'll always be able to see the road."

1. In what sense has Colleen "overcome the odds"?
2. What factors contributed to her decision not to drink?
3. What was her fear when she first decided to become a nondrinker?
4. What would Colleen probably do if she were at a party and her friends pressured her to drink and wouldn't take no for an answer?

Is Advertising Effective?

Advertisers spend over $1 billion a year promoting alcoholic beverages. They want to paint an image of alcohol as an aid in successful and problem-free relationships, working situations, and recreational opportunities. Advertisers would not spend that kind of money if the ads did not accomplish their purpose.

It is rare to see a sporting event these days that is not sponsored in part by a liquor or beer company. Car races, boat races, and tennis events are just a few examples.

The brand names of alcohol are in abundance on college campuses where basketball and football scoreboards are sometimes donated to a school just to make the name of the company or product visible.

One of the most effective advertising gimmicks is having the consumer buy products with the name of the company on them. T-shirts and hats are examples of this type of promotion. By wearing the product, a person actually provides free advertising for the company.

You would probably have great difficulty remembering any advertising messages against drinking. While there are some, most are not nearly as appealing as the pro-drinking ads sponsored by the producers of alcoholic products. You need to learn to differentiate the facts from the implied messages in the ads.

You and Your Decisions about Drinking

Drinking alcohol in any form has no place in your life. It is unhealthy, unsafe, and in most places, illegal. As you apply your decision-making skills to the question of drinking or not drinking, you will see that the negative consequences far outweigh any positive benefits. You can live a fun-filled, active, and productive life without drinking alcohol.

CONFLICT RESOLUTION

While fewer teens are trying illegal drugs these days, nine out of ten say they've tried alcohol. The difference is due mostly to positive messages about alcohol in advertising. Many of these messages are aimed directly at young people. There's clearly a conflict between what's good for the alcohol industry and what's good for teens.

Make up a public service announcement for television that shows the risks of alcohol use by teens.

LESSON 2 REVIEW

Reviewing Facts and Vocabulary

1. Identify four reasons young people choose not to drink.
2. What facts make drinking a special problem for teenagers?
3. What does *alcohol-impaired driving* mean?

Thinking Critically

4. **Analysis.** Describe three ways that alcohol is costly to our society.
5. **Analysis.** Select a current magazine and count the number of ads for alcohol products. Select one ad and list the number of facts stated. What are the implied messages? Which message is the strongest? Why do you think purely factual ads are not used?

Applying Health Knowledge

6. How might you react in a healthy way at a party where most people are drinking beer and wine coolers?
7. What might you say to a younger brother or sister you caught drinking beer with friends after school one day?

ALCOHOL: A SERIOUS PROBLEM

LESSON 3 FOCUS

TERMS TO USE

- Fetal alcohol syndrome (FAS)
- Blood alcohol concentration (BAC)
- Alcoholism

CONCEPTS TO LEARN

- The use of alcohol can lead to birth defects, driving accidents, and alcoholism.
- Blood alcohol concentration is affected by several factors.

ATTITUDES AND BEHAVIORS TO EVALUATE

- Self-Inventory, page 474.
- Building Decision-Making Skills, page 475.

For some people alcohol becomes a serious problem—one that changes their lives and the lives of those around them. In some cases the use of alcohol becomes life threatening.

Alcohol and Pregnancy

In recent years scientists have found a link between heavy drinking by pregnant females and birth defects in the babies born to them. This condition, which involves both mental and physical abnormalities, is called **fetal alcohol syndrome (FAS).** FAS is a leading cause of mental retardation in the United States.

FAS babies tend to be shorter and lighter in weight than normal, with impaired speech, cleft palate, general weakness, slow body growth, facial abnormalities, poor coordination, and heart defects.

Mental retardation, poor attention span, nervousness, and hyperactivity are also common in children born with FAS. All of these symptoms are present in some babies, while others may be affected by only some of the problems.

The alcohol the pregnant female drinks moves into her blood, then across the placenta through the umbilical cord into the blood of the unborn child. Any effects felt by the pregnant female as a result of drinking are also experienced by the unborn child.

Unfortunately, the unborn child cannot get rid of the alcohol as an adult can, so the alcohol remains in the baby's body much longer. If the pregnant female drinks three to four times a week, chances are the infant never rids itself of alcohol.

FAS is completely preventable. It does not occur in babies of nondrinking pregnant females. The public is becoming increasingly aware of the dangers of FAS. Each female, knowing the risks, must make the choice—to drink or not to drink.

In 1988 the United States Senate passed a bill that, in part, approved a label that warned of drinking during pregnancy. The warning reads: "According to the Surgeon General, women should not drink alcoholic beverages during pregnancy because of the risk of birth defects."

Drinking and Driving

The most serious and widespread problem involving drinking and the law is that of alcohol-impaired driving. This has become a serious problem for Americans of all ages. It is a problem for the nondrinker as well as the drinker—the nondrinker can easily become a victim in a crash caused by an alcohol-impaired driver.

For teenagers, alcohol-impaired driving is a particular problem. Alcohol-impaired driving is the leading cause of death among teenagers aged 15 to 19.

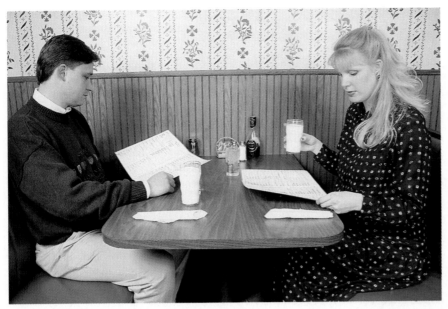

This woman is protecting her unborn child by not drinking any alcohol.

What Effect Does Alcohol Have on Driving?

Driving experts and medical researchers have tested the effects of alcohol on driving and have found that drinking at any level

- reduces the ability to judge distances, speeds, and turns.
- reduces the ability to judge accurately one's own capabilities and limitations.
- increases the tendency to take risks.
- slows reflexes.
- adds to forgetfulness of taking precautions such as using signals when turning.
- reduces the ability to concentrate.

For these reasons, only one who has had no alcohol to drink should drive. Others should always refuse rides with anyone who has had any alcohol to drink.

DWI (driving while intoxicated) and *DUI (driving under the influence)* are two terms for the same situation. Driving while intoxicated means that the person's blood alcohol concentration level exceeds the limit allowed by law in that state.

KEEPING FIT

Drinking and Its Consequences

Increasingly, underage drinking and drinking and driving are being targeted as major social problems. Consider these facts:
- Every state now has a minimum drinking age of 21.
- In more and more states,

drivers' licenses are revoked, or taken away, when drinking and driving violations occur.
- Sobriety checkpoints are becoming more numerous, as are the fines for drinking and driving violations.

- Fines are high and going up. According to a Gallup poll of almost 10,000 people, the average fine for a DUI or DWI is now more than $1,300.

BAC	Approximate Alcohol Consumed in a Two-Hour Period	Effect on a 100-Pound Person
0.05%	1 to 2 ounces liquor 1 to 2 12-ounce beers	Mild impairment in reaction time and judgment, careless behavior, some loss of coordination and self-control.
0.1%	3 to 4 ounces liquor 3 to 4 12-ounce beers	Substantial impairment in muscle coordination, perception, and judgment. Emotions and inhibitions are relaxed.
0.2%	5 to 6 ounces liquor 5 to 6 12-ounce beers	Increased loss of self-control, difficulty in thinking clearly, impaired memory. Unpredictable emotional behavior. Entire motor area of brain is depressed. Slurred speech, staggered walk. Simple tasks, like buttoning a coat, become difficult to impossible.
0.3%	7 to 8 ounces liquor 7 to 8 12-ounce beers	Body thrown into state of confusion, sense organs seriously affected—double vision, hearing impaired, distances difficult or impossible to judge—may be in a stupor, walking is difficult and dangerous to person.
0.4%	9 to 10 ounces liquor 9 to 10 12-ounce beers	Brain can barely function, nervous system shuts down, may experience vomiting or uncontrolled urination, unable to move, may slip into unconscious state.
0.5%	More than 10 ounces liquor More than 10 12-ounce beers	Coma, brain unable to control body temperature—respiratory failure due to paralysis of breathing centers of brain. When this occurs, death will soon follow.

The Blood Alcohol Concentration

The amount of alcohol in a person's blood is expressed by a percentage called the **blood alcohol concentration (BAC).**

The chart on this page describes the effects of alcohol on the body at various BACs. This is based on a 100-pound (45-kg) person and the amount of alcohol consumed over a 2-hour period. Factors that affect the amount of alcohol in a person's blood include the following:

- gender
- the person's metabolism
- the amount of alcohol, not the number of drinks, a person consumes
- whether or not the person eats before or while drinking
- how much the person weighs
- how much time elapses after drinking stops or between drinks

Each state has determined the legal acceptable limit of alcohol in the blood. In most states, driving while intoxicated is defined as having a 0.1 percent BAC.

The Costs of DWIs

There are many problems that are created for the individual who is stopped for alcohol-impaired driving. Here are some:

- immediate confiscation of driver's license
- arrest and a trip to jail
- court appearance
- fine
- possible suspension of driver's license
- possible mandatory jail sentence
- cost of bail to get out of jail
- higher insurance rates
- possible lawsuits

Efforts to Reduce DWIs

Because of the seriousness and extent of the alcohol-impaired driving problem, several efforts are being made to reduce it. Mandatory chemical tests for blood, breath, or urine exist in some states. Refusal to submit to a test can mean automatic suspension of one's driver's license.

Organizations such as MADD, Mothers Against Drunk Driving, and SADD, Students Against Driving Drunk, have been powerful forces in making the public and state legislators aware of the problem. Stricter enforcement of existing laws, tougher new laws, banning of open containers in cars, and abolishment of drive-through liquor stores are a few of the contributions that these organizations have made to the reduction of the problem of alcohol-impaired driving.

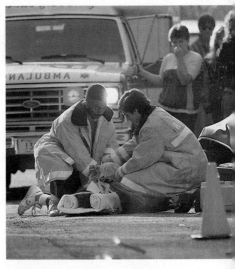

Alcohol-impaired driving is the leading cause of death among teens.

Alcoholism

Alcoholism, or addiction to alcohol, is a physical and psychological dependence on alcohol. It is a disease that may have a hereditary link. People with alcoholism are called alcoholics. They may have one or a combination of these behaviors:

- They cannot keep from drinking.
- They cannot manage tension without drinking.
- They cannot stop drinking once they have started.

Stages of Alcoholism

There are three clearly defined stages of alcoholism. They happen over a period of time. The time span can be long or short, depending on the individual and the age at which he or she started drinking.

Stage One. Alcoholism typically begins with social drinking, often to relax or to relieve stress. Gradually, this kind of drinking becomes necessary to manage stress. A physical and psychological dependency on alcohol develops. The person begins to drink and to become intoxicated regularly. The drinker cannot remember with whom he or she was drinking or what was said or done after each drinking episode. Often at this stage the drinker makes excuses and tries to rationalize his or her drinking behavior.

Stage Two. Gradually, the person reaches a point where he or she cannot stop drinking. Physical and mental problems become evident. At this stage of the disease, defensive behavior is evident. The drinker denies or tries to hide the problem. The body has developed a tolerance, and more alcohol is necessary. Drinking becomes the central event in the person's life. Performance on the job, at school, or at home decreases. Frequent absences from school, work, or other commitments occur.

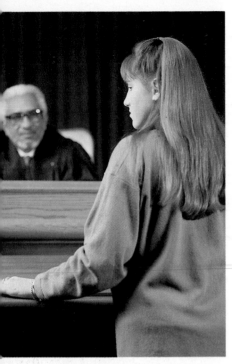

Teens who drink and drive may have their driver's licenses suspended, pay heavy fines, and even go to jail.

HEALTH UPDATE

LOOKING AT THE ISSUES

Alcohol, Advertising, and Adolescents

Recent polls show that up to 73 percent of the American public thinks that there is a direct link between alcohol advertising and teen drinking. Companies that produce and distribute alcoholic beverages claim there is no connection.

Analyzing Different Viewpoints

ONE VIEW. Some people claim that the constitutional rights to freedom of speech and freedom of the press should allow people to advertise their products how and where they want as long as they meet federal regulations and are willing to pay for the advertising.

A SECOND VIEW. Others argue that people will drink if they want to, regardless of whether or not beer commercials are shown on television or liquor ads fill billboards. They point out that even though cigarette and liquor commercials have been banned from TV, people continue to use these products, which are now advertised on billboards and in some magazines rather than on TV screens.

A THIRD VIEW. Others, alarmed by the vast number of teens who drink, call for strong measures, including pulling all beer advertising from television, particularly during sporting events that draw vast numbers of teen viewers.

A FOURTH VIEW. United States Surgeon General Antonia Novello believes that many alcohol advertisements are geared specifically to teens, that they try to sell a life-style message that is inaccurate and unhealthy, and that such messages need to be regulated more fully. She points out that many of the industry guidelines, which are voluntary, are not followed. She also charges that the television networks have relaxed their advertising standards. She says it is very confusing for teens when the law says not to drink while advertisers promote it.

Exploring Your Views

1. Do you believe alcohol products should be advertised on television? On billboards? Why or why not?
2. Does it seem to you that teens are targeted by alcohol producers and distributors? If so, how?
3. Do you ever feel caught in the middle of the drink/don't drink messages that the media send your way?
4. What do you think would be the most effective means of getting teens who drink to understand the dangers of drinking and to choose a healthy life-style that is alcohol-free?

Stage Three. In the final and worst stage of the disease, the drinking is visible. It can no longer be denied, and it is also uncontrolled. Alcohol becomes a constant companion. The alcoholic becomes aggressive and is isolated from friends and family. Malnutrition becomes a problem because the drinker overlooks his or her need for nutritional foods. The body is addicted to the drug. If the alcoholic stopped drinking, he or she would experience the withdrawal symptoms associated with alcoholism, called delirium tremens (DTs). They consist of hot and cold flashes, tremors, nightmares, hallucinations, and fear of people and animals. DTs need prompt medical attention.

Although alcoholism cannot be cured, it definitely can be treated and arrested. As many as two-thirds of all alcoholics recover with proper treatment. The goal of the various programs to treat alcoholism is to stop or control the intake of alcohol. Several sources are available to help people who have a drinking problem. Help is also available for the families and friends of people who have a drinking problem. These are discussed in Chapter 25.

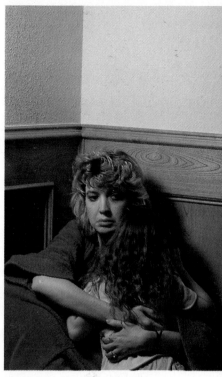

The heavy use of alcohol is often a cause of serious family problems. Alcohol is often a factor in spousal abuse, child abuse, and abuse of the elderly.

ALCOHOLISM AND THE FAMILY

One of the most tragic results of having an alcoholic in the family is what happens to the other family members. Here are some of the facts:

- There is prevalence of alcohol dependency in spousal and child abuse.
- Children of alcoholics are at greater risk of developing alcohol dependency than children of nonalcoholics.
- One in every eight Americans is the child of an alcoholic.
- Children of alcoholics exhibit symptoms of depression and anxiety more than children of nonalcoholics.
- Alcohol dependency and alcohol abuse are major factors in marital separation and divorce.

LESSON 3 REVIEW

Reviewing Facts and Vocabulary

1. What does *BAC* stand for, and what does it mean?
2. List three effects drinking alcohol at any level has on driving.
3. What are six factors that affect the amount of alcohol in a person's blood?

Thinking Critically

4. **Synthesis.** Explain why alcoholism is a problem for both drinkers and nondrinkers.
5. **Evaluation.** Do you think the Surgeon General and the United States Senate were justified in passing the bill to require a warning label on alcoholic beverages? Defend your answer.

Applying Health Knowledge

6. Interview five people. Ask each, "What is the cause of alcoholism?" Share your findings with the class. What do people believe about alcoholism?
7. Write a 30-second radio announcement warning of the dangers of fetal alcohol syndrome.

Self-Inventory

Are You in Trouble with Alcohol?

HOW DO YOU RATE?

Number a sheet of paper from 1 through 20. Read each item below and respond by writing *yes* or *no* for each item. Total the number of *yes* responses; then proceed to the next section.

1. Have you ever had a drink containing alcohol?
2. Have you ever had more than one drink in a two-hour period?
3. Do you drink on a regular basis (every weekend, every day, at all parties, and so on)?
4. Do you drink to escape problems?
5. Do you drink to feel more comfortable with people?
6. When you get angry at other people, do you immediately think of taking a drink?
7. Have other people commented on your drinking?
8. Do you get angry when other people bring up your drinking or when one of your classes deals with alcohol or other drug use?
9. Do you gulp drinks or drink until the supply is gone?
10. Do you find it difficult to say no to your friends when they encourage you to drink?
11. Do you hide your use of alcohol from others?
12. Do you lose time from school or work because of your drinking?
13. Are your grades suffering because of your drinking?
14. Have you lost or changed friends since you started drinking?
15. Do you choose your friends because they drink?
16. Do you avoid situations and places where you know there will be no alcohol?
17. Is there alcoholism in your family?
18. Have you ever ridden in a car driven by someone who had been drinking?
19. Have you ever driven a car or operated other equipment after having had one or more drinks?
20. Have you ever turned down the opportunity to be the designated driver because you wanted to drink instead?

HOW DID YOU SCORE?

Give yourself 1 point for every *yes* response. Find your total and read below to see how you scored. Then proceed to the next section.

0 to 2
You do not have a problem with alcohol.

3 to 5
You could be on your way to a problem with alcohol.

6 to 8
Chances are you already have a problem with alcohol.

9 or more
You have a serious problem with alcohol and should get help now.

WHAT ARE YOUR GOALS?

If you do not drink at all, keep up the good work! Try using the following goal-setting process to help you stay alcohol-free:

1. The steps I can take to help me stay alcohol-free include ____.
2. To help another friend stay or get alcohol-free, I plan to ____.

If you ever drink and drive or ride with a driver who has been drinking, begin the following goal-setting process:

3. The steps I need to take to refuse rides with drinking drivers include ____.
4. The steps I need to take to stop driving after drinking include ____.
5. My timetable for making these changes is ____.

If you drink at all, use the following goal-setting process:

6. The way that I will stop drinking and avoid potential problems will be to ____.
7. My timetable for stopping drinking will be ____.
8. The people or program I will turn to for suggestions and support in stopping drinking include ____.
9. My rewards for stopping drinking will be ____.

Building Decision-Making Skills

Allison's parents have gone away for the weekend, leaving her at home with specific instructions not to have anyone in the house. Allison invited her boyfriend and another couple over anyhow, but her boyfriend told some of his friends he was going to Allison's and the word "party at Allison's" got around quickly. She heard kids talking but didn't try to discourage it, because she thought she could control it and didn't want to be "uncool." Over 100 people, including some strangers, showed up, complete with beer and loud music. Things are getting rowdy, and some neighbors are at the door asking what's going on. What should Allison do? Some of her choices include:

A. Tell the neighbors she didn't invite anyone and ask them to help clear everyone out, knowing that some kids will probably resist forcefully.

B. Call the police.

C. Get her boyfriend and his friends to clear everyone out.

D. Let it go until someone else calls the police.

WHAT DO YOU THINK?

1. **Situation.** More than one decision needs to be made. What are they?

2. **Choices.** Think about what Allison should say to the neighbors. What are her choices?

3. **Consequences.** What are the advantages of each choice?

4. **Consequences.** What are the disadvantages of each choice?

5. **Consequences.** How are her parents probably going to react?

6. **Consequences.** What is the worst possible outcome of this situation?

7. **Decision.** What should Allison say to the neighbors?

8. **Decision.** What should Allison do after she talks to the neighbors?

9. **Evaluation.** Have you ever been in a similar situation? If so, what did you learn from it that you could apply to this situation? What advice would you give Allison?

Heidi and Kim, who are sophomores, agreed to go to the basketball game in the next town with two seniors. Kim had been trying to get her date to ask her out for weeks and was really excited about the evening. Since her parents weren't so excited, Heidi and Kim asked the guys to pick them up at the mall. After they got out of town, the guys opened beers for everyone from a fresh twelve-pack. The guys had smelled of beer when they first got into the car but said they hadn't been drinking. What should Heidi and Kim do?

A. Ask to be let out at a pay phone and call their parents to come for them.

B. Take the beer away and not let the guys drink any more.

C. Find a new way home when they get to the game.

D. Turn down the beer, knowing the guys will probably drink it if they don't.

E. Offer to drive, since Heidi just got her license. In fact, insist on it.

WHAT DO YOU THINK?

10. **Situation.** What risks are involved in this situation?

11. **Choices.** What other choices do Heidi and Kim have?

12. **Consequences.** What are the advantages of each choice?

13. **Consequences.** What are the disadvantages of each choice?

14. **Consequences.** What would Heidi's and Kim's parents probably want them to do?

15. **Decisions.** How do you think Heidi and Kim should handle this situation?

16. **Evaluation.** Have you ever been in a similar situation? How did you handle it? Would you handle it any differently today? Explain your answer.

REVIEW

Using Health Terms

On a separate sheet of paper, write the term that best matches each definition given below.

LESSON 1

1. Phrase that means food or beverage that has no nutritional value.
2. Condition in which liver tissue is replaced by scar tissue.
3. Chemical process in which yeast acting on sugar and starches produces alcohol.
4. An indicator of the concentration of alcohol in a beverage.
5. Type of alcohol in beer, wine, and liquor.
6. The process of changing alcohol to water, carbon dioxide, and energy.
7. The effect of mixing other drugs or medicines with alcohol.

LESSON 2

8. Driving under the influence of alcohol.

LESSON 3

9. A person who is driving and whose BAC exceeds the legal limit.
10. Birth defects caused by the consumption of alcohol by a pregnant female.
11. Addiction to alcohol.
12. People who have alcoholism.

Building Academic Skills

LESSON 2

13. **Math.** In 1990 alcoholism and problem drinking cost the economy over $136 billion. Do some research to find the most current population figure for the United States. Estimate and then calculate how much each U.S. citizen would have to pay to cover that expense. What percentage would each U.S. citizen be paying? How much would your entire family have to pay?

LESSON 3

14. **Reading.** Gather several ads for alcoholic beverages and brochures against drinking. Identify the stated and implied messages. Summarize your findings in writing.

Recalling the Facts

LESSON 1

15. Why is alcohol considered a drug?
16. What are the following symptoms an indication of: jumpiness, sleeplessness, sweating, poor appetite, tremors, convulsions, and hallucinations?
17. What are five immediate effects of alcohol?
18. What are four long-term effects of alcohol?
19. Why is it dangerous to drink after taking medicines?

LESSON 2

20. In what ways does alcoholism cost the economy every year?
21. How might family influence one's drinking behavior?
22. List four difficulties that problem drinkers may face.

LESSON 3

23. What are some of the problems children with fetal alcohol syndrome may encounter?
24. Describe the three stages of alcoholism a person may go through.
25. What are some symptoms of alcohol withdrawal?
26. Which of the following statements is true?
    a. Alcohol-impaired driving is the leading cause of death among 15- to 19-year-olds.
    b. Fetal alcohol syndrome is a leading cause of mental retardation in the United States.
    c. Driving under the influence of alcohol reduces one's ability to judge distances, speeds, and turns.
    d. Defensive behavior is common in the first stage of alcoholism.
    e. People in stage three of alcoholism suffer from DTs.
    f. Malnutrition becomes a problem in stage three of alcoholism.
27. Name at least five problems that someone stopped for alcohol-impaired driving may face.

REVIEW

Thinking Critically

LESSON 1

28. **Synthesis.** It is especially hazardous to use alcohol in cold climates. Give some reasons to support this statement.

29. **Synthesis.** List current slang terms that relate to alcohol or alcohol use. What can you infer about the role of alcohol in your environment from your list?

LESSON 2

30. **Evaluation.** Why do you suppose the average American drank less alcohol in 1991 than in 1980?

31. **Evaluation.** What responsibilities should people who sell alcohol to minors have?

LESSON 3

32. **Synthesis.** Penalties for drunk driving have become more severe. What reasons can you give for this trend?

33. **Evaluation.** Suppose you and a friend were on your way home from a football game and someone driving drunk hit you. Your friend was killed and you were badly hurt. How do you think you would feel toward the driver who hit you? What do you think should happen to that driver? How would you feel if you found out it was that driver's third DWI?

Making the Connection

LESSON 1

34. **Music.** Write a musical jingle encouraging students not to drink. Record the words and music.

LESSON 3

35. **Language Arts.** Interview a police officer in your community. What is being done to reduce the number of accidents caused by people who drive while intoxicated? Have the efforts worked? What age-group presents the most serious problem? How can teenage drivers help fight this problem? Summarize your interview in writing.

Applying Health Knowledge

LESSON 1

36. Look at the labels of medicines currently in your home. Which of these expressly state that alcohol should not be consumed while the medicine is in use?

LESSON 2

37. What are some ways a teenager can meet the needs to belong, to feel loved, and to be important without the use of alcohol?

38. Give examples to illustrate two situations that problem drinking has affected the economy.

LESSON 3

39. Find out what the legal acceptable limit of the blood alcohol concentration is in your state. How many 12-ounce beers is this for a 100-pound person? How many ounces of liquor is it?

40. Why do you think people who drink at parties try to get everyone else to drink also? What would you do in a situation in which your friends would not take no for an answer from you?

41. You are getting ready to leave a party. Your only way of getting home is with your friend who has had too much to drink. What would you do?

Beyond the Classroom

LESSON 2

42. **Parental Involvement.** Survey three popular magazines to determine which magazines have the most advertisements for alcohol. Determine the target market for each of the magazines. Discuss with your parents the conclusions that can be drawn from your survey.

LESSON 3

43. **Further Study.** Find out how MADD or SADD got started and what impact it has had.

ILLEGAL DRUGS

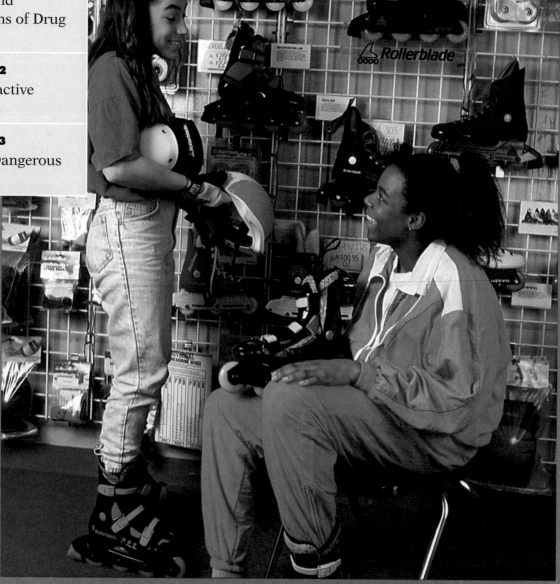

COSTS AND PROBLEMS OF DRUG USE

A s you know, the term *drug* is used to refer to dangerous and illegal substances, including alcohol and tobacco. Medicines sold on the street for purposes other than those intended by the manufacturer also become dangerous, illegal drugs.

The growing use of illegal drugs and medicines acquired illegally has captured the interest and attention of American families in the 1990s more than ever before. Almost daily in the newspaper, on television or the radio, there are stories about physical, mental, and social health problems resulting from illegal drug use.

Costs of Drug Use

The cost of using drugs affects almost everyone—not just the people who use drugs. Think about the number of drug-related crimes and deaths you read or hear about. Consider the effects of drugs in the work force in terms of lost productivity caused by absenteeism and accidents. Also consider the rising costs of consumer products and health care that result from drug use. Everyone pays a price for drug use.

Consider the cost to you and what happens if someone you know at school or at your job uses drugs. Drug use can

- hinder concentration,
- decrease memory function,
- affect attentiveness to tasks by causing either a drowsy, relaxed state or a highly anxious feeling,
- increase the possibility of making poor judgments and decisions,
- affect mood, and
- affect the senses and limit the ability to function.

Learning about the dangerous effects of drugs as well as ways to promote a healthy life-style is important in reducing or eliminating drug use and its costs.

Problems of Drug Use

People of all ages use drugs for many reasons. Some may use drugs because they feel pressure from others to do so. Others seek a good feeling, or high, in an attempt to ease boredom or forget problems. Still others use drugs because they have become addicted and have lost the power to choose. Unfortunately, drug use cannot make problems go away. In addition, using drugs can damage a person's health. Anyone who uses drugs will likely have one or more of the following problems:

LESSON 1 FOCUS

TERMS TO USE

- Physiological dependence
- Tolerance
- Withdrawal
- Psychological dependence
- Addiction

CONCEPTS TO LEARN

- The cost of using drugs affects almost everyone.
- Using drugs damages a person's health.

ATTITUDES AND BEHAVIORS TO EVALUATE

- Self-Inventory, page 492.
- Building Decision-Making Skills, page 493.

Overcoming The Odds

Ben is 16 and rather shy. "I've never been one to talk in public much, but I figured this was pretty important. The reason is because I know there are thousands more out there just like me who have friends in deep trouble with drugs, and nobody knows what to do about it." Ben continues, "Three of us—good friends from way back—watched what was happening to our friend, who I'll call Josh. He's this football fanatic, OK? He lives for it. So the coach told him if he could get some weight on and increase his strength, he'd be a starter on the team in the fall. So first he started to lift weights more. Then he started to use steroids. Pills. Sure we read all about steroids in health class and knew the dangers—on paper. But it's a different story when you see somebody you know real well starting to act differently, starting to go down the tube. We all just sat and watched it happening and didn't know what to do. I guess mostly what we did at first was either ignore it or razz him about it . . . till it got out of hand."

Ben goes on. "All of a sudden Josh just bulked up. Sure he was working out in the weight room a lot. That could account for some of the increase. But most of the rest of us were working out, too, and we didn't look like him. Then Josh started to have headaches and act edgy a lot. He got this awful acne. He had to use the bathroom all

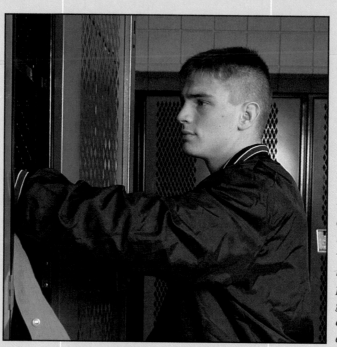

the time. He had this killer breath. All that was weird enough. But then, he started to behave weird, too. He got paranoid. He was either down or up. Sometimes he acted like he was going to take over the world. Other times, he just retreated. And then, there was the temper. He got really mean sometimes—even with us.

"Early this fall, some of us went away with the other peer helpers on a weekend training retreat. One of the things we talked about was what to do if you have a friend who is in trouble with drugs. I realized I had to do something."

Ben talked to the peer helper advisor. She suggested some ways Ben and his friends might approach Josh. She urged them to tell Josh's parents that he needed help. She also gave them some telephone numbers for counseling and drug treatment centers that might be able to help. Ben continues, "So three of us ended up going to talk to Josh about the steroids. We told him how he'd changed, what we thought the drugs were doing to him, and that we were there because we were worried about him. We were prepared that he might get angry, and he did. But we expected that and didn't react to it. We told him where he could get help. We also told him that if he didn't, we'd probably have to involve some adults. That felt really weird. I don't know if what we did will help or not. It's been only a couple of weeks."

1. What are some of the reasons confronting a friend with a drug problem is so difficult?
2. What are the possible benefits of such a confrontation—both to the drug user and to the person who does the confronting?

Types of Drugs	Effects
Stimulants Amphetamines	Results include excitation, restlessness, rapid speech, irritability, convulsions, insomnia, hallucinations, severe mental disorders, anorexia, malnutrition, and/or death.
Ice	Lethargy, severe depression, paranoia, and possible cardiopulmonary effects are likely to occur.
Cocaine	Negative effects include irritability, depression, mental disorders, damage to lining of nose and blood vessels when sniffed, seizures, heart failure, stroke, and death. When taken during pregnancy, cocaine can lead to abruptio placenta, miscarriages, and fetal death. Infants exposed perinatally may have long-lasting effects that include tremors, seizures, learning problems, a delay in or difficulty bonding, and failure to thrive.
Crack (a crystallized derivative of cocaine)	Crack is an extremely addicting form of cocaine with the same effects and problems, including insomnia, agitation, and paranoia. Users experience a very short period of intoxication for 5 to 10 minutes.
Depressants Barbiturates	Effects include decreased alertness, confusion, drowsiness, irritability, poor coordination, lack of judgment, loss of appetite, sleep disorders, nausea, addiction, and possible death.
Tranquilizers Valium	Use may lead to dependence and withdrawal symptoms that include convulsions, tremors, cramps, and overdose.
Narcotics Methadone Opium Morphine Heroin Codeine	Use may result in decreased alertness, confusion, stupor, slurred speech, nausea, vomiting, unconsciousness, and possibly death.
Hallucinogens PCP (phencyclidine)	Use may cause perceptual distortions, confusion, agitation, impaired memory, anxiety, loss of coordination, delusions, panic, irrational thought patterns, violent behaviors, and/or long-term developmental consequences.
LSD	Delusions, illusions, hallucinations, increased panic, severe mental disorders, or death may result from use.
Cannabis Marijuana Hashish	Drug combines stimulant, hallucinogenic, and depressant effects. The effects of intoxication, or high, may last 48 hours, long after the individual considers him- or herself no longer under the influence. User may experience reduction of inhibitions, panic, impaired memory, paranoia, loss of concentration, loss of coordination, loss of interest, loss of ambition, goals, and motivation, changes in perception, sterility, impaired heart function, lowered resistance to infection, lung cancer, psychological dependence, delayed sexual development, and lung damage caused by exposure to the smoke. Fetal marijuana syndrome may result from use during pregnancy, causing low birth weight and developmental abnormalities of infants exposed to marijuana before birth.

DRUGS AND THEIR EFFECTS

continued

Anabolic steroids	Severe acne, nausea, vomiting, diarrhea, hair loss, deep depression, excitation, power delusion episodes, aggressive behavior, uncontrolled violence, heart disease, hypertension, stroke, kidney damage, and abnormal liver function are among the negative effects. May also cause sexual underdevelopment or delays. In males, problems may include atrophy of genitalia, sterility, and stunted growth. In females, a decrease in estrogen, deepening of voice, a masculine build, and an increased risk of cancer.
Inhalants Solvents Gasoline Model glue Felt-tip markers Aerosols Insecticides Freon	The easily available household compounds are most frequently abused. Use may cause poor coordination, stupor, impaired thought processes, unconsciousness, violent behavior, hallucinations, and damage to liver, kidneys, and bone marrow. Single use may cause permanent brain damage.

- **Physiological dependence.** The body develops a chemical need for a drug. Physiological dependence is determined when a person experiences tolerance and withdrawal. **Tolerance** occurs when the body adjusts to the effects of the drug. Larger doses of the drug are needed to achieve the same effect. **Withdrawal** is characterized by symptoms that occur when a person stops using a drug to which he or she is physiologically dependent. These symptoms can include nervousness, insomnia, severe nausea, headaches, vomiting, chills, and cramps and, in some instances, even death.
- **Psychological dependence.** A person believes a drug is needed in order to feel good or to function normally.
- **Addiction.** An addict has a physiological or psychological dependence on a drug. Negative effects of drug use will vary with each individual. Some people have very serious effects with first use while others may experience harmful effects only after chronic use. The earliest consequences are frequently behavioral or social, which may be the most critical health concern. Drug use is a learned behavior. It is important, then, not to begin using drugs. The chart on pages 481 and 482 gives an overview of the drugs you will study in this chapter.

LESSON 1 REVIEW

Reviewing Facts and Vocabulary

1. Tell how physiological dependence is related to addiction.
2. Explain the term *drug*.

Thinking Critically

3. **Analysis.** Explain the difference between tolerance and withdrawal.

4. **Synthesis.** List three costs of drug use and give examples of how each cost might affect you.

Applying Health Knowledge

5. Write a one-page report telling ways you would help reduce the costs of drug use in your school or community.

PSYCHOACTIVE DRUGS

Like medicines, drugs are grouped according to their effects on the body. Many of the substances that will be discussed in this lesson promote health when used in a controlled medical situation. However, when not used for medical purposes, these substances can be very dangerous. They can cause irreversible harm and even result in death.

Psychoactive drugs affect the central nervous system and alter normal functioning of the brain, resulting in mental or behavioral changes. Stimulants, depressants, narcotics, and hallucinogens are psychoactive drugs. The first three have medicinal value. Hallucinogens have no medical use.

Stimulants

Stimulants speed up the central nervous system. They cause increased heart and respiratory rates, high blood pressure, dilated pupils, and decreased appetite. In addition, users may experience sweating, headaches, blurred vision, dizziness, and sleeplessness. Extremely high doses can cause irregular heartbeat, tremors, loss of coordination, and even physical collapse. Inhalation or injection of stimulants can cause a sudden increase in blood pressure that can result in stroke, high fever, or heart failure.

Psychological effects of stimulant use include moodiness, restlessness, and anxiety. Chronic users can experience hallucinations, delusions, and paranoia. These symptoms disappear when drug use ceases.

Amphetamines

Amphetamines are stimulants that have an effect similar to that of the sympathetic nervous system. They speed up the heart and breathing. They cause anxiety, sleeplessness, and loss of appetite. Medical use of amphetamines has declined greatly in recent years. They may be used in the treatment of narcolepsy, a disease that results in an uncontrollable need to sleep, as well as in some cases of brain damage resulting from senility. Some people use amphetamines illegally to stay awake and alert, to feel high and euphoric, to improve athletic performance, to lose weight, and to offset the effects of depressant drugs. Tolerance to amphetamines can develop. Psychological dependence also can result. The user can experience depression as the effect of the drug wears off.

Methamphetamine. Methamphetamine is an amphetamine that has been used medically in treating narcolepsy, Parkinson's disease, and obesity. When used illegally, this drug, which is also called crank, speed, or ice, may cause a person to be paranoid and violent. Because crank is made in labs, it is readily available. Crank can be smoked; snorted or sniffed up the nostrils; injected; or swallowed. The effects of this drug are long-lasting. Food and water become unimportant after taking crank. Seizures and death can result.

Cocaine

Cocaine is a white powder made from the coca bush, which grows in parts of South America. Cocaine was once widely available in the United States. In fact it was once an ingredient in a well-known soft drink. The drug was even used as a local anesthetic in the mid- and late nineteenth century. Other chemicals with stronger anesthetic effects and fewer side effects have almost eliminated cocaine's medical usefulness. Cocaine use and possession is now illegal under state and federal laws.

Cocaine is a rapid-acting, powerful stimulant. Its effects, which include increased heart rate, blood pressure, and respiration, can last from 20 minutes to several hours. The feelings of confidence that come from cocaine use are often followed by a letdown. Regular use can lead to depression, edginess, and weight loss. Physiological dependence occurs because the user wants to avoid the letdown feeling. As cocaine use increases, so does the danger of paranoia, hallucinations, and psychological dependence.

Cocaine is used in many ways. When snorted, the drug is absorbed into the bloodstream through the mucous membranes of the nasal cavity. It constricts, or contracts, the many little blood vessels in these membranes, reducing the blood supply to the nose and causing it to become dry. Repeated cocaine use can cause tissue damage in the nose and even holes in the nasal septum, the wall dividing the two halves of the nose.

Cocaine use can cause malnutrition and, especially among those with cardiac problems, an increase in the risk of heart attack. Even in healthy individuals who are not heavy users of cocaine, the drug may disturb the electrical impulses of the heart and cause death. An additional risk of cocaine use is the possibility of being infected with HIV when injecting cocaine with a shared needle.

Crack. Crack is a form of cocaine that can be smoked. Processing converts cocaine into lumps or rocks. This kind of cocaine is known as freebase. Preparing freebase may involve the use of dangerous solvents and can result in injury or death from an explosion or fire.

Crack is extremely addictive. Because it is smoked, its effects are felt within 10 seconds. The physical effects of crack include dilated pupils, increased pulse rate, elevated blood pressure, insomnia, loss of appetite, hallucinations, paranoia, and seizures. Crack users may develop a sore throat, hoarseness, and lung damage.

Using crack can cause death by cardiac or respiratory failure. Compared with other forms of cocaine, crack users are at increased risk because of the extreme dangers of this drug.

Depressants

Depressants, or sedatives, are drugs that tend to slow down the central nervous system. Depressants relax muscles, relieve feelings of tension and worry, and bring on sleep. They slow down the heart and breathing rates and reduce blood pressure. Depressants can easily cause physical and psychological dependence.

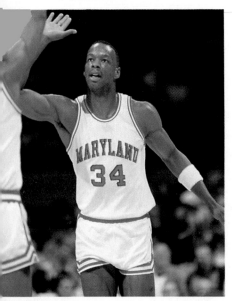

Len Bias, a star college basketball player, had just signed a major contract with the NBA when he went out celebrating—used crack and didn't live to tell about it.

Babies born to mothers who use depressants illegally during pregnancy may be physically dependent on them and show withdrawal symptoms at birth. Birth defects and behavioral problems among these infants also are common.

Combining depressants and alcohol has a synergistic effect and increased health risks to the person who does this. Results include depression of the central nervous system and death.

Sedative-Hypnotics

Sedative-hypnotics are a type of depressant. They induce sleep and reduce anxiety. Motor coordination and judgment can be impaired. When these drugs are used in excess, the respiratory and cardiovascular systems are depressed. Sedative-hypnotics can produce physiological and psychological dependence.

Barbiturates. Barbiturate use can result in mood changes, more than normal sleep, or even a coma. Barbiturates are rarely used for medical purposes such as treating insomnia. They are used illegally to give a feeling similar to intoxication and to counteract the effects of stimulants.

Tranquilizers

Tranquilizers are depressants that reduce muscular activity, coordination, and attention span. Antianxiety tranquilizers, such as Valium, are used medically to relieve anxiety, muscular spasms, sleeplessness, and nervousness. Valium helps a person relax and have a feeling of well-being. However, when tranquilizers are used in excess, physiological and psychological dependence occurs. Withdrawal from Valium causes severe shaking. In severe cases, coma or death can result.

Antipsychotic tranquilizers are used to treat severe mental disorders, such as schizophrenia. These tranquilizers can help control violent behavior by decreasing brain activity. They reduce muscle tone and activity as well as blood pressure and pulse.

Narcotics

Formerly, the term *narcotic* referred only to drugs made from the opium poppy flower. These drugs were called opiates. Narcotics now also include medicines used to relieve pain.

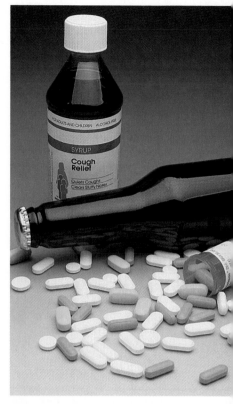

Medicines combined with alcohol can be deadly.

K E E P I N G   F I T

Driving and Marijuana

You've probably heard of people arrested for driving drunk getting DUIs (Driving Under the Influence) or DWIs (Driving While Intoxicated). But driving under the influence of marijuana can also be very dangerous. Marijuana puts added "blindfolds" on a driver by

- interfering with the perception of distance,
- interfering with the perception of depth,

- impairing thinking and judgment skills,
- slowing reflexes, thus affecting one's ability to brake and negotiate curves,
- impairing the ability to stay in the proper lane.

Some medicines made from opium have valuable medical uses in relieving pain and suffering. For example, morphine is used to relieve pain, and codeine is used to stop severe coughing. Both cause drowsiness and can result in physiological dependence. Drugs made from opium can cause stupor or sleep and can result in coma or death.

Heroin

Heroin is made from morphine and has no medical use in the United States. It is an illegal drug. Using heroin depresses the central nervous system and slows breathing and pulse rate. Coma or death may occur with large doses. Tolerance develops very quickly with this drug. Pregnant females who use heroin risk having babies born who are addicted. Retardation and delayed growth of these babies' muscular and nervous systems can result. Withdrawal from this drug is very painful. As with any drug that is injected, there are risks of HIV infection from using contaminated needles.

Treatment for heroin use often involves methadone—a synthetic narcotic. *Synthetic* means made from laboratory chemicals. Methadone depresses the central nervous system, causing drowsiness, and blocks the craving for heroin. The use of methadone, however, is dangerous and must be monitored by qualified medical personnel. Methadone also is addictive. Using too much can result in a deep coma.

Hallucinogens

Hallucinogens, or psychedelics, first became popular during the 1960s. These drugs alter mood, thought, and the senses, including vision, hearing, smell, and touch.

PCP

Phencyclidine (PCP), or angel dust, is a powerful and dangerous hallucinogen. It is prepared synthetically. PCP is considered to be one of the most dangerous drugs.

Users report that PCP makes them feel distant and detached from their surroundings. Time seems to pass slowly; body movements slow down. Muscle coordination is impaired, and the sensations of touch and pain are dulled. PCP can make the user feel strong and powerful. This

---

K E E P I N G   F I T

Dealing with the Dealers

What can you do when drugs are taking over your neighborhood and you feel unsafe?
- Call the police.
- Report license plate numbers of dealers.
- Get involved in a community

effort to rid your neighborhood of drugs.
- Let people know you are not interested in drugs.
- Protect yourself by staying away from trouble spots and from those dealing drugs.

- Keep reminding yourself that the fancy cars the dealers drive are temporary rewards. Many dealers wind up in prison, addicted, or dead by the time they reach their 20s.

---

feeling has resulted in tragic deaths, serious accidents, and acts of violence.

While overdoses of PCP can cause death, most PCP-related deaths are caused by the strange, destructive behavior the drug produces in the user. PCP users have drowned in shallow water because they were so disoriented they could not tell where they were or which direction was up. Others have died in fires because they were disoriented and had no sensitivity to the pain of burning.

Using PCP repeatedly makes it difficult to remember specific facts; it impairs speech, sometimes causing the user to stutter. Judgment and concentration are impaired long after the user has stopped taking the drug. Long-term users may experience anxiety, depression, and violent behavior. Serious mental problems have also resulted from PCP, causing users to need psychiatric care and, sometimes, institutional care.

The effects of PCP are widely unpredictable and vary from person to person. Once taken, PCP remains in the body long after the initial effect has worn off. A flashback, or recurrence of the effect of the drug, may occur at a later time.

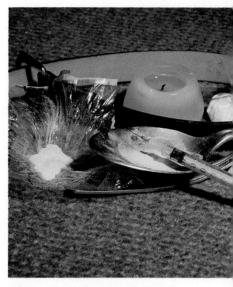

All illegal drugs are dangerous. Sharing needles adds other risks—HIV infection and AIDS.

LSD

Lysergic acid diethylamide (LSD) is probably the drug responsible for initiating an awareness of hallucinogens in American society. Use of LSD during the 1960s and the resulting tragedies—deaths from a false sense of security or hallucinations—received much publicity. Deaths resulted when people thought they could fly or could stop a train by standing on train tracks.

Current use of hallucinogens is illegal, although during the 1960s and 1970s, LSD was tried in different types of therapy. All medicinal use was stopped because the results were inconsistent and unpredictable.

LSD causes an increase in heart rate and a rise in blood pressure. The user may experience chills, fever, loss of appetite, or nausea. Bad experiences may lead to panic, anxiety, or accidental suicide. Flashbacks can occur even after use has stopped. Furthermore, much of the LSD currently being sold is mixed with potentially lethal substances like strychnine.

LESSON 2 REVIEW

Reviewing Facts and Vocabulary

1. Explain the effects of psychoactive drugs.
2. How do antipsychotics help in the treatment of severe mental disorders?
3. Describe what a flashback is and list with which type of drugs flashbacks occur.

Thinking Critically

4. **Analysis.** How do the effects of stimulants differ from those of narcotics?

5. **Synthesis.** What might happen if a person took alcohol with a tranquilizer?

Applying Health Knowledge

6. Make a poster that warns of the dangers of cocaine.

OTHER DANGEROUS DRUGS

LESSON 3 FOCUS

TERMS TO USE

- Marijuana
- Hashish
- Inhalants
- Designer drugs
- Look-alike drugs
- Anabolic steroids

CONCEPTS TO LEARN

- Marijuana is a hallucinogen but also has the effects of a depressant and a stimulant.
- Inhalants are not meant for human consumption.
- Anabolic steroid use has serious side effects.

ATTITUDES AND BEHAVIORS TO EVALUATE

- Self-Inventory, page 492.
- Building Decision-Making Skills, page 493.

The following types of drugs—marijuana, inhalants, designer drugs, and steroids—are additional dangerous drugs.

Marijuana

The scientific name for **marijuana,** a hemp plant, is *Cannabis*. The leaves and flowers of marijuana are smoked, eaten, or drunk for intoxicating effects. Scientists have been able to identify over 400 chemicals in marijuana.

The chemical that produces the psychoactive effect is delta-9-tetrahydrocannabinol (THC). Scientists measure the strength of marijuana by testing how much THC it contains. THC does not dissolve in water, and it is not easily flushed out of the body. It may take many weeks after heavy use for the body to excrete it. When THC enters the blood, some is stored in fatty tissue. The highest concentration of fat cells in the body is in the brain cells, liver, lungs, kidneys, and reproductive organs. In these cells, marijuana acts as a poison. It prevents the proper formation of DNA, proteins, and other essential building blocks for cell growth and cell division.

Hashish (hash) is the dark brown resin collected from the tops of the cannabis plant. Hash is stronger than marijuana because it contains more THC. Hash affects a user more strongly than marijuana. Both marijuana and hashish are illegal.

Marijuana is a hallucinogen but also has the effects of both a depressant and a stimulant. The effects of using marijuana include a calm state with a sensitivity to sight, touch, and sound. Time seems to pass slowly. Visual perception can change. Images may be seen. Marijuana lowers body temperature, but increases the heart rate and blood pressure. It stimulates the appetite. It reduces a person's control over behavior. Some people may become talkative and giddy, others quiet and withdrawn. The effects vary from person to person and can be influenced by a person's mood and surroundings.

Regular marijuana users tend to have personality problems that include loss of willpower and motivation, lack of energy, and paranoia. They tend to lose interest in activities that used to be important to them. Marijuana users may become apathetic and lethargic, withdrawing from academic and social activities. These problems, if not present before the beginning of regular marijuana use, develop and intensify as a result of regular use. Marijuana users often develop psychological dependence on the drug, wanting the feelings they experience to continue.

Studies have shown that marijuana affects memory, making it more difficult to recall and to pay attention. Concentration and coordination are impaired. Reaction time is slowed. Marijuana use definitely impairs driving ability. Drivers under the influence of marijuana react slower and make more accident-causing mistakes than drivers who are not under the influence. Since some of the effects of marijuana—delayed reaction time and poor concentration—seem to last longer than the actual high, a person may not think he or she is driving under marijuana's influence. Research is still going on to determine whether marijuana destroys certain cells in the brain, causing permanent damage.

Research shows that marijuana smokers may be more susceptible than nonsmokers to infection by viruses, bacteria, and other pathogens. Marijuana smoke contains more cancer-causing chemicals than cigarette smoke. Studies have shown that marijuana interferes with the cells in the lungs that destroy disease-producing bacteria, making the user more susceptible to infections from bacteria. Because marijuana users often inhale unfiltered smoke deeply and hold it in the lungs, marijuana is damaging to the respiratory system. Deep, long breaths associated with smoking marijuana allow more time for harmful particles and gases to act on the lung cells. Smoking marijuana causes a narrowing of the respiratory passages, making breathing more difficult.

Regular use of marijuana lowers the level of testosterone in the blood. Testosterone is responsible for the development of male secondary sex characteristics. Sperm production can decrease with marijuana use. Females should avoid marijuana use especially during pregnancy. Some studies show that marijuana use during pregnancy results in decreased birth weight and a condition similar to fetal alcohol syndrome.

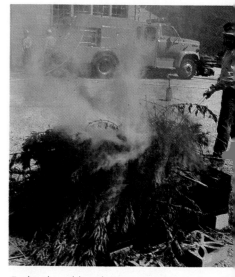

Federal and local governments are taking steps to destroy marijuana crops wherever they are found.

Inhalants

Inhalants are substances with fumes that are sniffed and inhaled to give a hallucinogenic high. Included among the inhalants are glue, spray paints, aerosols, and gasoline. Most inhalants depress the central nervous system and produce effects similar to those of alcohol. Immediate effects of inhalants include nausea, sneezing, coughing, nosebleeds, fatigue, lack of coordination, and loss of appetite. A person who regularly sniffs an inhalant has trouble keeping his or her balance, has a glassy stare, and finds it hard to talk. Judgment is impaired, and the behavior of the user may resemble the behavior of someone who is drunk.

Since inhalants were never meant to be taken into the body, any time they are not used according to the purpose for which they were made is considered illegal drug use. Heavy use of inhalants can result in fatigue, liver and kidney damage, changes in bone marrow, and permanent brain damage. High concentrations of inhalants can cause suffocation. "Clowning around" under the influence of an inhalant has been the cause of many accidental deaths.

Designer and Look-Alike Drugs

To avoid using illegal substances, street chemists make drugs with synthetic substances. These drugs are called **designer drugs.** One of the most well-known designer drugs is called ecstasy, or MDMA. Ecstasy's chemical composition is similar to that of methamphetamines and mescaline. It is a combination stimulant and hallucinogen. Use of this drug gives a feeling of euphoria and results in long-term damage to brain cells.

FINDING HELP

Many young people need treatment for drug and alcohol addiction, but the cost of that treatment is sometimes prohibitive. But now students in Little Rock, Arkansas, have complete insurance coverage for drug and alcohol treatment thanks to a new experimental approach. The district's 26,000 students in grades K through 12 now have 100 percent coverage. The program, which grew out of a community coalition, will include education, early intervention, treatment, and family therapy for young people with chemical dependency. The program is being financed by a grant and local fund-raising efforts.

Look-alike drugs are made from legal substances to look like illegal drugs. With these drugs the user never knows exactly what he or she is getting. Using these kinds of drugs or mixing them with other drugs is very dangerous.

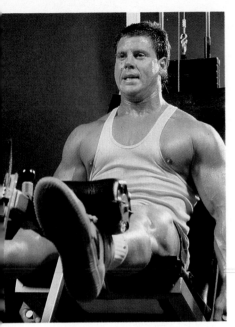

Exercise is a healthy way to build muscle. Taking steroids is unhealthy and illegal.

CONFLICT RESOLUTION

Mike never saw anyone dealing drugs in his neighborhood—until yesterday. Then, he saw a neighbor pass a bag of white powder to a stranger in a car. Mike is pretty sure it was a cocaine deal. Mike wants his neighborhood to be safe, but he's afraid to report what he saw to the police. His neighbor might retaliate if Mike turns him in.

What should Mike do?

HEALTH UPDATE

LOOKING AT THE ISSUES

Drug Testing

According to the National Institute on Drug Abuse, on any given day in the United States, 25 percent of workers between the ages of 18 and 40 would test positive for drugs. Some experts estimate that drug use costs employers over $60 billion a year in decreased productivity, absenteeism, and accidents. Therefore, in the interest of health, safety, and economics, many companies are now testing employees for drug use, but the practice is stirring heated debate.

Presently, drug testing is used in hospital emergency rooms for suspected drug overdoses and when arrests for driving violations suggest drug use. Some schools are now suggesting random drug testing for students.

Analyzing Different Viewpoints

ONE VIEW. Some groups claim that randomly testing people for drug use without just cause is an invasion of their rights, including their right to privacy.

A SECOND VIEW. Others believe that drug testing should be restricted to those who are in jobs where public safety is involved—such as pilots or bus drivers— or to cases where there is just cause, such as after an accident where drug use is suspected.

A THIRD VIEW. Some people claim that widespread drug testing deters the use of drugs, and that, considering the size of the drug problem in the United States, such testing is needed.

A FOURTH VIEW. Others say that drug testing is one way to get those who use drugs to confront their problem and get help and treatment.

A FIFTH VIEW. Still other people argue the tests are not always accurate and can have severe consequences for the individual who incorrectly tests positive. These consequences include job loss or a damaged reputation.

A SIXTH VIEW. Some people believe that random drug testing is not enough—that to stop the drug problem in the United States, everyone in the workplace as well as in schools should be tested.

Exploring Your Views

1. Who, if anyone, do you think should be tested for drugs? Why? In what kinds of situations?
2. Do you think this testing should be random or "across-the-board"?
3. When people do test positive for drugs, what do you think should happen to them? Why?
4. What do you think about schools testing students for drugs? Why?
5. What other means of identifying and getting help for students in trouble with drugs can you suggest?

Moderate doses of any one of these substances can produce nervousness, restlessness, insomnia, or increased blood pressure and heart rate. Regular use of look-alikes, and their use in combination with other drugs, can lead to the same behavior found with frequent use of amphetamines.

The use of look-alikes is hard to diagnose. This makes treatment very difficult. If look-alikes are taken with other drugs, such as alcohol, serious reactions can occur. If a user is admitted to an emergency room, the medical staff may not be able to treat the patient successfully because no one can know for sure what drugs the user took.

Anabolic Steroids

Anabolic steroids are synthetic derivatives of the male hormone testosterone. When used as medicine, these drugs help build muscles in patients with chronic diseases. They also have been used to treat bone diseases, burns, hormonal imbalances, and as protection for blood cells during treatment for cancer.

These drugs are used illegally by some athletes to enhance performance. Because steroids help the body synthesize protein for muscular growth, athletes who use them recover more quickly in practice or after a game. Use also increases aggressiveness and strength. Teens who want to look more muscular sometimes use steroids because steroids help make muscles stronger and bigger. This use of steroids is illegal and dangerous.

Steroid use has serious side effects, including high blood pressure, acne, and increased risk of liver damage, heart disease, and stroke, as a result of clogged arteries. Males can experience baldness, depression, aggressiveness, a decrease in sperm production and testicle size, and an increase in breast growth and body and facial hair. Females can experience breast shrinkage, growth of facial hair, and baldness. Teens who use steroids are at special risk because the reproductive and skeletal systems can be permanently affected. Steroid use causes mood swings and violent behavior. The super aggressive behaviors experienced are termed "'roid rages." The user exhibits behaviors that would never have occurred without using the drug. Because steroids can be taken by injection, risk of infection with HIV exists from shared needles.

HELP WANTED

Drug Enforcement Officer

The "army" needs you—the one fighting the war on drugs, that is. Your working conditions will be terrible and your hours long. You will face danger and will deal with the lowest of the low life. However, the opportunity for satisfaction is great, as you make a difference in one of the most important battles of our times. Integrity is a must as are physical fitness and some acting ability. You need solid policework skills, which you may have gained from a combination of classroom training and experience. We will be glad to consider your particular background.

For more information contact your local office of the U.S. Drug Enforcement Agency.

LESSON 3 REVIEW

Reviewing Facts and Vocabulary

1. Explain the dangers of using inhalants.
2. Relate how designer drugs came into being.

Thinking Critically

3. **Analysis.** Compare the immediate and long-term effects of marijuana use.

4. **Evaluation.** What do you think about steroid use for professional athletes? On what did you base your position?

Applying Health Knowledge

5. Develop a list of strategies that might be effective for reducing drug use in your community.

Self-Inventory

What Is Your Attitude About Drug Use?

HOW DO YOU RATE?

Number a sheet of paper from 1 through 20. Read each item below, and respond by writing *yes* or *no* for each item. Then proceed to the next section.

1. I avoid any type of drug use.
2. I have been encouraged to try drugs.
3. I choose friends who avoid drug use.
4. Some of my best friends use drugs.
5. I feel comfortable saying *no* to friends who want me to use drugs.
6. Most of my friends use drugs at parties.
7. When using an inhalant, such as spray paint, for its intended purpose, I am in a well-ventilated area.
8. I sometimes take medicines that are not prescribed for me.
9. I belong to an organization that promotes a drug-free life-style.
10. I get angry when someone tries to tell me not to use drugs.
11. I stay away from areas where I know drugs are used.
12. I have covered for someone who uses drugs.
13. Whenever possible I avoid peers who use drugs.

14. I sometimes attend parties when I know drugs will be available.
15. I know where to get help for drug problems and would feel comfortable passing the information along to someone who needed it.
16. I frequently am in areas where drugs are sold.
17. I want to remain in control of my actions at all times.
18. I think I would like the experience of getting high.
19. I understand the dangers involved in using drugs and want to avoid the high risks.
20. I think it would be fun to watch others get high.

HOW DID YOU SCORE?

Give yourself 1 point for every *yes* answer to an odd-numbered item. Give yourself 1 point for every *no* answer to an even-numbered item. Total the points, and find your score below. Then proceed to the next section.

19 to 20
Excellent. Your attitudes and behaviors related to drugs are commendable.

15 to 18
Good. Your attitudes and behaviors related to drugs are positive, but limited in scope.

11 to 14
Fair. You need to change your attitudes and behaviors.

Below 11
Needs Improvement. You need to get help to change your behavior and thoughts about drugs. Your health may be in danger.

WHAT ARE YOUR GOALS?

If you received an *excellent* or *good* score, complete the statements in Part A. If your score was rated *fair* or *needs improvement*, complete Parts A and B.

Part A

1. I plan to learn more about drug use and preventing drug use by ____.
2. I want to learn more about drug use because ____.
3. My timetable for accomplishing this is ____.
4. I plan to share my information with others by ____.

Part B

5. The attitude or behavior toward drugs I would most like to change is ____.
6. The steps involved in making this change are ____.
7. My timetable for accomplishing this is ____.
8. The people or groups I will ask for support and assistance are ____.
9. My rewards for making this change will be ____.

Building Decision-Making Skills

Nikita's friends smoke a joint almost every day during lunch in the restroom at school. While Nikita seldom participates, she helps her friends by being a "lookout" for school officials who occasionally happen by. The friends insist they could never put up with their afternoon teachers without mellowing out. Nikita thinks the smoking habit is getting worse. She also thinks it is affecting her friends; they are barely passing their courses. Nikita doesn't use drugs and wishes that her friends would stop. What should she do? Some of her choices are:

A. Tell the school counselor about the situation and ask for help in dealing with it.

B. Tell her friends she's not going to take the risks of being the "lookout."

C. Tell her friends she doesn't want to have anything more to do with them.

D. Think about what is important to her and which decision coincides with her value system.

WHAT DO YOU THINK?

1. **Choices.** What are some other choices Nikita has?

2. **Consequences.** What are the positives and negatives of each choice?

3. **Consequences.** What risks are involved in this decision?

4. **Consequences.** How will Nikita's health triangle be affected by this decision?

5. **Decision.** How do you think Nikita should handle this situation?

6. **Evaluation.** Have you ever been in a similar situation? If so, how did you handle it? What did you learn? Would you handle a similar situation differently now? Explain your answer.

Tom has been approached in the restroom by a student council officer selling pot and cocaine. He feels he should report it, but since Tom has been in trouble before, he doesn't think the principal will believe his word against a student leader. Even though Tom has had his share of trouble, he doesn't do drugs. Tom has a good relationship with his math teacher but doesn't know whether or not to get him involved. Tom has several choices. Some of them include:

A. Tell the principal or the assistant principal.

B. Tell the math teacher and ask him to pursue it but keep Tom's name out of it.

C. Forget the situation. Stay away from the pusher and let him get caught on his own.

D. Write an anonymous letter informing the school administration and the police of the situation.

WHAT DO YOU THINK?

7. **Choices.** What other choices might Tom have?

8. **Consequences.** What are the advantages and disadvantages of each choice?

9. **Consequences.** What risks does Tom face?

10. **Consequences.** Who will probably be affected by his decision? Explain your answer.

11. **Evaluation.** Have you ever been unfairly stereotyped by others because of your appearance or because of previous experiences? Explain the situation and how you dealt with it.

REVIEW

Using Health Terms

On a separate sheet of paper, write the term that best matches each definition given below.

LESSON 1

1. A physiological or psychological dependence on a substance.
2. A chemical need for a drug.
3. The need for larger doses of a drug to achieve the same effect.
4. When a person believes a drug is needed in order to feel good.

LESSON 2

5. Drugs that affect the central nervous system and cause mental or behavioral changes.
6. Recurrence of the effect of a drug, often associated with PCP and LSD.
7. A smokable form of cocaine.
8. Drugs that slow down the central nervous system, relax muscles, relieve feelings of tension, and bring on sleep.
9. Tranquilizers used to treat severe mental disorders.

LESSON 3

10. Substances with fumes that are sniffed to give a hallucinogenic high.
11. Drugs that resemble the action but not the chemical makeup of a drug.
12. Synthetic derivatives of the male hormone testosterone.
13. A drug that is a hallucinogen but also has the effects of a depressant and a stimulant.
14. The dark brown resin collected from the tops of the cannabis plant.

Building Academic Skills

LESSON 1

15. **Reading.** Read a magazine article about an individual or family who has been affected by drugs. Summarize your conclusions about the impact of a life of drugs on the people around the individual.

Recalling the Facts

LESSON 1

16. How do average Americans learn about the growing drug problem in the United States?
17. What are some of the effects of drug use on the work force?
18. How does drug use contribute to rising consumer costs?
19. What are some reasons people give for using drugs?
20. List five problems an individual who uses drugs will likely experience.
21. Distinguish between physiological dependence and psychological dependence.

LESSON 2

22. What are psychoactive drugs?
23. What is the name of the drug commonly called crank, speed, or ice?
24. Explain the effects cocaine has on the nose.
25. What is freebase?
26. What is crack? Why is it so dangerous?
27. Define *stimulants* and give four examples.
28. What problems can result from regular cocaine use?
29. Define *depressants* and give two examples.
30. What may happen to babies born to mothers who use depressants during pregnancy?
31. What are tranquilizers?
32. Why are tranquilizers so popular?
33. Define *narcotic* and give five examples.
34. Define *hallucinogens*; give two examples.

LESSON 3

35. What health problems do look-alike drugs present?
36. What is THC? Where is it stored in the body? What parts of the body are most affected?
37. Why does hashish affect a user more strongly than marijuana?
38. Why is it dangerous to ride in a car with a driver who has been smoking marijuana?
39. Define inhalants and give five examples.
40. What are the risks of using steroids?
41. What are the dangers of inhalants?

REVIEW

Thinking Critically

LESSON 1

42. Analysis. Drug use takes an enormous toll on society, as well as on the individual. Explain this statement and provide several illustrations of the costs to both the individual and society.

LESSON 2

43. Synthesis. Drug use is not unique to the teenage culture. Many adults also use drugs. How might cocaine use affect the life of an adult user? How might it affect the children of the user?

44. Analysis. Talk with someone who was a young adult in the 1960s to learn more about the social climate of that time, especially the attitude toward drug use. What was his or her favorite music, dance, hairstyle, movie? What conclusions can you draw about life in the 1960s? How was the social climate of the 1960s similar to the social climate today? How was it different?

LESSON 3

45. Evaluation. The value of legalizing marijuana has long been debated. Take a stance and argue your position. You may need to find out more about this drug in order to make an intelligent argument. Support your opinion with facts.

Making the Connection

LESSON 1

46. Math. Find an article about drugs that has a chart or bar graph. Present the information in a different form, such as a pie chart.

LESSON 2

47. Language Arts. Work with classmates to write, edit, design, and print an informational leaflet, "Signs of Possible Drug Use." Distribute the leaflet with a school newsletter, at a parents' meeting, or at a shopping mall.

Applying Health Knowledge

LESSON 1

48. Write down three of your personal goals. Next to each goal write a statement about how involvement in drugs would interfere with your ability to reach your goal.

49. You have many learned behaviors. Make a list of five behaviors you practice and describe how you worked to learn each one. Then think of a behavior you have decided to change. Tell the process you followed to stop that behavior.

LESSON 2

50. Drug users often started experimenting occasionally with drugs and then became dependent on them. Explain how a change from experimentation to dependency can happen.

LESSON 3

51. Name some bacterial infections to which marijuana smokers may be more susceptible than nonsmokers.

52. What ramifications does the fact that marijuana lowers the level of testosterone have for a teenage male who uses marijuana heavily?

53. If you had a friend who told you he wanted to start taking steroids to develop his muscles, what advice would you give him?

Beyond the Classroom

LESSON 1

54. Parental Involvement. With your parents, read *Go Ask Alice* which is a true anonymous account of a 15-year-old's struggle with drugs . Discuss the thoughts and feelings you each had while reading this book.

55. Further Study. Read a newspaper from a major city in your area for a week. Clip each article that is somehow related to drugs or drug use. Draw conclusions based on these articles. Share your findings with your peers.

RECOVERING FROM ADDICTION AND CODEPENDENCY

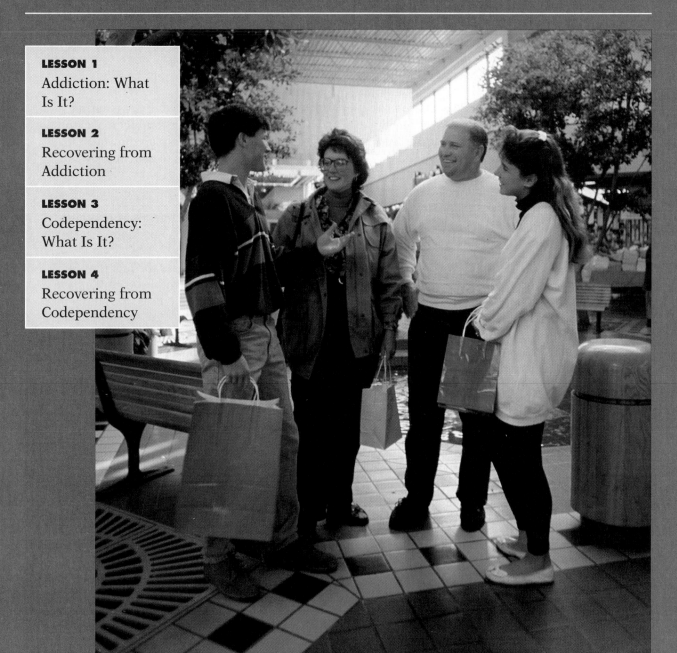

ADDICTION: WHAT IS IT?

Addiction is a complex matter. Like a jigsaw puzzle, an addiction is made up of many interlocking parts. These puzzle pieces may fit together differently in different people.

These days some experts are comparing alcohol and drug addiction to illnesses such as diabetes and cardiovascular disease. They have found that the tendency to develop these diseases may be inherited. However, the life-style decisions people make and the messages society gives about the use of alcohol and drugs also affect whether or not people become addicted.

Addiction

An **addiction** is a physiological or psychological dependence on a substance or activity. One can be addicted to alcohol, drugs, gambling—even food. In this chapter we will discuss addiction to alcohol and other drugs. **Physiological dependence** means that the body has become accustomed to a drug or drugs and needs these chemicals just to function. The body of an addict craves these substances. Physiological dependence is determined when a person experiences tolerance and withdrawal. Tolerance means the body becomes used to the effect of the drug. The body then requires larger doses of the drug to produce the same effect. Withdrawal occurs when the person stops taking a drug to which he or she is physiologically dependent and experiences physical symptoms.

Psychological dependence means a person comes to depend on the feeling received from a drug. Psychological dependence often involves denial, which means that the addict does not admit or does not realize that he or she is in trouble with alcohol or other drugs. The person believes that he or she can control the use of the drug and is not causing any harm.

ALCOHOLISM

Alcoholism, or addiction to alcohol, is considered a disease by the American Medical Association (AMA). Since 1987 **drug dependence,** or drug addiction, has also been considered a disease by the AMA. Both of these diseases are described as chronic, progressive, and potentially fatal. *Chronic* means that the diseases are ongoing, and *progressive* means that they get worse over time. *Potentially fatal* means that people can die from the disease.

The Addiction Continuum

Addiction is a process—a series of gradual changes that happen over time. This process happens more quickly to some than to others. Some

---

LESSON 1 FOCUS

TERMS TO USE
- Addiction
- Physiological dependence
- Psychological dependence
- Alcoholism
- Drug dependence
- Intervention

CONCEPTS TO LEARN
- An addiction is a physiological or psychological dependence on alcohol or other drugs.
- Alcoholism and drug dependence are considered diseases by the American Medical Association.
- Addiction is a series of gradual changes that happen over time.

ATTITUDES AND BEHAVIORS TO EVALUATE
- Self-Inventory, page 512.
- Building Decision-Making Skills, page 513.

- Each year in the U.S., between 5,000 and 10,000 children are born with fetal alcohol syndrome.
- Up to 100,000 children may be born each year with fetal alcohol effects, the less severe but still serious results of drinking alcohol during pregnancy.
- Exposure of a fetus to alcohol is now a leading cause of mental retardation in the U.S.

people get hooked on a drug from the first time they take a drink, a pill, or an injection. For other people, an addiction develops more slowly, perhaps over a period of many years. Others do not become addicted at all. For this reason it is difficult to know or predict exactly when a person becomes addicted.

ADDICTION: THE DOWNWARD SLIDE

These steps show the way an addiction to alcohol or other drugs might develop.

Step 1: First use/occasional use
- Takes first drink or uses other drug for the first time
- Likes the way it feels and reduces stress
- Uses the drug in social settings

Step 2: Occasional trouble with drug
- Shows mood swings or personality changes (may happen on the first use)
- Has greater tolerance than others—for example, can outdrink others without seeming drunk
- May cry, get violent, or show high-risk behaviors while drinking and using drugs
- May have blackouts, not remembering what was said or done

Step 3: Regular use of drug
- Finds that tolerance increases—needs more of a drug and may crave it more frequently
- Tries to control drug use but cannot
- Feels guilty after binges, or episodes
- Hangs out with others who drink or use drugs
- Denies problem; gets angry when others suggest a drinking or drug use problem

Step 4: Multiple drug use
- May combine or switch drugs for new and stronger effects or to assure supply
- May become cross-addicted, or hooked on more than one kind of drug

Step 5: Increasing dependency
- Needs drug just to function
- Finds that drug no longer has same effect; needs drug just to stop shaking or feeling sick
- Loses interest in family, friends, school, job, sports—everything but drugs

Step 6: Total dependency
- Suffers major loss because of addiction, such as getting thrown out of school, losing a relationship, causing a car crash, being hospitalized, getting arrested
- Feels physically and emotionally defeated

K E E P I N G   F I T

The Gene Scene

Studies published in 1991 support the idea that there is a gene or family of genes at least in part responsible for alcoholism and other drug dependencies.

This idea is not accepted by everyone. Research does show that children of alcoholic parents are statistically at a greater risk than others of becoming alcoholics. However, the role of heredity versus environment remains unclear to many on this issue.

Knowing your family's medical history can provide important clues about your health and possible risks.

Sarah W. is 17. Her dad is an alcoholic, and last fall, her dad's drinking seemed to get worse. He started the day with whiskey and ended it with beer. He stayed home from work a lot. Whenever he drank, he seemed to change. "The slightest thing could set him off," she says. "Then he'd yell, slam doors, and threaten Mom, my brother, or me. A couple of times he slapped my brother Mark around, and once, he banged my head against the wall. It was really scary. I would lie awake nights listening to my mom yelling or crying or my father bad-mouthing my brother. It was always a bad scene, and it was ripping me up inside."

Finally, Sarah stopped having her friends over. She couldn't eat or sleep either.

Then, last winter, Sarah had a great health teacher named Mrs. Quintana. In her class, Sarah learned that alcoholism is a disease. She learned how it not only affected her dad but was affecting everyone in her family—that they all, not just her dad, needed help. She finally got up the courage to call a good friend whose mom was a recovering alcoholic, and she asked her what she should do.

The next week her friend took Sarah to her first Alateen

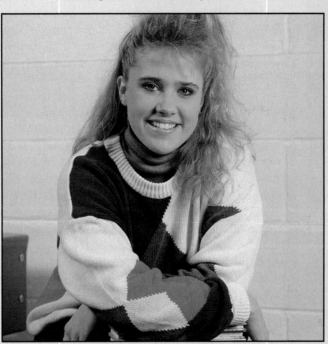

meeting. She was uncomfortable at first but says she soon felt like she belonged. "It was so great to learn that I'm not alone in this," she says. "What a relief to know I didn't need to keep it all a secret anymore and that I don't have to spend my whole life worrying about my dad's drinking."

Soon Sarah's mom started going to Al-Anon, and they both stopped covering up for her dad. Recently, they confronted her dad with just how bad the situation had gotten, and now her dad is in recovery, too. "True, my older brother is still drinking and using drugs," Sarah says, "but now I know there's help out there for him, too, when he's ready. I didn't use to know that. I didn't use to know that at all."

Sarah says she feels really good about herself and her own life these days and proud that her decision to help herself has begun to help her whole family. "I'm starting to learn that I'm not responsible for anybody's behavior except my own. I've also learned that with alcoholism in the family, I'm at risk of becoming an alcoholic myself, so I feel more committed to not drinking than a lot of my friends. The biggest change, though, is that I don't feel so numb. I feel more alive. I used to feel so ashamed, so afraid, so shut off from life. Yes, there are still scary times, but mostly I have hope now. And my dad, well, he's doing so much better. We jog together before dinner every night and talk. We joke around and call it our 'happy hour.' Life is really so much better around here since he quit drinking and agreed to get help."

1. In what ways does Sarah's story illustrate that alcoholism is a family disease?
2. Why should the first step in getting help for a family member's addiction be to get help for oneself?
3. Why do you think Sarah's brother's chances for recovery might be better than average?

Intervention

Many families rely on a process called intervention. **Intervention** means interrupting the addiction continuum before the alcoholic or addict hits bottom. The process begins with meetings of family members and other significant people involved in the life of the chemically dependent person. These meetings take place without his or her knowledge. A certified drug and alcohol counselor and someone from a support group such as Alcoholics Anonymous usually oversee these meetings. Family members learn about addiction and the ways in which they have become affected by it. They do list work—listing all of the episodes they can remember when the person's drinking and drug use were involved and how it made them feel. They rehearse what might happen at the actual intervention—a surprise meeting with the alcoholic or addict when the list work is presented. Often this meeting forces the alcoholic or drug addict to face just how bad his or her addiction is and just how unmanageable his or her life has become because of it. The group presents the alcoholic or addict with a plan for immediate treatment. If the person refuses to get this needed help, the family, boss, or others taking part in the intervention process tell the person what steps they plan to take in response to the refusal to get help. For example, a wife might say, "If you will not get help, I will move out"; or a boss might say, "If you drink again at work, you're out of a job." Such ultimatums let the chemically dependent person know that all enabling has stopped and the person must now face the consequences of his or her addiction.

Imagine addiction to alcohol or other drugs as a downward slide. An addiction can begin with the first use of alcohol or other drug. Unfortunately, an addiction often ends at the bottom end of the continuum with irreversible damage to the body and mind—or with death. It is this side of addiction that has become a major health problem in the United States.

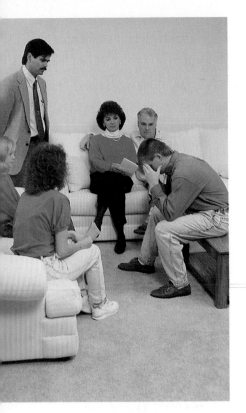

During an intervention, evidence of addiction is presented to the person with the drug problem.

LESSON 1 REVIEW

Reviewing Facts and Vocabulary

1. Define the term *addiction*.
2. How are alcoholism and drug dependence described by the American Medical Association?

Thinking Critically

3. **Analysis.** Compare physiological and psychological dependence.

4. **Synthesis.** What explanations can you give for why some people become addicts and some people do not.

Applying Health Knowledge

5. Draw an addiction continuum. Think about someone you know or know of who may have an addiction to alcohol or other drugs. Where would you place this person on the continuum? Which characteristics of the downward slide seem to apply to this person?

RECOVERING FROM ADDICTION

Getting well again is known as **recovery.** Recovery from alcohol or drug addiction means learning to live an alcohol- or drug-free life. In addition to the physical aspects, there are also mental and social aspects to deal with for successful recovery from an addiction.

The Recovery Continuum

Like addiction, recovery is a process. It happens over time. It happens at different rates and in different ways for different people. Yet there are certain characteristics common to most recovery stories.

Imagine recovery on a continuum as you did for the addiction process. The first steps in recovery are to recognize that there is a problem with alcohol or other drugs and to make the decision to give them up. The next step is to actually remove these drugs from the body. This process is called **detoxification** and should take place under medical supervision. In addition to regaining physical health, recovery also involves restoring one's mental health by learning to build healthy relationships and by taking responsibility for one's own life.

People in recovery describe themselves as recovering rather than being recovered. This is because the recovery process is ongoing. The biochemical and perhaps genetic conditions that first set them up for addiction remain in their bodies and brains whether or not they use drugs. Alcoholism and drug dependence are therefore considered lifelong diseases. They cannot be cured. They can, however, be kept from progressing further.

Experts on the addiction and recovery process used to believe that people had to hit bottom, or suffer some major loss as a result of their

Experts recommend total abstinence for a recovering alcoholic.

LESSON 2 FOCUS

TERMS TO USE

- Recovery
- Detoxification
- Relapses
- Total abstinence
- Alcoholics Anonymous (AA)

CONCEPTS TO LEARN

- Recovery is a series of gradual changes that happen over time.
- There are many treatment options available for someone with an addiction who wants to obtain help.

ATTITUDES AND BEHAVIORS TO EVALUATE

- Self-Inventory, page 512.
- Building Decision-Making Skills, page 513.

- People in recovery sometimes develop transfer addictions. That means they go from being addicted to one substance to being addicted to another substance or behavior. For example, recovering alcoholics sometimes develop eating disorders or become compulsive gamblers.

- People in recovery do not concentrate on the fact that they will have to live a lifetime without drugs. Instead, they talk about staying sober or clean one day at a time.

drinking or drug use, before they would decide to get well. Now it is generally recognized that people can begin the recovery process at any point on the downward slide into addiction—even before they suffer major losses.

Most experts in the field of addiction recommend total abstinence for the recovering alcoholic and addict. **Total abstinence** means not using any mood-altering drugs including alcohol. Long-term studies show that attempts at controlled drinking and drug use usually fail. Even small amounts of alcohol or other drugs can send an addict back into addiction.

Many people in recovery manage to stay drug-free for the rest of their lives. Others may have **relapses,** or slips—periodic returns to drinking and drug use. Yet despite how far down the addiction continuum a person goes or how many times that person relapses, the choice of and chance for recovery are always there.

RECOVERY: THE UPWARD CLIMB

The following scale shows how a person's recovery from alcoholism or other drug dependency might progress:

- Decides to get help
- Actually asks for or goes for help
- Has medical evaluation, or checkup
- Detoxes (gets drug out of the system)
- Learns about the disease
- Finds that physical health improves
- Sees appearance improve
- Experiences improvement in mental health
- Gains emotional control
- Rebuilds or makes healthy relationships
- Sets and achieves new goals
- Rebuilds self-esteem
- Continues to stay drug-free
- Helps others with addictions to recover
- Takes responsibility for own life
- Continues lifelong adventure in recovery

Treatment Choices: Where to Go for Help

When someone wants help with an addiction, a first step in getting help may be to talk with someone whom that person trusts, preferably someone knowledgeable about addiction.

Counseling

A parent, teacher, school counselor, or peer counselor may be a place to start. A person in trouble with alcohol or other drugs might also call one of the toll-free drug and alcohol hot lines, the National Council on Alcoholism, or a drug and alcohol treatment center. Someone there would connect the caller with a counselor who specializes in drug and alcohol counseling.

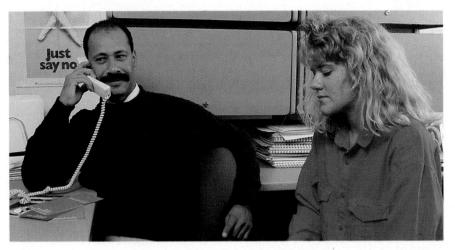

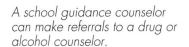

A school guidance counselor can make referrals to a drug or alcohol counselor.

Support Groups

A support group is a group of people who share a common problem and work together to help one another and themselves cope with and recover from that problem. Regular attendance at such support groups is the most popular form of ongoing treatment for addictions. Support groups such as **Alcoholics Anonymous (AA)** have played a major role in helping people to get and stay alcohol- and drug-free. At meetings, which are held frequently all over the world, members provide support and help one another stay sober or otherwise drug-free. Such meetings are confidential; members can remain anonymous because no one has to give his or her last name. They are also free of charge. Each AA office can direct people to local AA meetings or to other support groups such as Narcotics Anonymous or Cocaine Anonymous.

Alcohol and Drug Treatment Centers

Alcohol and drug treatment centers offer a wide range of services to addicts who want to recover. Many centers specialize in treating teens with addictions or have special units solely for adolescents.

Some treatment centers are privately owned, but there are also state and community alcoholism and mental health clinics that offer professional care at a low cost or free of charge. Since drug and alcohol dependence are considered diseases, some health insurance plans may cover at least some of the costs.

Culturally Speaking

Busted

A group of young African Americans who are aspiring to be actors and actresses have produced an antidrug film, *Busted*, for the Partnership For a Drug-Free America. The Partnership wanted to "unsell" kids on drugs. So they tried something new. *Busted* is a 10-minute film that is shown before feature films aimed at teen audiences. During *Busted*, at a test run in a Harlem theater, the audience became so involved they were actually talking to the girl in the film encouraging her to choose her longtime, straight friends over those who use drugs. The Partnership hopes this scene will be repeated in real life as well.

K E E P I N G   F I T

Tips for Killing the Craving

After an addicted person goes through withdrawal he or she may still crave the drug for some time. A person newly into recovery may lessen such cravings by
- keeping in mind that a person only has to stay drug-free one

day at a time,
- eating fruit or drinking juice when cravings hit,
- avoiding places, people, or behaviors that he or she associates with drinking or drugging,
- getting lots of exercise,

- finding a sober friend whom the person can call to talk over problems and get reinforcement for staying drug-free,
- getting lots of sleep.

HEALTH UPDATE

LOOKING AT THE ISSUES

Health Threats to Unborn Babies

When a pregnant female is addicted to alcohol or other drugs, her baby can be born addicted. The health consequences of the baby's addiction and withdrawal can be severe and long lasting. In some states, mothers who give birth to babies addicted to cocaine and crack are now being charged with endangering—even though those drugs are given indirectly to the babies before they are actually born.

In 1989, a young female from Florida became the first mother convicted of delivering drugs to her baby while pregnant. She delivered those drugs through the umbilical cord by using them herself. Found guilty, she was sentenced to 1 year in a drug rehabilitation program and 15 years of probation. This conviction was later overturned.

Analyzing Different Viewpoints

ONE VIEW. Some people think that pregnant females who use drugs are unfit to be parents at all and should have their children removed from them by the courts.

A SECOND VIEW. Others believe such females should be placed in prison just as other parents who commit life-threatening child abuse sometimes are.

A THIRD VIEW. Still others think that these females have a disease and should be sentenced to treatment, followed by close observation and drug testing. People with this view believe that by getting these females into treatment, they have a better chance at becoming responsible, drug-free parents.

Exploring Your Views

1. Which of these views seems most reasonable and fair to you? Why?
2. Do you think that children who are born addicted should be taken from their mothers? Temporarily? Permanently? Should they be put in foster care or put up for adoption? Should they be given back to the mothers when the babies are out of medical danger? When the mothers are in recovery for addiction? How far into recovery? Give reasons for each of your answers.
3. Should females also be prosecuted, or charged, with child abuse when they drink, smoke, or use other addictive drugs? Should they be charged only when their babies are born addicted to or showing harmful side effects from these drugs? Why or why not?

Detox Units. In some hospitals or treatment centers, there are medical detox units for alcoholics and addicts undergoing the detoxification process. During this process, which usually lasts from three to seven days, the person is under a doctor's care and may be given some medication to ease the sometimes dramatic symptoms of withdrawal. Some people go directly from detox to ongoing involvement in a support group.

Inpatient or Residential Treatment Centers. People generally stay in this kind of facility for a month or more. Such centers, often in peaceful and attractive surroundings, offer a time away from the person's usual environment so that full concentration on recovery can take place. The first few days are spent in detox. After that, people spend a month or more taking part in drug and alcohol education, individual and group counseling, and support group meetings.

Outpatient Treatment Centers. Outpatient treatment involves getting treatment for a few hours each day at a nearby treatment center but spending the rest of the time in one's regular surroundings and activities. This approach to treatment allows people to go to work or school and to live at home during the treatment process. It is less expensive than inpatient treatment, but it takes place over a longer period of time. For people with mild to moderate withdrawal symptoms, outpatient treatment is now being used even for the detoxification process.

Continuing Programs. Many inpatient and outpatient rehabilitation centers have long-term programs of counseling and support for people in recovery who have gone through their standard short-term treatment programs. These usually involve follow-up sessions, individual and group counseling, and family system therapy—counseling that gets the whole family involved in the recovery process.

Halfway Houses. Halfway houses, sometimes called continuing-care facilities, offer people housing, counseling, and support meetings as they are recovering from a severe addiction. People are generally admitted to halfway houses only after having completed at least a 28-day program of recovery at a treatment center. They stay for six months to a year as they learn coping and living skills they will need when they return to society. Residents are also sometimes channeled into vocational rehabilitation or job training programs.

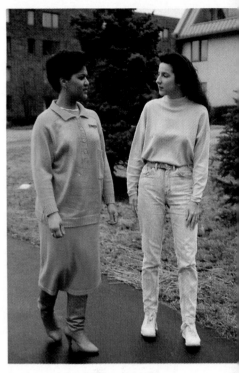

At a residential treatment center, full concentration on recovery can take place.

LESSON 2 REVIEW

Reviewing Facts and Vocabulary

1. For what reasons do people in recovery describe themselves as recovering rather than being recovered?
2. Use the words *total abstinence* and *relapse* in a short paragraph that describes the dangers of trying controlled drinking.
3. Outline some of the treatment choices for an alcoholic who wants to recover.

Thinking Critically

4. **Analysis.** Compare inpatient and outpatient treatment centers.

5. **Evaluation.** Why do you think recovery includes more than just physical detoxification?

Applying Health Knowledge

6. Make a booklet that lists and describes alcohol and drug treatment services available in your community.

LESSON 3

CODEPENDENCY: WHAT IS IT?

LESSON 3 FOCUS

TERMS TO USE
- Codependency
- Enabling

CONCEPTS TO LEARN
- Codependency means being overly concerned with other people's behavior and problems.
- Codependents learn rigid roles to play.

ATTITUDES AND BEHAVIORS TO EVALUATE
- Self-Inventory, page 512.
- Building Decision-Making Skills, page 513.

Being overly concerned with other people's behavior and problems and feeling driven to fix and control those problems is known as **codependency.** People who live with or are close to alcoholics and drug addicts and show this kind of behavior are called codependents. Their codependency is sometimes also referred to as co-addiction.

Common Traits of Codependents

Though each person who exhibits codependent behavior does so in a unique way, codependents share many traits in common:

- They feel like they have to fix other people's problems, particularly those related to another's drinking and drug use.
- They feel lost, bored, or bad about themselves when not rescuing someone in trouble.
- They feel responsible for other people's feelings, actions, and happiness.
- They have difficulty having fun, relaxing, or taking good care of themselves.
- They constantly seek others' approval.
- They do not meet their own needs and may not even know what their own needs are.

Enabling: Hurting by Helping

One of the most common traits of codependency is enabling. **Enabling** means trying to protect the person having trouble with alcohol or drugs from facing the consequences of his or her drug-related problems. Codependent people enable an addict by lying for him or her; lending money, which may be used to purchase more drugs or alcohol; or making excuses for him or her. Enabling is not healthful caring. Such actions do not help the addict. They just make it more comfortable and possible for the alcoholic or addict to keep on drinking or using drugs.

What Codependency Is Not

Codependent people are not physically addicted to a drug the way an addict is. Though codependency is often referred to as an addiction, it is neither an addiction nor a disease in the physical sense. It is, instead, a very damaging emotional and social preoccupation, or obsession, which often can have physical consequences. This type of obsession is different from drug addiction.

Codependents can suffer from a variety of stress-related mental or physical disorders, from depression and eating disorders to high blood pressure and digestive disorders.

Addiction as a Family Disease

In a family where there is alcoholism or other drug dependence, both addicts and codependent family members are hurting and need help. That is why alcoholism and drug dependence are sometimes referred to as family diseases. They affect everyone in the family.

People in a family with drug or alcohol dependency experience terrible shame, fear, disappointment, guilt, and anger. They are embarrassed to admit these feelings, not realizing that millions of other families suffer from the effects of drug dependency.

Roles in Families with Addiction

In a healthful family system, rules are flexible and members play many roles based on changing situations and needs. In families with drug dependency, codependents instead learn to cope by acting out rigid, unchanging roles such as these:

- Main enabler. This role is usually played by the husband or wife. He or she may be a responsible caretaker who nags, blames, controls, rescues, and covers up for the alcoholic or addict in the family.
- The good child or hero. This role may be assumed by the oldest child in the family. He or she often gets straight As, wins awards, and tries to bring esteem to the family with his or her achievements.
- The troublemaker. This person may use drugs, fail in school, or show other self-destructive behaviors. The troublemaker's goal is to hold the family together by keeping it focused on his or her bad behavior.
- The sensitive child. This person may be the youngest in the family. He or she may be overly aware of everyone else's emotions, and despite hurting deeply inside, always puts on a smile. This child works to keep family peace. This child may also play the role of family clown.
- The invisible child. This person may withdraw from the family altogether, not wanting to add to the family's problems. He or she may try to live in a fantasy world or be very passive, adjusting to anything that happens without complaint.

Regardless of what role or roles family members play, they all make the alcoholic or drug addict the center of their lives. They adjust their needs, emotions, and behaviors to the unhealthy demands, behaviors, and emotions of the addicted person. In the process they, too, become unhealthy.

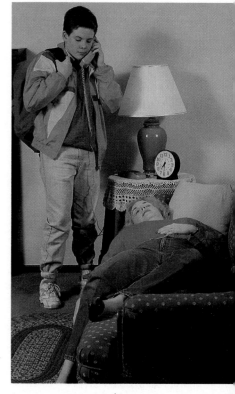

Lying to a parent's boss to cover up a drinking problem is an example of enabling behavior. It permits the individual to continue drinking.

K E E P I N G   F I T

Excuses, Excuses

An enabler is someone who shields the addict from the consequences of his or her behaviors. In addition, the enabler may "buy the addict's line"—or believe the chemically dependent person's rationalizations—that he or she is drinking or drugging because of other great problems. For example, the addict might convince the enabler that he or she needs to drink or smoke because of stress at school or work, financial worries, other illnesses, broken relationships, and so on. What enablers and addicts do not realize is that continuing the addictive behavior creates problems and creates stress rather than relieving them.

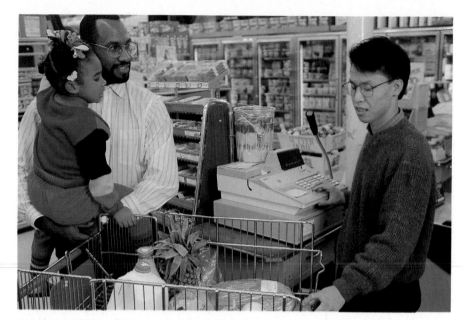

Family members often put their life on hold hoping an addiction will go away. Some teens may delay going to college to help meet family expenses.

The Codependency Continuum

As a family member's alcoholism or addiction progresses, his or her family's codependency also gets worse. It, too, is a downhill process. The rage, sadness, excuses, and disappointment increase. People get sick. Violence may occur. Some family members may become overly involved in others' problems, taking the focus off themselves. Other family members may simply withdraw. In either case, family members put their lives on hold hoping the addiction will go away, but it does not. In turn, they may scream, cry, beg, threaten, nag, retreat, leave, come back, or even use alcohol or other drugs to avoid their pain. Like the alcoholic or addict, they may also be in denial, not realizing or being able to admit just how bad things at home have become.

LESSON 3 REVIEW

Reviewing Facts and Vocabulary

1. What is meant by the term *codependency*?
2. List some common traits of codependents.
3. Give three examples of enabling behavior.

Thinking Critically

4. **Synthesis.** Suggest ways that a family member could be supportive to an alcoholic family member and not be considered codependent.

5. **Analysis.** In what ways are chemical dependency and codependency similar? In what ways are they different?

Applying Health Knowledge

6. Write a skit or make a drawing in which you show the roles in families with drug or alcohol dependency. Include the dependent person actively drinking or using drugs. Show how everyone else in the family reacts to this behavior, each according to his or her role.

RECOVERING FROM CODEPENDENCY

There are many ways for families with chemical dependency to get help. These days more families are seeking and getting that help.

The Recovery Continuum for Codependents

Just as addiction is not hopeless, neither is codependency. The downward slide into codependency, like that of addiction, can be turned around and changed into a process of recovery. Like recovery from chemical dependency, recovery from codependency takes time and effort. Different people may recover at different speeds and in different ways. Whatever anyone's timetable for recovery, the personal and family rewards can be great.

RECOVERY FROM CODEPENDENCY: THE UPWARD CLIMB

A codependent's recovery might progress like this:
- Hits an emotional bottom as a result of involvement with someone else's addiction
- Desires and goes for help
- Gets educated about the diseases of addiction
- Accepts the disease concept and his or her part in that disease
- Stops trying to control others, including the addict
- Focuses on self instead of the addict
- Begins to pay attention to personal appearance
- Experiences improvement in own physical, mental, and social health
- Rebuilds self-esteem
- Helps family become more flexible; aids in the process of redefining once-rigid roles
- Continues to attend support group meetings, helping other codependents and self
- Takes full responsibility for own life

Strategies for Getting Well

There are many ways that a person from a family with addiction as well as the addicted family member can get help. The first step is to admit that there is a problem. The next step is to reach outside the family system for help. This can seem like an impossibility to many people since families of active alcoholics and drug addicts have usually lived by the unspoken rules—"don't talk, don't trust, and don't feel."

Reaching outside the family for the first time can feel like a betrayal. However, it is a healthy step to take, and a sense of relief often results. Whatever the risks are in seeking outside help, not seeking it holds

LESSON 4 FOCUS

TERMS TO USE
- Al-Anon
- Alateen

CONCEPTS TO LEARN
- The first step to recovery is admitting that there is a problem.
- Seeking outside help is an important step in recovering from codependency.

ATTITUDES AND BEHAVIORS TO EVALUATE
- Self-Inventory, page 512.
- Building Decision-Making Skills, page 513.

Fifteen-year-old David lives a secret life that no one at school knows about. He never invites friends home because his dad's an alcoholic. David's not only ashamed about this, but he's terrified his friends will witness one of the "scenes" his dad makes when he gets drunk. These "scenes" often result in physical abuse. When David and his mom get hurt and develop bruises, they lie about their cause. They also lie to his dad's boss about why he misses so much work.

How are David and his mom supporting his dad's alcoholism?

What could they do to resolve the conflict in their own lives as well as help his dad stop drinking?

greater risks. Continuing to adapt to an unhealthy family system can be far more damaging to everyone involved.

Sometimes only one person in a chemically dependent family seeks and gets outside help. Because of this, that person may feel very lonely. When everyone in the family seeks help and assumes responsibility for his or her own role in the family, recovery can occur more quickly.

Interventions can hasten the speed with which the alcoholic or addict gets into a treatment program. It also can speed up the rate of recovery for the co-alcoholics or co-addicts in the family. Sometimes intervention fails. In families where this happens the alcoholic or addict will continue to drink or take drugs. However, the rest of the family can work on being healthy again.

Abstinence, or staying away from all alcohol and other drugs, is particularly important for the child of an alcoholic or drug addict. Research indicates that having a chemically dependent parent does not necessarily mean a person will also become chemically dependent. However, research shows that a child of an alchoholic or drug addict has a better than average risk of developing an addiction.

Counseling

Many codependents need professional care. Individual and group counseling may be available with a psychiatrist, psychologist, social worker, or therapist trained in chemical dependency and codependency. Family therapy is often recommended and may help the family even if the alcoholic or addict refuses to participate.

Support Groups

There are many support groups for people involved in the lives of alcoholics and other drug addicts. The most widely known of these groups is **Al-Anon.** Like Alcoholics Anonymous, Al-Anon is a worldwide self-help organization. It welcomes family members and friends of alcoholics. It is open for the codependent whether or not the chemically dependent person decides to get well. Like AA meetings, Al-Anon meetings offer a support system for coping and a structured program for regaining emotional and social health. The program encourages detachment—the process of pulling back or separating from involvement with

---

K E E P I N G   F I T

Smashing Stereotypes

There are many unfair stereotypes about people who suffer from addictions. What is your mental picture of a typical alcoholic? Is the person of a particular race, age, sex, or socioeconomic group? The fact is that alcoholism is an equal-opportunity disease that strikes people of all races, ages, sexes, and classes. Though some ethnic groups seem to be at greater risk for developing the disease, all groups are represented in statistics for active addiction and recovery from those addictions.

someone else's addiction and refusing to let that addiction rule one's life any longer. Al-Anon meetings are free, and what is said at the meetings remains confidential.

Other support groups such as Codependents Anonymous, the National Association for Adult Children of Alcoholics, The National Association for Children of Alcoholics, and Children of Alcoholics offer information and support at both national and local levels

Alateen, an offshoot of Al-Anon, is for teens and preteens between the ages of 12 and 20, whose parents or other family members or friends have drinking problems. Like Al-Anon, its members come together to share their experiences and discuss how the addiction of someone close to them has affected their lives and how they can cope and recover. Information about Al-Anon and Alateen can be found by calling the local Al-Anon office listed in the phone book. Other similar programs such as Nar-Anon and Coc-Anon are available to help families and close friends of narcotics and cocaine addicts.

Family Programs

When an alcoholic or drug addict enters a rehabilitation or treatment center, the family is usually included in at least part of the program. During weekend visits or in a three- to seven-day program of their own, family members learn about the disease of addiction, how they have been affected by it, and how they can recover and support the recoveries of others in the family.

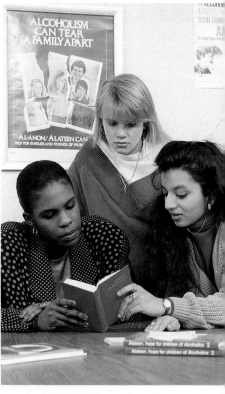

Alateen is a support group for teens who have a family member with a drinking problem.

LESSON 4 REVIEW

Reviewing Facts and Vocabulary

1. Where might the family of an addict or alcoholic turn to get treatment information?
2. Why is it important to seek help outside the family?
3. Give two examples of support groups often used by codependents.

Thinking Critically

4. **Analysis.** For what reasons do you think it is difficult for people to confront close friends with drinking and drug use problems?
5. **Analysis.** Why do you think it is possible for a codependent to recover even if the chemically dependent person in his or her life does not?

6. **Analysis.** Is there a danger that overinvolvement with support groups can keep someone from taking full responsibility for his or her life? Explain your reasoning.

Applying Health Knowledge

7. Write what you would say to a close friend or relative who was deeply depressed or otherwise upset by a parent's addiction. How would you guide that person for help?
8. Set up a Recovery Resource Table at your school. Provide information about local recovery resources for people suffering from chemical dependency and for those suffering from codependency.

Self-Inventory

How Codependent Are You?

HOW DO YOU RATE?

Number a sheet of paper from 1 through 15. Read each item below and respond by writing *yes* or *no* for each item. Total the number of *yes* and *no* responses. Then proceed to the next section.

1. Do you live with a person who is addicted to drugs or alcohol?
2. Do you have a close friend who is an addict?
3. Are your life and emotions totally wrapped up in the addiction of this person you care about?
4. Do you spend a great deal of time, energy, or money trying to fix this person's problems?
5. Has your involvement with his or her addiction affected your appetite, sleep habits, or mental or physical health?
6. Do you ever lie or cover up for the person when his or her drinking or drug use results in trouble?
7. Do you feel overly responsible for other people's feelings, behavior, and happiness?
8. Do you feel comfortable, happy, or useful only when you are trying to rescue someone in trouble?
9. Do you focus on others' needs before focusing on your own?
10. Do you try to control people, situations, and outcomes?

11. Are you compulsive? Do you overdo it in such areas as work or exercise, not knowing when to stop?
12. Do you feel you have to please everyone?
13. Do you avoid arguments at all costs?
14. Are you loyal to others even when they hurt you?
15. Are you uncomfortable when the tables are turned and someone asks you how *you* are feeling?

HOW DID YOU SCORE?

Give yourself 1 point for every *yes* answer and 0 points for every *no* answer. Find your total, and read below to see how you scored. Then proceed to the next section.

0 to 4
Good. You are concerned with what others think of you, but you probably are not codependent.

5 to 9
Fair. You are showing symptoms of codependence that may lead to further problems.

10 to 15
Watch out! There is a good chance that you are codependent.

WHAT ARE YOUR GOALS?

If you received a *good* score, complete the statements in Part A. If your score was rated *fair* or *watch out!* complete Parts A and B.

Part A

1. I plan to learn more about the subjects of codependency and recovery from codependency in the following ways: ____.
2. My timetable for completing this is ____.
3. I plan to share my information with others by ____.

Part B

4. The codependent behavior I would like to change or improve is ____.
5. The steps involved in making this change are ____.
6. My timetable for making this change is ____.
7. The people or groups I will ask for support or assistance are ____.
8. My rewards for making this change will be ____.

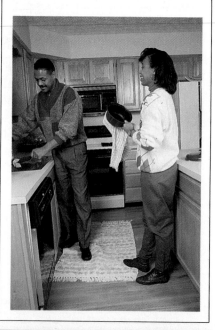

Building Decision-Making Skills

Craig's younger brother has been admitted to a drug rehabilitation center. This program encourages counseling for the entire family. Craig loves his brother, but feels he and his brother now have very little in common. As a star athlete and president of his local Youth-to-Youth chapter, Craig is very antidrug and is embarrassed by his brother's problem. He'd like to avoid the counseling. What should Craig do? Some of his choices include:

A. Tell his parents why he doesn't want to go.

B. Find excuses, such as football or basketball practice, to keep away during the scheduled counseling sessions.

C. Realize that his brother's problem does not reflect on him and that as president of Youth-to-Youth, he should be involved in helping people overcome their problems.

D. Do it just to help his brother and his family.

E. Find out why he is embarrassed by his brother's problem with drugs.

WHAT DO YOU THINK?

1. **Situation.** Why do you think Craig feels embarrassed?

2. **Choices.** What other choices does Craig have?

3. **Consequences.** What are the costs and benefits of each choice?

4. **Consequences.** How will his brother, parents, the counselors, and Craig's friends feel about Craig if he participates in the counseling? How will he feel about himself if he participates?

5. **Consequences.** How will other people involved feel about Craig if he doesn't participate in counseling?

6. **Consequences.** What's the worst thing that could happen if Craig participates in the counseling? What's the best thing that could happen?

7. **Decision** What should Craig do? Explain your reasoning.

8. **Evaluation.** Have you ever been in a situation in which it was easier to respond positively to a stranger than to someone close to you with the same problem? How did you handle that situation?

Janet's older sister uses alcohol, pot, and cocaine. Janet loves her sister very much and wishes she could get her to give these drugs up as she has said so many times she would like to do. She is also into prostitution, theft, and selling drugs to support her habit. Janet is afraid of the people her sister associates with in these activities. She is not only afraid of what might happen to her sister but also what might happen to herself and their mother and younger sister. Their mother is a single parent who works long hours trying to support them. She may not be able to cope with this additional burden. What should Janet do?

WHAT DO YOU THINK?

9. **Choices.** What possible solutions can you come up with for Janet?

10. **Consequences.** What do you think the chances of success for each approach are? What are the costs of each approach?

11. **Consequences.** What risks exist for the older sister and for the rest of the family?

12. **Decision.** What do you think Janet should do? How should she go about implementing her plan?

13. **Evaluation.** What situations have you dealt with in which you felt too young and powerless to help? How did you handle the situation? What was the outcome? Who did you find to help? What advice would you give to others who find themselves in a similar situation?

REVIEW

Using Health Terms

On a separate sheet of paper, write the term that best matches each definition given below.

LESSON 1

1. Physiological or psychological dependence on alcohol or drugs.
2. When a person's body has a need for a certain substance.
3. When a person comes to depend on the feeling received from a drug.

LESSON 2

4. The process of removing alcohol or other drugs from one's body.
5. The act of going without alcohol or other drugs.
6. Periodic returns to drinking alcohol and using drugs.
7. The ongoing process of getting well again.

LESSON 3

8. Role of a responsible caretaker who blames, controls, or covers up for the alcoholic or addict in the family.
9. People who are overly concerned with other people's behavior and problems.
10. Role played by a family member to get the family to focus on his or her bad behavior.
11. The act of trying to protect the alcoholic or drug addict from the consequences of his or her own actions thereby helping the addict to continue the self-destructive behavior.

LESSON 4

12. An organization for teens and preteens whose parents or other family members have drinking problems.

Building Academic Skills

LESSON 1

13. **Reading.** Many articles and books are available that deal with drug and alcohol dependency. Read one and summarize it in writing. Identify cause-and-effect relationships described in the article.

Recalling the Facts

LESSON 1

14. How does the American Medical Association describe the diseases of alcoholism and drug dependence? Explain what these terms mean.
15. Why is denial an important part of psychological dependence?
16. What is at the beginning of an addiction continuum? What is at the end?
17. How long does it take for one to become addicted?

LESSON 2

18. What is meant by the statement "Recovery is a process"?
19. What is it about an addict that causes his or her recovery process to be considered ongoing?
20. Why do experts on alcohol and drug addiction recommend total abstinence for the addict?
21. What happens at a detoxification unit? How long does detoxification usually take?
22. Besides regaining one's physical health, what factors are involved in an addict's recovery?
23. What is a halfway house? How does this facility help in the treatment of an addict?
24. What services do continuing programs provide for people in recovery?

LESSON 3

25. Name and describe three roles a codependent may play in a family with addiction.
26. List some emotions people in a family living with an addict might experience.
27. How might being a codependent adversely affect a person's physical and mental health?

LESSON 4

28. What part might a family play in an addict's recovery program?
29. Why is intervention important?
30. What is Al-Anon? What is a major purpose of this organization?

REVIEW

Thinking Critically

LESSON 1

31. **Synthesis.** What might cause a person to experiment with drugs or alcohol? How could this be avoided?

32. **Evaluation.** Cigarette ads were banned from television in the 1970s. Do you think ads for alcohol should be banned? Support your answer.

LESSON 2

33. **Synthesis.** Most experts recommend that recovering addicts totally abstain from the substance(s) they have used. How long do you think the addict would have to abstain? What effects on the addict's future might this have?

LESSON 3

34. **Evaluation.** Years ago people often hid the problem of addiction within a family and suffered in silence. How are things beginning to change? What do you think is causing the change? How is this change for the better?

LESSON 4

35. **Evaluation.** Why do you suppose many codependents need professional help?

36. **Analysis.** How does Alcoholics Anonymous compare with Al-Anon?

Making the Connection

LESSON 2

37. **Art.** Design and paint a large two-panel mural. On one half, paint images that suggest addiction to alcohol or other drugs. On the other half, paint images that suggest recovery.

38. **Art/Music.** Make a sculpture or write a song about the *down* escalator of addiction and the *up* escalator of recovery.

39. **Language Arts.** Rehearse in writing what you would say if you were to confront someone close to you who was in trouble with drugs.

Applying Health Knowledge

LESSON 1

40. Watch television for one hour during a sporting event. Record the number of commercials aired that sell alcohol. How is the use of alcohol depicted? Discuss the influence these commercials could have on you and your peers.

41. Your friend wants to experiment with drugs and wants you to join him or her. What will you tell your friend? Explain your answer.

LESSON 2

42. Your friend lives in a single-parent household. His parent is an alcoholic who drinks in the evening and on weekends. What kind of treatment program do you think is best suited for your friend's parent?

43. Why do you suppose detoxification often takes place under medical supervision?

LESSON 4

44. Your friend and his younger sister live with alcoholic parents. You can see that their lives are very difficult because of their parents' actions. How can you help your friend?

Beyond the Classroom

LESSON 1

45. **Parental Involvement.** In recent years, programs have been developed encouraging young people not to get started with alcohol or drugs. With your parents, find out what similar programs are available in your community and what it takes to get involved in them.

46. **Community Involvement.** Research two support groups for addicts and codependents within your community. Interview a facilitator from each group to learn all you can about the program. If no group presently exists, research the need for such a group in your area.

COMMUNICABLE DISEASES

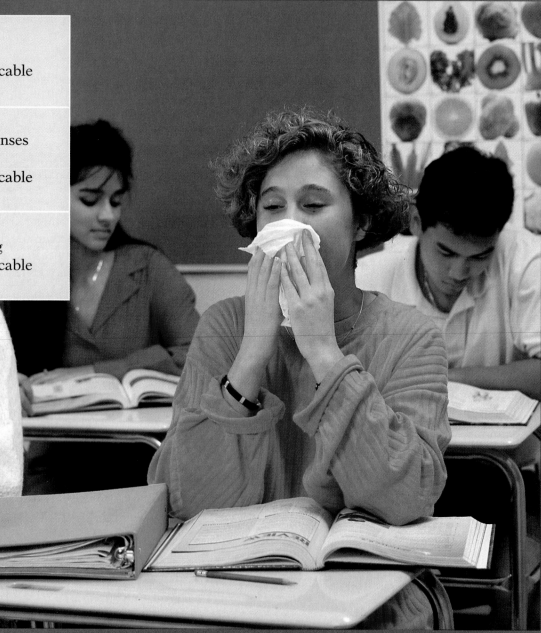

CAUSES OF COMMUNICABLE DISEASES

Many of the most common diseases are caused by tiny microorganisms called pathogens. Pathogens infect, or invade, the body and attack its cells and tissues. Some bacteria, rickettsias, fungi, protozoans, certain types of worms, and all viruses are pathogens.

Diseases caused by the direct or indirect spread of pathogens from one person to another are called **communicable diseases.**

Bacteria

Bacteria are one-celled microscopic organisms that rank among the most widespread of living things. Some bacteria are so small that a single grain of soil may contain over 100 million of them. Of course, most bacteria do not cause disease.

In order to live, all bacteria must have a food supply, as well as suitable temperature, moisture, and darkness. Some bacteria digest nonliving food materials, such as milk and meat. These organisms are called **saprophytes.** If the food supply is a living plant or animal, the microorganism is called a **parasite.** The plant or animal that the parasite feeds on is called a **host.**

Resident Bacteria

Many kinds of bacteria, called **resident bacteria,** live in your mouth and intestines and on your skin. These help protect you from harmful bacteria.

Lactobacilli, found in the gastrointestinal tract, produce lactic acid from simple carbohydrates. Coliform bacilli, found in the intestines, help break down carbohydrates and combat disease-causing bacteria.

As you will read later in this chapter, the resident bacteria form one line of defense against disease. They cause disease only if they move to a place in the body where they do not belong. For example, if bacteria from your mouth move into your middle ear, you may develop an ear infection.

The Spread of Bacteria

Most diseases caused by bacteria begin when microorganisms not usually present in the body invade the body. When these bacteria enter the body, they multiply at a rapid rate through cell division. A fully grown cell divides, forming two new cells. If conditions are good, this division can repeat itself at intervals of 20 minutes. That may not sound like much, but calculate what this multiplication rate can mean.

LESSON 1 FOCUS

TERMS TO USE
- Communicable diseases
- Saprophytes
- Parasite
- Host
- Resident bacteria
- Viruses

CONCEPTS TO LEARN
- Pathogens cause communicable diseases.
- Communicable diseases have various modes of transmission.
- The common cold is preventable, but not curable.

ATTITUDES AND BEHAVIORS TO EVALUATE
- Self-Inventory, page 532.
- Building Decision-Making Skills, page 533.

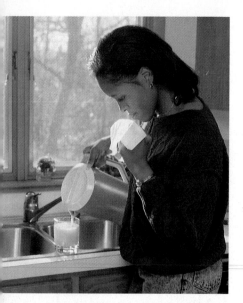

Cold symptoms may include fever, sneezing, a runny nose, a cough or sore throat, and headache.

If a single bacterial cell divides, 30 minutes later the 2 cells become 4. After 30 more minutes (1 hour elapsed), the 4 cells become 8. In just 15½ hours, there would be more than 4 billion bacteria!

Obviously, if this multiplication continued for long, the bacteria would soon take over completely. Because the bacteria must compete with one another for food, competition kills many of them, which helps control their numbers.

Toxins

Some other bacteria cause disease by producing certain poisons called toxins. Botulism, a type of food poisoning, results from this type of bacteria. Bacteria that normally live in the soil can enter the body through a wound and produce a poison that affects muscles and nerves in the body. Tetanus, or lockjaw, is an example of the actions of such bacteria.

Bacterial diseases include certain types of pneumonia and food poisoning, diphtheria, tetanus, tuberculosis, strep throat, syphilis, and gonorrhea. We will discuss some of these diseases in greater detail in this unit.

THE COMMON COLD

Colds are caused by viruses that are spread through the air, through water, or by any direct or indirect contact with a contagious person. Once you have been exposed to a cold virus, it usually takes one to two days for the symptoms to appear.

The cold virus is most contagious the day before symptoms appear. Symptoms can include a mild fever, aching, sneezing, congestion, a runny nose, a cough, a mild sore throat, and a headache.

At present there is no cure for the common cold. Getting rest, drinking liquids, and maintaining good nutrition are the best methods of treating the cold virus. Americans spend millions of dollars each year on over-the-counter cold remedies. Some of these may help relieve the symptoms, but many are useless and some may even be harmful.

Although it may be difficult to prevent colds, you can keep your body healthy so that it can better resist infection. Good nutrition, regular exercise, adequate sleep, and good health care all contribute to prevention. Controlling stress levels and relaxing also help ward off infections.

Not smoking is another way you can help prevent infections. People who smoke get more colds, and their colds tend to last longer.

Colds can be dangerous. Call a doctor if any of these symptoms last two or more days:

- a fever of 101°F (38°C) or higher
- a sore throat with a 101°F (38°C) fever
- pain in the chest or shortness of breath
- continued coughing
- pain in the back of the throat or in the ears
- any of the above, even after taking over-the-counter medicines

Viruses

Viruses are small, simple lifelike forms—from one-half to one-hundredth the size of some bacteria. These organisms are also one of the human body's worst enemies. Scientists had not actually seen viruses until the 1930s, when the high-powered electron microscope was developed. Using an electron beam instead of light and a photographic plate instead of the human eye, the electron microscope made the study of viruses possible.

An examination of viruses reveals that they are not cells. They have no nucleus, no cytoplasm, and no cell membrane. The virus particle consists of nucleic acid, a complex chemical that is an acid present in the cells of all organisms.

Viruses at Work

All viruses are parasites, requiring living cells for survival and reproduction. Viruses are highly specific in the kind of cells they invade. Only certain viruses invade animal cells, and these various viruses can attack only specific types of cells. For example, the rabies virus can enter only brain cells, polio viruses attack only the nervous system, and cold viruses enter only the cells lining the respiratory system.

Viral hepatitis is caused by a virus that affects the liver. Mumps and mononucleosis are caused by viruses that infect glandular tissues. Smallpox, chicken pox, shingles, and warts are infections caused by viruses that attack the skin tissues.

When a virus enters the body, it attaches itself to a cell and releases its nucleic acid into the host cell. The substance disrupts the cell's activities and causes it to begin producing more viruses identical to the one that attached itself to the cell wall. These viruses then spread to other body cells, where the process is repeated.

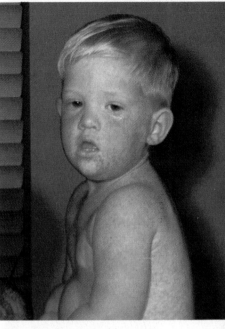

One disease caused by a virus is measles.

Rickettsias

Rickettsias are organisms that are considered intermediate, that is, somewhere between a virus and a bacterium. They are smaller than bacteria. Most of them grow in the intestinal tracts of insects, which then carry them to their human hosts. A rickettsia requires a living cell in order to grow and multiply.

Bloodsucking insects, such as lice, mites, and ticks, carry rickettsias to humans. Typhus fever and Rocky Mountain spotted fever are diseases caused by these organisms.

K E E P I N G   F I T

Don't Let Strep Get You by the Throat

Streptococcal bacteria are the cause of strep throat. The classic strep infection can cause a severe sore throat, fever, and a general feeling of illness. However, a newly mutated strain of strep is becoming more common. The bacteria that cause this ferocious kind of strep have also been linked to rheumatic fever, which can lead to permanent heart damage. This new strain of strep, first reported in 1987, has also been linked to skin rashes and shock-like symptoms. About 10,000 cases of this severe strep are reported annually.

If you have a persistent sore throat or skin infections, see a physician. Most strains of strep can be treated.

Overcoming The Odds

Dave Clowes is a saddle-maker. He loves to ride horses. As a teenager, he was a weight lifter and an award-winning gymnast. He is also one of the millions of people who contracted polio in the 1940s and 1950s before there was a vaccine to prevent it. Today, one of his legs is smaller than the other and he walks with a cane, but Dave is healthy and enjoying life. He says, "I was a year old when I got polio. I spent nine months in the hospital. A doctor told me years later that polio could be no worse than the flu, it could affect people as it did me, or worse. The point is that it affected different people in different ways. I remember having a brace when I was a little kid. The thing about me was that I never thought about it much. It wasn't as if I'd ever known differently, so it didn't feel like I had to overcome anything."

He continues, "I started lifting weights when I was thirteen. All of a sudden, I was stronger than everybody else, and I enjoyed that. I got involved in gymnastics in the eighth grade. I applied myself to that and got pretty good at it. I tied for metropolitan champ in the AAU, the American Athletic Union. I tied for first place on the rings one year. I went to the AAU junior nationals that same year, and I got third on the rings. That was really fun.

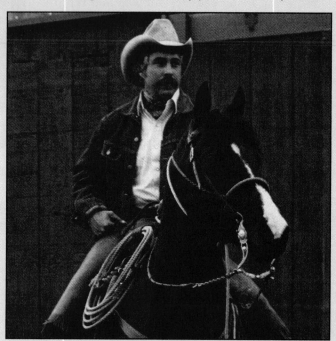

"Back in the 50s, when everyone else had to line up for the polio shots (the Salk vaccine), I didn't get them because they thought I was immune. Then they found out there were three different strains of the disease, so I ended up having to take sugar cubes when I was in college." The sugar cubes contained the oral polio vaccine approved in 1961. This vaccine, called the Sabin vaccine, is still given today.

Decades after their initial polio infections, many people are suffering from recurring polio symptoms. "My doctor warned me about post-polio syndrome, but I don't worry about it," Dave says. "My friend with a bad back says I'm healthier than he is. We're all victims of some disease—or of ourselves. If you have a problem, it's your problem, not somebody else's, and it's your responsibility to do something about it. I did it. I overcame it. And I have a beautiful wife, two stepsons, a business, horses, five acres. I've done okay in life."

1. Dave realized what he could do and worked to excel at it, rather than dwelling on what he couldn't do. Do you take this approach, or do you dwell on your limitations?
2. One reason Dave was able to accept his disability was that he had never known any other way. How might a sudden change in health or ability later in life make it harder to adjust?
3. Why is it important to remember that diseases affect different people in different ways?

Fungi

Fungi are living organisms that cannot make their own food. Many feed off dead animals, insects, and leaves. Fungi are, therefore, saprophytes. They prefer dark, damp environments. Two of the most common fungi are yeast and mushrooms.

Disease-producing fungi invade mainly deep tissues of the hair, nails, and skin. Fungi cause infections of the scalp, such as ringworm, and of the feet, such as athlete's foot. Pathogenic fungi can also cause brain inflammation and serious lung infection.

Protozoans

Protozoans are single-celled organisms that are larger than bacteria and have a more complex cellular structure. Most protozoans are harmless. The disease-producing protozoans are most common in tropical areas that have poor sanitation. Protozoans cause malaria, African sleeping sickness, and amoebic dysentery, a severe intestinal infection.

Other Pathogens That Can Cause Infections

Certain flatworms and roundworms, while not microorganisms, are regarded as pathogens and cause diseases in the human body. Disease-producing flatworms include flukes, which can invade the blood, intestines, liver, or lungs, and tapeworms, which live in the intestines. Pathogenic roundworms can infect the intestines, muscles, and fluids under the skin. You may have heard of trichinosis, a disease caused by an intestinal roundworm. Trichinosis is usually transmitted when a person eats improperly cooked pork.

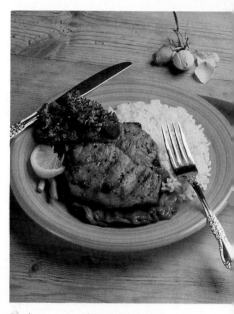

Trichinosis, a disease caused by an intestinal roundworm, can be transmitted when a person eats pork that has not been cooked properly.

LESSON 1 REVIEW

Reviewing Facts and Vocabulary

1. What is a communicable disease?
2. Name six types of pathogens that cause disease.
3. How are viruses different from other pathogens?

Thinking Critically

4. **Analysis.** Compare a parasite and a saprophyte. Give an example of each.
5. **Synthesis.** How might a communicable disease influence one's mental health?

Applying Health Knowledge

6. Contact a local veterinarian to find out about parasites (such as ticks and fleas) that affect pets. How do these microorganisms work? How can they be stopped from causing illness or discomfort to pets or people? How does warm weather affect the problems associated with fleas and ticks? Share your findings with your class.
7. On one side of a poster board, make a collage of ads for cold remedies. On the other side, create your own ad for preventing the common cold through good health habits.

BODY DEFENSES AGAINST COMMUNICABLE DISEASES

You may know someone who seems to get colds or flu a lot. Why do some people get these diseases often and others do not? How does anyone get a communicable disease? How does your body respond when a pathogen enters?

Ways Pathogens Are Spread

Pathogens are spread in many ways. As you learn the ways they can be spread, you can practice habits that help promote your health.

Indirect Contact

Many communicable diseases spread as a result of indirect contact with an infected person. The common cold, strep throat, and pneumonia are diseases that can be spread through the air. The pathogens that cause these diseases are in the tiny droplets of moisture expelled when a person coughs or sneezes. Anyone near the infected person can breathe in the pathogens in the airborne droplets.

Certain pathogens are spread when an uninfected person touches objects that an infected person has used. These objects can include eating utensils, combs, or toothbrushes. They also can include needles used to inject drugs that are shared with an infected person.

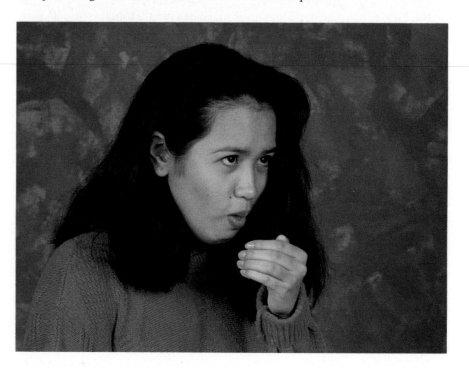

Pathogens are expelled into the air when a person coughs or sneezes.

Direct Contact

Pathogens may be spread when an uninfected person comes into direct physical contact with an infected area on another person. Some skin rashes can be spread in this way. Sexually transmitted diseases are also spread when an infected person with sores comes in contact with an uninfected person.

Contact with Animals

Animals spread many serious diseases. When an insect, such as a mosquito, bites an infected person, the insect may take pathogens into its own body. The pathogens then continue their development within the insect.

When the insect later bites an uninfected person, it injects some of the pathogens into that person's body, thus spreading the disease. Some communicable diseases, such as rabies, are spread by contact with infected mammals and birds.

Your Immune System

Though you cannot see them, your body is exposed each day to millions of pathogens. Pathogens are in the air you breathe, and they cling to the surfaces you touch. Your body is constantly fighting pathogens that enter your body. When they enter your body, pathogens attack your body cells and use these cells to grow and multiply. The end result of such an attack is an infection.

Most of the time, your body manages to stay free of infection because of your immune system. Your immune system includes two main types of defenses. One type of defense is nonspecific resistance. Another type of defense is specific resistance. Both types work together to protect your body against pathogens that could harm you.

Nonspecific Resistance

Body defenses that are nonspecific respond in the same way each time your body is invaded by a foreign substance. Your body's nonspecific defenses include mechanical mechanisms, chemical barriers, cells, and inflammatory response.

Mechanical Mechanisms. Mechanical mechanisms form barriers to help keep pathogens out of the body. Your body's main mechanical mechanism is your skin. Unbroken skin helps prevent pathogens from entering body tissues. The tough dead cells that make up the outer layer of skin form a very effective barrier. Mucous membranes in your mouth, nose, and bronchial tubes produce a sticky substance called mucus that traps pathogens. Some mucous membranes have cilia, tiny hairs, that also trap pathogens, which are then expelled when you cough or sneeze. Tears and saliva are other mechanical barriers that help carry pathogens away.

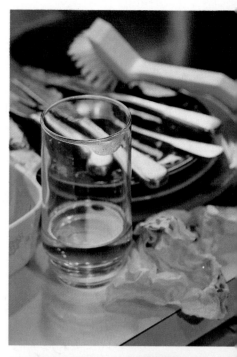

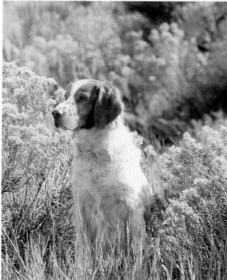

Pathogens may be spread by sharing eating utensils—or even from your pet.

Chemical Barriers. Chemicals on the surface of cells can kill pathogens or prevent them from entering the body. Such chemicals can be found in tears, saliva, and sweat. The acidic digestive juices of the stomach also are chemical barriers. These juices destroy pathogens that are swallowed with food. Other chemicals cause body changes that help cells inside the body fight pathogens.

Cells. Certain types of white blood cells, called phagocytes, travel through blood and group together to destroy foreign substances. This action is called phagocytosis. **Phagocytosis** is the process by which phagocytes engulf and destroy pathogens. **Neutrophils** are one type of phagocyte that are most actively involved in the process of phagocytosis.

Inflammatory Response. After bacteria enter the body or cause damage to body tissue, chemical mediators are released. These cause the blood vessels to dilate and allow increased blood flow. Increased blood flow brings phagocytes to the area to leave the blood and enter the tissues. This process continues until the pathogens are destroyed. Once the pathogens are destroyed, tissues can be repaired. Symptoms of inflammation confined to a specific area include heat, redness, and swelling, which result from increased blood flow. Pain can result from swelling.

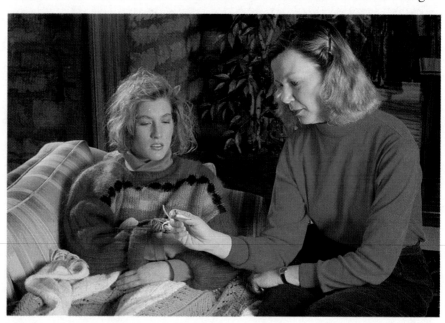

Fever is another way that the body fights infection by speeding up the activities of the immune system.

K E E P I N G   F I T

The Spread of Disease

- Rumors are rampant about how disease-carrying organisms are spread—toilet seats, kissing, casual contact. All pathogens are different, so there is no single set of rules for all. Many pathogens need warm, moist, dark environments to survive. Once these organisms leave the body, they die quickly.
- Many other organisms are resilient and can last a long time outside the body.
- Antiseptics, such as household disinfectants, inhibit the growth of bacteria and can be used to clean skin, wounds, and inanimate objects. Germicides, such as bleach, also kill bacteria.

Should Animals Be Used for Medical Research?

Many people and organizations believe that the use of laboratory animals for medical research is critical. Animal-rights advocates, however, claim that such testing is not only unnecessary but also cruel and inhumane. This heated debate goes on.

Analyzing Different Viewpoints

ONE VIEW. Those who support the use of laboratory animals for medical research maintain that various medical procedures or medicines must first be tested on animals to see if they will be safe and effective when used on humans. They state that animal research has led to a great many important medical advances for humans. Dogs were used in the perfecting of coronary artery bypass surgery. Mice have been used in the development of vaccines for various communicable diseases and are even now being used to test how some vaccines might trigger defenses in humans. Those in favor of using animals in biomedical research caution that if funding is cut for research, many humans suffering from diseases will not get the treatment, medi-

cations, or cures that might be available to them if testing were to continue.

A SECOND VIEW. Many animal-rights advocates say that they are not against all animal research if the aim of such research is truly to aid human beings in the treatment or prevention of diseases rather than to make money for medical companies. Some animal-rights advocates add that more humane, less painful methods of testing than those presently used must be developed and implemented. They also claim that some animal testing, such as that for cosmetics, is completely unnecessary, since such products are not needed for improved health.

A THIRD VIEW. Some people are opposed to any use of animals for research. They claim no human has the right to harm another living creature for any purpose.

Exploring Your Views

1. Do you favor the use of animals for medical research? Why or why not?
2. Are there any limitations or conditions that you would put on that research?

Culturally Speaking

Spreading Diseases

Many human activities may unwittingly spread diseases. Some activities simply allow diseases to be carried to new populations. People and animals traveling by air may be infected with a disease, although they have no symptoms. Sometimes pathogens actually "catch a ride" to new areas in cargo shipments.

Other human activities spread disease by causing favorable environments for some disease carriers. Building highways and clearing land for farming have caused new mosquito breeding grounds in parts of South America, Asia, and Africa.

Specific Resistance

The general response of your nonspecific defenses is not always enough to protect your body from disease. Another defense mechanism is specific resistance. This defense gives specific protection against specific types of pathogens. When this happens, another body defense goes to work. This defense is the cells that not only fight off pathogens but also keep a record of them in case they enter the body again.

Tomorrow night is the senior prom, and Gloria's been looking forward to it for weeks. Everything was going to be perfect—until she woke up this morning with a sore throat. Now Gloria's mom thinks she should stay home from the prom so she won't "spread her germs." Gloria thinks that going to the last social event of her senior year is more important than protecting her date from a sore throat.

What do you think Gloria should do?

MONONUCLEOSIS

Mononucleosis is a communicable disease common among young people that is characterized by abnormal shapes of lymphocytes. It spreads primarily through direct contact, such as kissing. Symptoms include chills, fever, sore throat, fatigue, and swollen lymph nodes. Complete bed rest is needed. Treatment and recovery can take three to six weeks.

Lymphocytes. **Lymphocytes** are a type of white blood cell that fights pathogens. Lymphocytes travel through your body along two networks of vessels. One of these networks is your blood vessels. The other network is your lymph vessels, which are a part of your lymphatic system. Your lymphatic system also includes your spleen, tonsils, thymus gland, lymph, and lymph nodes. This system is part of your body's defense system. Lymphocytes multiply in the spleen, tonsils, thymus gland, and lymph nodes.

The immune system uses two major types of lymphocytes—T cells and B cells. T cells and B cells originate in bone marrow, the soft material at the core of your bones. T cells move through blood vessels and mature in your thymus gland. B cells mature in red bone marrow. Both T cells and B cells travel between your blood and your lymph tissues.

T cells and B cells both fight specific pathogens. Imagine that pathogens that cause a particular disease have entered your body. Your immune system searches your lymph nodes for the right T cell and B cell to fight those particular pathogens. When the right T cell and B cell are found, your body begins producing many copies of these cells to ensure that enough lymphocytes are on hand to attack the pathogens.

T cells and B cells work in different ways. There are many types of T cells, and these different types have different functions. Some T cells kill pathogens. Other T cells regulate other cell functions. B cells are stimulated by T helper cells, one type of T cell, to make antibodies. **Antibodies** are proteins that destroy or neutralize pathogens in your body. The antibodies for a particular pathogen remain in your blood to become active if you encounter the specific pathogen again.

LESSON 2 REVIEW

Reviewing Facts and Vocabulary

1. How are pathogens spread?
2. List the body's nonspecific defenses.
3. Explain the term *antibodies*.

Thinking Critically

4. **Analysis.** Explain why the presence of antibodies is often used to determine if an individual has a communicable disease.
5. **Analysis.** Compare B cells and T cells.

Applying Health Knowledge

6. In small groups make up a game or activity that explains ways your immune system works. Exchange completed projects with classmates as a review for this lesson.

PREVENTING COMMUNICABLE DISEASES

What can you do to protect yourself from being infected by disease? You have several choices. You can avoid contact with pathogens and you can avoid spreading pathogens to others. Follow these guidelines to reduce the spread of infection.

- Bathe or shower every day to keep your skin, hair, and nails clean.
- Avoid sharing eating or drinking utensils.
- Store and prepare food in a safe way to prevent food poisoning.
- Wash your hands after using the bathroom, after changing diapers, and before preparing or serving food.
- If you know you are sick, avoid giving your illness to someone else. Get medical treatment for your illness. Cover your mouth when you cough or sneeze to prevent spreading the germs. Use tissues only once and dispose of them immediately in a waste container.
- If you are well, avoid contact with people who are sick.

There are three other ways to protect yourself from communicable diseases. You can become immune by having the disease. You can be immunized by injection if a vaccine is available, and you can practice biofeedback.

Immunity

As you have read, immunity is the body's natural resistance to many pathogens. Certain pathogens cannot live in the body, while others are quickly destroyed if they enter the body.

One important feature of the body's immune system is that it remembers the pathogens it meets. This gives the body long-term protection—immunity—against many communicable diseases. For example, if you had chicken pox, your immune system remembers the chicken pox virus. If the virus enters your body again, cells designed specifically to combat the chicken pox virus will attack it immediately. In most cases, the virus does not get a chance to make you sick again.

This immunity your body develops to protect you from disease is called **active immunity.** Some types of immunity last a lifetime; others last only a short period of time. A single virus causes chicken pox, so once a person has had the disease, the body is usually protected against chicken pox for life. However, many different kinds of viruses cause the common cold. Because the body is continually exposed to different pathogens, immunity to colds is limited.

Vaccines Provide Active Immunity

Through the use of vaccines, the body can develop active immunity against a disease without actually having had the disease. **Vaccines** are

LESSON 3 FOCUS

TERMS TO USE
- Active immunity
- Vaccines
- Vaccination
- Passive immunity
- Biofeedback

CONCEPTS TO LEARN
- You can protect yourself from communicable diseases by avoiding contact with pathogens.
- There are many strategies to help prevent communicable diseases.

ATTITUDES AND BEHAVIORS TO EVALUATE
- Self-Inventory, page 532.
- Building Decision-Making Skills, page 533.

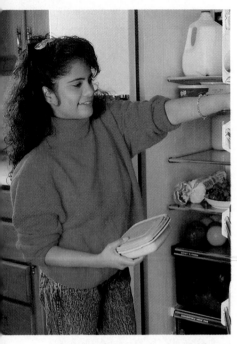

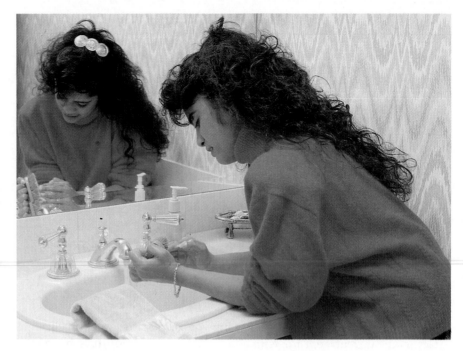

Storing food properly and keeping your hands clean are two ways to prevent becoming infected with a communicable disease.

preparations that usually are composed of dead or weakened viruses. Vaccines provide immunity by causing the body to produce antibodies against the pathogen. The vaccine contains substances that are strong enough to cause the production of antibodies, but not strong enough to cause the disease. Through the process of **vaccination,** a vaccine is injected into the body.

The first vaccine was developed by Dr. Edward Jenner in 1798. In an effort to control the deadly smallpox disease, he injected people with pus from the sores of an animal with cowpox. (The cowpox and smallpox viruses are closely related.) People developed a mild case of cowpox but also developed an immunity to smallpox. Jenner's technique has been refined, and vaccinations are now used to protect people from a variety of crippling or fatal diseases.

At birth, babies carry in their blood small amounts of the antibodies that protected their mothers. Babies are thus protected from the same diseases as their mothers. This immunity lasts for a few months after birth until the baby can produce antibodies of its own. The temporary immunity that the infant acquires from the mother is called **passive immunity.**

Types of Vaccines

Some of the major types of vaccines include live-virus vaccines, killed-virus vaccines, and toxoids.

Live-Virus Vaccine. Some vaccines are made from weakened viruses. By using mechanical means or chemicals and growing the virus over and over until it is very weak, scientists develop a live-virus vaccine. In this weakened state, the virus cannot cause a disease, but the virus does stimulate the production of antibodies in the body. Measles, rubella, and oral polio vaccines all contain live viruses.

Killed-Virus Vaccine. Another type of vaccine is the killed-virus vaccine. Scientists use mechanical means or chemicals to kill the viruses. The killed-virus vaccine causes the body to produce antibodies, but it is not as powerful as the live-virus vaccine. Because it is less powerful, people need booster shots of killed-virus vaccines. Booster shots are injections given to add strength to the antibody in guarding against infection.

Toxoids. Diphtheria and tetanus are diseases caused by bacteria that release a toxin. Scientists have discovered that by chemically treating bacteria toxins, they can make very effective vaccines. The treated toxins, called toxoids, stimulate the production of antibodies and establish active immunity against diphtheria and tetanus.

Reactions to Vaccines

Vaccines are as safe as medical scientists can make them. However, vaccinations sometimes cause minor reactions, usually in the form of a mild fever or skin rash. On rare occasions more serious reactions may occur. Yet the risks from vaccines are far less than the risks from the diseases themselves.

Immunization for All

Immunization is more than just a good idea—the law often requires it. Each state has its own laws governing immunizations and school attendance. In most states, students cannot enter kindergarten without up-to-date immunizations. Several states now enforce laws that prevent teenagers from attending school without complete immunization. Why, do you think, are immunizations so important in the school setting?

Some communicable diseases are more common than others. Diseases that were once dreaded can now be controlled through immunizations. Some of these diseases have been completely eradicated. However, because some diseases are no longer the threat they used to

DID YOU KNOW?

- Lyme disease is named for the town in Connecticut where symptoms were first noted. This illness is caused by tick-borne bacteria. In most cases, symptoms include a circle of reddened skin around a pale area where the tick had attached itself. After a few days, similar rashes appear on the body along with fever and flulike symptoms. If treated with antibiotics within ten days, recovery can be complete. If treatment is not received, second stage symptoms include temporary paralysis of the face, headache, stiff neck, and vomiting. The third, untreated stage of Lyme disease results in chronic arthritis that affects and damages the joints.
- Prevention is the best means of avoiding Lyme disease. Wear long sleeves and pants when in the woods. Light colors make it easier to spot ticks. Check your dog for ticks. They can also get Lyme disease from ticks.

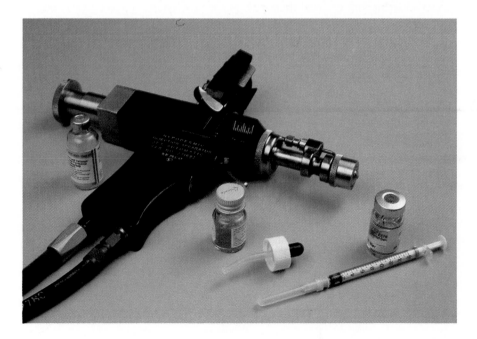

Vaccines may be administered with a "gun," or with a conventional needle.

be, people have become lax in obtaining immunization, and isolated cases of some diseases, such as polio, are being reported. An immunization program is essential, just as is the practice of simple biofeedback.

Biofeedback

One way to keep checking on yourself is through **biofeedback**—biological feedback about your body. Biofeedback is the process of becoming aware of physical events in your body that you normally are not aware of, with the intent of gaining voluntary control of such events.

Simple and basic examples of biofeedback include the following:

- weighing yourself
- taking your pulse when exercising
- taking your temperature when you are sick

Biofeedback provides a means for receiving feedback on functions of your body that are involuntary—that is, functions under the control of the autonomic nervous system. These functions include those of the brain, the heart, and the circulatory system.

Other Uses of Biofeedback

Besides the personal methods of biofeedback, other methods can be used to help restructure many body malfunctions. Using sophisticated instrumentation, muscle tension, brain waves, skin temperature, skin resistance, and other physical processes can be regulated.

The implications of biofeedback in preventive medicine are tremendous. Changes to the body's balanced healthy state can be prevented or overcome by consciously reestablishing normal body conditions. Biofeedback is used clinically to manage stress, to relieve migraine and tension headaches and anxiety disorders, to rehabilitate the neuromuscular system, and to ease gastrointestinal disorders.

Biofeedback Instruments

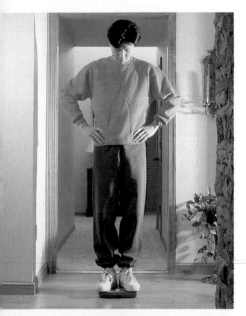

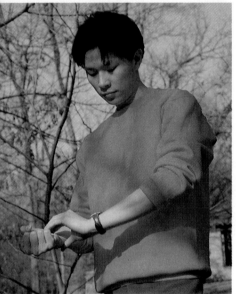

Weighing yourself regularly and taking your pulse before and after exercising are two examples of biofeedback.

The principal instruments used in biofeedback training are as follows:

- Electromyogram (EMG). The feedback of bioelectric information from the muscles regarding muscle tension.
- Electroencephalogram (EEG). The feedback of bioelectric information from the brain regarding changes in the brain-wave status.

K E E P I N G   F I T

What to Do for Colds: Getting the Cold Facts

- Drink plenty of liquids.
- Get lots of sleep and rest.
- Wash your hands frequently to prevent spreading the virus.
- Use a humidifier or a vaporizer. When using a vaporizer, keep it clean to avoid infections.

- Don't take aspirin. You may have flu. Aspirin should never be taken when you have flulike symptoms. Instead, take an aspirin substitute.
- If you develop a severe earache, a sore throat, a fever of 101°F or

more, wheezing, difficult breathing, or a deep cough, consult a physician. You may have more than a cold. Also call your physician if you cough up greenish phlegm or blood.

- Thermal trainer. The feedback of changes in skin temperature, a result of blood flow.
- Electrodermal response (EDR). The feedback of changes in skin resistance, a result of perspiration.

Biofeedback may become increasingly popular in the future. However, the simple disease-prevention steps that we all take day after day are also invaluable.

HEPATITIS

Hepatitis is a disease involving an inflammation of the liver. There are two main types—viral hepatitis and toxic hepatitis. The two most comon forms of viral hepatitis are hepatitis type A and hepatitis type B.

Hepatitis A results from eating food or drinking water that has been contaminated with the virus. Symptoms include weakness, loss of appetite, vomiting, and jaundice—a yellowish discoloration of the skin. Symptoms usually appear three to four weeks after exposure to the virus and last from two to six weeks.

A person who has been exposed to the hepatitis virus receives a shot of gamma globulin, a protein fraction of blood rich in antibodies. If this vaccine is administered within a week of exposure to the hepatitis virus, the disease can be prevented.

Hepatitis B virus is found in all body fluids of an infected person, especially blood. Hepatitis B used to be transmitted through blood transfusions from an infected donor. However, tests that detect the virus in the blood have helped eliminate this means of transmission. Contaminated medical instruments, sexual contact with an infected person, and hypodermic needles shared by drug users are the main ways hepatitis B is spread. Symptoms usually appear six to twelve weeks after the infection. The treatment is the same for types A and B. Bed rest is prescribed for both.

Toxic hepatitis results from exposure to certain chemicals. The chemicals can enter the body by being swallowed, inhaled, injected, or absorbed through the skin. Symptoms will depend on the particular chemicals causing the hepatitis.

DID YOU KNOW?

- A body temperature of 99.6°F (37.5°C) or higher is considered a fever. The body can tolerate only a slight variation from normal body temperature.
- A fever causes dehydration, lethargy, nausea, headache, and loss of appetite.
- In teens and adults, fevers higher than 103°F (39.5°C) have mental effects, such as confusion, irritability, and even delirium.
- Caffeine stimulates body metabolism and raises body temperature. When you feel feverish, avoid caffeinated drinks and caffeine-containing medicines.

LESSON 3 REVIEW

Reviewing Facts and Vocabulary

1. Define *active immunity* and *passive immunity*.
2. How can biofeedback benefit a person?
3. Name three major types of vaccines.

Thinking Critically

4. **Synthesis.** What are some major factors that would lessen the effectiveness of the body's immune system?
5. **Analysis.** When the polio vaccine first was introduced, some people actually contracted the disease from the vaccine. Explain how this could happen.

Applying Health Knowledge

6. Develop an information pamphlet on a common communicable disease. Include symptoms, mode of transmission, prevention, and treatment.
7. In recent years some groups have challenged the right of government to make laws requiring immunization of children before they enter school. If you were given the task of explaining the need for such laws, what would you say? Limit your response to two paragraphs.

Self-Inventory

Your Disease-Prevention Efforts

HOW DO YOU RATE?

Number a sheet of paper from 1 through 20. Read each item below and respond by writing *M* if the statement describes you *most of the time*, *S* if the statement describes you *some of the time*, and *N* if the statement *never* applies to you. Total the number of each type of response. Then proceed to the next section.

1. I keep my immunization records up-to-date.
2. I stay away from people who currently have a cold or the flu.
3. I eat a balanced diet daily.
4. I get at least eight hours of sleep each night.
5. I exercise aerobically at least three times a week.
6. I do not smoke.
7. I avoid using towels others have used.
8. I avoid using other people's combs and brushes.
9. I take a few minutes each day to relax.
10. I stay home at least the first day that symptoms of illness appear.
11. I listen and respond to my body's message that it is tired or that something may be wrong.
12. I wash my hands before every meal, before preparing food, and after using the bathroom.
13. I shower or bathe regularly.
14. I do not share eating utensils or glasses with other people.
15. I cover my mouth when I cough or sneeze.
16. I avoid walking barefoot in locker rooms and shower rooms.
17. I avoid eating dairy products and poultry that might not have been refrigerated.
18. I advise my parents to make sure that our pets have their shots.
19. I put food waste in closed containers.
20. I support efforts to enforce public health laws for immunization and for reporting communicable diseases.

HOW DID YOU SCORE?

Give yourself 4 points for each *most of the time* answer, 2 points for each *some of the time* answer, and 0 points for each *never* answer. Find your total, and read below to see how you scored. Then proceed to the next section.

60 to 80
Excellent. Your disease-prevention efforts are outstanding. Congratulations.

40 to 59
Good. You are doing very well in your efforts to prevent communicable diseases.

20 to 39
Fair. Disease prevention is not important enough to you. Some effort will be beneficial to you and others.

Below 20
Needs Improvement. Be careful. You may be spreading communicable diseases to yourself and to others. Now is a good time to start taking better care of yourself.

WHAT ARE YOUR GOALS?

If you received an *excellent* or *good* score, complete the statements in Part A. If your score was *fair* or *needs improvement*, complete Parts A and B.

Part A

1. I plan to learn more about disease prevention by ____.
2. My timetable for accomplishing this is ____.
3. I plan to share my information with others by ____.

Part B

4. The behavior I would most like to change is ____.
5. The steps involved in making this change are ____.
6. The people or groups I will ask for support and assistance are ____.
7. My rewards for making this change will be ____.

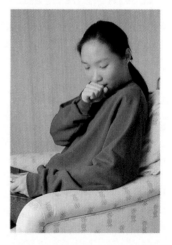

Building Decision-Making Skills

Lavonda is a major contributor to the school's select choir, which has a major performance tomorrow. This morning she noticed she had symptoms of chicken pox. What should Lavonda do?

A. Don't tell anyone and go ahead with the performance because it means so much to both her present happiness and future opportunities. She is a critical part of the group and doesn't want to let the other members of the group down.

B. Tell the teacher and let her decide, based on what is best for the group.

C. Tell her mother and let her decide. It may be that she doesn't really have chicken pox or that she isn't contagious or that no one else in the group is susceptible.

D. Go to the doctor and let him or her decide.

WHAT DO YOU THINK?

1. **Situation.** Why does a decision need to be made?

2. **Situation.** How much time does Lavonda have to make this decision?

3. **Choices.** What other possibilities exist for Lavonda?

4. **Consequences.** What risks are involved in this decision and to whom?

5. **Consequences.** What are the advantages of each approach to this problem?

6. **Consequences.** What are the disadvantages to each approach?

7. **Consequences.** What obligation does Lavonda have to the other members of the group both healthwise and musically?

8. **Consequences.** How will Lavonda's health triangle be affected by this decision?

9. **Decision.** What do you think Lavonda should do? Why?

10. **Decision.** How should Lavonda implement this decision?

11. **Evaluation.** Have you ever been in this type of situation? What process did you use to make your decision? Was it effective? What did you learn that could be applied to this situation?

Marco is captain of the school's wrestling team. In past years he has gotten strep infections from the mats, resulting in an athletic department policy that the mats be washed before every practice and match. The new coach is a "drill sergeant type" who believes wrestlers should be tough and worry only about getting in the maximum training time. On several occasions he has started practice without washing the mats. Marco's teammates have asked him to talk to the coach. What should Marco do?

A. Tell the guys to quit complaining and be tough.

B. Talk to the coach but say it's on behalf of his teammates.

C. Tell the coach he and his teammates are concerned about not only their health but the possible effects an absence would have on the team's success.

D. Go to the administration with the problem and ask for anonymity.

E. Wait and see if strep becomes a problem.

WHAT DO YOU THINK?

12. **Situation.** Why does a decision need to be made?

13. **Choices.** What other choices does Marco have?

14. **Consequences.** What are the advantages and disadvantages of each choice?

15. **Consequences.** Does Marco have different obligations as a result of being captain? If so, what are they?

16. **Consequences.** What are the risks involved in this situation?

17. **Decision.** How do you think Marco should handle this situation?

REVIEW

Using Health Terms

On a separate sheet of paper, write the term that best matches each definition given below.

LESSON 1

1. Disease-producing organisms.
2. A type of bacteria that digest nonliving food materials.
3. Bacteria that live off plants or animals.
4. Poisons.
5. Small, simple lifelike forms—smaller than bacteria.
6. Organisms that are somewhere between viruses and bacteria and that grow in the intestinal tracts of insects.
7. Simple organisms that cannot make their own food, such as yeasts and mushrooms.

LESSON 2

8. White blood cells that travel through blood and destroy foreign substances; part of nonspecific resistance.
9. The process in which pathogens are engulfed and destroyed.
10. Body defense that gives specific protection against specific pathogens.
11. Cells that multiply in the spleen, tonsils, thymus gland, and lymph nodes.
12. Cells that are stimulated to make antibodies.

LESSON 3

13. The body's ability to resist disease.
14. Preparations that may be composed of dead or weakened viruses.
15. The injection of a vaccine into the body in order to provide immunity to a disease.

Building Academic Skills

LESSON 2

16. **Writing.** Look up information about a communicable disease that was not mentioned in this lesson. Write a newspaper article telling about this disease, i.e., how it is transmitted and how the body defends itself.

Recalling the Facts

LESSON 1

17. What do bacteria need to survive?
18. What are resident bacteria, and what purpose do they serve?
19. Although resident bacteria are generally helpful bacteria, they can be harmful. How can they become harmful?
20. Bacteria can multiply fast enough to take over one's body in a short time. What usually prevents this from happening?
21. Suppose you are planting some flowers and you cut yourself on one of the tools you are using. What disease could result if soil containing bacteria enters the open wound?
22. Name eight different bacterial diseases.
23. How does a virus work?

LESSON 2

24. List ways indirect contact spreads pathogens.
25. Explain nonspecific resistance.
26. Explain how chemical barriers work and where they can be found in the body.
27. Describe the role of chemical mediators during the inflammatory response.
28. List symptoms of inflammation confined to a specific area.
29. Explain specific resistance.
30. What tissues are part of your lymphatic system?
31. Describe how antibodies are made and their role in the blood.

LESSON 3

32. What are some behaviors that will help a person avoid communicable diseases?
33. In what two ways can a person become immune to a communicable disease?
34. If the body is able to remember a virus that has invaded it and fight against it in the future, why do people not develop an immunity to colds?
35. Name and briefly describe three types of vaccines.
36. In what ways might a person contract hepatitis?

REVIEW

Thinking Critically

LESSON 1

37. **Analysis.** Many people think they can catch a cold by becoming chilled, getting caught in the rain, or not dressing warmly enough in cold weather. Analyze why people might think this way.

38. **Synthesis.** Interview four people who are 35 or older about polio. What were some of the myths about this disease that existed during their youth? How do these myths compare to some early impressions about AIDS? Write some generalizations about why myths develop and how they affect people.

LESSON 2

39. **Analysis.** Compare and contrast the function of phagocytes during nonspecific resistance and lymphocytes during specific resistance.

LESSON 3

40. **Evaluation.** In the past, people usually visited a physician only when they were sick. Now many insurance policies reimburse people for wellness checkups. In your opinion, is this a good or bad practice? Support your answer.

Making the Connection

LESSON 1

41. **Social Studies.** Write a one-page report about a protozoan-caused communicable disease, such as malaria, sleeping sickness, or amoebic dysentery. How did the disease affect people in the past? Is it still affecting people today? If so, in what way? How is the disease treated?

LESSON 3

42. **Physical Education.** Talk with a coach or physical education teacher about what process the school follows to try to decrease the incidence of athlete's foot transmission in the locker rooms.

Applying Health Knowledge

LESSON 1

43. Discuss how a disease can affect a person's mental, social, and emotional health.

44. For many years Ellis Island in New York City harbor was a clearinghouse for millions of immigrants who came to the United States. Find out about the disease-prevention efforts that were carried out with the immigrants. Draw some conclusions about the effectiveness of these efforts.

LESSON 2

45. Your brother works at a day-care center. He says that the children there are always passing colds and flu to each other. What could you share with him about the spread of pathogens?

46. Make a chart with three columns. At the top of each column, write one of the following: indirect contact, direct contact, and contact with animals. List several examples of communicable diseases known to be spread in this way.

LESSON 3

47. Antibacterial soap is now available in many stores. What is the benefit of this kind of soap? What is a drawback?

48. Each year, as flu season approaches, a flu vaccine is made available. Who is usually advised to receive this vaccine? Why do you suppose this is?

49. Find out what the law is in your state regarding immunizations.

Beyond the Classroom

LESSON 1

50. **Further Study.** Find out how parasites such as ticks and fleas affect pets.

LESSON 3

51. **Further Study.** Find out more about Jonas Salk and A. B. Sabin. What was the difference in their discoveries? What impact did they have on public health?

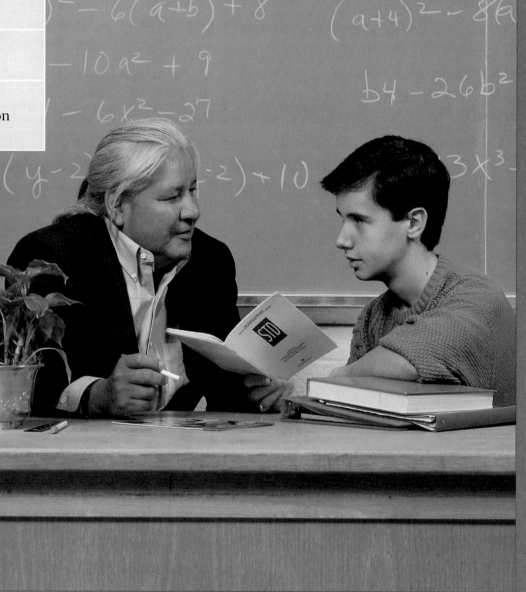

GONORRHEA

A sexually transmitted disease (STD) is a communicable disease that is spread from person to person through sexual contact. While many of the common communicable diseases are being controlled, rates of STDs are rising steadily. STDs represent a serious threat to the health of all Americans, but particularly to young adults.

Nearly 3 million adolescents contract an STD each year. One in four of sexually active adolescents will become infected before graduating from high school. Although epidemics of STDs do occur in the United States, there are ways to control and even prevent these diseases completely. The first step is to remain sexually abstinent until marriage. Next, obtain accurate information about such diseases and recognize inaccurate information.

People often fail to seek medical attention for an STD. A social stigma exists about STDs, and some people are embarrassed. Others are not willing to take responsibility for their actions. Still others just will not believe that they could have an STD. Through denial and rationalization, they ignore the signs and symptoms. In many cases, symptoms are not obvious, and the person does not know that he or she has the disease.

Gonorrhea is a disease caused by bacteria that live in warm, moist areas of the body, primarily in the lining of the urethra of the male and in the cervix of the female. The bacteria are transmitted during sexual contact. A person cannot pick up the pathogens from towels or toilet seats because the bacteria cannot live outside the body.

Gonorrhea is one of the most frequently reported communicable diseases in the United States. Despite the fact that gonorrhea is a treatable disease and can be cured, about 2 million cases of it are reported in the United States each year. There is no way of knowing how many unreported cases there are.

LESSON 1 FOCUS

TERMS TO USE
- Sexually transmitted disease (STD)
- Gonorrhea (gahn•uh•REE•uh)
- Pelvic inflammatory disease (PID)

CONCEPTS TO LEARN
- There are immediate and long-term consequences when one gets gonorrhea.
- The symptoms of gonorrhea are often difficult to detect, especially for females.
- The seriousness of gonorrhea warrants diligent protection and immediate treatment.

ATTITUDES AND BEHAVIORS TO EVALUATE
- Self-Inventory, page 550.
- Building Decision-Making Skills, page 551.

Symptoms of Gonorrhea

Symptoms of gonorrhea are not always obvious. This is true particularly in the female, who may never know that she has gonorrhea. The symptoms may not be present or may be so slight that an infected person does not notice them.

In the female, symptoms may include a slight discharge from the vagina, a burning sensation during urination, abnormal menstruation, and abdominal pain or tenderness. In the male, symptoms may include a whitish discharge from the penis and a burning sensation during urination. The lymph nodes in the groin may also become enlarged and tender.

These symptoms usually appear between three days and three weeks after sexual contact with an infected person. These symptoms may go away on their own, but the disease is still present in the body.

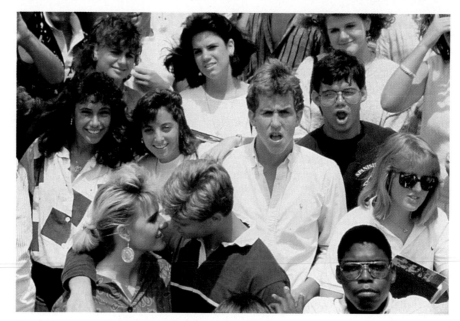

The only way to be absolutely certain that you won't become infected with an STD is to practice abstinence.

Diagnosis and Treatment

Gonorrhea can only be confirmed by a medical diagnosis. This involves a laboratory culture at the sight of the infection. In a male, gonorrhea is diagnosed by examining discharge from the penis under a microscope. In a female, a culture test of the vagina is done to make the diagnosis. This involves taking a sample of cells from the vagina and examining them under a microscope. The Pap smear, which is a test for cervical cancer, does not test for gonorrhea.

Most cases of gonorrhea can be quickly and easily cured if diagnosis is made early. Antibiotics, such as penicillin or tetracycline, are usually used for treatment. However, there presently is a new strain of gonorrhea that is resistant to penicillin. With this particular strain, a different antibiotic is used to treat it. Follow-up visits to the health clinic or doctor's office also are suggested to be sure treatment is effective.

The body does not build an immunity to gonorrhea or any other sexually transmitted disease. So being cured of gonorrhea does not protect a person from getting the disease again. Furthermore, since a different pathogen causes each of the more than 50 different sexually transmitted diseases, a person can have more than one sexually transmitted disease at the same time. There is only one sure means of preventing gonorrhea or other sexually transmitted diseases—avoiding sexual contact.

Problems from Untreated Gonorrhea

If gonorrhea is not diagnosed and treated, the disease can spread in the body. In a small number of infected persons, the bacteria will enter the blood and spread throughout the body. This incidence causes high temperature, sores on the skin, and pain in the joints. Sometimes the joints, heart valves, and meninges will become infected.

In both males and females, untreated gonorrhea can lead to infertility—the inability to reproduce. In the male, this can result from scarring from the infection, which obstructs the epididymis and the vas deferens.

This blocks the passage of sperm. The urethra can also be affected. In the female, the infection can move from the uterus to the Fallopian tubes. Scarring of both tubes can block the pathway of ova. Pelvic inflammatory disease can also result. **Pelvic inflammatory disease (PID)** is a painful infection of the Fallopian tubes, ovaries, and/or the uterus. If PID progresses, it also causes scar tissue to develop on the Fallopian tubes and results in infertility. Symptoms of PID include pain and tenderness of the lower abdomen and high temperature and chills. Because the incidence of PID is increasing, better diagnostic measures are needed for this situation.

In pregnant females, having gonorrhea increases the chance of premature labor and stillbirth—the birth of a dead fetus. If a female has gonorrhea when she gives birth, the bacteria that cause the disease can enter the baby's eyes. The baby can develop an eye infection that can lead to permanent blindness. For this reason, most physicians treat all newborn babies with special eye drops shortly after birth.

PROBLEMS WITH CHRONIC PID

Chronic PID can lead to temporary or permanent infertility. It also can lead to ectopic pregnancy. An ectopic pregnancy occurs when a fertilized ovum implants outside the uterus.

Even if the Fallopian tubes are partially blocked due to PID, fertilization can occur. However, a fertilized ovum may not be able to pass through the Fallopian tube to the uterus. In this situation, the fertilized ovum may implant at various places in the reproductive system of the female. The most common site is in the Fallopian tubes. As the embryo develops in this type of pregnancy, the wall of the Fallopian tube can rupture. Major internal bleeding results and surgery is needed to remove damaged tissue. Often the Fallopian tube cannot be repaired. If this type of pregnancy is not diagnosed and treated early, the mother may die.

LESSON 1 REVIEW

Reviewing Facts and Vocabulary

1. What are the symptoms of gonorrhea?
2. What is PID?
3. How is gonorrhea diagnosed and treated?

Thinking Critically

4. **Evaluation.** Do you think that giving someone an STD should be considered a criminal offense? Explain your answer.

5. **Analysis.** How might it be possible for a person to have more than one STD at a time?
6. **Analysis.** Why are sexually transmitted diseases a serious threat to one's total health?

Applying Health Knowledge

7. In small groups, role-play how you would give advice to a friend who complains of having symptoms of an STD and is embarrassed to go to the doctor.

SYPHILIS

Caused by a small bacterium called a spirochete, **syphilis** is a disease that attacks many parts of the body. While syphilis is not as common as gonorrhea, it is one of the most dangerous of all the sexually transmitted diseases.

Historically, syphilis is supposed to have first been brought to the Old World 500 years ago by Christopher Columbus's crew. In 1494 syphilis appeared in Europe. It is likely that some of the crew or passengers on Columbus's ships had contracted the disease and brought it back to Spain on the return voyage after the discovery of the New World. It was present among Native Americans in the New World, but in a milder form. In Europe the disease took the most destructive form. With the introduction of penicillin in the late 1940s, syphilis cases in the United States declined by 99 percent. Beginning in 1985, however, the number of cases rose sharply and has now reached its highest level in 40 years.

Syphilis is dangerous because, when left untreated, it can damage vital organs, such as the heart, the liver, the kidneys, and the central nervous system, including the brain. It can cause heart disease, blindness, paralysis, and insanity.

Symptoms of Syphilis

Syphilis develops in stages. Symptoms appear and then go away on their own. However, if treated in the early stages, the disease can be cured.

Primary Stage

The first sign of syphilis is a **chancre,** a reddish sore at the place where the pathogen enters the body, usually on the genitals. It is a painless sore that appears within 10 to 90 days after contact with an infected person. The chancre lasts 1 to 5 weeks and will then go away, even if not treated. However, the disease continues to develop in the body.

Secondary Stage

The pathogen, if not treated early, will be circulated in the blood. Within one to six months after contact, the highly contagious second stage of syphilis appears. This is commonly characterized by a nonitching rash on the chest, back of the arms, and legs. In females, the rash is most often found on the outer edges of the vagina. Sores may develop from the rash. These sores will likely give off a clear liquid filled with the infectious spirochetes. Some swelling may occur in the lymph nodes under the arms and around the groin. Fever, sore throat, and a generally sick feeling are also common symptoms. Without treatment, these symptoms will disappear, but the disease continues to develop.

Dangerous Liaisons: STDs and Lawsuits

There are an estimated 12 million new cases of STDs reported annually in the United States. The physical, emotional, and social costs of these diseases can be very high. The legal and financial costs can also be very high. Increasingly, people infected by partners who did not tell them of their known STD are taking these partners to court. Some people who have intentionally infected others have even ended up in jail.

Analyzing Different Viewpoints

ONE VIEW. Many people believe that anyone who knows he or she has an STD has an obligation to inform all sexual partners. Some people with this view also believe that if such a person does not inform his or her sexual partners, a lawsuit for medical bills and damages is justifiable if the partners become infected.

A SECOND VIEW. Some people state that anyone infected with an STD who knowingly has sex with someone without disclosing the presence of his or her STD should be charged with a crime—whether or not infection results. Such charges range from reckless endangering (for having sex under such conditions even if the partner does not become infected) to aggravated assault or attempted murder (when sex is used intentionally to harm another through infection).

A THIRD VIEW. There are also people who maintain that anyone who has sex outside of marriage is asking for trouble and has taken the risk of contracting an STD by being sexually active. They state that those infected made the decision to have sex and therefore should at least share the responsibility for getting an STD.

Exploring Your Views

1. What do you think is one's responsibility regarding sexual relations when a person knows he or she has an STD?
2. What do you think a person should do if he or she is infected by someone with an STD who knew he or she had it but did not disclose this information?
3. Do you think anyone planning to have sex should ask the prospective partner about his or her sexual history?
4. What is one sure way teens can make sure they do not contract or pass on STDs?

DID YOU KNOW?

- Syphilis is sometimes called "pox," "lues," "syph," or "bad blood."
- There are now more than 50,000 syphilis cases a year. That is the highest rate of syphilis since the 1940s.
- The number of cases of syphilis in the United States is increasing by 14 percent a year.
- The Earl of Condom, personal physician to King Charles II of England, was asked to make a protective prophylactic to prevent the king from getting syphilis. His protective sheath was made from sheep intestine.

Latent Stage

The third stage of syphilis usually begins about two or more years after the initial infection. All signs disappear, leading the individual to think that he or she is cured or never had the disease.

It is in this stage that syphilis begins to attack the heart and blood vessels and the central nervous system. The damage to these areas is slow and steady. Even though people have reached the latent stage, they can relapse into the second stage. Sores will reappear.

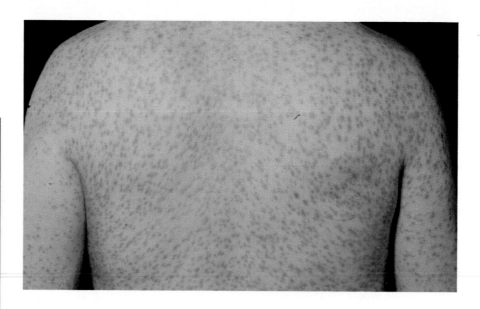

Culturally Speaking

"Shadow" Disease

The origins of syphilis are not clear. Some suggest an American origin because there are no indisputable references to syphilis in European literature until after the American voyage of Columbus. Some skeletal remains of Native Americans dated before Columbus's voyage also show evidence of the disease. On the other hand, early accounts of leprosy in Europe describe symptoms that might be syphilis rather than leprosy. For example, there is reference to spread by sexual contact, and treatment with mercury. Mercury was the first recorded treatment for syphilis. Syphilis has been called the "shadow disease" and the "great imitator" because its symptoms can be mistaken for other diseases.

Neurosyphilis Stage

If untreated, syphilis moves into the neurosyphilis stage within 10 to 30 years. When the symptoms of this stage occur, the heart, skin, brain, and spinal cord are affected. A person loses the ability to coordinate muscular movements and may experience blindness or insanity. The central nervous system is affected resulting in a loss of mental abilities. A person in this stage of syphilis may experience paralysis and convulsions. Syphilis can be treated but not cured in this stage.

Diagnosis and Treatment

While gonorrhea is detected by means of a microscopic slide exam, the test for syphilis, called the Venereal Disease Research Laboratory, or VDRL, is a blood test. The presence of the spirochete in the blood or in sores indicates the presence of the disease. Some states require that couples who plan to marry be tested for syphilis.

Penicillin is the main drug used in the treatment of syphilis. Doctors strongly recommend follow-up to be sure the disease has been cured. However, no matter how effective the treatment is, it cannot undo any harm that has already been done. Early treatment of syphilis is crucial.

Syphilis has no immunity. One may become reinfected at any time. If a person goes through too many treatments, the body may become

K E E P I N G   F I T

STDs—A Major Problem

Most STDs could be completely eradicated if people practiced responsible health behaviors. Ignoring signs of a disease is not being responsible. Responding to symptoms, seeking treatment, and following medical care instructions will combat this serious epidemic.

But the best way teens can combat this serious health problem is by having no sexual contact. It is not only okay to say no—it is healthy.

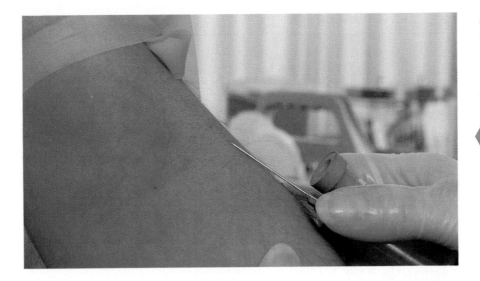

Many states used to require a blood test for syphilis before they issued marriage licenses. This practice was not effective in preventing the spread of syphilis.

immune to penicillin as a means of treatment. As in the case of all STDs, the only sure means of prevention is practicing abstinence.

Congenital Syphilis

A pregnant female who has syphilis is likely to transfer the infection to her unborn child. This condition is called **congenital syphilis.** *Congenital* means "existing at or dating from birth." The unborn child can develop syphilis any time after the fourth month of pregnancy. The mother's chances of having a miscarriage—the body's natural expulsion of a fetus prematurely—are greater if she has syphilis. In addition, her chances of having a stillborn baby are doubled.

If the baby is born, symptoms of congenital syphilis begin to appear within three to four weeks. If syphilis is diagnosed early enough in the mother, penicillin treatment will usually protect the fetus.

CONFLICT RESOLUTION

When leaving Health class, Kara heard some of her classmates continuing the class discussion about syphilis. A few were saying that getting syphilis doesn't seem to be a big deal, since it can be cured when treated in an early stage. They also think that once cured, a person need never worry about syphilis again. However, Kara knows that her cousin got syphilis twice, because he thought being cured gave him immunity to this disease.

What can Kara tell her classmates to convince them that getting syphilis is a big deal?

LESSON 2 REVIEW

Reviewing Facts and Vocabulary

1. What is a chancre?
2. How is syphilis diagnosed and treated?
3. What is congenital syphilis?
4. If syphilis can be treated and cured, why is early treatment critical?

Thinking Critically

5. **Analysis.** Compare complications resulting from syphilis to complications resulting from gonorrhea.

Applying Health Knowledge

6. Investigate the prevalence, spread, and treatments of syphilis in another period of history. Follow the case of one famous syphilis sufferer from the period, such as Christopher Columbus, King Henry VIII of England, or Al Capone. Write your findings in the form of a research paper, a medical report written from the point of view of a doctor from that period, or a journal entry from a patient's experience.

OTHER COMMON STDs

LESSON 3 FOCUS

TERMS TO USE
- Herpes 2
- Dormant
- Nongonococcal urethritis (NGU) (nahn•gahn•uh•KAHCK•ul yur•i•THRYT•uhs)
- Chlamydia (kluh•MIHD•ee•uh)

CONCEPTS TO LEARN
- There are many myths and misconceptions centered around STDs.
- The number of STDs and the number of individuals affected are increasing.
- All sexually transmitted diseases require medical attention.

ATTITUDES AND BEHAVIORS TO EVALUATE
- Self-Inventory, page 550.
- Building Decision-Making Skills, page 551.

Other serious diseases transmitted through sexual contact are herpes 2, nongonococcal urethritis (NGU), and chlamydia. Acquired immune deficiency syndrome (AIDS), also a sexually transmitted disease, will be discussed in Chapter 28. Cures are available for NGU and chlamydia, but at present no cures or vaccines exist for herpes 2 or AIDS.

Herpes 2

Herpes simplex type 1 virus is a virus that causes herpes 1, cold sores on or around the mouth. Herpes simplex type 2 virus is a virus that causes genital herpes, blisterlike sores in the genital area. Genital herpes is sometimes called **herpes 2.** It is transmitted by sexual contact and is, at present, an incurable STD. An estimated 30 million Americans have genital herpes. The Centers for Disease Control and Prevention has declared the number of cases of this STD to be at an epidemic level.

Recently, medical professionals have decided not to distinguish between herpes 1 and herpes 2, because it is possible to find a type 2 infection on the mouth and a type 1 infection on the genitals. However, for the purpose of this text section, the infection that affects the genitals that is transmitted through sexual contact is described as herpes 2. It has certain characteristics.

Symptoms

Symptoms of herpes 2 include painful, itching sores in or around the genitals. Sores usually appear 2 to 20 days after contact with an infected person. They may last as long as three weeks. Other symptoms include fever and a burning sensation during urination. With the help of moisture and friction, the herpes 2 virus can spread to other areas of the body. This is why a person who has herpes 2 is told not to rub the skin and to keep it dry.

Diagnosis and Treatment

Herpes 2 is diagnosed by a medical examination of genital sores and verified by lab tests. Currently, no cure exists for herpes 2, but there are medications that treat the symptoms.

The blisterlike sores of herpes 2 go away, but the virus remains in the body. Blisters may reappear at any time. When the blisters are present, the disease can be transmitted to another person.

One of the problems with this virus is that the disease may be contagious for a period of time before the blisters appear and after they disappear. There is no sure way of knowing when the disease is in its contagious state. This makes controlling its spread very difficult.

Although the symptoms of herpes 2 disappear, the virus remains in the body in such a state that it may be reactivated and cause another rash. After the healing from the initial outbreak has taken place, the virus can enter nerve endings near the initial rash. The virus then moves away from the surface of the skin, thus escaping the body's defenses. It moves to nerve-cell bodies near the spinal cord, where it becomes **dormant,** or inactive. The dormant herpes 2 virus can remain in this state indefinitely without causing damage.

Some people never have another outbreak of the virus, while others experience periodic outbreaks. Different factors, which are very individual, influence recurring outbreaks. Stress is one factor thought to bring on recurrences.

Infected females should have regular Pap smears, because herpes 2 infections have been linked to the development of cervical cancer cells. A pregnant female infected with herpes 2 may infect her developing baby. Death or deformity may result to the baby if infected before birth. There also is a chance the baby may acquire the virus during delivery while passing through the birth canal. If herpes develops and is untreated, the baby may suffer permanent damage or die.

A pregnant female should inform her doctor if she knows or suspects she has herpes 2. A doctor may choose to perform a cesarean delivery—birth by surgical means—to avoid risk to the baby.

One of the problems in preventing the spread of herpes 2 is that an infected individual may be contagious even before the blisters appear.

Nongonococcal Urethritis (NGU)

Nongonococcal urethritis (NGU) is a disease caused by several different kinds of bacterialike organisms that infect the urethra in males and the cervix in females. This STD is called nonspecific, because the specific cause of it has not yet been discovered. Like all STDs, NGU is transmitted through sexual contact.

Symptoms and Treatment

Males notice symptoms of NGU more than females do. In males, there may be a discharge from the penis anywhere from one to three weeks

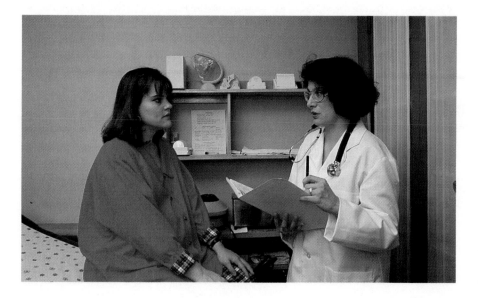

A pregnant female should inform her doctor if she suspects she has an STD.

Disease	Description	Cause	Symptoms	Treatment
Vaginitis	A common inflammation of the female genitals. Can be carried by males. Many types exist.	Microscopic organisms	Female—severe itching, discharge. Male—few or no symptoms.	Antibiotics
Moniliasis	Yeast infection	Fungus	Thick, white, cheesy discharge, general itching and irritation.	Antibiotics
Trichomoniasis	A vaginal infection that can lead to urethra and bladder infections. Males are rarely infected, but they can be carriers.	A protozoan parasite	Female—yellowish discharge, strong odor, irritation, itching. Male—slight or no symptoms.	Prescription medicine
Genital warts	Pink or reddish warts that have cauliflowerlike tops.	A virus	Warts appear on genitals 1 to 3 months after infection.	Application of a prescription skin medication
Infestation of pubic lice	Tiny insects called lice attach themselves to skin and hair in the pubic area. Lice feed on blood and cause intense itching.	Lice, insects that are parasites resemble tiny crabs	Intense itching, small nits (eggs) on pubic hair, small spots of blood on underwear.	Special medicated shampoo
Scabies	Infestation of skin by mites that cause red, swollen itchy bumps on the skin.	Tiny insects called mites that burrow into the skin	Itching in the genital area 4 to 6 weeks after infection. Mites can be spread to forearms or fingers.	Hot baths and medicated creams

K E E P I N G   F I T

Symptoms of STDs in Males

General symptoms of STDs in men include:
- difficult or painful urination
- penile discharge
- soreness inside the penis

- sores in the genital area
- itching genitals
- flulike symptoms
- painless rash on hands, feet, or body

The most important thing to do when such symptoms are present is to get medical attention as soon as possible.

after infection. Males may also experience a mild burning during urination. Females may have a vaginal discharge and pain in the lower abdomen.

NGU can be treated and cured. Treatment consists of an antibiotic, usually tetracycline.

Chlamydia

Chlamydia is the most prevalent STD in the United States today. Annually, about 4 million cases are reported, which is 2 million cases more than gonorrhea. Chlamydia is an infection that affects the vagina in females and the urethra in males. If the infection is not treated, serious damage can be done to other reproductive organs. Chlamydia is a common cause of sterility. Chlamydia is caused by a special type of bacteria that has been only recently recognized.

Symptoms

In males, the symptoms include pain and burning during urination and an unusual discharge from the penis. These symptoms usually occur one to three weeks after exposure. If left untreated, chlamydia can result in chronic inflammation of the urethra.

In females, the symptoms are not always obvious. If symptoms do occur, they may include an unusual discharge from the vagina, pain in the pelvic region, and painful urination. If left untreated, chlamydia can cause pelvic inflammatory disease (PID). PID is a painful infection of the ovaries, Fallopian tubes, and/or uterus.

A pregnant female who has chlamydia can spread it to her baby during delivery. In infants, the disease can cause eye infection, blindness, and sometimes pneumonia.

Treatment

Chlamydia is diagnosed through a laboratory test. Certain antibiotics can cure chlamydia. However, if scar tissue has already formed, treatment cannot undo that damage. Chances of sterility in the male and in the female will remain.

K E E P I N G   F I T

Symptoms of STDs in Females

General symptoms of STDs in women include:
- abnormal discharge from the vagina
- difficult or painful urination
- warts, blisters, sores, bumps, or rashes in the pubic area
- itching in the pubic area
- unusual bleeding from the vagina
- stomach cramps not associated with menstruation
- flulike symptoms
- rash on hands, feet, or body
- painful intercourse

The most important thing to do when such symptoms are present is to get medical attention as soon as possible.

Overcoming The Odds

Andrea is 18. "There's only one simple way to put it," she begins. "I have genital herpes—a very common sexually transmitted disease—something I thought I'd never get. I'm just your average high school senior, thinking a lot about the future, involved with my friends, active in school activities, all of it. I didn't do any more or worse than some of my friends, but here I am now paying for it."

Andrea continues, "I first noticed something wasn't right when I got this weird itching, then those painful sores. They were like blisters. It hurt when I went to the bathroom. After a while, they broke open and they became even more painful. I figured it was just some passing thing. But I did have swollen glands, a fever, and I felt like it was maybe the flu. Then the sores went away and I just brushed the whole thing off. Then, around exam time, when the pressure was on, the sores came back. I felt lousy. They hurt. Then I got the call."

The call was from her second boyfriend. He informed

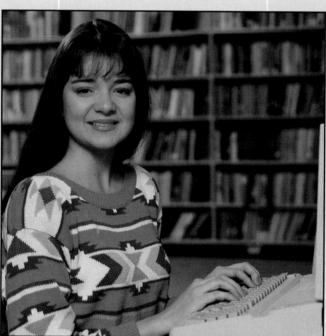

her that he had been tested, and genital herpes had been confirmed. "It was really the most awful and embarrassing phone call of my life," Andrea says. "But he said he knew he had to tell me. His sores were recent, so he said he figured I'd given it to him, that I'd had it first, and that I'd better call my first boyfriend and tell him. He hung up, and I just wanted to throw up. Then I cried.

"After a while, I made that awful second call to the other guy. He just laughed it off. I

was so angry. I can't even look at him in school.

Then I used the anger to take action for myself. I finally got up the courage to go to the clinic. They told me there were no antibiotics I could take because it is not a bacterial infection. There is no cure.

They also told me the disease would stay with me for the rest of my life. I had it, and whenever it was active, I could pass it on. They also said that if I have children someday I may have to have a cesarean section so my babies won't get the infection. They said stress could cause a flare-up, so now when I'm under stress, I'm really stressed because I don't want those lesions back."

1. Why was Andrea surprised that she got herpes?
2. Why was it important that all the sexual partners involved be informed that one of them had tested positive for the disease?
3. If you had been Andrea, how would you have felt about the first phone call? If you were she, would you have made the second phone call? Why or why not?

Other STDs

There are several other diseases that are spread through sexual contact. Some are more serious than others, but they all require medical attention. The chart on page 546 provides a description of some of the more common ones. You will notice that two of the conditions listed in the chart can be acquired in ways other than sexually.

Treatment

Treatment for sexually transmitted diseases is an important personal responsibility. Having an STD is not like having a cold. It will not simply go away if a person waits long enough. In fact, it is possible for a person to have more than one STD at the same time. The individual must do something about it. No one else can do it for that person.

It is understandable that a person may feel embarrassed about having an STD. However, a person who seeks treatment from a private doctor or a public health clinic is guaranteed by law that all information will remain confidential. It is important for the infected person to notify all people with whom he or she has had any sexual contact. A doctor or a public health clinic can help a person make these decisions.

If you think you have an STD, it is important that you get immediate medical help.

Why is it important that an individual infected with an STD notify all of his or her sexual partners?

Prevention of STDs

Sexually transmitted diseases are different from other diseases. The body does not build up an immunity to any STD. No vaccination is available to prevent these diseases. Since STDs are spread by sexual contact with an infected person, the only sure way not to contract an STD is not to be sexually active. More and more young people are recognizing this choice as the only alternative to contracting STDs and experiencing their crippling effects. Abstinence is the only choice that is 100 percent effective in preventing the spread of STDs.

LESSON 3 REVIEW

Reviewing Facts and Vocabulary

1. What is chlamydia?
2. Why is NGU called nonspecific?
3. What is the best way to prevent STDs?

Thinking Critically

4. **Analysis.** Explain how good general health practices can be helpful in preventing STDs.
5. **Analysis.** What reasons can you give for chlamydia being so common?

6. **Evaluation.** Have the current practices for controlling STDs been effective? Explain your answer. What would you do differently?

Applying Health Knowledge

7. Many states now require screening for some STDs before granting a couple a marriage license. Do you agree with mandatory screening? Why or why not? State your position in a letter that could be sent to your local newspaper.

Self-Inventory

STDs: Where Do You Stand?

HOW DO YOU RATE?

Number a sheet of paper from 1 through 10. Read each item, and respond by writing *agree* or *disagree* for each statement. Total the number of each type of response. Then proceed to the next section.

1. Being in good health will keep a sexually active person from getting an STD.

2. A sexually active person can have only one STD at a time.

3. There is no known way to prevent the spread of STDs.

4. Untreated STDs usually go away in time.

5. Health problems associated with STDs are usually more serious in males.

6. STDs are basically a problem for adults.

7. Having only one sexual partner will prevent a sexually active person from getting an STD.

8. Once the symptoms of an STD have disappeared, the disease has been cured.

9. Having an STD is a private matter, so a sexually active person should not have to tell his or her partner if he or she has an STD.

10. All STDs can be treated and there are known cures for all of them.

HOW DID YOU SCORE?

Give yourself 1 point for each *disagree* answer and 0 points for each *agree* answer. Find your total, and read below to see how you scored. Then proceed to the next section.

9 to 10
Excellent. You are up-to-date in your knowledge of STDs, you have a healthy attitude about STDs, and how to protect yourself.

7 to 8
Good. You have a healthy attitude about STDs, but you could learn more about how the spread of STDs might be prevented.

Below 7
Needs Improvement. You need to learn more about STDs and how they are spread to protect yourself and others.

WHAT ARE YOUR GOALS?

If you received an *excellent* or *good* score, complete the statements in Part A. If your score was *needs improvement*, complete both Parts A and B.

Part A

1. I plan to rethink some of my attitudes and decisions about STDs after I ____.

2. My timetable for accomplishing this is ____.

3. I plan to share my knowledge with others by ____.

Part B

4. I plan to learn more about STDs by ____.

5. The steps necessary to do this are ____.

6. My rewards for making this change will be ____.

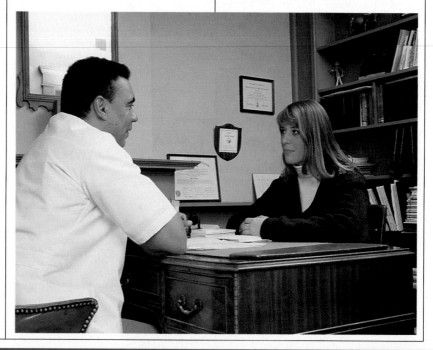

Building Decision-Making Skills

O ne of Angel's former boyfriends has just told her he has herpes. He suggests that because of their sexual contact she should see a doctor in order to be tested for the disease. In the meantime, Angel has had several other boyfriends but she has not had sex with any of them. Angel is embarrassed. She does not want her reputation to suffer by having people find out that she may have a sexually transmitted disease. What should Angel do?

A. Put the whole thing out of her mind and pretend it never happened.

B. Don't panic. Get medical attention immediately but don't tell anyone else until she gets the results of the test.

C. Share the news with someone she can trust so that she will have some emotional support.

D. Tell her current boyfriend if it turns out that she has the disease.

E. Protect her reputation by keeping the results of the test secret.

WHAT DO YOU THINK?

1. **Situation.** What should Angel do to get the facts about her situation?

2. **Situation.** Why does Angel need to make a decision?

3. **Situation.** Why is Angel in this situation?

4. **Situation.** Who is involved? Who will be affected?

5. **Situation.** How much time is there to decide?

6. **Choices.** What alternatives does Angel have?

7. **Choices.** What factors should Angel consider in making her decision?

8. **Consequences.** How will Angel's decision affect her former boyfriends, her current boyfriend, her parents, her friends, and the people who have respected her in the past?

9. **Consequences.** How will Angel's decision affect the various sides of her health triangle?

10. **Consequences.** Are there any legal obligations involved in Angel's situation? What are they?

11. **Consequences.** How will Angel's decision affect her self-esteem and her plans and goals for the future?

12. **Consequences.** How might Angel's decision affect her ability to bear healthy children?

13. **Decision.** What decision do you think would be best for Angel?

14. **Evaluation.** In an age when sexual activity is obviously increasing, do you think the stigma attached to sexual diseases has changed? Do you think it should?

15. **Evaluation.** Should past sexual experiences and exposure to STDs be discussed by teens who are currently going out together?

16. **Evaluation.** Have you ever known anyone who had been involved in a situation involving moral and legal obligations? What did the individual do? Do you think it was a good decision? Why or why not? How would you handle such a situation in the future?

B etsy's older sister, Sue, is about to get married. Her fiancé just told Sue he has an STD. What should Sue do?

WHAT DO YOU THINK?

17. **Choices.** What are several choices Sue has?

18. **Consequences.** What are the advantages of each choice?

19. **Consequences.** What are the negative consequences of each choice?

20. **Consequences.** What are the health risks to Sue and to her fiancé?

21. **Decision.** What do you think Sue should do? Explain your answer.

22. **Decision.** How should Sue go about implementing her decision?

REVIEW

Using Health Terms

On a separate sheet of paper, write the term that best matches each definition given below.

LESSON 1

1. A communicable disease that is spread from one person to another through sexual contact.
2. The inability to conceive children.
3. The birth of a dead fetus.

LESSON 2

4. A sexually transmitted disease that is caused by a bacterium called a spirochete.
5. Existing at or dating from birth.
6. The body's natural expulsion of a fetus prematurely.

LESSON 3

7. A virus that causes cold sores on or around the mouth.
8. A virus that causes blisterlike sores in the genital area.
9. Birth by surgical means.
10. A term used to describe a disease for which the exact cause has not yet been discovered.

Building Academic Skills

LESSON 1

11. **Writing.** Abstinence is the only 100 percent effective method of avoiding STDs. Write an editorial or letter to the editor of your school newspaper explaining the health issues of STDs and encouraging your fellow students to remain abstinent or to return to abstinence.

LESSON 3

12. **Reading.** Use the context clues in the following sentences to define the word *dormant*.

    The quiet volcano had been dormant for years, but no one knew how long it would remain inactive. Some believed it would erupt at any moment.

Recalling the Facts

LESSON 1

13. In what part of the body do the bacteria that cause gonorrhea usually live?
14. How long might it take symptoms of gonorrhea to occur after sexual contact with an infected person?
15. If the symptoms of gonorrhea occur and later disappear, does it mean that the person is free of the disease? Explain.
16. What is the only sure means of preventing gonorrhea?
17. Why can a person get the same STD more than once?
18. How is it possible for a person to have more than one sexually transmitted disease at the same time?
19. How can gonorrhea lead to sterility in males? In females?
20. What is the major danger to a baby born to a woman who has gonorrhea?

LESSON 2

21. Why is syphilis a dangerous disease?
22. What effect did the introduction of penicillin have on the number of syphilis cases in the United States?
23. Where on the body is the first sign of syphilis, a chancre, likely to be found?
24. How long after sexual contact with an infected person will a syphilitic chancre appear?
25. How long after initial infection does the third stage of syphilis begin?

LESSON 3

26. How long after sexual contact with an infected person will the symptoms of herpes 2 usually appear?
27. Why is it important for women to have regular Pap smears?
28. What special risks do babies of females with herpes 2 experience?
29. What part of the body does nongonococcal urethritis (NGU) affect?

REVIEW

Thinking Critically

LESSON 1

30. Synthesis. Make a chart similar to the one in Lesson 3 and complete information for gonorrhea. Do some additional research to fill in any information not provided in the text.

LESSON 2

31. Synthesis. Add syphilis to the chart you began in item 30 above.

32. Synthesis. Some states have a law requiring couples who apply for marriage licenses to be tested for syphilis. What is the purpose of such a law? Why is such a law not as effective in controlling the spread of syphilis as it might have been fifty years ago?

33. Synthesis. Develop a law of your own that you think would be effective in the control of syphilis. Explain your thinking.

LESSON 3

34. Synthesis. The only known way to prevent any kind of sexually transmitted disease is to abstain from sexual contact. What strategies can you suggest that would be effective in "selling" this concept to teens who are already sexually active?

35. Analysis. Why is a person who has many different sexual partners more likely to contract a sexually transmitted disease than a person who has only one sexual partner? Explain your answer.

Making the Connection

LESSON 1

36. Math. Do some research on the number of cases of gonorrhea during 5-year intervals from 1950 to the present. Present your findings in a bar graph. Develop a comparable bar graph for population increases during the same period. Compare the two graphs.

Applying Health Knowledge

LESSON 1

37. Contact your local health department to find out about the relationship between gonorrhea and arthritis and gonorrhea and heart trouble. Share your findings with the class.

38. Design a booklet entitled "Gonorrhea Alert" that summarizes the major points presented in the lesson.

LESSON 2

39. What steps could public health agencies take to further control the spread of syphilis? What steps could individuals take?

40. Why is it inadvisable for females with syphilis to become pregnant? When can an unborn baby develop syphilis during pregnancy?

LESSON 3

41. If an individual is diagnosed as having a sexually transmitted disease, who should he or she tell in order to prevent further spread of the disease?

Beyond the Classroom

LESSON 1

42. Parental Involvement. Ask your parents or other adults at home how they learned about STDs. Ask about the quality of that information. Talk with them about the best ways for young people to learn about STDs.

LESSON 3

43. Further Study. Use a dictionary to find the etymology, or origin, of the words *gonorrhea, syphilis,* and *herpes.* Which of these words has an alternate spelling and what is it?

44. Community Involvement. Find out what kinds of assistance are available to help people who have STDs in your community. Prepare a report to share your findings with your classmates.

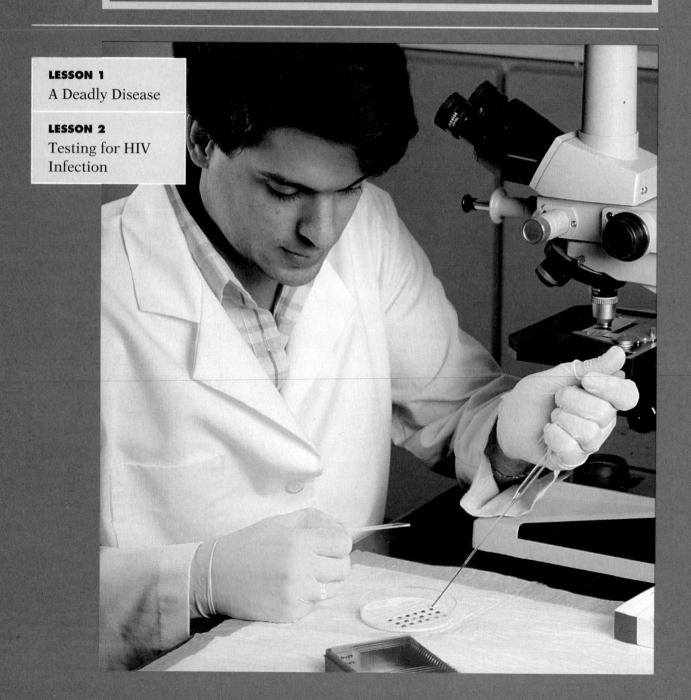

CHAPTER

28

AIDS

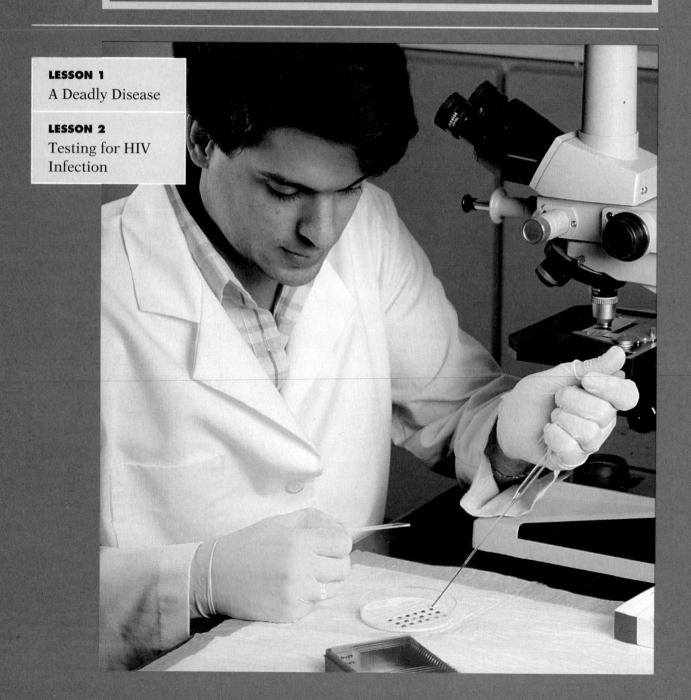

LESSON 1
A Deadly Disease

LESSON 2
Testing for HIV
Infection

A DEADLY DISEASE

Today more Americans are infected with STDs than at any other time in history. The most serious of these diseases is AIDS. Since the first cases were identified in the United States in 1981, AIDS has touched the lives of millions of families. This deadly disease is unlike any other in modern history.

What Is AIDS?

Acquired immune deficiency syndrome (AIDS) is a fatal communicable disease with no effective treatment or known cure. AIDS is the final stage of infection caused by the **human immunodeficiency virus (HIV).** When HIV enters the body, it attacks the body's immune system.

How Does HIV Affect the Body?

In order to understand how HIV attacks the body's immune system, it is necessary to review the function of lymphocytes. HIV causes specific changes in the functions of the lymphocytes, which differ from changes caused by other kinds of viruses.

Lymphocytes and Antibodies

As you know, **lymphocytes** are white blood cells made in bone marrow. Lymphocytes move throughout your lymphatic system between blood and lymph tissue, and help your body fight pathogens, disease-causing organisms. There are two major types of lymphocytes—B cells, which mature in bone marrow and T cells, which mature in the thymus gland. T helper cells, a type of T cell, stimulate B cells to produce antibodies. **Antibodies** are proteins that help destroy pathogens that enter the body.

When HIV enters the body, it enters certain cells, including T helper cells. Here HIV reproduces its genetic material, which causes more T helper cells to become infected and to be destroyed. This decrease in the number of T helper cells affects the ability of the immune system to fight pathogens. As a result, many illnesses can occur in the body. Indicator illnesses are those illnesses associated with a person who has AIDS. These include opportunistic infections, which are infections a healthy immune system would usually be able to fight. A person is said to have the disease AIDS when he or she is infected with HIV, has a low T helper cell count, and has one or more indicator illnesses.

Origin of HIV

There are many theories as to where HIV originated and how it spread to the United States. It is thought that the virus spread as people

LESSON 1 FOCUS

TERMS TO USE
- Acquired immune deficiency syndrome (AIDS)
- Human immunodeficiency (IM•yuh•noh•di• FISH•uhn•see) virus (HIV)
- Lymphocytes (LIM•fuh•syts)
- Antibodies

CONCEPTS TO LEARN
- AIDS is the final stage of infection caused by the human immuno-deficiency virus (HIV).
- To date HIV is known to be transmitted only through blood, vaginal secretions, semen, and breast milk.
- Specific behaviors are known to transmit HIV from an infected to an uninfected person.
- HIV is not transmitted through casual contact.

ATTITUDES AND BEHAVIORS TO EVALUATE
- Self-Inventory, page 564.
- Building Decision-Making Skills, page 565.

traveled. It is also known that the virus assumes many different forms within the body.

The first group of people in the United States diagnosed with AIDS were male homosexuals. Many people then believed AIDS was a disease only homosexuals could contract. This is not true. Anyone who participates in behaviors known to spread HIV is at risk of becoming infected, regardless of age, race, or sexual orientation.

How HIV Is Transmitted

There are many myths about how HIV is or is not spread. The fact is, HIV must enter a person's bloodstream to infect the person. HIV has been found in body fluids such as blood, semen, and vaginal secretions of infected persons. Small concentrations have also been found in saliva, sweat, tears, feces, urine, and breast milk. To date, HIV is known to be transmitted only through blood, vaginal secretions, semen, and breast milk. Certain behaviors and situations are known to transmit HIV from an infected to an uninfected person because the exchange of body fluids is involved.

Behaviors Known to Transmit HIV

About 93 percent of adults and teenagers testing positive for HIV have acquired the virus through sexual intercourse or IV drug use. These two actions are high-risk behaviors for HIV infection.

Sexual Intercourse. HIV can be transmitted during any form of sexual intercourse. During intercourse, secretions containing HIV can enter a partner's blood through tiny cuts in the body. The risks of HIV infection increase with the number of sexual partners a person has or by having sexual contact with someone who has had many sexual partners. Having an STD that results in sores and bleeding or discharge also increases the risks of HIV entering the blood.

Contaminated Needles. If a person who is infected with HIV injects drugs into his or her veins with a syringe, drops of that person's blood are left on the needle. If another person uses the same needle, it is very likely that the infected blood will be passed to this person's blood. Sharing any needle, including one used to inject steroids, make tattoos, or pierce ears, puts a person at risk of becoming infected with HIV.

Situations Known to Transmit HIV

HIV is carried in the blood. Any transfer of blood from one person to another is a potential risk for HIV infection.

Blood Transfusion. Prior to March 1985, before donated blood was tested for HIV, people who received blood transfusions were at risk of being exposed to HIV. All blood donated in the United States is now tested for the presence of HIV antibodies. This testing has almost eliminated the risk of receiving contaminated blood or blood products from a transfusion. There is no risk when donating blood because disposable needles are used. These needles are used only one time.

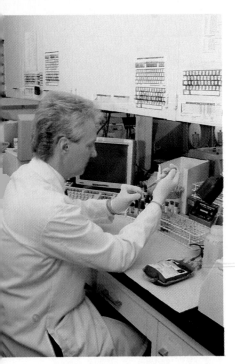

Blood that is donated in the United States is tested for the presence of HIV antibodies.

CONFLICT RESOLUTION

Assume you have a friend who is infected with HIV.

Would you advise your friend to tell other classmates and teachers about the infection or keep the infection a secret?

How would you convince your classmates and teachers that they are a greater health risk to your friend than your friend is to them?

Overcoming The Odds

Henry Nicols is 18. He loves to swim, do karate, backpack, and hike. He is an Eagle Scout. He is also a hemophiliac, and he has AIDS.

Henry begins, "I was diagnosed with hemophilia when I was just 18 months old. Hemophilia is an inherited bleeding disorder that prevents blood from clotting. So when I get a cut or a bruise, I need a blood transfusion. I've had more than 300 transfusions over the years." It was one of those transfusions that infected Henry with HIV. Because of his condition, sports were out. But illness did not stop Henry from being active. "I swim quite a bit, and I started taking karate classes about three years ago. I've also been involved with the Boy Scouts for a long time."

He continues, "In 1985, when they developed a test for HIV infection, I was taking part in an experimental test of a new medicine for hemophilia. As part of the program, they tested my blood for HIV. It was positive. They called my father and asked if he wanted to know the results. At first my father said "no," but later, he changed his mind. He waited a week before telling my mother. He waited two more weeks before telling me and my sisters."

Neither HIV nor AIDS has stopped Henry, however. In fact, he has turned his illness into a passionate mission to educate other young people about the disease. He explains. "The highest rank in scouting is the Eagle Scout Award," he says. "To get it, you have to

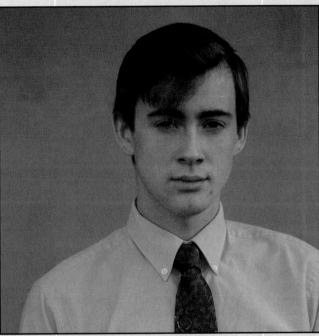

complete a number of requirements, and one of them is an Eagle Scout Project. The project has to be a service to the community and has to demonstrate leadership. I chose speaking about AIDS and educating other young people about the disease as my project. I earned the badge in July. But I didn't feel I should end it there. I talk in high schools and colleges across the country now. The support is usually overwhelming. There's very little negative reaction."

There has been some prejudice, though, Henry says, "but mostly in the form of ignorance. For example, in our scout troop, one of the mothers didn't want her son eating out of the same potato chip bag as I.

"My family has been behind me 100 percent. This has brought us closer together. Some people figure they have a long time to tell their parents they love them or to make up for mistakes. We know better.

"I have very good self-esteem," he continues. "I think family support helped me to feel good about myself and what I'm doing."

In closing, Henry says with great seriousness and directness, "You have to change the way you think about HIV, AIDS, and those infected. You need to recognize that not everyone with AIDS contracted the virus through high-risk behavior. And you must take action to avoid high-risk behaviors. That may mean changing your behavior. It should mean choosing abstinence."

1. How can ignorance about AIDS or any other disease be a form of prejudice?
2. If you knew you had a terminal disease, how might you live your life differently?

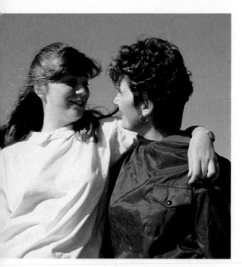

HIV is not transmitted through casual contact.

Before, During, and After Birth. A pregnant female who is infected with HIV can pass the virus to the baby in blood exchanged through the umbilical cord. A baby also could be infected with HIV during birth if the virus enters a cut on the baby's body. A nursing baby could receive HIV while breast-feeding.

Teenagers at Risk

Teenagers are at primary risk for contracting HIV. The Centers for Disease Control and Prevention (CDC) is part of the United States Department of Health and Human Services. The CDC gathers statistics regarding disease throughout the world. According to the CDC:

- Over one-fifth of the people with AIDS are in their 20s. Most of these people probably became infected with HIV as teenagers.
- As of March 30, 1993, 1,167 cases of AIDS had been reported among teenagers.
- AIDS is the seventh leading cause of death among 15- to 24-year-olds in the United States.

A teen who chooses to abstain from sexual intercourse and who does not use intravenous (IV) drugs virtually eliminates the risk of HIV infection. In addition, abstaining from the use of alcohol and other drugs, which can impair a person's judgment in regard to sexual activity and drug use, can also reduce the risk of HIV infection. Making responsible decisions means protection from HIV infection.

How HIV Is Not Transmitted

Fear of AIDS has caused people to react negatively and sometimes violently toward people known to be infected with HIV. Ignorance feeds this fear. Remember, HIV is transmitted in body fluids. It is not an airborne pathogen.

HIV cannot be transmitted through casual contact. Casual contact includes sharing towels, combs, eating utensils, bathroom facilities, or having close physical contact, such as touching or hugging. In studies of families who have a member infected with HIV, no incidence of the virus spreading to other family members through casual contact has been found. In addition, according to the Centers for Disease Control and Prevention, HIV is not spread through an insect bite.

How Infection with HIV Can Be Prevented

Although AIDS is not curable, being infected with HIV is preventable. Knowledge is the first step in prevention. Because HIV and AIDS research is ongoing, scientists are learning more and more about HIV and AIDS. New information is continually being updated and changing what is known about HIV infection.

Facts about HIV infection and AIDS can be obtained from a variety of sources. Newspapers, professional journals, and health news reports on television and radio often report the latest scientific findings. The Centers for Disease Control and Prevention, as well as state and local health organizations, are excellent resources for accurate information about HIV infection and AIDS. Parents, teachers, school counselors, church leaders, and doctors also can be sources or provide guidance about where to find information.

The second step in preventing HIV infection is applying information learned. This includes avoiding those behaviors known to transmit HIV—sexual intercourse and using illegal IV drugs. Teens who practice abstinence, or voluntarily refrain from sex, help prevent the spread of HIV to themselves and to others. Teens who avoid using drugs and the people who use them, do the same.

Saying no to behaviors known to transmit HIV may not be easy, especially when the person you are saying it to is someone whose friendship you value. Using refusal skills may help you save both your friendship and your health.

Unfortunately, despite the life-threatening risks involved, some persons will continue to participate in behaviors known to increase their risk of HIV infection. You may feel a responsibility to share the information you know about HIV infection and AIDS, or have someone you know talk with them. Each person must accept responsibility for decisions he or she makes about behaviors, including the ones that involve risks of HIV infection.

LESSON 1 REVIEW

Reviewing Facts and Vocabulary

1. What is AIDS?
2. What is the function of T helper cells?
3. Explain the ways HIV is known to be transmitted.

Thinking Critically

4. **Evaluation.** Do you think an individual infected with HIV is responsible for informing others of the infection? Why or why not?

5. **Synthesis.** Why is AIDS a serious threat to public health?

Applying Health Knowledge

6. Design a poster that tells teens how to avoid HIV infection.

TESTING FOR HIV INFECTION

Presently, testing for HIV is required for people who donate blood, body organs and tissue, and for those who join the armed forces. Testing is recommended for State Department Foreign Service employees and people in the medical profession. It also is recommended for people who have practiced behaviors known to transmit HIV. Because of the stigma associated with HIV infection and AIDS, results of tests for HIV are kept confidential.

Detecting HIV Antibodies

As you know, when a pathogen enters the body, the immune system produces antibodies to fight and destroy the pathogen. The immune system does produce antibodies to fight HIV, but these antibodies are not effective in preventing HIV infection. However, finding these antibodies in the blood indicates a person is infected with HIV.

ELISA and Western Blot

In 1985 the ELISA test was developed to detect the presence of antibodies for HIV. **ELISA** means enzyme-linked immunosorbent assay. ELISA is a test for HIV infection, not a test to determine the disease AIDS. ELISA is used for screening donated blood. ELISA also is used on persons who suspect they are infected with HIV because of behaviors they have chosen. One ELISA is given. If a person tests positive, two more tests are done. If after the three tests, two or three are positive, then the Western blot is done to confirm the test results. The **Western blot** is a more expensive test to use but is very specific in identifying HIV antibodies.

Test Results. A positive test means that the person has HIV antibodies in his or her blood. This person is infected with HIV although he or she may show no signs of the disease. In fact a person infected with HIV can feel and look fine. However, this individual can still infect others when practicing behaviors known to transmit HIV. A person can be infected with HIV for 10 to 12 years or longer before showing signs of infection. Many people who have the disease AIDS actually became infected with HIV years earlier.

A negative test means that there were no HIV antibodies in the sample of blood. It does not mean, however, that the person is uninfected. After being infected, it may take the body anywhere from two weeks to six months or longer to develop HIV antibodies. If a person concerned about possible exposure to HIV does test negative, he or she should be retested in six months. During that six-month period, behaviors known to transmit HIV must be avoided. If the second test is negative, the person is probably not infected with HIV.

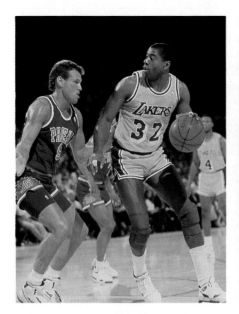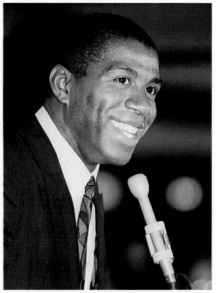

Symptoms of HIV Infection

Although symptoms of HIV infection may not appear for 6 months to 10 to 12 years, a person infected with HIV will eventually develop the disease AIDS. A person infected with HIV will experience many signs and symptoms before a diagnosis of AIDS is made. Symptoms include fever, rash, headache, body aches, swollen glands, and the decreasing ability to fight pathogens. T helper cell count decreases. In a later stage, thrush appears. This fungal infection results in white spots and sores in the mouth and infections on the skin and in mucous membranes.

Diagnosis of AIDS

Diagnosis of AIDS is based on several factors, including a positive test for HIV antibodies and the presence of an opportunistic infection. As mentioned earlier, these illnesses result from a breakdown of the immune system. A person who has been diagnosed with AIDS may live only a few months or for several years. AIDS patients die from the effects of opportunistic infections. Several opportunistic infections are associated with AIDS. **Pneumocystis carinii pneumonia (PCP)** is a

---

KEEPING FIT

Volunteering Helps

What can you do to help in the AIDS crisis?
- Work to educate fellow teens about AIDS and how to prevent it. Organize an AIDS awareness week at your school.
- Work to organize a fund-raiser

for a local AIDS hospice or AIDS education program.
- Consider becoming an AIDS buddy, doing food shopping and other chores for people who are too sick to do these things for themselves.

- Check yourself for any judgments or prejudices you may have about people with AIDS. Do you really know and believe that you cannot get AIDS from casual social contact?

form of pneumonia with symptoms that include difficulty in breathing, shortness of breath, fever, and persistent cough. **Mycobacterium avium intracellulare (MAI)** is the leading cause of wasting syndrome, a gradual deterioration of all body functions. It is characterized by fatigue, sudden high fever, severe night sweats, cramps, and weight loss.

HEALTH UPDATE

LOOKING AT THE ISSUES

Testing for HIV

Questions surrounding this issue include whether these tests should be voluntary or mandatory, who should be tested, and if those with positive test results should be identified.

Analyzing Different Viewpoints

ONE VIEW. Many health-care professionals call for mandatory testing for HIV in patients undergoing surgery, pregnant women, and IV drug users. Why? Because such persons could put others at risk. For example, surgeons operating on infected patients could become infected.

A SECOND VIEW. Other people believe that HIV testing should be voluntary. The Centers for Disease Control has recently proposed widespread voluntary tests for hospital patients. Under these proposals, patient test results would be kept confidential.

A THIRD VIEW. Some people claim that health-care workers should be tested. New federal guidelines urge testing for health-care workers such as surgeons or dentists who may have blood-to-blood contact with patients. The American Medical Association (AMA) is opposed to mandatory testing for health-care workers, but it is calling for routine, voluntary screening for doctors at risk either because of their work or their life-styles. The AMA would also ask HIV-positive doctors to stop performing invasive surgical procedures.

A FOURTH VIEW. Some people are calling for mandatory testing for everyone. They state that no safety precautions are foolproof. They fear that some health-care workers infected with HIV may continue to practice, putting patients at risk because they are afraid of losing their jobs and medical benefits if they disclose that they are infected.

A FIFTH VIEW. Others maintain that mandatory testing infringes on the right to privacy. They state that testing health-care workers is discriminatory, because the risk of infection from health-care workers is small.

A SIXTH VIEW. Others think that taking precautions such as disposing of needles, wearing gloves and masks, and avoiding contact with body fluids are safeguards enough, so that in most cases not even voluntary testing is necessary.

Exploring Your Views

1. Who do you think should be tested for HIV?
2. Should that testing be voluntary or mandatory? Explain your answer.
3. If you had to be admitted to the hospital, would you agree to voluntary testing for HIV? Why or why not?

AIDS dementia complex is a progressive disorder that destroys brain tissue of a person with AIDS. Symptoms range from mild confusion to inability to control one's muscular movement.

Research and Treatment

There is no cure for HIV infection or AIDS. However, since 1981 the world's scientific community has made great progress in AIDS research. Scientists have gained enough information to develop experimental treatments and possible vaccines. Through concentrated efforts in researching HIV, scientists' understanding of the immune system has increased. It is hoped this knowledge will help advance the fight against this disease.

Medical Research

In March 1987 the medicine zidovudine (AZT) was approved for use in treating persons infected with HIV. AZT slows the multiplication of HIV and seems to help delay the onset of opportunistic infections. It also can help reduce the severity of some AIDS symptoms and prolong life. AZT does not cure AIDS. With estimated annual costs of treatment ranging from $2,000 to $4,000 per patient, AZT is an expensive medicine. Almost half of all AIDS patients must stop taking AZT because it damages their bone marrow. Other medicines, ddI and ddC, have also been approved for use. These medicines also delay the onset of serious illnesses. However, both can cause side effects.

A variety of approaches is being used in an attempt to discover a vaccine against the AIDS virus. A main focus has been finding a protein that will cause the body's immune system to produce effective HIV antibodies. Experimental vaccines have been developed through gene splicing. Only time will tell whether the antibodies produced by the vaccines can protect the body against HIV.

LESSON 2 REVIEW

Reviewing Facts and Vocabulary

1. What determines a diagnosis of the disease AIDS?
2. List two medicines currently being used to treat AIDS.
3. What precautions should a person take whose first test for HIV antibodies is negative?

Thinking Critically

4. **Analysis.** Compare and contrast the ELISA and Western blot tests.

5. **Synthesis.** Why do you think the number of AIDS cases continues to increase?

Applying Health Knowledge

6. Develop a one-minute public service announcement (PSA) to inform others about the spread of HIV. Submit the PSA to your school office to be read over the intercom during announcements.

Self-Inventory

Are You at Risk?

HOW DO YOU RATE?

Number a sheet of paper from 1 through 15. Read each item below and respond by writing *true* or *false* for each item. Then proceed to the next section.

1. I have not used illegal drugs, including alcohol, in the past.
2. I do not use illegal drugs, including alcohol, now.
3. I have abstained from sexual intimacy in the past.
4. I abstain from sexual intimacy now.
5. I keep informed about HIV infection and AIDS.
6. I can say no to something I do not want to do or do not feel ready for.
7. I am not easily influenced by peer pressure.
8. I like myself and feel good about the decisions I make.
9. I do not use needles, including tattoo needles, razors, or other items that have been used by someone else.
10. I have not received a blood transfusion prior to 1985.
11. I have not been treated for an STD in the past.
12. I avoid those behaviors that can transmit HIV.
13. I know who to talk to and where to get information when I have questions about HIV infection and AIDS.
14. I know how HIV is not transmitted.
15. If I suspect I have an STD, I will see my physician for treatment.

HOW DID YOU SCORE?

Give yourself 2 points for each *true* response and 0 points for each *false* response. Find your total, and read below to see how you scored. Then proceed to the next section.

25 to 30
Excellent. You do not take unnecessary risks, and you use decision-making skills in addressing problems. You like yourself and feel comfortable with your decisions. You are not easily influenced by others.

19 to 24
Good. You use decision-making skills in solving some of your problems. However, you would be wise to look at your behavior to see whether some risks you are taking could prevent you from achieving your goals.

0 to 18
Watch out! You take too many risks and do not use decision-making skills in solving problems. You are taking risks that could cause you to contract STDs or HIV infection and to be involved in situations that could harm you for the rest of your life.

WHAT ARE YOUR GOALS?

Select one area in which your behavior needs improvement. Then complete each statement below.

1. I plan to learn more about HIV infection and AIDS by ____.
2. My timetable for accomplishing this is ____.
3. I plan to share my information with others by ____.
4. The attitude or behavior about HIV infection I would most like to change is ____.
5. The steps involved in making this change are ____.
6. My timetable for accomplishing this is ____.
7. The people or groups I will ask for support and assistance are ____.
8. The benefits I will receive for making this change are ____.

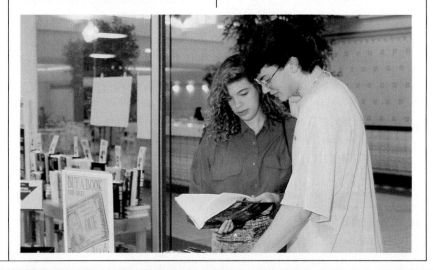

Building Decision-Making Skills

M eredith's neighbor Jansen goes to school at the state university. The last time Jansen was home, he told Meredith that he was being treated for an ear infection at the university's health center. He also told her that there were rumors that there was a doctor on staff at the health center who was infected with HIV. He said that the doctor who treated him was the one rumored to be HIV-infected. Jansen said he is scheduled to go back to this doctor to see if the infection has been cleared up and if he would need another prescription for antibiotics. Jansen is concerned about being treated by this doctor. What should Jansen do?

A. Not worry about the office procedure unless either the doctor's or Jansen's body fluids are involved.

B. Make sure the doctor wears gloves and a face mask while treating Jansen.

C. Make an appointment to see another doctor on the health center's staff.

D. Cancel the appointment and treat the ear infection with any remaining antibiotics and OTC medicines.

WHAT DO YOU THINK?

1. **Situation.** What possible risks are involved in this situation?

2. **Choices.** What other choices can you think of for Jansen?

3. **Consequences.** What are the costs and benefits of each choice?

4. **Consequences.** Who will be affected by Jansen's decision?

5. **Choices.** Where might Jansen go for more information? Whom should he talk with about this situation?

6. **Decision.** What do you think Jansen should do? Explain your answer.

7. **Evaluation.** Have you ever been involved in something that posed a risk of harming your health? How did you handle the situation?

T risha's little brother Vince, who is a freshman, just found out that he is infected with HIV. Because Vince has hemophilia, his blood does not clot properly. As a result he may bleed excessively from a minor injury. Vince can receive a clotting factor through injections or transfusions. Unfortunately, Vince obtained HIV through a transfusion years ago. The word about Vince has now spread throughout their small town. There has been a negative reaction to his returning to school. Fear and misunderstanding are widespread. Trisha has overheard some very harmful statements from her friends. She doesn't know how to handle this. She has considered five options.

A. Take the offensive, challenging her friends and school officials to show some understanding of the disease and compassion toward her brother.

B. Stay out of it and let the professionals, and the lawyers if necessary, handle the matter.

C. Try to convince her brother that he would be better off being tutored at home.

D. Suggest to her parents that they move to another state where they can start over and lead normal lives.

E. Finish her senior year as quietly as possible and go off to college where she can be away from the problem.

WHAT DO YOU THINK?

8. **Choices.** What other choices does Trisha have?

9. **Consequences.** What are the probable consequences of each choice?

10. **Consequences.** How honest should Trisha be with her brother and family about her feelings in each case? Explain your answer.

11. **Decision.** What do you think Trisha should do?

12. **Evaluation.** Would your opinion in these two cases change depending on which side of the situation you were on?

REVIEW

Using Health Terms

On a separate sheet of paper, write the term that best matches each definition given below.

LESSON 1

1. The final stage of infection caused by HIV.
2. White blood cells that are made in bone marrow.
3. Lymphocytes that mature in the thymus gland.
4. Proteins that help destroy pathogens in the body.

LESSON 2

5. A test that is very specific in identifying HIV antibodies.
6. A term that describes an infection that results from a breakdown of the immune system.
7. The leading cause of wasting syndrome, characterized by fatigue, sudden high fever, night sweats, cramps, and weight loss.
8. A progressive disorder that destroys brain tissue of a person with AIDS.
9. Medicine that slows the multiplication of HIV and seems to help delay the onset of opportunistic infections.

Building Academic Skills

LESSON 1

10. **Writing.** Write a narrative composition describing the life of a person who becomes infected with HIV.

LESSON 2

11. **Writing.** Write a composition titled, "People Who Should Be Tested for HIV." Include reasons for your choices.
12. **Math.** According to the CDC, 872 cases of adolescents with AIDS had been reported through June 1992. The following are some of the causes with the number of cases: IV drug use—112; hemophilia—267; receipt of blood transfusion or tissues—55. Determine what percentage of the total each of these cases represents.

Recalling the Facts

LESSON 1

13. What is the connection between HIV infection and AIDS?
14. How does HIV attack the body's immune system?
15. Where do lymphocytes move and what function do they serve?
16. Name the two major types of lymphocytes and tell where they mature in the body.
17. What is the function of T helper cells?
18. In what kinds of cells does HIV reproduce its genetic material?
19. What happens when T helper cells become infected and are destroyed?
20. Through which body fluids is HIV known to be transmitted?
21. AIDS is not curable, but it is preventable. What are the best methods of prevention?
22. Name two ways teens can reduce their risk of HIV infection.
23. How can using alcohol and illegal drugs increase a person's risk of HIV infection?
24. What role does sexual intercourse play in the spread of HIV?

LESSON 2

25. For what groups of people is HIV testing now required?
26. What are the two main tests for detecting HIV? Which is more specific?
27. Which HIV test is used for screening donated blood?
28. How long may it take the body to develop antibodies to HIV after being infected?
29. How long can HIV stay in the body before a person shows signs of infection?
30. What are the advantages and disadvantages of the medicine AZT in treating AIDS patients?
31. What does a positive test for HIV mean? A negative test?
32. Which of the following are AIDS researchers hoping to find in order to cure people who are suffering from AIDS: a vaccine, a surgical operation, a new vitamin?

REVIEW

Thinking Critically

LESSON 1

33. **Analysis.** Indicate which of the following behaviors are known to transmit HIV from an infected to an uninfected person.
    a. sexual intercourse
    b. shaking hands
    c. kissing with the mouth closed
    d. sharing contaminated needles
    e. sharing bathroom facilities
    f. eating at the same table
    g. receiving a blood transfusion
    h. being stung by a wasp
    i. donating blood
    j. breast-feeding a baby

34. **Evaluation.** Do you think all health-care providers should be tested for HIV? Do you think the results should be made known to a provider's patients? Why or why not?

35. **Evaluation.** Why do you think many people are uninformed about HIV infection and AIDS?

LESSON 2

36. **Synthesis.** Design a care facility for people with AIDS. Describe the physical, mental, and social services that would be provided.

37. **Evaluation.** Do you feel that people who are known to have AIDS should be legally banned from entering the United States? Why or why not?

38. **Evaluation.** Do you believe that people should be required to undergo a test for AIDS before being considered for employment? Why or why not?

39. **Evaluation.** Do you think required HIV testing for groups such as organ donors is an invasion of privacy? Explain.

Making the Connection

LESSON 1

40. **Language Arts.** Write a letter to someone who is afraid of becoming infected with HIV. Explain behaviors and situations known to transmit HIV and how the virus is prevented.

Applying Health Knowledge

LESSON 1

41. Your friend Sam will be undergoing surgery in a few months that will require several blood transfusions. How much risk does Sam run because of this? How can Sam minimize the risk of receiving blood contaminated with HIV?

42. How can having sex only in a marital relationship minimize the risk of contracting AIDS?

LESSON 2

43. Why is confidentiality an important aspect of HIV testing?

44. Your friend has been engaging in behaviors that could lead to HIV infection. He has had his blood tested for HIV antibodies, and the result has been negative. What should he do next?

Beyond the Classroom

LESSON 1

45. **Community Involvement.** Where can a person get information about HIV infection and AIDS?

46. **Community Involvement.** Interview five people in your neighborhood. Ask them what they think are the five primary causes of infection with HIV. Are their ideas based on fact or fiction?

47. **Community Involvement.** Find out what organizations in your community are helping people with AIDS. Make a list of these organizations and tell what specific steps each is taking to help AIDS patients.

LESSON 2

48. **Further Study.** At the present time, AIDS is an incurable disease. Many diseases of the past were also incurable until medical researchers found a way to combat them. Choose one of the following diseases and write a report on its history: polio; tuberculosis; pneumonia; bubonic plague; malaria.

CHAPTER 29

NONCOMMUNICABLE DISEASES

LESSON 1
Cardiovascular
Diseases

LESSON 2
Treating and
Preventing Heart
Disease

LESSON 3
Cancer

LESSON 4
Diabetes

LESSON 5
Arthritis

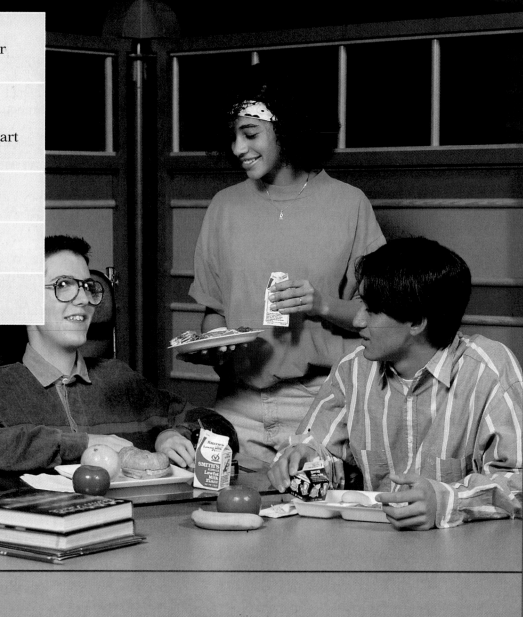

CARDIOVASCULAR DISEASES

There are many diseases that are not caused by pathogens. These are **noncommunicable diseases,** meaning diseases that are not transmitted through contact with others. The diseases that are perhaps most closely related to one's life-style are **cardiovascular diseases**—those of the heart and blood vessels. Cardiovascular disease is the number one killer in the United States.

Over half of all Americans die of some form of cardiovascular disease. The importance of this statistic to young people is great because many cardiovascular diseases are the result of life-style choices and health habits that people adopt early in life.

Learning about cardiovascular diseases is also important because knowing how to recognize these diseases, what to do in an emergency, and where to get help may mean the difference between life and death.

Hypertension

Blood pressure is the force of blood against the walls of blood vessels as blood flows through the cardiovascular system. The force is created by the contraction of the heart muscle and the resistance of the vessel walls. Normal blood pressure varies with age, height, weight, and other factors. If a person's blood pressure stays above his or her normal pressure, the person has high blood pressure, or **hypertension.**

Approximately 60 million people have some elevation of blood pressure, and many of them do not know it. Hypertension has been detected in children as young as 6 years old.

Hypertension can be a silent mysterious killer. It is silent, because in early stages there may be no symptoms that alert a person that medical attention is needed. It is mysterious, because in more than 90 percent of all cases the cause is unknown, and because no cure exists. Since there is no cure, prolonged hypertension can result in major complications, such as stroke, heart attack, heart failure, or kidney failure.

Causes

In many cases the exact cause of hypertension is not known. However, many factors have been identified as being related to it. For example, people in highly stressful environments seem to be more susceptible to hypertension. Another factor is heredity. Children of parents who have hypertension will most likely also have high blood pressure.

Another factor that has definitely been identified as a contributor to hypertension is excessive sodium intake. What is excessive? The recommended daily allowance is 3 grams of sodium. One teaspoon of salt provides about 2 grams of sodium. The average American consumes two to three times this amount. Some people have a natural sensitivity to sodium, which elevates blood pressure.

LESSON 1 FOCUS

TERMS TO USE
- Noncommunicable diseases
- Cardiovascular diseases
- Hypertension
- Arteriosclerosis (ahr•TIR•ee•oh•skluh• ROH•suhs)
- Atherosclerosis (ath•uh•ROH•skluh• ROH•suhs)
- Angina pectoris (an•JY•nuh PEK•tuh•ruhs)
- Fibrillation (FIB•ruh•LAY•shuhn)
- Stroke

CONCEPTS TO LEARN
- Cardiovascular diseases have serious consequences to a person's life.
- Many cardiovascular diseases are related to a person's habits and life-style.

ATTITUDES AND BEHAVIORS TO EVALUATE
- Self-Inventory, page 592.
- Building Decision-Making Skills, page 593.

High blood pressure, hypertension, is called a silent killer.

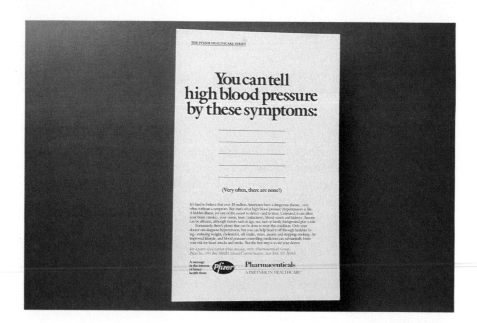

As you know, sodium is essential for cellular function, but the body needs it only in small amounts. Most foods contain some sodium without adding table salt. Table salt provides more than enough sodium for almost everyone. You can reduce your sodium intake by checking food labels and limiting foods high in sodium. Taste your food before salting it, and try to substitute other seasonings.

Treatment

Hypertension cannot be cured, but 90 percent of cases can be controlled with medicine and by diet. Diet controls, besides limiting sodium intake, include maintaining desirable weight, reducing sugar consumption, and reducing intake of foods high in cholesterol and saturated fats. Regular exercise also helps reduce blood pressure.

Diseases of the Arteries

At birth the lining of the blood vessels is very smooth. Over the years fatty deposits, called plaque, build up along the inner lining of the arteries. This buildup is due mainly to dietary choices.

Arteriosclerosis

Arteriosclerosis is a condition in which the walls of arteries become thick and lose their elasticity. The condition is commonly called hardening of the arteries. It is by far the most common cause of death in the United States.

Atherosclerosis is a form of arteriosclerosis. Fatty deposits gradually collect in blood vessels. These deposits clog the vessel so that blood flow is affected. As blood flow is slowed, blood tends to thicken. This can result in the formation of a thrombus, or blood clot. In some cases, an embolus may develop. An embolus is a blood clot that moves from the point where it was formed. Fatty deposits, a thrombus, or an embolus can block a blood vessel. If a coronary vessel becomes blocked, the heart

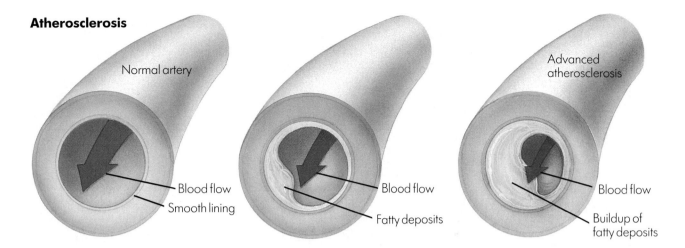

Atherosclerosis

Normal artery

Blood flow
Smooth lining

Blood flow

Fatty deposits

Advanced
atherosclerosis

Blood flow

Buildup of
fatty deposits

muscle is deprived of the normal supply of oxygen. The result is a heart attack.

As fatty deposits collect along artery walls, the flow of blood is seriously affected.

Diseases of the Heart

Heart disease, or heart attack, is a common way to refer to a number of disorders that involve the heart and blood vessels.

Heart Attack

A heart attack occurs because the heart muscle cells are not getting the oxygen and nutrients they need. Any part of the heart that does not get nourishment dies. The severity of the heart attack is determined by how much heart tissue dies.

The heart can keep functioning if the damaged area is not too great. Scar tissue will gradually form over the damaged area, and other arteries will assume the work of the blocked ones. However, because scar tissue is not elastic, it does not contract when the heart does, so the heart is never again able to function at its highest capacity.

A heart attack can occur at any time; it usually is sudden and happens without warning. However, immediate response to the early signs of such an attack can mean the difference between life and death. These early signs include discomfort in the center of the chest. The sensation may be one of pressure, fullness, squeezing, or aching. The distress may extend into one or both arms, the neck, jaw, upper abdomen, and even

---

K E E P I N G   F I T

Reducing the Risks of Cardiovascular Disease

- People who smoke a pack of cigarettes a day are twice as likely to have heart attacks as nonsmokers. The risk increases with the amount smoked. Cigarette smoking also

increases a person's risk of having a stroke.
- After quitting smoking, the risk of heart attack becomes the same as that of a nonsmoker.
- Consuming a diet high in fat is

a risk factor in atherosclerosis. Reduce your intake of cholesterol and fat simply by cutting down on butter, mayonnaise, beef, pork, and lamb.

Electrical shock may be given to someone with ventricular fibrillation.

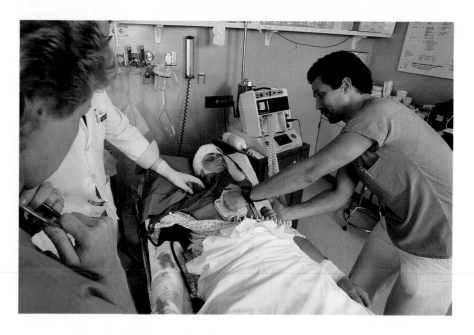

DID YOU KNOW?

- Your risk of having a heart attack may have less to do with your overall cholesterol level and more to do with the ratio of its two components: HDL, the good cholesterol, and LDL, the bad cholesterol.
- According to the National Heart Lung and Blood Institute, people 20 years of age and older should have an LDL of less than 130 and an HDL of 40 or more.
- The best ways to raise your HDL level are by losing weight, if you are overweight, and getting regular aerobic exercise.
- For cholesterol levels that do not respond to exercise and dietary changes, there are medications that can lower overall cholesterol levels.

the back. Nausea, vomiting, sweating, and shortness of breath may also accompany the attack.

A person can easily mistake some of these signs for other problems, such as heartburn or indigestion. Self-diagnosis in this case could be fatal. A person with these symptoms should seek medical attention immediately.

Angina Pectoris

Many people who have atherosclerosis experience a condition known as angina pectoris. In the case of **angina pectoris,** pain and tightness or pressure in the chest occur as a result of the heart's not getting enough oxygen. People who have never had a heart attack may experience angina pains, which are intense attacks of chest pain. Medication can relieve the pain. In addition, these people may have to limit their physical activity to avoid the pain.

Fibrillation

Fibrillation is a rhythmic disturbance that occurs when the muscle fibers of the heart contract in an uncoordinated manner. The rhythm is irregular and is usually at a very fast rate.

KEEPING FIT

Reducing the Risks of Cardiovascular Disease

Don't watch ball games, play them. Even though watching games can be exciting, the games you watch do nothing for your heart, lungs, or weight. But the ball games you play—softball, football, tennis, handball, racquetball, basketball or volleyball—do help. Stop being a fan and start being a player. You'll find that the game is far more exciting from the inside!

When this condition occurs in the ventricles, it is called ventricular fibrillation. If not corrected it is usually fatal because the ventricles stop pumping blood efficiently out of the heart. Doctors can sometimes correct ventricular fibrillation by sending a powerful jolt of electricity into the heart muscle. The treatment is successful if the heart muscle responds by resuming normal rhythm.

Fibrillation can occur in the atria, the upper chambers of the heart. Although this is a serious condition, blood can continue to flow into the ventricles and be pumped out if the ventricles are still functioning.

Cardiac Arrest

Cardiac arrest occurs when the heart stops completely. In the case of cardiac arrest, circulation stops, and the brain can live for only about five minutes.

If cardiac arrest occurs in the hospital, the doctors and hospital staff will attempt external heart massage first. If that procedure does not revive the heart, electrical shock may be administered.

If cardiac arrest occurs, medical help is needed immediately. The victim's life may be saved if someone administers cardiopulmonary resuscitation (CPR) until medical help is available. This lifesaving skill, explained in Chapter 36, forces blood out of the heart and into the arteries. It includes mouth-to-mouth resuscitation, so that the victim gets oxygen. Only someone properly trained in the technique should administer CPR.

Stroke

A **stroke** occurs when the blood supply to a part of the brain is cut off and, as a result, the nerve cells in that part of the brain cannot function. In order to function, brain cells must have a continuous and ample supply of oxygen and nutrients. If brain cells are deprived for five minutes, they will die. The nerve cells of the brain control most of our body movements and the way we receive and interpret sensations.

Any part of the body can be affected by a stroke—it all depends on what area of the brain was deprived of oxygen and nutrients. Because the brain controls the body's movement, a stroke may affect any part of the body. Suppose an artery is blocked in the area of the brain that controls speaking. Then speech will be affected. If the blocked area controls leg muscles, then those muscles will be affected. Even memory can be affected.

Sometimes a stroke will have little effect on the person. At other times the effect will be severe. Some people recover quickly, while others may not recover at all.

Interference with blood supply to the brain may be due to a number of causes. It is not always possible to determine the particular cause of a stroke.

Cerebral Thrombosis

One of the most common causes of stroke is the blocking of a cerebral artery by a thrombus that forms inside the artery. This condition is known as cerebral thrombosis. Sometimes the thrombus occurs in one of the four neck arteries that supply the brain with blood.

A clot is not likely to occur in a healthy artery. One may occur in an artery that has been damaged by atherosclerosis.

Cerebral Embolism

A cerebral embolism occurs if an embolus becomes wedged in one of the cerebral arteries. The result is an interference with the flow of blood to the brain.

Cerebral Hemorrhage

A diseased artery in the brain can burst and flood the surrounding brain tissue with blood. This condition is called a cerebral hemorrhage. The brain cells that the artery nourished do not get the food and oxygen they need. A cerebral hemorrhage is more likely to occur when a person suffers from a combination of atherosclerosis and high blood pressure.

Warning Signs of a Stroke

Following are the major signs of a stroke:

- sudden, temporary weakness or numbness of the face, arm, and leg on one side of the body
- temporary loss of speech, or trouble in speaking or understanding people
- temporary dimness or loss of vision, particularly in one eye
- unexplained dizziness, unsteadiness, or sudden falls.

If you notice one or more of these signs, be sure to tell your doctor.

LESSON 1 REVIEW

Reviewing Facts and Vocabulary

1. What factors are associated with hypertension?
2. How does atherosclerosis develop?
3. Define *thrombus* and *embolus*.

Thinking Critically

4. **Evaluation.** Why do you think that the non-communicable diseases have replaced the communicable diseases as the leading causes of death?
5. **Analysis.** How is a heart attack different from a stroke?

Applying Health Knowledge

6. If you or someone you know is in a high-risk group for heart disease, what life-style changes could you suggest to reduce the risks of heart attack? Design a poster that lists those factors that could be changed to reduce the risks of developing cardiovascular disease or suffering a heart attack.
7. Research a recent discovery or development in heart surgery. Write a one-page descriptive report on your findings.

TREATING AND PREVENTING HEART DISEASE

In recent years amazing advances have been made in treating heart disease. However, medical professionals still believe that preventive measures are the best solution.

Instruments and Techniques

An **electrocardiogram** (EKG or ECG) produces a graph of the electrical activity of the heart. The resulting pattern indicates the heart activity and rhythm. An EKG can help detect the nature of a heart attack and how the heart is behaving. It can indicate if the heart is beating regularly or irregularly, fast or slow, and if the heartbeat is weak or strong.

Phonocardiography involves placing a microphone on a person's chest to record heart sounds and signals, transferring them through photography to graph paper. A professional can then examine the tracings for heartbeat irregularities.

Coronary angiography is a procedure that is used to help evaluate the extent of coronary artery disease. This procedure uses a catheter, which is a thin, flexible tube that can be guided through blood vessels to certain body organs. When checking the vessels and chambers of the heart, the catheter is first inserted into an artery or a vein in either an arm or a leg. Then it is threaded to the aorta and through a coronary artery. When dye is injected into the catheter, X rays can be taken with a fluoroscope. A **fluoroscope** is similar to an X-ray machine except that it gives a moving image instead of a still photograph. This moving image allows narrow or obstructed areas of the heart to be detected.

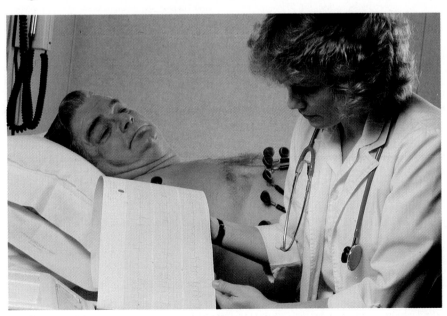

An EKG is a recording of the electrical changes during a cardiac cycle, which is a complete heartbeat.

Recently ultrasound, or high-frequency sound waves, has been used with catheters to collect images of the heart.

If the doctor detects a blocked artery, then balloon angioplasty can be performed at the same time. **Balloon angioplasty** involves threading a balloon-tipped catheter through the body to the site of the blockage. As the balloon is inflated, it pushes the plaque against the artery wall, opening a path for the blood to flow through.

Open-Heart Surgery

In 1952 the first successful open-heart surgery was performed by an American surgeon, Dr. F. John Lewis. He used ice to lower body temperature and to slow circulation to lessen the heart's need for oxygen. A heart-lung machine performs the job of the heart and lungs for several hours during such an operation. The development of this machine has resulted in many advances in open-heart surgery.

Coronary Bypass Surgery

In 1967 a surgical technique for treating heart disease—coronary bypass surgery—was introduced to the medical profession. **Coronary bypass surgery** creates detours around obstructed or narrowed coronary arteries so that more blood can reach the heart.

In this operation a portion of a vein is removed from the patient's leg. One end of the vein is connected to the coronary vessel below the blocked area. This allows blood to flow to the area that was not getting enough blood.

Heart Transplants

Imagine having your heart completely removed and another one put in its place. In South Africa in 1967 Dr. Christiaan Barnard first used

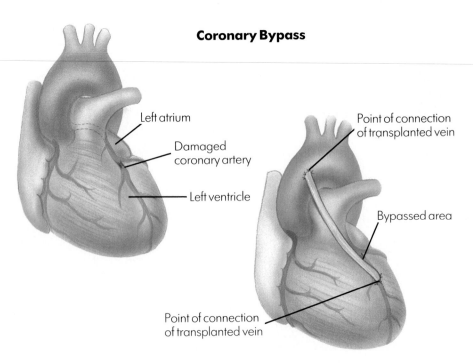

Coronary Bypass

Left atrium

Damaged coronary artery

Left ventricle

Point of connection of transplanted vein

Bypassed area

Point of connection of transplanted vein

the heart transplant procedure. Most patients died within the first year, however, mainly because their bodies rejected the organ.

The Artificial Pacemaker

The heart has a natural pacemaker responsible for initiating electrical impulses that cause the heart to beat. When something interferes with this natural pacemaker, regular, strong heartbeats are not initiated.

An artificial pacemaker is a small unit that is implanted in the chest muscle and wired to the heart. It transmits an electrical impulse to the heart, causing the heart to beat. Many pacemakers are battery-operated, and the batteries must be replaced every four to five years. In the 1970s surgeons began using nuclear-powered and rechargeable battery-powered pacemakers.

Heart Valve Surgery

Valves control the proper flow of blood through the heart. Defective valves may be present at birth or develop later in life. A valve may be too tight, in which case the flow of blood is restricted. Or, a valve may not close tightly enough, which can cause blood to flow backwards.

A common surgical procedure involves replacing a defective valve. Three types of valves can be used to surgically replace a nonfunctioning valve. One type is a valve from a pig's heart and functions like a human valve. Another is a transplanted human valve. The third is a cage-ball valve, which involves a heat-treated carbon ball enclosed in a tiny stainless steel cage. This valve is sewn into the heart and allows blood to pass in only one direction. The pressure from the blood as it tries to flow backward forces the ball into the mouth of the cage, closing the valve.

Artificial Hearts and Blood Vessels

In the United States in 1982 a man whose heart was expected to collapse within hours was given the first artificial heart as a stopgap measure until a human transplant was arranged. Experiments involving the development of an artificial heart are still ongoing.

Some scientists are now working on a device that would duplicate the work of the left ventricle. This part of the heart often wears out before

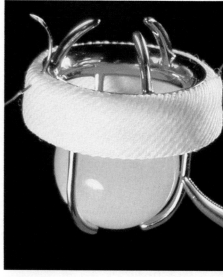

A cage-ball valve allows a normal flow of blood through the heart.

■ Heart disease claims about a million Americans each year.
■ According to the Harvard Medical School, about 300,000 people undergo bypass surgery each year in the United States.
■ Each coronary bypass procedure and follow-up costs more than $20,000.
■ Death rates from this type of bypass surgery range from 1 to 2 percent in major medical centers.
■ The risk of heart attack can be reduced by 2 percent for every 1 percent reduction in blood cholesterol.

the other parts. The device would pump blood into the aorta for distribution throughout the body. Presently, experiments are being done on artificial blood vessels. If the research is successful, 300,000 to 500,000 people may benefit from these artificial vessels each year.

Prevention of Heart Disease

So far, the focus has been on identifying heart disease—its causes and signs, its care and treatment. These are all important areas and many lives have been saved through scientific and medical advances.

However, prevention offers the most promise. To help prevent cardiovascular diseases, it is necessary to look at the risk factors associated with contracting these diseases. A risk factor is a characteristic that has been shown to increase the chances of contracting a disease.

Obviously, you have no control over the factors of age, sex, race, and family medical history. However, you can significantly lower your risk by paying attention to the factors over which you do have control.

■ People who smoke a pack of cigarettes a day are twice as likely to have heart attacks as nonsmokers. The risk increases with the amount smoked. Smoking also increases a person's risk of having a stroke.
■ Within two years of giving up smoking, the risk of heart attack drops significantly. Within 10 to 15 years, the ex-smoker's risk of heart attack is no greater than that of a nonsmoker.
■ Diet is an important factor in atherosclerosis. Reduce your intake of cholesterol and fat by cutting down on butter, mayonnaise, and fried foods. Choose a diet with plenty of vegetables, fruits, and grain products.
■ Being overweight or obese is a contributive factor to heart disease. A middle-aged overweight person is two to three times more likely to have heart disease than a person of normal weight.
■ Sodium intake is directly related to hypertension. You can control it by not adding salt to food and limiting your intake of salty foods.
■ People who exercise regularly reduce their risk of heart disease.
■ Managing stress in your daily life can be an important factor in reducing your risk of heart disease.

LESSON 2 REVIEW

Reviewing Facts and Vocabulary

1. How does an artificial pacemaker work?
2. Define and describe *balloon angioplasty.*
3. List at least seven ways of treating heart disease.

Thinking Critically

4. **Analysis.** Compare two types of artificial valves used during surgery.

Applying Health Knowledge

5. Investigate the kinds of chemicals that are injected during cardiac catheterization. What purpose does each serve? Are there any health risks associated with using these chemicals?
6. Heart transplants and artificial hearts are in the news almost daily. Look for articles in newspapers and magazines about this subject. Display the articles on a classroom bulletin board.

CANCER

Cancer is the second leading cause of death among adults in the United States. Cancer is not one disease, but many diseases, and it is difficult to define cancer by using only one definition. Generally, all **cancers** constitute abnormal, uncontrolled cell growth. Cancer cells are more powerful than normal cells because they can travel beyond their environment and invade other cells. In the process of growth, the cancer cells take over and destroy normal cells and tissues.

Cell division produces new cells; however, some cell divisions result in abnormal cells. Abnormal cells reproduce by dividing, but not at a controlled rate as do normal cells. The uncontrollable division of abnormal cells produces more abnormal cells.

As these cells reproduce and multiply, a mass of tissue, called a **tumor,** develops. Some of these tumors are **benign,** that is, noncancerous. They do not spread to healthy tissue or other parts of the body. Other tumors are **malignant,** or cancerous. Malignant tumors invade and eventually destroy surrounding healthy tissue.

Cancer cells can break away from a malignant tumor and move through lymph or blood vessels to other parts of the body. New tumors, called secondary tumors, can then develop. This process of cancer cells spreading is called **metastasis.** Once a tumor has metastasized, it is very difficult to control. This is the reason early detection of cancer is so important. The sooner cancer is detected, the better the odds are of curing it. Today, half of all cancer cases are curable.

Types of Cancer

About 100 different kinds of cancer affect humans. Cancers are classified in two ways: by the part of the body where the cancer cells first develop, and by the type of body tissue within which the cancer begins.

Cancers that develop in epithelial tissue, tissue that forms the skin and linings of body organs, are called carcinomas. Sarcomas are cancers that develop in connective and supportive tissues such as bones, muscles, and tendons. Lymphomas are cancers that develop in the lymphatic system. Hodgkin's disease is a type of lymphoma.

Diagnosing Cancer

During a physical examination, a doctor can detect many types of cancer. This is one reason regular physical exams are important. If a tumor is found, a physician may do a biopsy. A **biopsy** is the removal of a small amount of tissue that is examined for the presence of abnormal cells. A doctor can check for cervical cancer in women by ordering a Pap smear. The Pap smear detects unusual cells or potentially cancerous tissue long before any symptoms might appear.

LESSON 3 FOCUS

TERMS TO USE
- Cancers
- Tumor
- Benign
- Malignant (muh•LIG•nuhnt)
- Metastasis (muh•TAS• tuh•suhs)
- Biopsy
- Melanoma
- Chemotherapy

CONCEPTS TO LEARN
- There are several warning signs of cancer.
- Early diagnosis of cancer is important so that appropriate treatment can begin.
- An increasing number of kinds of cancer are curable.
- Life-style, environment, and genetic factors can increase an individual's risk of developing cancer.

ATTITUDES AND BEHAVIORS TO EVALUATE
- Self-Inventory, page 592.
- Building Decision-Making Skills, page 593.

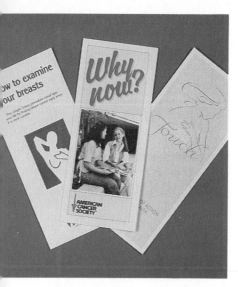

Regular self-examinations help prevent cancer. Your doctor will have pamphlets that show you how.

Identification of colon and rectal cancer has improved as a result of two developments: the fecal occult blood test and the flexible fiberoptic endoscope. The development of the computerized axial tomography (CAT) scan and magnetic resonance imaging (MRI), two techniques that provide clearer, more detailed images than ordinary X rays, are also used to detect cancer.

Cancer's Warning Signs

Early detection of cancer is the most critical factor in treating or curing the disease. The individual should be alert to the seven warning signs of cancer.

- **C**hange in bowel habit. Either loose stools, or constipation.
- **A** sore that does not heal.
- **U**nusual bleeding or discharge (as from the uterus, bladder, bowels, or with coughing).
- **T**hickening or a lump in the breast, or elsewhere (let your doctor decide what the lump means).
- **I**ndigestion or difficulty in swallowing.
- **O**bvious change in a wart or mole.
- **N**agging cough or hoarseness.
  Other symptoms include fatigue and unexplained weight loss.

Carcinogens

Carcinogens are substances that cause cancer. Carcinogens include many chemicals, such as those in tobacco smoke. Asbestos is also a known carcinogen. Radiation from X rays, exposure to the ultraviolet rays in sunlight, and certain viruses are also cancer-causing substances. Some dietary factors such as contaminated water may also be substances. Not everyone is equally susceptible to the same carcinogen. You can control your exposure to, and ingestion of, many carcinogens.

Despite the documented dangers of exposure to the sun, millions of Americans continue to bask in it and increase their risk of developing **melanoma,** or skin cancer. People who work out-of-doors and people who have fair skin are particularly susceptible to skin cancer. This is the reason those people need to use sunscreen lotions that protect the skin from the ultraviolet rays of the sun.

Although radiation is often used in the treatment of cancer, it is in itself a cancer-producing agent in humans. The overuse of X rays in past years exposed people unnecessarily to potential harm from radiation.

K E E P I N G   F I T

Avoiding Unnecessary Cancer Risks

Many cancer specialists recommend that people follow these guidelines to avoid unnecessary cancer risks:
- Maintain an ideal weight.
- Limit your consumption of preserved foods.
- Limit your consumption of prepared meats.
- Avoid artificial sweeteners.
- Limit foods with artificial flavors and colors.
- Increase dietary fiber and bulk.
- Limit your time in the sun.
- Avoid using all forms of tobacco.

We are constantly being exposed to the cosmic rays in the universe, so any unnecessary exposure through X rays is unwise. When considered absolutely necessary in medicine, X rays are used in diagnosis.

Our quality of health is directly related to the air we breathe. Lung cancer has shown the greatest increase of any form of cancer in the past 35 years. The increase in lung cancer is due essentially to smoking tobacco. In addition, air pollution caused by industrial wastes and automobile exhausts is a source of lung cancer concern.

The decision about cigarette smoking is an individual one. Air pollution from industrial sources is really a matter of community responsibility.

DIFFERENT TYPES OF CANCER

Body-Site Type	Organ(s) Most Often Affected	Occurrence
Skin cancer	Skin	Most common type in United States
Digestive system	Colon and rectum	Second most common type in United States
Respiratory system	Larynx and lungs	Occurs mainly in males; increase in incidence of lung cancer in females
Breast	Breast	Occurs mostly in females
Reproductive system	Males—prostate gland, testicles Females—cervix, ovaries, uterus	
Blood and lymph system	Bone marrow, lymph	Occurs in males and females

Treatment of Cancer

Treatment of cancers is directed at confining and killing the cancerous cells. At present, this is accomplished by three basic approaches: surgery, radiation, and chemotherapy.

Surgery

Surgery has been a standard method used for removing tumors and affected areas. Today with improved surgical techniques cancer patients have a longer life expectancy and an improved quality of life. For example, amputation used to be standard practice for treating cancer of arm and leg bones. One way doctors can successfully treat many patients is by removing the diseased bone tissue and transplanting healthy bone tissue from another part of the patient's body.

Radiation

Radiation energy from cobalt or radium can penetrate a tumor. The energy destroys the tumor cells by damaging DNA in the nuclei. DNA is responsible for cell division.

With radiation therapy there is always the risk of causing damage to normal cells near the cancerous area. However, with today's more sophisticated equipment, doctors are able to aim radiation more directly at tumors while sparing surrounding healthy cells.

Radiation therapy is very successful in arresting certain kinds of cancer, such as cervical cancer. It is also very helpful in areas of the body where surgery is difficult, such as the head and neck.

Chemotherapy

Chemotherapy is the use of anticancer medications in the treatment of cancer. The goal of chemotherapy is to destroy malignant cells without excessive destruction of normal cells.

Anticancer medicines interfere with cell division of the cancer cells. The idea is that if the medicine can break up the process of growth, the cancer will not spread.

Unfortunately, some unpleasant side effects, such as nausea and vomiting, occur with the use of these strong medicines. However, new

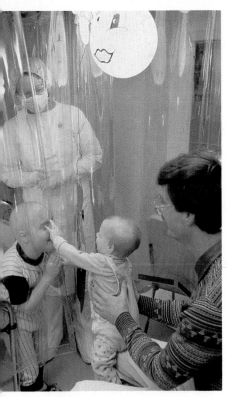

Someone undergoing bone marrow transplantation is carefully protected from possible infection.

HEALTH UPDATE

LOOKING AT THE ISSUES

Do Electromagnetic Fields Cause Cancer?

Sometimes research results are contradictory or inconclusive, and they may take years, even decades, to sort out. An example of one such debate is whether or not there is a link between electromagnetic fields (EMFs) and cancer. EMFs are emitted from power lines, computer monitors, microwave ovens, other home appliances, or any time an electric current passes through a wire.

Analyzing Different Viewpoints

ONE VIEW. Many people believe that claims of the dangers of EMFs are unfounded, even hysterical. They say the exposure from standard power lines and appliances is minimal.

A SECOND VIEW. Some people believe that exposure to EMFs can be linked to birth defects, high incidences of miscarriage, and even increased cancer rates.

A THIRD VIEW. Some people and organizations remain unsure and cautious. Many experts feel the evidence is unclear and more studies are needed to make definitive claims about the EMF/cancer link.

Exploring Your Views

1. When you hear about controversial health issues that are not yet resolved, how do you usually handle the situation?

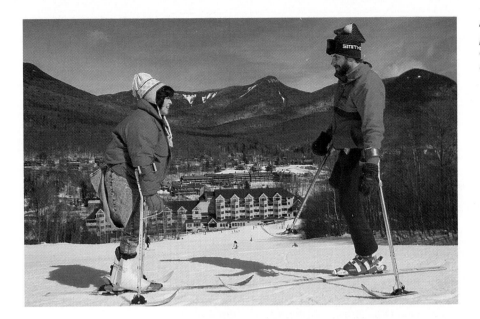

Many former bone cancer patients resume physical activities despite their disabilities.

techniques are allowing physicians to administer chemotherapy more safely and with fewer complications.

Efforts to Combat and Prevent Cancer

The United States began its war against cancer in 1971 when President Richard Nixon signed into law the National Cancer Act. The National Cancer Act established 15 comprehensive cancer centers around the country and greatly increased funding for research and treatment. Since 1971 federal spending for cancer research and treatment has totaled more than $21 billion.

Cancer is being attacked on many fronts. In some cases, we are winning the war. More cancer patients are living longer, better lives; more types of cancer are now curable; diagnosis has greatly improved and so have the three forms of treatment. Most importantly, scientists are learning more about why normal cells become cancerous and how to fight them.

Four main resources have contributed to the control of cancer.

- Education—for medical professionals and the public
- Research programs
- Public interest and support
- Organizations—such as the American Cancer Society and the National Cancer Institute

Prevention is possible in the case of some cancers, but not all. By avoiding exposure to harmful chemicals and excessive radiation, an individual can greatly reduce the risk of some forms of cancer.

There is evidence that there is a relationship between diet and cancer. However, no single vitamin or food has been proven to prevent cancer. Foods rich in vitamins A and C may help lower the risk for certain cancers. Choose to eat a variety of foods including dark green and yellow vegetables as well as cauliflower, broccoli, cabbage, carrots, and other foods high in fiber.

DID YOU KNOW?

- About half a million Americans die from cancer each year—about one every 63 seconds.
- It is predicted that by the year 2000, cancer, not heart disease, will be the number-one killer in the United States.
- According to the American Cancer Society, 49 percent of people with cancer are still alive 5 years after the diagnosis.
- About 90 percent of lung cancer cases in men and 79 percent of cases in women are attributable to cigarette smoking.

Overcoming The Odds

Lea Ann Baldwin is 17. She used to play basketball and loved to bike and run—until she got sick. "I never understood why everyone else could run and run and why I couldn't." She soon discovered the reason. Lea Ann had leukemia. At Minneapolis Children's Hospital she was diagnosed with chronic myelogenous leukemia on her fifteenth birthday. "They said I'd have between five and six years to live unless I had a bone marrow transplant, the only possible cure.

"My whole family was tested to see if their HLA type (tissue type) matched mine, and none of them matched. My name was put on a computer list at the Red Cross and they searched for a match. I was lucky because they found my donor in a couple of months. A boy named Jason was ten days ahead of me in the transplant process. He would prepare me for what to expect. . . . That really helped."

Lea Ann wanted to make her hospital stay as happy and home-like as possible. "My mom brought sheets that made my room so colorful. I also covered the walls with posters. I painted my windows. I went wild."

Lea Ann goes on to describe the transplant process. "First

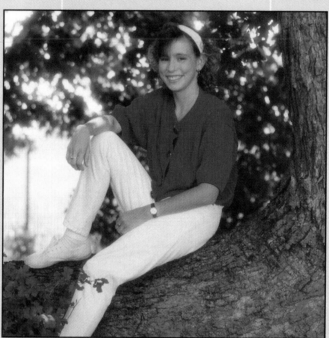

you have five days to get used to everything. Then for three days you have massive doses of chemotherapy and radiation. It's the worst three days of your life. You can't eat. You throw up. You get mouth sores. After the three days, the donor donates the bone marrow. The donated marrow for me was flown in a cooler and brought to the hospital by cab. They checked it, and put it into an IV. The whole process took only about an hour, and I was awake. They told me that afterward I'd feel like I'd been kicked in the lower back by a horse. After twenty-eight days, they gave me a biopsy to see if the other person's marrow was growing in my bones, and at that point I had 50 percent bone marrow, which was a good sign. My last checkup,

my 2-year checkup, showed 100 percent donor bone marrow, which is great. They now say I'm cured.

"The donor who donated marrow to me is 31. She's a doctor of immunology, and that's special to me. Her name is Judy Scheppler, and I have not met her, but I really want to. We were a great match, even better than identical twins. I don't know if I'm quite ready to call her yet. I will eventually. She saved my life. It's just that I'm not sure what to say. Thank you just doesn't seem to cover it."

Lea Ann encourages everyone who can to become a donor. "Then everyone who needs a transplant will be able to get one."

1. What factors helped Lea Ann to face her health struggles?
2. Lea Ann made her environment colorful and homey. Doing so gave her a sense of control. What steps can you take to shape your environment so that you feel more in control of it and more positive about it? How might taking these steps affect your self-esteem?
3. What does it mean to you to have control over the things that affect your health and your life?

Today early diagnosis and treatment remain the most effective ways of treating all types of cancer. Although many cancer researchers hope for a vaccine that could prevent some types of cancer from occurring, the discovery of a vaccine is probably 20 years or more away. Meanwhile, scientists are learning more about the role of heredity in families that experience multiple cases of the same type of cancer. New ways to treat the disease by enhancing the body's immune system are also being studied.

CANCER QUACKERY

In the United States, laetrile is an illegal drug that contains cyanide, a potentially lethal poison, as well as many impurities. Laetrile is available in Mexico and some people from the United States go there in the hope of finding a cure. Drugs like laetrile will always be available as long as cancer exists, because people want to be free of pain, either from the cancer itself or from the effects of chemotherapy.

When a person reaches a terminal stage, he or she is more likely to try anything. People involved in cancer quackery can influence a desperate person and make money.

As long as we have no known cure for cancer, there will be many drugs, treatments, and devices that people will sell to unknowing and desperate people. Sometimes the cancer patients convince themselves that such unproven practices work, often because they want to believe it. Also, cancer patients tend to have periods when they seem to improve. The patient often interprets this as a sign that the unproven practice or drug is actually working. Sadly, these people invest money in worthless attempts to cure their cancer. Valuable time is wasted. They may delay getting medical assistance that could provide them with the only real chance they might have for cure and survival.

DID YOU KNOW?

- Donated bone marrow can mean the difference between life and death for many leukemia patients and patients with other fatal blood and genetic diseases. Often, family members donate marrow. However, sometimes family members cannot or will not donate their marrow or their marrow is not a match.
- The chances of finding a marrow match outside the family, however, are low. Matches are most likely to be found within a person's ethnic group.

LESSON 3 REVIEW

Reviewing Facts and Vocabulary

1. What is the difference between normal cells and cancerous cells?
2. Why is early diagnosis and treatment of cancer so important?
3. Define *benign* and *malignant*.

Thinking Critically

4. **Evaluation.** Use the library to locate a magazine article about the controversies surrounding animal testing in medical research, particularly in cancer research. Explain the different viewpoints. What do you think about the use of animals for medical research?

Applying Health Knowledge

5. Interview someone in your school or neighborhood who has successfully undergone cancer treatment. Get details about the treatment, any side effects, and time required. Summarize your findings in a one-page report.

DIABETES

LESSON 4 FOCUS

TERMS TO USE
- Diabetes
- Glucose
- Insulin
- Type I diabetes
- Type II diabetes

CONCEPTS TO LEARN
- Metabolism of carbohydrates is the main source of energy for body cells.
- The release of energy from carbohydrates is a function of insulin, a hormone produced by the pancreas.
- There are two classifications of diabetes—type I and type II.

ATTITUDES AND BEHAVIORS TO EVALUATE
- Self-Inventory, page 592.
- Building Decision-Making Skills, page 593.

Diabetes is one of the leading health problems in the United States and a leading killer of adults. It affects an estimated 12 million Americans, and the number seems to be increasing. Many people have diabetes and do not know it.

About 700,000 new cases of diabetes occur each year. Persons with diabetes are more prone to suffer from heart disease and stroke; more prone to blindness; and more prone to kidney disease than persons who do not have diabetes.

Diabetes lessens the chance of a female's maintaining a full-term pregnancy and increases the frequency of birth defects in babies. The economic toll of diabetes in hours of work lost and in medical costs is over $20 billion annually.

How Diabetes Affects the Body

Diabetes is a chronic disease that affects the way body cells convert food into energy. Diabetes can be controlled but as yet cannot be cured. In the normal digestive process carbohydrates are changed to a sugar called **glucose,** absorbed into the blood, and delivered to body cells. Normally, with the help of **insulin,** a hormone produced in the pancreas, glucose is converted into energy for use by the cells. In the case of diabetes, this process is interrupted.

Diabetes develops either because no insulin or insufficient insulin is produced or because the insulin produced is not used efficiently. When glucose is unable to enter the cells, it accumulates in the blood until the kidneys filter out some of the surplus and it is passed off in urine. High sugar content in urine and in blood is one of the surest signs that a person has diabetes.

Types of Diabetes

The National Diabetes Data Group has established two classifications of diabetes: type I, insulin-dependent diabetes, and type II, noninsulin-dependent diabetes.

Type I, Insulin-Dependent Diabetes

Type I diabetes (formerly called juvenile-onset diabetes) occurs most often before the age of 15 and accounts for about 10 percent of all cases of diabetes. Type I usually appears abruptly and progresses rapidly. Symptoms of type I diabetes include frequent urination, abnormal thirst, unusual hunger, weight loss, irritability, weakness, fatigue, nausea, and vomiting.

Because the pancreas produces little or no insulin, these patients must take daily injections of insulin to stay alive. Before the discovery of

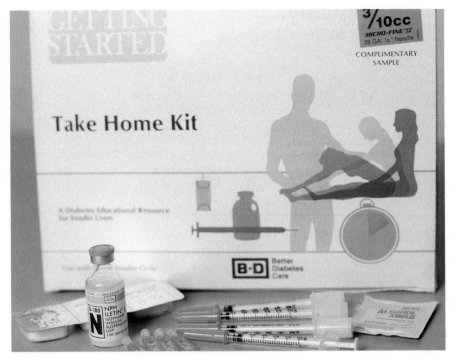

This diabetes kit is for use at home.

insulin, persons with type I diabetes usually lived no more than two years after diagnosis. Today, because of advanced methods of treatment, many persons with diabetes live near-normal life spans.

Type II, Noninsulin-Dependent Diabetes

Type II diabetes (formerly called adult-onset diabetes) occurs usually in adults over 40 years of age. This is the more common form of diabetes and accounts for about 90 percent of all cases of diabetes. In type II diabetes, the pancreas produces some insulin, but because of a cell receptor defect, the cells cannot use the insulin effectively.

Type II diabetes can usually be controlled by diet and exercise. In some cases, oral medications or injections of insulin are also required. Problems related to circulation are common in this type of diabetes. Because the onset of type II diabetes is gradual, the disease often goes undetected for years. Symptoms of type II diabetes include excess

KEEPING FIT

Diabetes and Exercise

Research continues to support the fact that regular exercise helps to prevent or control a variety of diseases. Now studies suggest that regular exercise not only helps to control blood sugar levels in cases of diabetes, but it can also help prevent the disease. As little as 20 minutes of moderate aerobic exercise 3 times a week can help prevent diabetes. So can controlling one's weight.

DIABETIC EMERGENCIES

Type of Emergency

Low blood sugar

Signs
- Staggering, poor coordination
- Irritability, belligerence, hostility
- Pale color
- Sweating
- Stupor or unconsciousness

Possible Causes
- Delayed or missed meals
- Too much insulin, by overdose or error
- Extreme exercise

Treatment
- Look for diabetic identification bracelet or necklace.
- The diabetic may carry candy or special quick-sugar commercial preparations in plastic soft-tipped containers. Squeeze the contents into the person's mouth.
- If the person can swallow without choking, offer any food or drink containing sugar, such as soft drinks, fruit juice, or candy. Do not use diet drinks!
- If the person does not respond in 10 to 15 minutes, take him or her to a hospital.

Type of Emergency

High blood sugar

Signs
- Thirst
- Very frequent urination
- Flushed skin
- Vomiting
- Fruity or winelike odor of breath
- Stupor or unconsciousness

Possible Causes
- Insulin forgotten or omitted
- Stress, such as illness or injury
- Overindulgence in certain foods or beverages

Treatment
- Look for diabetic identification bracelet or necklace.
- If unsure, contact a physician.
- Take the person to a hospital.

weight, drowsiness, blurred vision, tingling or numbness in hands and feet, skin infections, and itching and slow-healing cuts.

Type II diabetes has been linked to heredity, obesity, and inactivity. About 80 percent of all patients are overweight at the time they are diagnosed. People can prevent many cases of type II diabetes if they maintain a desired weight and keep physically active.

LESSON 4 REVIEW

Reviewing Facts and Vocabulary

1. In one sentence, describe diabetes.
2. How can a person help prevent type II diabetes?
3. What is a sure sign that a person has diabetes?

Thinking Critically

4. **Evaluation.** Is the presence of sugar in urine an effective test for diabetes? Explain.

Applying Health Knowledge

5. Find out why people with diabetes should wear emergency medical symbols.
6. Ask people who have diabetes to speak to your class about the effect of diabetes on lifestyle.

ARTHRITIS

The term *arthritis* means "inflammation of a joint." **Arthritis** covers at least 100 different conditions that cause aching, pain, and swelling in joints and connective tissue throughout the body. It can and does occur at all ages, from infancy on. The National Center for Health Statistics estimates that about 37 million people have arthritis severe enough to require medical care. Arthritis costs the national economy over $18 billion yearly in lost wages and medical bills. It is likely that someone you know has arthritis, since it affects one in seven people and one in three families. The two most common kinds of arthritis are rheumatoid arthritis and osteoarthritis.

Rheumatoid Arthritis

Rheumatoid arthritis is the most serious type of arthritis and is mainly a destructive and disabling inflammation of the joints. It affects primarily the joints of the hands and arms, the hips, and the feet and legs. Rheumatoid inflammation also attacks connective tissue throughout the body, and this causes symptoms such as fever, fatigue, and swollen lymph glands.

Rheumatoid arthritis causes the joints to stiffen, then swell and become tender. The inflammation can do progressive damage inside the joint if it is not diagnosed and properly treated.

What Rheumatoid Arthritis Does

The area where two bones meet is enclosed in a capsule, containing fluid. The capsule has an inner lining called the synovial membrane.

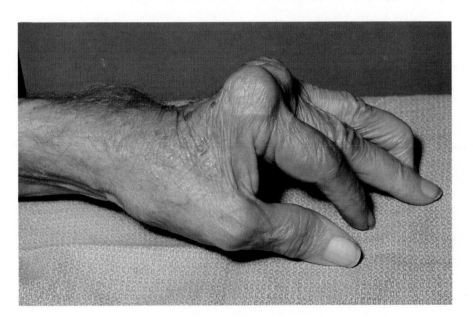

LESSON 5 FOCUS

TERMS TO USE
- Arthritis
- Rheumatoid arthritis
- Osteoarthritis (AHS•tee•oh•ahr•THRYT•uhs)

CONCEPTS TO LEARN
- Arthritis can affect people of any age.
- Treatment programs are available to ease the discomfort of arthritis.

ATTITUDES AND BEHAVIORS TO EVALUATE
- Self-Inventory, page 592.
- Building Decison-Making Skills, page 593.

Rheumatoid arthritis causes joints to stiffen and swell.

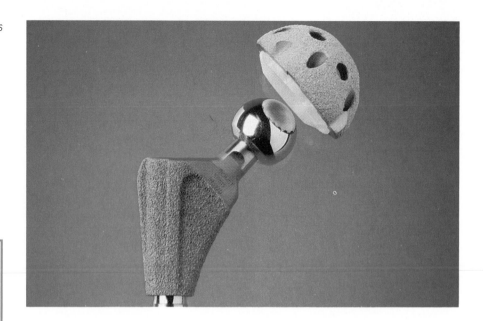

A hip joint damaged by arthritis can be replaced with an artificial joint.

Inflammation starts here, causing the membrane to swell and spread to other parts of the joint. Outgrowths of inflamed tissue invade the cartilage surrounding the bone ends, eventually eroding the bone tissue. Finally, scar tissue can form between the bone ends and sometimes change to bone, so that the joint becomes fused, and immovable.

Inflammation can also lead to distortion of the joint. This is most apparent when the disease attacks the hands. The fingers become drawn back and angled sideways, so that the hands are deformed and difficult to use properly in performing common daily tasks. These conditions can develop at any age. With proper treatment started early, some of the symptoms can be relieved.

Treatment of Rheumatoid Arthritis

Scientists do not know the cause of rheumatoid arthritis, and at the present time there is no cure for it. Treatment programs are designed to relieve pain, reduce inflammation, prevent damage to joints, prevent deformities, and keep joints movable and functioning properly.

A full treatment program for rheumatoid arthritis may include the following: medication (aspirin is the most frequently used anti-inflammatory medicine), rest, exercise, good posture, splints, walking aids, heat, surgery, and rehabilitation.

K E E P I N G   F I T

Understanding People with Chronic Diseases

If you are close to someone who is chronically ill, remember these guidelines.
■ Offer help when it is needed or asked for. Allow the chronically ill person to be as independent as possible.

■ Be patient. Imagine what it would be like to be in the other person's place.
■ Don't always focus on the other person's condition. Talk about yourself, your own life, the outside world.

■ Don't underestimate the power of touch. Just holding a hand or giving a hug can do a lot for someone who is ill.
■ Don't forget humor.

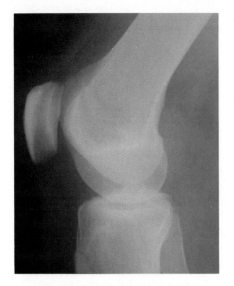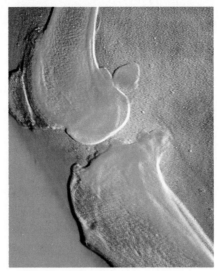

Osteoarthritis

Osteoarthritis is the most common type of arthritis, affecting about 16 million people. It results from wear and tear in the mechanical parts of a joint. Unlike rheumatoid arthritis, inflammation is rarely a problem. Osteoarthritis affects primarily the weight-bearing joints of the knees and hips.

In osteoarthritis, the cartilage becomes pitted and frayed and, in time, may wear away completely. Bone ends then become thicker and bony spurs may develop. As a result, surrounding ligaments and membranes become thickened, changing the whole structure and shape of the joint.

Aching and soreness around the joints, especially when a person moves, are the major symptoms of osteoarthritis. Although there is no cure, treatment can slow down and even control the disease process.

Aches and pains in or around joints can mean different things. Early detection and diagnosis of arthritis is essential and can prevent unnecessary damage and pain. Yet, arthritis specialists report that people suffering from arthritis wait an average of four years after their first symptoms appear before seeking assistance.

> ### DID YOU KNOW?
>
> - Joints that are damaged by severe arthritis, other disease, or injury can be replaced by artificial ones. Joints that can now be replaced include ankles, elbows, fingers, hips, knees, and toes. Most recipients of joint replacement have this surgery to reduce pain and improve joint function because of arthritis.

LESSON 5 REVIEW

Reviewing Facts and Vocabulary

1. What are the early signs of arthritis?
2. How is arthritis treated?

Thinking Critically

3. **Analysis.** Compare rheumatoid arthritis and osteoarthritis.
4. **Synthesis.** What effect could arthritis have on physical, social, and mental health?

5. **Synthesis.** Develop a short oral presentation that could be used to get people with arthritis to seek medical treatment.
6. **Analysis.** Explain why people with arthritis would be very susceptible to quackery.

Applying Health Knowledge

7. Invite a physical therapist to your class to discuss rehabilitative therapy for people with arthritis. Summarize the main points in writing.

Self-Inventory

Risky Business!

HOW DO YOU RATE?

Number a sheet of paper from 1 through 18. Read each item below and respond by writing *yes* or *no* for each. Total the number of each type of response. Then proceed to the next section.

1. I avoid sitting or standing near people who are smoking.
2. I put salt on my food.
3. I smoke cigarettes.
4. I avoid eating fried foods.
5. I limit the amount of fat in my diet.
6. When I am in sunlight during midday, I use a sunscreen lotion.
7. I use smokeless tobacco products.
8. I exercise aerobically at least three times a week.
9. I eat foods high in fiber.
10. Fresh fruits and vegetables are a major part of my diet.
11. I avoid long exposure to dust, fumes, and industrial chemicals.
12. I limit my intake of foods high in cholesterol.
13. When I get upset, I take some action to relax.
14. I keep my weight under control.
15. I wear protective clothing when I am in the sun for long periods of time.
16. I use some effective ways to relax.
17. I avoid smoke-filled rooms.
18. I eat a lot of greasy foods.

HOW DID YOU SCORE?

Give yourself 1 point for each of these items you answered *yes:* 1, 4, 5, 6, 8, 9, 10, 11, 12, 13, 14, 15, 16, 17. Give yourself 1 point for each of these items you answered *no:* 2, 3, 7, 18. Find your total and read below to see how you scored. Then proceed to the next section.

17 to 18
Excellent. You are doing a great job of reducing your risk of getting heart disease and cancer.

15 to 16
Good. You are certainly on the right track, doing many positive things to protect yourself. Keep moving forward.

9 to 14
Fair. Obviously you are doing some things to protect yourself, but not as much as you could possibly do.

Below 9
Look out! It is time you realized that there is much that you should be doing to reduce your risk of heart disease and cancer.

WHAT ARE YOUR GOALS?

If you received an *excellent* or *good* score, complete the statements in Part A. If your score was rated *fair* or *look out!*, complete Parts A and B.

Part A

1. I plan to learn more about reducing my risks by ____.
2. My timetable for accomplishing this is ____.
3. I plan to share my information with others by ____.

Part B

4. The behavior toward heart disease and cancer I would most like to change is ____.
5. The steps involved in making this change are ____.
6. My rewards for making this change will be ____.

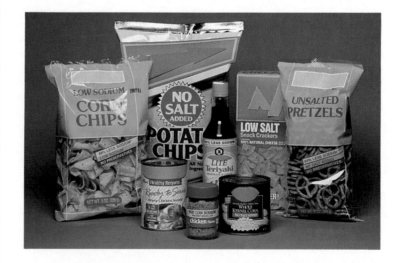

Building Decision-Making Skills

E ven though Paige's grandfather had a heart attack over a year ago, she is still concerned about his health. He is trying hard to follow his doctor's orders of regular exercise, and he is taking his medicine faithfully. However, Paige is concerned about his diet. She knows that certain foods do not promote a healthy heart, and her grandparents have not changed their eating habits. Paige's grandmother says she is too old to change her habits and if you cannot enjoy a good meal, then why live? She thinks she'll die in a few years anyway. Paige has tried hard to convince her grandmother that choices a person makes can affect the quality of life, but she will not listen. Paige lives close to her grandparents, so she sees them often. What should Paige do next?

WHAT DO YOU THINK?

1. **Choices.** What choices does Paige have?
2. **Consequences.** What are the advantages and disadvantages of each choice?
3. **Consequences.** What risks are involved in this decision?
4. **Consequences.** How might Paige feel about each choice now and several years from now?
5. **Decision.** What should Paige do?
6. **Evaluation.** What do you do when you cannot convince someone you love and respect about the benefits of an idea that is new to them?

D iabetes runs in Rachel's family. Both her father and his brother have this disease. Now Rachel's aunt was just diagnosed as having type II diabetes. She is very worried. She has seen how this disease has affected older family members. One relative lost a leg, and another lost his eyesight. As a result Rachel's aunt is afraid to eat much of anything. She has lost a lot of weight and looks too thin. Rachel is concerned about her aunt. What should Rachel do?

WHAT DO YOU THINK?

7. **Situation.** Why does a decision need to be made?
8. **Choices.** What could Rachel do to help her aunt?
9. **Consequences.** What are the advantages of each choice?
10. **Consequences.** What are the disadvantages of each choice?
11. **Decision.** What do you think Rachel should do?

B ill and Linda have been going together for over a year. Both of them like to have fun and have many friends. They are anticipating the school dance that is coming up in two weeks. Bill and Linda will be meeting a group of friends there. Today in the cafeteria, many were talking about the upcoming dance. Sally told Linda that her brother, Marcus, was coming home from college the weekend of the dance. Sally asked Linda if she would like to go with Marcus to the dance. Sally knows that Linda goes with Bill, but said, "I just thought that since Bill is in a wheelchair because of his arthritis, you might want to go with someone who might be more fun at a dance." What should Linda do?

WHAT DO YOU THINK?

12. **Choices.** What are Linda's choices?
13. **Consequences.** What are the advantages and disadvantages of each choice?
14. **Decision.** What do you think Linda should do?
15. **Evaluation.** What do you usually do when you find yourself in a position where you must deal with negative stereotypes?

REVIEW

Using Health Terms

On a separate sheet of paper, write the term that best matches each definition given below.

LESSON 1

1. High blood pressure.
2. A condition that occurs when a blood vessel in the brain is blocked.
3. Diseases of the heart and blood vessels.
4. Diseases that are not transmitted by contact with others.

LESSON 2

5. Responsible for initiating electrical impulses that cause the heart to beat.
6. A procedure in which a damaged or nonfunctioning organ is removed and replaced with one from a donor.

LESSON 3

7. A mass of tissue formed by cells multiplying faster than normal.
8. Cancer-causing substances.
9. Cancerous.
10. Abnormal, uncontrolled cell growth.
11. Noncancerous.

LESSON 4

12. A form of sugar produced by the digestion of carbohydrates.

LESSON 5

13. Inner lining of capsule where two bones meet.
14. A condition in which cartilage becomes pitted and may eventually wear away completely.

Building Academic Skills

LESSON 1

15. **Writing.** Keep a log of your sodium and fat intake and your activity level for one week. Analyze your diet and activity level and write a one-page paper, evaluating your potential risk for heart disease based on your log and making specific suggestions for improvement.

Recalling the Facts

LESSON 1

16. What are the early signs of a heart attack?
17. How long can the brain live once the heart has stopped?
18. What happens as a result of plaque buildup in the arteries?
19. What might hypertension lead to?
20. What are the signals that indicate a stroke may be occurring?

LESSON 2

21. What are two developments in the treatment of heart disease currently being studied?
22. What can a person do to lower his or her risk factor for heart disease?
23. What causes high blood pressure?

LESSON 3

24. Where can carcinogens be found? Give three examples of carcinogens.
25. What factor is the leading cause of lung cancer?
26. What are strategies for treating cancer?
27. What is an advantage of chemotherapy over surgery or radiation in the treatment of cancer?
28. What benefits were realized from the National Cancer Act? When was it signed into law, and under whose administration?
29. What kind of cancer can be detected by a Pap smear?
30. What are seven warning signs of cancer?

LESSON 4

31. Who is most likely to suffer from type I diabetes and what are its symptoms?
32. Who is most likely to suffer from type II diabetes and what are its symptoms? Why might a case of type II diabetes go undetected for several years?

LESSON 5

33. Why is early diagnosis of arthritis vital?
34. What are the goals of treatment of rheumatoid arthritis? What might treatment of rheumatoid arthritis involve?

REVIEW

Thinking Critically

LESSON 1

35. Synthesis. What kind of life-style is associated with the development of hypertension? Why do hypertension and atherosclerosis increase the risk of stroke?

36. Synthesis. Explain how a stroke, which causes the death of brain cells, can cause paralysis of a leg or similar loss of motor function elsewhere in the body.

LESSON 3

37. Synthesis. How is early detection of cancer related to the likelihood of cure and to the increase in reported cancer cases?

38. Evaluation. Why do you think people knowingly expose themselves to carcinogens and so increase their risk of developing cancer later in life? Consider carcinogens such as ultraviolet rays on the skin from sunbathing and nicotine in the lungs from smoking cigarettes. What role does age play in such risky behaviors?

LESSON 4

39. Synthesis. Although persons with diabetes can die because of too much or too little sugar in their blood, they are more likely to die from heart or kidney disease that has progressed over many years. Why? What is the connection between diabetes and these other life-threatening illnesses?

LESSON 5

40. Evaluation. What can you do to help prevent osteoarthritis?

Making the Connection

LESSON 2

41. Language Arts. Research the history of one of the treatments for heart disease. How did the treatment develop? How long was research done before the treatment was tried on humans? How effective has this particular treatment been?

Applying Health Knowledge

LESSON 1

42. One of the factors related to hypertension is a highly stressful environment. Stress occurs as a result of good and bad events. List events or activities you consider stressors. Include both kinds of stressors on your list.

43. Why do you think noncommunicable diseases have replaced communicable diseases as the leading causes of death?

LESSON 2

44. Talk to someone who has survived a heart attack. Find out how his or her life has changed.

45. Many foods are now labeled with words such as *low-fat, low-cholesterol, low-sodium,* and *lite.* Are these labels encouraging people to buy certain products? Are they misleading? Do they provide people with a false sense of security? Explain.

LESSON 3

46. If someone you loved was diagnosed with cancer and wanted to go to Mexico for laetrile treatment, how would you react?

LESSON 4

47. What would you do if you knew your insulin-dependent brother had intentionally not taken his insulin?

LESSON 5

48. Arthritis affects one in seven people and one in three families. Do the people you know typify this statistic? Explain.

Beyond the Classroom

LESSON 1

49. Further Study. Find out what is a recommended daily sodium intake. Then read the labels of the food you consume most often to estimate about how much sodium you consume in an average day. Include estimates of table salt you use.

GLOBAL ENVIRONMENTAL ISSUES

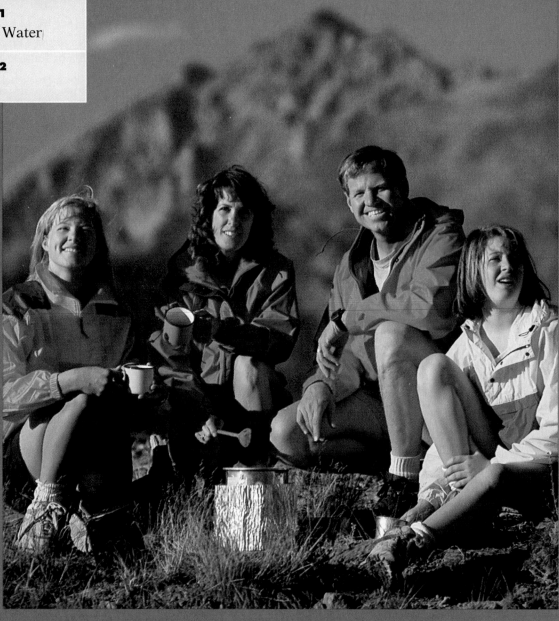

AIR AND WATER

You do not have to leave your home to see that the planet is in trouble. Almost any newspaper or newsmagazine carries headlines and articles about the health—or illness—of our world. Reports about acid rain, oil spills, global warming, droughts, famine, destruction of rain forests, and other disasters often fill the pages. Television reports show forests that are being destroyed and deserts that are expanding. There are scenes of the world's lakes, rivers, oceans, and air that are being degraded and polluted.

In every country increasing numbers of individuals and groups of people are becoming aware of environmental problems and are working to change things for the better. Let us review some of the environmental issues throughout the world, including what is being done to help protect and restore the planet.

Global Air Pollution

In just five days in 1952, one of London's smogs killed more than 4,000 people—a tragedy that still holds the record as the worst air pollution disaster in the world. London smogs were caused by a combination of fog and pollution. The pollution was mainly sulfur dioxide released when sulfur-containing coal and oil were burned in homes and power plants. After the tragedy the whole city, like many others in the United Kingdom, was declared a smoke-free zone. No one was allowed to burn a coal fire unless a preprocessed sulfur-free fuel or a more efficient smoke-eating stove was used. Industrial chimneys were required to be higher and to have built-in dust precipitators to remove some of the worst of the pollution. London smog is now mostly a thing of the past, and there have been no serious outbreaks of air pollution in London since the early 1960s.

Unfortunately, the story in developing nations of the world is another matter. There, many people continue to depend on coal or, more often, wood or charcoal for their cooking and heating needs. Controls either have not been introduced or have been difficult to carry out.

Photochemical Smog

Smog in the United States is an entirely different problem. It was first noticed in the early 1940s when residents of Los Angeles began to detect a tint in the air coupled with a stinging sensation in their eyes. Comparing their problems with what they knew of London, local authorities blamed sulfur dioxide and took steps to reduce it. However, the smog got worse.

Researchers named this new pollution **photochemical smog.** It occurs when vehicle exhausts, activated by sunlight, combine with other hydrocarbons in the atmosphere. One of the other hydrocarbons is the fumes from the fuel itself.

CONFLICT RESOLUTION

Theresa Bennett lives with her mother and three-year-old sister in an old apartment building. In health class, Theresa learned that lead paint in old buildings is a possible cause of brain damage in young children. She and her mother are concerned that her sister may be at risk, but they can't convince their landlord to repaint their apartment. They feel trapped because they can't afford to move to a newer apartment. Theresa has considered organizing the other tenants and reporting the situation to city inspectors.

What other options can you think of to resolve Theresa's conflict?

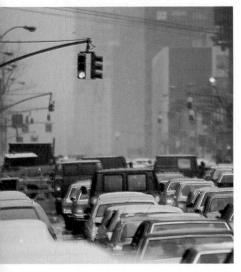

Photochemical smog is a big problem in large cities.

Photochemical smog is found in many parts of the world, especially where there is dense traffic and a warm, sunny climate. In all of these places visibility is seriously reduced, and sometimes as little as one-tenth of the available sunlight actually penetrates the smog and reaches the ground.

Lead

Another toxic chemical pollutant in the atmosphere is lead—which spews from the exhausts of cars and other vehicles. Lead is still used as an anti-knock agent in gasoline in many parts of the world. In some urban areas toxic levels have been found in the bloodstream of traffic police officers and other outdoor workers. Scientists also have found that pigeons living in urban areas have as much as 10 times more lead in their blood than birds who live in rural areas.

Current research is being done on the long-term effects of lead poisoning. It is known that toxic effects of lead include loss of appetite, anemia, damage to the nervous system and, possibly, brain damage leading to a lowering of intelligence levels in young children.

Acid Rain

Air pollutants rarely go away; some return to the earth in rain, as in the case of sulfur and nitrogen from vehicles, industry, and home heating. Since the 1950s the acidity of rainfall in some parts of the world has increased dramatically. Acid rain can be 4 to 40 times more acidic than normal rainwater, sometimes as acidic as lemon juice or vinegar.

In industrial regions of England and Germany, acidic pollutants are damaging lakes, streams, and large tracts of forests. These pollutants are also becoming a serious problem in heavily industrialized parts of Asia, Latin America, and Africa.

Acid rain is spread over the earth by air currents. It is associated with depletion or total elimination of fish in lakes and **estuaries,** or ecosystems where seawater mixes with fresh water from rivers, streams, and runoff from the land. Besides damaging crops and forests, acid rain also damages steel and stone structures, outdoor artworks, and even nylon stockings.

Some responses to local air pollution standards have added to acid rain problems in other parts of the world. For instance, very tall smokestacks are sometimes added to power plants and smelting plants for dumping acid-laden smoke high in the atmosphere so that winds can distribute it elsewhere. For example, the world's tallest smokestack, which is in Ontario, Canada, accounted for 1 percent of the annual worldwide emissions of sulfur dioxide.

It is important to realize that Canada is not alone in this situation. In fact, Canada presently receives more acid deposits from industrialized regions of the northeastern United States than it sends across its southern border. Most of the acidic pollutants in Finland, Norway, Sweden, the Netherlands, Austria, and Switzerland are blown there from industrialized regions of western and eastern Europe. As you can see, prevailing winds do not stop at national boundaries; the problem of air pollution is of global concern.

Damage to the Ozone Layer

The ozone layer in the lower atmosphere absorbs most of the ultraviolet wavelengths from the sun. Unfortunately, this layer is being changed by the effects of man-made chemicals. In addition, each spring an ozone hole appears over the Antarctic. It extends over an area about the size of the continental United States.

Presently there is a large increase in skin cancers, which is believed to be related to increases in ultraviolet radiation from the sun. Cataracts may become more common because of the radiation; and the immune system may be weakened, making people more vulnerable to some viral and parasitic infections. In addition, reduction in the ozone layer may adversely affect the world's populations of **phytoplankton,** microscopic organisms, such as green algae, found in open, sunlit waters. These organisms are the basis of food webs in freshwater and marine life and are a factor in maintaining the composition of the atmosphere.

Chlorofluorocarbons.   The causes of ozone reduction are being debated in the scientific community. To be sure, large volcanic eruptions, such as the recent eruptions of Mount Pinatubo in the Philippines, and cyclic changes in solar activity have serious effects. However, the major factor in ozone reduction is **chlorofluorocarbons (CFCs),** which are compounds of chlorine, fluorine, and carbon. They are odorless and invisible and are widely used as propellants in aerosol spray cans and as coolants in refrigerators and air conditioners. They are also used in making industrial solvents and plastic foams. CFCs enter the atmosphere slowly and resist breakdown.

The United States, Canada, and many other countries have reduced or banned the use of CFCs. Nonaerosol use of CFCs throughout the world has increased.

The Greenhouse Effect

Before the Industrial Revolution fossil fuels such as coal, oil, and gas were locked up within the earth's crust. Virtually all of the carbon dioxide that was released by people came from wood fires. Today carbon dioxide is being sent into the atmosphere from a whole range of sources, including human and animal respiration and decay, forest clearance, open fires, stoves, central heating, power station burners, and cars and other vehicles.

K E E P I N G   F I T

Protection Against Air Pollution

Protect yourself during pollution emergencies or when pollution levels are high:
- Avoid strenuous outdoor activities.

- Do not smoke.
- If you exercise outdoors, work out early in the morning when the concentration of pollutants in the air is lowest.

- Eat well-balanced meals; good nutrition enables your body to better handle toxic substances.

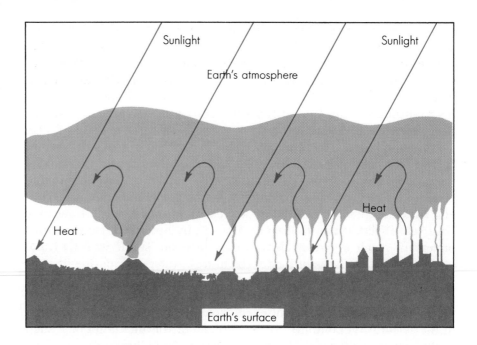

In the greenhouse effect, large quantities of carbon dioxide, caused by the burning of fossil fuels, form a cloud around the earth. Heat is kept near the surface, thus causing higher temperatures and humidity.

Although it makes up only a tiny fraction of the earth's atmosphere, carbon dioxide is vitally important because it regulates the amount of heat that the earth absorbs from the sun. The more carbon dioxide there is, the better an insulator the atmosphere becomes. It reflects heat that normally would escape from the earth into space. As current carbon dioxide levels rise, a growing proportion of the solar radiation is becoming trapped inside the earth's atmosphere and is being reflected back to the earth's surface. This condition, known as the greenhouse effect, results in higher temperatures, more water vapor, and steam.

There are about as many opinions on the results of the greenhouse effect as there are scientists studying it. One view is that the earth will get increasingly warmer. Other scientists predict that the results will be more complex and that some parts of the world might even get colder.

Global Water Pollution

Many people do not have enough water, or if they do, it is contaminated or too salty. There are about 336 million cubic miles (1,400 million cubic km) of water on the earth, but 97 percent of it is seawater—nearly all of it permanently held in the oceans. The rest is fresh water; and at any one time about 77 percent of it is stored in ice caps and in glaciers. A little over 22 percent is groundwater stored beneath the surface of the earth, and about 0.035 percent is held in the atmosphere. Surprisingly, surface water, such as the water in rivers and lakes, accounts for only 0.33 percent of all the fresh water on the earth.

In arid areas of the world, there may be no rain at all in some years. The tropics, by contrast, are deluged with water every day during the rainy season. The distribution of rainfall is so uneven over the earth's surface that one-third of all surface water is carried into the sea by only 15 rivers. The Amazon River carries 15 percent of this amount.

Each year the growing world population makes increasing demands on the world's water supply. Industry, mining, power generation, agriculture, and irrigation call for vast amounts of water. For example, about half the food being produced today grows on irrigated land. Water is piped into agricultural fields from groundwater or from lakes and other sources of surface waters. Many of these groundwater sources, which took thousands of years to create, are being used up or polluted.

Unfortunately, many people have taken water for granted over the years. Just as it was assumed that our vast atmosphere could absorb, dilute, and detoxify whatever was dumped into the air, it was believed that our water supplies had an unlimited capacity to wash away anything that was thrown into them. Tons of untreated sewage, solid garbage, and barrels full of toxic industrial wastes have ended up in streams, lakes, rivers, and oceans all over the world. For many years, this practice seemed to work. The "dilution solution to pollution" appeared to be a good one. Now, however, we know this solution is not effective.

The dumping of raw sewage into the world's rivers and oceans occurs almost everywhere you find human populations. Around the Mediterranean 70 percent of the coastal cities dump untreated sewage directly into the sea. In India the sacred Ganges River is among the most revered of rivers, yet it is the most polluted. The Hindu religion views the Ganges as bringing spiritual cleanliness through daily immersion rituals. In the meantime billions of gallons of raw sewage are dumped into the river each year. Although many Americans may not be aware of it, or prefer not to admit it, many of the cities in the United States dump raw or inadequately treated sewage, solid garbage, and industrial and hospital wastes into our oceans and waterways.

Despite efforts to provide more people with water and sanitation, the number of people without clean water increased during the past decade by 100 million. One of the greatest threats posed by contaminated water is the spread of water-borne diseases, such as cholera, typhoid, and amoebic dysentery.

In some cases specific illnesses have been traced to chemical water pollutants. In Japan in the late 1950s, for example, large quantities of mercury-containing wastes were dumped into a bay by a fertilizer manufacturer. The mercury settled, was picked up by bottom-dwelling organisms, and traveled up the food chain to fish, livestock, pets, and people. Thousands of people were stricken with muscular paralysis, impaired vision, and mental retardation. Many died—all from eating mercury-contaminated seafood. Other chemicals, often leaking into water supplies from industrial plants, have been linked to bone disintegration and cancer.

KEEPING FIT

Chlorofluorocarbon Gases

Chlorofluorocarbon gases are gases used in spray cans to force out their contents. These chlorofluorocarbons float up into the air when they are released from the aerosol can. In the atmosphere, the chlorofluorocarbons release chlorine, which destroys ozone.

The first alert about the danger to the ozone layer was in 1974. However, not until 1978 did the United States ban the use of chlorofluorocarbons in aerosols.

Check for any aerosol cans in your home. Is their use absolutely necessary? Could you use a non-aerosol alternative?

It has become apparent that dilution of toxins and other pollutants will not solve pollution in the world's lakes, streams, and oceans. While it may still be possible to find patches of clean air, there are very few large bodies of clean water left in most parts of the earth.

Oil Spills

In 1989 the oil tanker *Exxon Valdez* emptied 10 million gallons (38 million l) of crude oil into the waters around Prince William Sound in Alaska. Over 800 miles (1,287 km) of what had been one of the earth's most unspoiled and picturesque coastlines had been fouled, perhaps permanently. The accident, the largest oil spill in U.S. history, followed closely on the heels of two other major oil disasters. In December 1988, Grays Harbor in the state of Washington was the site of a 300,000-gallon (1,136,400-l) accidental spill. In January 1989, a calamity began at the opposite pole when an Argentine ship struck a reef and began leaking 3,000 gallons (11,364 l) of fuel and crude oil each day into the previously fresh and clean waters surrounding the Antarctic Peninsula. Many other less publicized spills have occurred in recent years. In fact, hardly a day goes by without a spill of some sort.

Studies by the National Academy of Sciences and other groups have found that the largest single source of oil pollution in ocean regions is the discharging of tank flushings and gravel used to help stabilize a ship, such as a crude oil tanker. In the North Sea alone, it is estimated that 400,000 tons of oil are released into the water each year from offshore oil rigs and ships emptying their tanks at sea. Additionally, oil from blowouts of offshore wells contaminates the seas.

Evidence shows that crude oil not only fouls our water and beaches but also contains **carcinogenic,** or cancer-causing, substances or substances that are poisonous. Though our energy-hungry world demands petroleum, we need to acquire our fuel in environmentally responsible ways. In addition, by developing and using alternative forms of energy, the world can reduce its fuel consumption and slow down oil drilling, thus helping preserve our oceans and beaches.

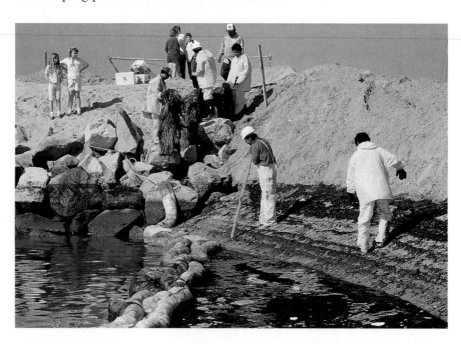

Oil spills harm our water, beaches, fish and wildlife.

LOOKING AT THE ISSUES

The Ozone Layer

Ozone is the protective layer around the earth that is needed to shield humans from the sun's ultraviolet light. The ozone layer is being destroyed by gases found in freon (used in refrigerators and air conditioners), Styrofoam (polystyrene foam), and propellants in some aerosol cans. How quickly is ozone being destroyed and what should be done about it?

Analyzing Different Viewpoints

ONE VIEW. According to the United Nations Environmental Program, the ozone situation is getting worse fast. U.N. scientists are predicting that at least 3 percent of the ozone layer could be destroyed within the next 10 years.

A SECOND VIEW. According to the Environmental Defense Fund, the depletion rate for ozone is much greater—in the 10 to 12 percent range over the next decade. The Environmental Protection Agency projects that for every 1 percent decrease in the ozone, 20,000 more people will develop skin cancer.

A THIRD VIEW. Others believe that such predictions of health catastrophe are overstated and hysterical and that technology can be created to deal with the problem effectively.

Exploring Your Views

1. What global steps do you think could be taken to ensure that the ozone layer will not be further destroyed?
2. What steps can you take to become active in environmental issues? How will doing so affect your self-esteem?

DID YOU KNOW?

- According to the Environmental Protection Agency, the use of pesticides has more than doubled in the past two decades.
- About 820 million pounds of pesticides are used by farmers every year.
- Despite spraying, about one-third of all United States crops are destroyed each year by a variety of pests.

LESSON 1 REVIEW

Reviewing Facts and Vocabulary

1. Write a public service announcement about air pollution, using the terms *photochemical smog, chlorofluorocarbons,* and *carcinogenic.*
2. What are CFCs, and what are they suspected of causing?

Thinking Critically

3. **Analysis.** Find out the major sources of air pollution in your area. Decide whether or not sufficient efforts are being made to reduce the problem.

4. **Synthesis.** Investigate which water pollution dangers appear to be the most prevalent in today's world. Prepare an oral report to describe the causes and effects of these dangers.

Applying Health Knowledge

5. Develop and administer a student survey to determine the student body's awareness of global air and water pollution.
6. Use the results of the above survey to write an article for the school newspaper about global environmental issues.

LAND

The health and future of the earth are in the hands of its people. A population explosion, along with increasing technology and a growing desire for more material goods, is challenging the future of our global environment.

The World's Growing Population

More than 1½ million people are born each week—about 240,000 each day, which is about 10,000 each hour. The total world's population is more than 5.4 billion people. During most of our existence as a species, human population growth has been slow. For example, it took half a million years for humankind to achieve a population size of 1 billion. The next 1 billion people were born between 1850 and 1930, a total of 80 years. The third billion arrived between 1930 and 1960, in only 30 years. The fourth billion came along even more quickly, between 1960 and 1975 in just 15 years. About 1.4 billion more have been born since 1975.

This incredible growth of the human population is occurring when at least one person in six is hungry or malnourished and without adequate housing. One in four lacks clean drinking water, and one in three lacks access to adequate sewage facilities or effective health care. In a given year between 5 and 20 million people now die of starvation and malnutrition-related diseases.

Human Population and Changes in the Land

A growing human population is changing the land. Human beings are covering the surface of the earth with new highways, buildings, factories, and landfills, clearing billions of acres of what were once wilderness areas or rain forests, and cultivating crops needed to feed additional people.

Disappearing Forests. The number of people in developing countries in Central America, Africa, and Southeast Asia is increasing rapidly. By some estimates, 90 percent of the total population growth is occurring there. These countries have been clearing their tropical forests on a massive scale, mostly for fuel, farm, and ranchland. **Deforestation,** or destruction of forests, means extinction for thousands of plant and animal species.

The world's great forests play major roles in the **biosphere,** the thin layer of soil, water, and air near the earth's surface. Forested watersheds are like giant sponges that absorb, hold, and release water gradually. By influencing the downstream flow of water, forests help control soil erosion, flooding, and sediment buildup in rivers, lakes, and reservoirs. Deforestation, especially on steep slopes, leads to loss of the fragile soil layer and disrupts the watershed. In the tropics, soil loss means long-term fertility loss as nutrients are quickly washed out of the system, leaving nutrient-poor soil behind.

Deforestation can also change regional patterns of rainfall as a result of altered rates of evaporation, transpiration (the exhaling of vapor from the surface of green tissues in plants), and runoff. Between 50 and 80 percent of the water vapor above tropical forests is released from the trees themselves. Without trees, annual precipitation declines and a region gets hotter and drier. The rain that does fall rapidly runs off the bare soil. As the local climate gets hotter and drier, soil fertility and moisture levels decline even more. Eventually, sparse grassland or even desertlike conditions may prevail where there had once been a rich tropical forest.

Clearing large tracts of tropical forests may also have global repercussions. These forests absorb much of the solar radiation reaching the equatorial regions of the earth's surface. When the forests are cleared, the land becomes shinier, so to speak, and reflects more incoming energy back into space. In addition, the trees of these forests help maintain the global cycling of carbon and oxygen through their photosynthetic action. When they are harvested or burned, the carbon stored in their biomass is released to the atmosphere in the form of carbon dioxide—and this may play a role in the greenhouse effect.

Almost half of the world's expanses of tropical forests has already been cleared for cropland, grazing land, timber, and fuelwood. Deforestation is greatest in Brazil, Burma, India, and Indonesia. At present rates of clearing and damage, only Brazil and Zaire will have large tracts of tropical forest in the year 2010; by 2035 those forests may also be gone.

Expanding Deserts. The world has always had deserts. Never before, however, have new ones been created as fast as now. Eighty percent of the productive land in the arid and semi-arid areas of the globe—or about one-third of Earth's surface—is believed to be affected by **desertification,** the conversion of grasslands, rain-fed cropland, or irrigated cropland to desertlike conditions, with a drop in agricultural productivity of 10 percent or more. The problem concerns both developed and developing countries. In the United States 10 percent of the land has already been affected, and a further 20 percent is threatened. About 2 billion acres worldwide have turned into deserts over the past 50 years. At least 44 million acres are still being transformed each year.

Today large-scale desertification is occurring mainly as a result of overgrazing on marginal lands. With a growing world population and an increasing requirement for food, scientists believe that food production must be increased by one-third by the end of the century simply to maintain present levels of nutrition. The desertification of once productive land poses a great threat to the health of the world's people.

Solid Waste. Resources are scarce in developing countries, and very few materials are discarded. However, in more affluent countries, a "throwaway" mentality often prevails. People use something once, discard it, and buy another.

Billions of tons of solid waste are dumped, burned, and buried annually in the United States alone. Instead of recycling most of these materials, as is done in natural ecosystems, people bulldoze them down the

Is there a better way to dispose of solid waste? Could some of these waste products be recycled?

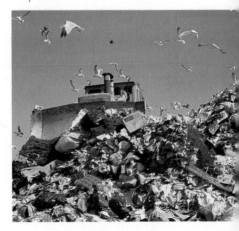

sides of canyons or dump them in wetlands, oceans, or landfills. There are only so many canyons; people must now deal with the pressing issues of solid waste disposal; air, water, and ground contamination; diminishing resources; and the growing unavailability of landfill space.

Technology and the Environment

There was a time when humankind took tens of thousands of years to accomplish much change. Then the intervals became just a few thousand years, then just a few hundred. Now these intervals are occurring in tens of years—or less—in terms of our capacity to alter our planetary living space. We have probably accomplished as much change in the years since 1950 as we did during the previous 2,000 years. One of the reasons for this decrease in time is the rapid increase in population.

Fossil fuels, such as petroleum and natural gas, have enabled people to develop agricultural technology that has brought about many changes, some good and some bad. For instance, modern farming has brought an abundance of food to people in many parts of the world. However, it has also resulted in the use of ever-increasing amounts of chemicals, such as pesticides and fertilizers. Some of these chemicals have contaminated parts of the world's food and water supplies. In addition, fertilizers, pesticides, tractor fuel, farm electricity, food processing, and food transportation all require fossil fuels—gasoline, oil, and natural gas.

Nuclear Energy. Today nuclear power plants dot the world's landscape. Industrialized nations that are poor in energy resources depend heavily on nuclear power. However, in many countries, plans to extend reliance on nuclear energy have been delayed or canceled. The cost, efficiency, environmental impact, and safety of nuclear energy are being seriously questioned. The overall net energy produced by nuclear reactors is relatively low, and the cost of constructing nuclear power plants is high—much higher than initially expected.

What about safety? Radioactivity escaping from a nuclear plant during normal operation is actually less than the amount released from a coal-burning plant of the same capacity. Nuclear plants do not add carbon dioxide to the atmosphere, as coal-burning plants do.

However, there is the potential danger of a meltdown. As nuclear fuel breaks down, it releases considerable heat, which is usually absorbed by

---

K E E P I N G   F I T

Conserving Energy

- Save energy by washing clothes in warm water and rinsing in cold instead of using the hot water cycle.
- Clean the lint trap in the dryer, and the dryer will run more efficiently.

- Try drying your clothes outside on a line.
- Put insulated wrap on the water heater but follow manufacturer's advice first.
- Insulate and weatherstrip your home.

- Draw curtains and shades at night to keep in heat when it is cold outside.
- In winter, set the thermostat lower; in summer, set the air conditioner higher or consider not using it at all.

---

water circulating over the fuel. The heated water produces steam, which drives electricity-generating turbines. If a leak should develop in the circulating water system, water levels around the fuel might drop. The nuclear fuel would heat rapidly, rising above its melting point. The melting fuel would pour onto the floor of the generator. There it would come into contact with the remaining water and instantly convert it to steam.

Formation of enough steam, along with other chemical reactions, could blow the system apart, releasing radioactive material into the surroundings. In addition, the overheated reactor core could melt through its thick concrete containment slab and into the earth, causing groundwater contamination.

All reactors have secondary cooling systems designed to flood the reactor if the initial cooling water is lost. In 1979 the Three Mile Island nuclear plant located in Pennsylvania underwent a partial meltdown. This was a result of the combination of equipment failure and human error. Some critics believe a meltdown was avoided only by luck. Others believe the incident proved the effectiveness of multiple backup safety systems in nuclear power plants.

In 1986 a meltdown occurred at the Chernobyl power station in the former Soviet Union. Radiation was released into the atmosphere, spreading to eastern Europe or beyond. A number of people died immediately; others died of radiation sickness weeks after the accident. Throughout Europe today people are still concerned about the long-term consequences. How long will the environment, including the land, water, produce, fish, and livestock, be contaminated? What are the risks of cancer from such exposure?

Nuclear Wastes. The Chernobyl incident underscores the consequences of nuclear accidents. What about routine nuclear wastes? Nuclear fuel cannot be burned to harmless ashes, as coal can. Nuclear wastes are a radioactive, extremely dangerous collection of materials. The decay rates of some nuclear wastes mean they must be isolated for 10,000 years or more.

The costs of simply cleaning up after currently operating nuclear facilities can range in the billions or trillions of dollars. The costs are so staggering that there remains the possibility that many sources of contamination will be abandoned because the money needed to adequately clean up the nuclear waste is not available.

War and the Planet

Battles among humans have probably always resulted in some damage to the environment. At no time in history has this been more true than today. Deliberate oil spills and the burning of hundreds of oil wells during the 1991 war in the Persian Gulf caused untold damage to the earth and its inhabitants.

The prospect of nuclear war is horrifying. Consequences would be measured in terms of billions of people who would be killed immediately and another billion who would die in the aftermath from radiation, starvation, and other effects. Many scientists predict that a nuclear war could bring about an effect called nuclear winter, which could lead to global extinction. They foresee that nuclear detonation would inject a

Drip Irrigation

In desert areas, lack of rain and minerals in the soil make it difficult to grow food. The Israelis developed a solution—drip irrigation. Water containing fertilizers is pumped into thin drip lines that lie along planted rows. Water drips out providing a slow, constant source of water. In 1984, an Israeli farmer shared this method with a U.S. Navajo tribe. Now Navajos use drip irrigation on many of their vegetables.

What are the advantages and disadvantages of nuclear power?

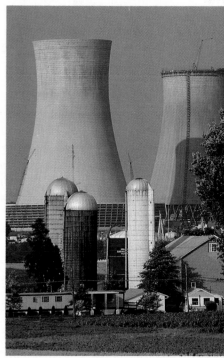

Overcoming The Odds

Shawn Gibbs is 18. He loves basketball and singing. He also has a special interest in the environment, but he did not develop this interest in the usual way.

Shawn begins, "When I was growing up, I lived with my mom, just me and my brother and my mom. Most of the time we lived with my grandmother. We didn't have very much. While my mom was at work working real hard, I took care of my brother a lot and did things around the house and we all did the best we could."

He goes on, "I wasn't doing real well in school—it was when I was in eighth grade. We came over some real hard times then. My mom was really struggling. So that eighth grade year I did really bad. We moved from the city, and I did better after that. I tried a lot harder. And when I came to my present high school, the associate principal, Mr. Arnell, helped me a lot and opened my eyes. In school I'd gotten into a fight with some guy. I had to do work as a punishment, and that is how I got involved with Mrs. Dean, a social studies teacher, and her environmental project. As my punishment, I had to go once or twice to the St. Jones River and pick up trash." Shawn had such a positive experience there by the river, however, that he continued to go there to work long after his punishment time had been served. "I liked it so much, to be out there by

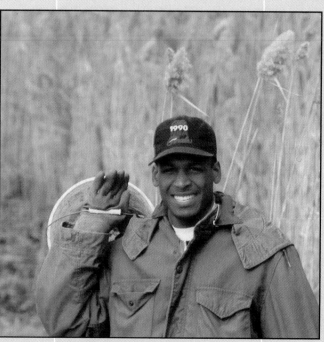

ourselves," he says. "It's beautiful out there. So I asked if I could go back. I made new friends out there and was with some old friends, too. We picked up two or three tons of trash. It was a big accomplishment. We were trying to save the river from the highway being built over it. We found a rare tree called a Bald Cypress. We found out that this kind of tree doesn't grow around here usually. We mostly picked up trash but we also took pictures of a blue heron and other animals in the area to show that there was wildlife to save and that we'd be killing them off or forcing them to move if we didn't save the area."

Shawn plans to continue caring for the environment. "I'll try to help the environment in the future as much as I can." He concludes, talking about how he first got involved with the river, "The thing that works for me is that out of something bad can come something good if you just hang in there."

1. How did Shawn first become involved in cleaning up the river? What personal and environmental benefits grew out of Shawn's initial punishment?

2. Shawn points out that "out of something bad can come something good." Can you apply this statement to your own life? If you can't apply it to your past, how might you apply it to some area of your life right now that seems bad but might eventually prove to be good?

huge dark cloud of soot and smoke over most of the earth, which would block out the sun. Much of the planet would be thrown into darkness, and temperatures would fall below freezing for months.

Natural Catastrophes

Although many of the recent assaults upon the earth have been caused by its human population, natural events cause major changes as well. Earthquakes, hurricanes, tornadoes, and volcanic eruptions affect the environment and its inhabitants. Some of these, such as volcanic eruptions, not only change the nearby environment but also can affect air quality and weather conditions over large parts of the world.

Addressing the Issues

Many environmental problems are basically social problems. They begin with people as the cause and end with people as the victims. People and nature need each other; by hurting one, we wound the other. Fortunately, there is action being taken to stop the destruction of our global environment. In some countries, governments or conservation groups have turned abandoned land into wildlife parks. A number of countries and international groups have been working together on a comprehensive plan to preserve tropical forests, and the plan is already being implemented. A few developing countries have been reevaluating their agricultural policies. Brazil has designated some of its tropical rain forest as unsuitable for agriculture. This region has been set aside for ecological research and for recreation.

The world's efforts must go into renewing the environment by reducing pollution and waste and bringing back at least part of the earth's natural clothing of vegetation. All nations—and individuals—must work to put an end to deforestation, desertification, acidification, contamination and erosion of the soil, and the destruction of living species.

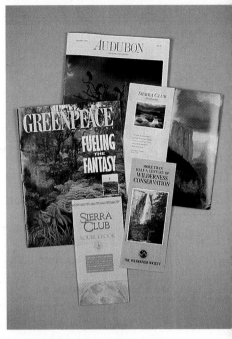

Many organizations are working to make people aware of environmental concerns.

LESSON 2 REVIEW

Reviewing Facts and Vocabulary

1. Explain the difference between deforestation and desertification.
2. Write a paragraph using the term *biosphere* in which you point out its relation to global environmental issues.

Thinking Critically

3. **Synthesis.** Find examples in newspapers and magazines of land pollution and its effects on the global environment. Write a summary of your findings.

4. **Analysis.** Use a current and an older world map to compare the growing effects of deforestation and desertification.

Applying Health Knowledge

5. Develop an exhibit depicting some aspect of excessive population and its effect on the earth.
6. Write a letter that could be sent to a national or international organization, such as the Red Cross, asking what students and families can do to assist victims of a natural catastrophe. Share the information with the class.

Self-Inventory

Environmental Alert Checklist

HOW DO YOU RATE?

Number a sheet of paper from 1 through 14. Read each item below, and respond by writing *often*, *sometimes*, or *never* for each item. Total the number of each type of response. Then proceed to the next section.

1. I avoid buying things just for the sake of having them.
2. I recycle whatever is possible when disposing of a product or package.
3. I reuse things instead of disposing of them and buying new things.
4. I consider what pollution and wastes were created in the manufacture of the things I buy.
5. I read labels and buy the least toxic products available.
6. I shop at secondhand stores, garage sales, consignment shops, and flea markets.
7. I avoid buying disposable items when longer-lasting alternatives are available.
8. I avoid short car trips by walking, riding a bicycle, or using public transportation.
9. I refuse packaging for products that are already packaged.
10. I read consumer information articles to learn about the quality, durability, and toxicity of the products I buy.
11. I ask that less wrapping be used for my order at fast-food restaurants.
12. I reuse paper and plastic bags that are brought home from the store.
13. I recycle aluminum cans, newspapers, glass jars, and plastic bottles.
14. I share old magazines, books, and items of clothing I no longer need or want.

HOW DID YOU SCORE?

Give yourself 2 points for every *often* answer, 1 point for every *sometimes* answer, and 0 points for every *never* answer. Find your total, and read below to see how you scored. Then proceed to the next section.

25 to 28
Excellent. You are serious about caring for the environment.

17 to 24
Good. You are doing some reusing, reducing, and recycling, but you could do more to protect the earth.

9 to 16
Fair. Get serious about doing your share of planetary house-keeping, and try to do more to make the environment a better place for all of us.

Below 9
Poor. Not only are you not helping to clean up the environment, you are contributing to its destruction.

WHAT ARE YOUR GOALS?

If you received an *excellent* or *good* score, complete the statements in Part A. If your score was *fair* or *poor*, complete Parts A and B.

Part A
1. I plan to learn more about saving the global environment by ____.
2. My timetable for accomplishing this is ____.

Part B
3. The behavior or attitude that I would most like to change is ____.
4. The steps involved in making this change are ____.
5. My rewards for making this change will be ____.
6. My timetable for making this change is ____.
7. The people or groups I will ask for help are ____.

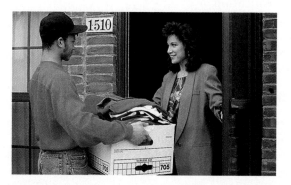

Building Decision-Making Skills

E lizabeth Tremain is a member of the high school environmental club. The club has decided that local and national environmental issues are so significant that it is going to take an active part in the next congressional election, based on how the candidates stand on these issues. The incumbent in the district is a friend of Elizabeth's parents, and Mr. and Mrs. Tremain have been active in supporting him and his party. However, his voting record has been unacceptable by the environmental club's standards. The club prefers to vote for his challenger, whose platform lines up with the club's views. This will be Elizabeth's first chance to vote in an election and be active in a campaign. How should Elizabeth vote?

WHAT DO YOU THINK?

1. **Situation.** Why does Elizabeth need to make a decision?

2. **Choices.** What choices does Elizabeth have?

3. **Consequences.** What are the advantages and disadvantages of each choice?

4. **Consequences.** How will Elizabeth's family feel about her decision? How will the rest of the community react? How will the congressman and his opponent react?

5. **Decision.** What should Elizabeth do?

6. **Decision.** How should Elizabeth explain her decision? What advice would you give her?

R ico's school and other community buildings have been common targets for graffiti. They have become environmental eyesores. Rico and his friends have been as guilty as anyone of contributing to this problem. The new principal, whom Rico likes, has called on students to help clean up the school and to come up with a solution to the graffiti problem. As Rico has matured, he has regretted his contribution to this problem and become interested in helping to "save the city."

WHAT DO YOU THINK?

7. **Situation.** Why does Rico face a dilemma?

8. **Choices.** In what ways can Rico affect the situation?

9. **Consequences.** How will Rico's old friends respond to his actions?

10. **Consequences.** How will the community respond to Rico's actions?

11. **Consequences.** How will students, especially those who are still a part of the problem, feel about students who are part of the solution?

12. **Decision.** What should Rico do? Why? How should he carry out his decision to get the most people on his side?

13. **Evaluation.** Have you ever been in a situation similar to Rico's? What did you do? Was your decision a good one, and how did you decide that?

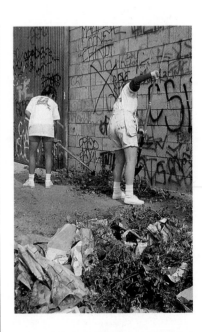

REVIEW

Using Health Terms

On a separate sheet of paper, write the term that best matches each definition given below.

LESSON 1

1. Air pollution that occurs when vehicle exhaust, activated by sunlight, combines with other hydrocarbons in the atmosphere.
2. Ecosystems where seawater mixes with fresh water.
3. Microscopic organisms, such as green algae, found in open, sunlit waters.
4. Contain chlorine, fluorine, and carbon.
5. Cancer-causing.

LESSON 2

6. The thin layer of soil, water, and air near the earth's surface.
7. A condition that occurs when an overheated nuclear reactor core melts through its concrete containment slab into the earth.

Building Academic Skills

LESSON 1

8. **Reading.** Identify cause and effect in the following sentence.
   Lead poisoning can lead to loss of appetite, anemia, damage to the nervous system, and possibly, brain damage leading to a lowering of intelligence levels in young children.
9. **Writing.** Air conditioning is one of the major sources of damage to the ozone layer. Write a composition of at least five paragraphs defending the use of air conditioning or persuading people to consider living without it.
10. **Math.** Imagine that all the earth's water is represented by one gallon of water. How much of that gallon would be the amount of water contained in rivers and lakes: about a cup, about half a cup, or less than two tablespoons?

Recalling the Facts

LESSON 1

11. What steps were taken to eliminate smog in the city of London?
12. What were the first signs of smog in Los Angeles in the 1940s?
13. What is acid rain?
14. List three effects of acid rain.
15. How can efforts to reduce air pollution in one place add to acid rain problems in other parts of the world?
16. How does the ozone layer protect people living on Earth?
17. What is the major cause of damage to the ozone layer?
18. What are the three main sources of chlorofluorocarbons?
19. What are the advantages of carbon dioxide in the atmosphere? The disadvantages?
20. Explain the meaning of the phrase "the dilution solution to pollution."
21. Name three water-borne diseases.
22. Name three effects of mercury poisoning.
23. List three ways water can become polluted, and explain the effects.

LESSON 2

24. How does an increasing population affect land use?
25. Why do people cut down forests?
26. What advantages for the environment do forests have over cleared land?
27. How does deforestation affect rainfall?
28. Explain the relationship between deforestation and the greenhouse effect.
29. What are the advantages and disadvantages of pesticides and fertilizers used by farmers?
30. What are the benefits and dangers of nuclear power plants?
31. How can an accident at a nuclear power plant affect the environment?
32. What is the cause of most environmental problems?
33. Who are the victims of most environmental problems?

REVIEW

Thinking Critically

LESSON 1

34. Analysis. How is London smog different from Los Angeles smog?

35. Evaluation. Describe two conflicting views on the greenhouse effect. Do some research on this topic and decide which view you agree with.

LESSON 2

36. Analysis. Label each of the following causes of environmental change *air, water,* or *land,* to indicate which part of the environment it has the most serious effect on.
   a. deforestation   **e.** oil spills
   b. desertification   **f.** smog
   c. volcanic eruptions
   d. vehicle exhaust emissions

37. Synthesis. How can a volcanic eruption affect air quality over a large part of the world?

38. Synthesis. Invent one or more new ways for society to dispose of trash or garbage. Be creative. Present your plan to the class. Draw pictures or diagrams to illustrate your presentation. You may work on this project with two or three classmates.

39. Evaluation. If you could pass one law to protect our environment and address the pollution problem, what would it be? How would you enforce it? Explain why you chose the law you did.

Making the Connection

LESSON 1

40. Science. Fill a shallow pan half full of water. Pour in one cup of salad or cooking oil. Devise several ways to remove the oil from the water. (You might try a lettuce leaf, cotton balls, a piece of absorbent fabric, a suction tube, or anything else you can think of.) Which of your cleanup devices worked best? What does this experiment tell you about the difficulty of cleaning up oil spills in the environment?

Applying Health Knowledge

LESSON 1

41. Describe the environmental advantages and disadvantages of living where you do. Consider how your area is affected by each problem described in this lesson.

42. Your aunt Hildegarde used to be a lifeguard on a Florida beach. She has been treated for cataracts and several cancerous moles. What may have caused these health problems? What advice would you give her?

LESSON 2

43. What could happen to the drinking water in an area served by a nuclear power plant if a meltdown occurred?

Beyond the Classroom

LESSON 1

44. Community Involvement. Find out how your community treats water before it is consumed. Report your findings to the class.

45. Further Study. Choose one of the pollution problems described in this lesson. Read at least five articles related to the problem. Write a report describing the problem, its causes, and possible cures.

LESSON 2

46. Further Study. Do some research on the deforestation problem in Brazil. Find out why Brazilian forests are being cleared and how deforestation in Brazil will affect Brazil and the rest of the world.

47. Parental Involvement. Observe and keep track of your trash for a week. Then talk to your parents about a family recycling plan. Identify the items you throw away that could be recycled, such as aluminum cans, plastic and glass bottles and jars, and newspapers. Decide which family members will be responsible for each kind of item and what will be done with the items to be recycled.

PROTECTING YOUR ENVIRONMENT

LESSON 1
Reducing Waste

LESSON 2
Being Informed and Involved

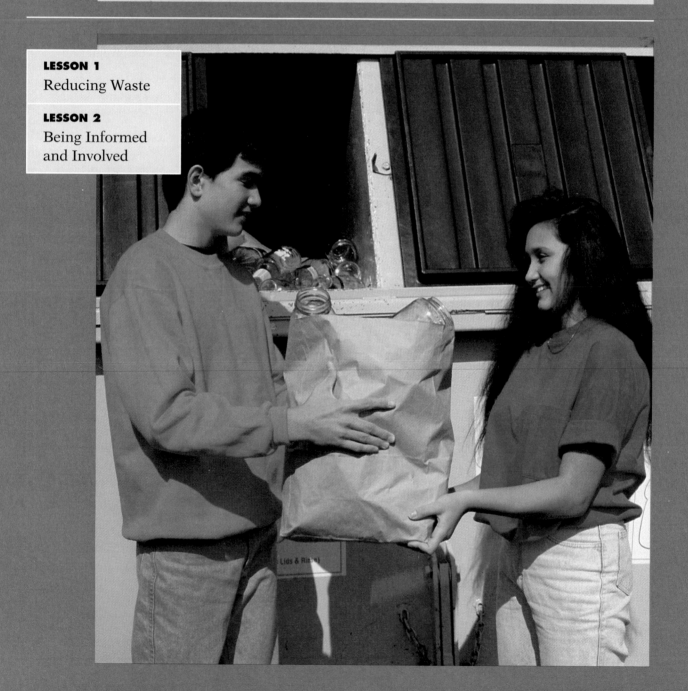

REDUCING WASTE

With so many people in the world, it may be hard for you to realize that you can make a difference in regard to environmental issues. Behaviors you choose can not only promote your personal health but also can help protect the environment. If you decide you have no responsibility to care for the environment, who will? Everyone has a responsibility to protect the Earth.

Conservation

Concern about preserving the environment, or **conservation,** is not new. After the Civil War there was great destruction of forests due to industrialization. Such events sparked the founding of our nation's two oldest environmental organizations, the Sierra Club and the Audubon Society. Both of these groups attempted to organize public opposition to the exploitation of the environment.

Theodore Roosevelt, the president of the United States between 1901 and 1909, is the president best known to support the cause of environmental conservation. He is known as the father of the national park system because of his great interest and love of nature. He is honored on the face of Mount Rushmore for his contributions to the preservation of our natural environment. Conservation is more than preserving national parks such as Yosemite or Yellowstone or our delicate wilderness.

Civilization and industrial development have resulted in life-styles that separate most people from direct contact with the resources that keep us alive. We buy food from stores, get water from faucets, and throw our waste in plastic bags. We sometimes take for granted our essentials in life.

Much responsibility and power in regard to conservation lies with you. You can help reduce waste and conserve precious natural resources by being aware of environmental issues. You also can protect the environment and conserve our resources by making good decisions as a consumer.

Guidelines for Saving Energy at Home

Energy conservation involves helping protect the environment and avoiding the use of irreplaceable resources. Of great significance to health is the fact that energy conservation reduces pollution of the environment.

About 70 percent of the energy we use at home is for heating or cooling. We use an additional 20 percent for heating water. The remaining 10 percent goes for lighting, cooking, and running small appliances.

Refer to the chart on page 616 to determine what you can do to conserve energy at home. Some of the actions may involve decisions that are not yours to make. You might discuss them with your family as ways to save money and conserve energy.

| **LESSON 1 FOCUS** |

TERMS TO USE
- Conservation
- Precycling
- Recycling

CONCEPTS TO LEARN
- You can practice conservation by not using irreplaceable resources.
- Precycling is making environmentally sound decisions at the store, thereby reducing waste before it occurs.
- Recycling is treating or changing waste so that it can be reused.

ATTITUDES AND BEHAVIORS TO EVALUATE
- Self-Inventory, page 628.
- Building Decision-Making Skills, page 629.

Action	Effect
Heating and Cooling	
In hot weather use exhaust fans when cooking, bathing, or doing laundry.	Reduces heat gain that would increase the need for artificial cooling.
Close window drapes at night.	Reduces heat loss.
Have at least 6 inches (15 cm) of insulation over the top floor ceiling and 3 inches (7.6 cm) on an exterior wall.	Helps keep hot air in and cold air out during the cold season and does the reverse during the hot months.
Keep doors and windows shut during the air-conditioning season. Close fireplace vents.	Reduces the strain on the air-conditioning unit.
Keep air conditioning at a constant temperature and on automatic control.	Reduces the load on the system.
During the heating season turn down the thermostat 5 or 10 degrees at night.	Provides savings of 9 to 15 percent on heating bills.
Keep windows near the thermostat tightly closed.	Saves energy by preventing variations in temperature near the thermostat, which would cause the unit to run hotter or colder.
Water	
Insulate the water heater.	Saves energy.
Wash clothes only when you have a full load.	Saves water.
Use less detergent than suggested by the manufacturer.	Reduces the amount of phosphates in the detergent from going into the environment.
Wash clothing in warm or cold, not hot, water; use cold-water detergents.	Reduces energy costs.
Wash the car with water in a bucket instead of using a hose.	Saves gallons of water.
Place a filled plastic bottle in the toilet tank to displace water.	Saves 1 to 2 gallons (4 to 8 l) of water per flush.
Place a faucet aerator on water faucets.	Reduces water flow up to 50 percent by mixing air with water as it leaves the tap.
Fix leaky hot-water faucets.	Saves energy costs of heating water.
Never leave hot water running unnecessarily.	Saves electrical or gas energy and water.
If you have a food disposal, run it using cold water rather than hot water.	Saves electrical or gas energy and water.
Lighting	
Use fluorescent bulbs when possible. They now come in compact sizes.	Saves energy because fluorescent bulbs last longer and use less energy.
Use one higher-watt bulb rather than two lower-watt bulbs in a two-bulb fixture.	Saves electrical energy.
Cooking	
If you have a gas stove at home, be sure that it has a blue flame in the pilot light.	Saves fuel; a blue flame is a sign of a more complete burn.
When you have a choice, cook on top of the stove rather than in the oven.	Saves energy and uses less heat.

Precycling

Precycling, a new concept in protecting the environment, is a strategy to help avoid many problems of waste and recycling. **Precycling** means making environmentally sound decisions at the store, thereby reducing waste before it occurs. This strategy means that you, as a consumer, would avoid buying unnecessary things that need to be disposed of or recycled.

It will not be possible for you to precycle everything that you buy because there may not be choices for every purchase you need to make. However, the more you precycle, the less trash you will generate.

Guidelines for Precycling

Some basic guidelines for precycling are as follows:

- Be selective about packaging. When you are about to buy something, look at the way it is packaged. Determine whether or not the package can be reused, refilled, or recycled.
- Choose products packaged in recyclable materials. This includes packages made of paper, glass, aluminum, or cardboard.
- Do not pay for overpackaging, or layers of unnecessary packaging. If the packaging is not necessary to protect the product, buy products with more simple packaging. You might also save money by choosing these products.
- Avoid buying plastic. Even plastic that can be recycled cannot be reused as many times as glass, aluminum, or cardboard.
- Avoid forms of polystyrene, such as Styrofoam. Styrofoam contains chlorofluorocarbons, gases that harm the ozone layer and that are released when Styrofoam crumbles. Styrofoam is not biodegradable.
- Avoid buying disposable items, such as razors, diapers, cups, and plates. These items often end up as waste in already overflowing landfills.
- Buy in large or bulk quantities. This not only saves money but also helps eliminate unnecessary packaging. Single-serving items, such as individual juice drinks, small packages of raisins, and individual candies, are very overpriced and overpackaged.
- Look for products in refillable containers. Many manufacturers package products so that the consumer can buy one container and just buy refills after that. This eliminates the need to buy unnecessary, additional containers.
- Say, "No bag, please," when making few or small purchases. Instead, use a cloth bag for shopping.

Recycling

Recycling involves treating or changing waste so that it can be reused. Recycling has become very popular in many communities as individuals are taking responsibility to help protect the environment. Recycling more products means less need for incineration and landfills.

Recycling pays off in many ways. Here are some examples:

- Recycling can produce six times as many jobs as when landfills and incineration are used.

Using a cloth bag for shopping eliminates the need for paper and plastic bags.

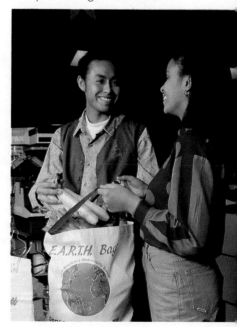

- Whatever does not have to be burned or buried is money saved.
- Recycling saves energy by requiring far less energy than using raw materials. For example, making a can out of recycled aluminum takes only 10 percent of the energy needed to make an aluminum can from its original source, bauxite ore.
- Recycling saves resources by reducing the need for foresting, mining, and drilling activities.
- Recycling preserves air and water quality because using recycled materials causes less pollution than when using raw materials.

According to the Institute of Scrap Recycling, producing a ton of paper from waste paper requires 64 percent less energy, needs 58 percent less water, results in 74 percent less air pollution and 35 percent less water pollution, and can result in 5 times more jobs than producing a ton of paper from virgin wood pulp. In addition, it saves 17 pulp trees and reduces solid wastes going into landfills.

Guidelines for Recycling

Not everything can be recycled. However, more than four out of five items of household waste can be recycled in some form.

Different recycling centers accept different products. To shorten handling time and conserve space that is used for recycling, most centers require that all items be clean, dry, sorted, and condensed. The following sections identify common recyclable products with guidelines for each. It is important to recycle, but it is more important to consider limiting your use of each of the following materials.

Aluminum.   Aluminum is one of the most expensive and polluting metals to produce. Fortunately, aluminum is totally recyclable. Recycling it saves money and prevents pollution. About 55 percent of all aluminum cans are recycled. Recycling aluminum is easy. Rinse cans and crush them to save space. You can include pie pans, frozen food trays, and foil in this group. In some states and national park areas, cans may be returned for a refund.

Batteries.   Dry-cell batteries range from the large flashlight type to the small batteries used in cameras, calculators, and watches. These items often are so small that they appear harmless, but they do contain toxic materials.

K E E P I N G   F I T

Organize a Cleanup

One way that you can help the environment is to do a beach cleanup. Each year in September, the Center for Marine Conservation sponsors the nationwide effort. The debris picked up not only makes beaches look cleaner, it also helps to save the lives of seabirds, fish, and mammals that might choke or be poisoned by litter. To organize a group for a local beach cleanup, write the Oceanic Society at 218 D Street SE, Washington, DC, 20003. If you do not live near a beach, organize a group cleanup at a local park, lakefront, zoo, or other public place.

When burned in incinerators, metals from batteries, such as cadmium, lead, mercury, zinc, and nickel, pollute the air. When thrown into landfills, they leak into groundwater supplies.

Battery recycling is not yet very popular in the United States, although it is common in Japan and Europe. Ask your local recycling center or waste management (trash pickup) company for more information. Try to buy rechargeable batteries. Auto batteries, containing lead, are dangerous. They can best be disposed of by taking them to a service station or an auto parts dealer for recycling or safe disposal.

Cardboard. This product, used primarily in boxes, is fully recyclable. Cardboard is in short supply, so it is highly valued. About half is recycled in the United States. To recycle cardboard, flatten boxes, tie them together, and take them to a recycling center.

Clothing and Household Items. You might throw away clothing after buying something new. What do you do with a broken radio you cannot get fixed? What happens to an old refrigerator? Recycle all clothing and household items you no longer want by donating them to a community organization that can use them.

Glass. Like aluminum, glass is 100 percent recyclable. Glass accounts for 10 percent of household waste. It is among the easiest materials to recycle. Old glass is melted down and added to new glass to be used again hundreds of times.

There are three types of glass: clear, green, and brown. Check with your recycling center to see which types it accepts. Glass should be separated according to color. It does not matter if it is broken or cracked. Usually, paper labels need not be removed.

Most recycling centers will not accept auto glass, window glass, plates, ceramics, or light bulbs. Bottles and jars are usually the most common glass products recycled. Glass should be well rinsed. Caps, stoppers, wires, or lids should be removed.

Oil. More and more people change their own car oil. Some do not dispose of it properly. Just one quart of oil from a car can contaminate 250,000 gallons (946,350 l) of drinking water. A single gallon (3.8 l) of motor oil can form an oil slick for nearly 8 acres (32,376 square m).

Used oil is very valuable. About 2½ quarts (2.4 l) can be extracted from 1 gallon (3.8 l) of used oil. This oil is valuable as lubricating oil, road oil, wood preservatives, and oil for starting fires. Take used oil to a service station, auto garage, or oil change shop for proper disposal.

Paper. More paper is consumed in the United States than in any other country. Of the 72 million tons (65.5 million t) produced each year, about one-fourth is recycled. That amount saves 200 million trees per year. Paper accounts for more than one-half of all household waste.

Even though there is a demand to recycle paper, not all paper is desired. Some recycling centers will not take yellow paper, brown bags, or junk mail. Newspaper is excellent to recycle and should be bundled with cotton string or placed in paper bags. Do not mix magazines, catalogs, books, phone directories, and junk mail with newspapers.

Reuse the backs of envelopes and paper from junk mail. Reuse paper bags from stores, and use rags instead of paper towels.

FINDING HELP

The Sierra Club works on hundreds of conservation issues at the local, regional, national, and international levels. To find out more about the organization—and the chapter or group nearest you—write to: Sierra Club Public Affairs 730 Polk Street San Francisco, CA 94109

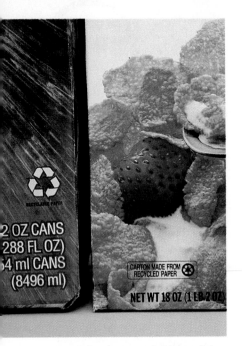

Look for the recyclable and the recycled symbols when making purchases.

Plastics. Only a small percentage of plastics can be recycled. Unlike paper, glass, and aluminum, plastics can be recycled only a limited number of times, so try to buy beverages in glass or aluminum containers. Remove lids; then wash and squash plastic bottles you recycle.

Tin Cans. Tin cans are steel cans with a thin coating of tin inside of them. In the United States 30 billion tin cans are thrown away each year. Tin cans should be separated from aluminum cans when being recycled.

Tires. Almost one tire for each American is thrown away each year. Old and worn tires are a major source of litter, and they present a major fire hazard. Old tires can be recycled and used as padding for play equipment, as gardening containers, and as bumpers. Parts of the rubber also can be used in roads, playground surfaces, and running tracks. You should give your business to tire stores and service stations that recycle old or worn tires. Keep your tires properly inflated to extend their use. Doing so also saves gas.

Yard Waste. Leaves, grass clippings, and other yard wastes represent about 20 percent of all waste that ends up in landfills. Yet these materials can be of use, and recycling them can save money.

One option is to keep lawn mower blades sharp and high. Doing so enables grass to develop strong, healthy roots. Clippings can be left on the lawn to act as a natural fertilizer.

Composting is another option for yard waste. Composting refers to the biological decomposition of organic waste material under controlled conditions. Compost can be used as a soil conditioner, mulch, or plant cover. Food and yard waste can all be used in compost. A florist or gardener can give you details on how to start a compost pile.

Identifying Recycled and Recyclable Products

Using recycled products and products that can be recycled not only reduces waste but also reduces pollution and energy costs. To identify recycled packaging, look for one of these three indicators:

- the recycled symbol on the package
- a statement such as: "This package made from recycled materials."
- a gray interior such as that found in cereal and cake mix boxes

Recyclable products also carry an identifying symbol.

KEEPING FIT

Becoming a Concerned Shopper

When going grocery shopping, show your environmental consciousness by
- bringing your own cloth or mesh shopping bag
- asking the grocery checker to pack your food in biodegradable paper bags
- buying products with limited packaging
- buying milk in cartons rather than plastic containers
- buying rechargeable batteries
- buying bulk and unpackaged goods instead of packaged goods
- buying locally grown and seasonal produce
- avoiding single-serving containers

Jason, the Sludge-Detecting Robot

Industries and individuals have been dumping chemicals and other pollutants into waterways for years. Medical waste washing up on beaches has become a widespread problem in the United States. Drinking water is threatened with pesticides, hazardous wastes, solid wastes, and toxic chemicals. Many United States waterways now have thick black sludge on their bottoms sometimes referred to as "black mayonnaise." Originally, it was assumed that such sludge buildup would only occur in shallow or landlocked waterways. But now the evidence is mounting that sludge is even accumulating on the ocean floor.

Scientists know that ocean dumping may have serious consequences for the environment, and they are studying what the potential long-term health and environmental hazards of this dumping may be. One way that they are doing this is with Jason, a sludge-detecting robot working on the ocean floor off the coasts of New Jersey and New York. The robot, attached by fiber optic cables, is operated by a scientist on a research ship who watches the robot on a video screen and moves a joystick to make the robot perform various operations. Using a variety of monitors and video screens, scientists aboard the ship study the remote-controlled robot's movements 9,000 feet below the water's surface as it moves across the ocean floor scooping up sediment and water samples. The samples will be studied to determine the long-term damage of the millions of tons of sewage and other pollutants that have been dumped into the ocean.

DID YOU KNOW?

- At least 35 states in the United States now have comprehensive recycling programs.
- Recently, a controversy has started about the use of juice boxes and whether or not they are recyclable. Some states have already banned them. Others are beginning to try to recycle them, turning them into, among other things, plastic timber used in building park benches and decks.

LESSON 1 REVIEW

Reviewing Facts and Vocabulary

1. How does recycling contribute to protecting the environment?
2. Define *precycling* and tell how consumers benefit from doing this.

Thinking Critically

3. **Analysis.** Compare precycling and recycling. Include examples of both.
4. **Analysis.** Why do you think only 10 percent of recyclable household products are actually recycled?

5. **Evaluation.** Why do you think recycling is more popular today than it was 25 years ago?

Applying Health Knowledge

6. Find out how to make a compost pile. How can doing this save money?
7. How would driving a car a few extra years be a good example of precycling?
8. Write a report on recycling efforts in your community. Evaluate the success of these efforts.

BEING INFORMED AND INVOLVED

LESSON 2 FOCUS

TERMS TO USE
- Biodegradable (by•oh•di•GRAYD•uh• buhl)
- Organic

CONCEPTS TO USE
- Your personal health is related to environmental health; you can become an informed environmental consumer.
- There are many current environmental issues.
- You can become involved in protecting the environment.

ATTITUDES AND BEHAVIORS TO EVALUATE
- Self-Inventory, page 628.
- Building Decision-Making Skills, page 629.

Business people, government leaders, and individuals like yourself make decisions that affect the environment. It is important to look ahead to consider the effects those decisions have on future generations.

Sometimes in the past, short, quick answers were given to problems. Some of these answers caused new problems that, in time, proved to be greater than the original ones later on. The development of pesticides, the gasoline combustion engine, and nuclear power are all examples of inventions that were immediately beneficial to human life but later resulted in other problems to the environment.

Be Aware as a Consumer

Your personal health is related to environmental health. It is important to choose products that are safe for you and the environment.

There are a growing number of terms used on product labels to attract consumers who are interested in shopping for environmentally safe products. As a consumer, become aware of and familiar with the following terms:

- *Nontoxic* is a term that is meant to imply a product is not harmful or poisonous to humans. However, it could be harmful to plant and animal life, or the product's packaging could be harmful. What could happen to such a product when it becomes waste?

- When an item can eventually be broken down by microorganisms, it is **biodegradable.** The time for this process to occur can vary greatly. Some products may take up to several hundred years or more to decompose.

- You see the term *natural* on the packaging of many products. There are many natural ingredients that can also be dangerous and even poisonous. For example, lead and mercury are both natural and poisonous.

- The word **organic** means a product is derived from living organisms without the use of chemicals. For example, organic food is grown with fertilizer of plant or animal origin. Chemical fertilizers are not used. While some states have defined this term, there is no legal requirement to meet this claim. All living matter and even hazardous chemicals can properly be called organic.

- Consider the phrase *environmentally safe.* Does it refer to the contents of the package, the package itself, or both? Remember, almost everything has some impact on the environment.

Many common household products or chemicals for the yard are toxic. Disposing of them down a drain or in the ground could result in toxic chemicals reaching nearby water sources.

The Environmental Protection Agency (EPA) can give you advice about which products to avoid and can suggest safe alternatives. This

Overcoming The Odds

Meg Chandler is 15. She keeps a journal and is thinking about a career in journalism in the future. She is on the newspaper staff at her school, and she has a part-time job working in a shoe store. But her real interest for the past several years has been working with Kids Against Pollution, an organization devoted to getting young people involved in helping to protect the environment.

She begins, "I became involved in environmental issues when I was in the sixth grade. That's when Kids Against Pollution was first started by the fifth grade class of Mr. Byrne. He asked me to help him with a presentation to the board of education about banning the use of Styrofoam in the town's three schools. After that, I became involved in making presentations in front of state legislators on issues like Earth Day 2000 and making environmental education mandatory."

Meg's environmental efforts are not just public ones. They are also private and personal. "I try to implement environmental awareness in my day-to-day routines," she says, "by buying only cleaners that are packaged in environmentally conscious ways and products that do not contain ingredi-

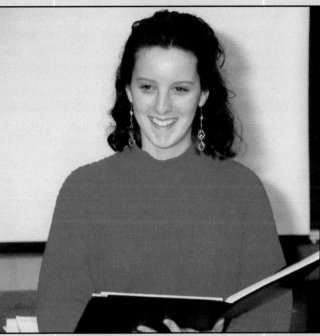

ents that are particularly harmful to the environment. A lot of it is also common sense, like turning off lights when you leave the room or turning off the water when you're not using it. The Earth is running out of resources," Meg says, "and facing the environmental problems in our world are odds that all of us have to overcome."

She goes on, "One particular set of odds stacked against people like me and others in Kids Against Pollution is simply the fact that we are just kids. But we also have the odds stacked in our favor because we are kids. We're open to new ideas. We aren't jaded about the situation we live in. We have a wonderful advantage because from the beginning we are being taught

to be environmentally conscious, and these lessons are more likely to stick with us for the rest of our lives.

"Working with Kids Against Pollution has dramatically increased my self-confidence," Meg says. "It's shown me I can accomplish things. There are now over 1000 chapters of Kids Against Pollution, and several in foreign countries, too."

Meg concludes, "If you are like most teenagers, you are probably underestimating what you can do. One thing that I wish I could say to every kid in America is not to underestimate yourself—that if you see something that you would like to change, then by all means give it your best shot."

1. How did one individual's concern for the environment grow? How did many individuals pooling their commitment, energy, and talent make an even greater difference?
2. How has Meg's involvement in Kids Against Pollution affected her self-esteem?
3. What are your primary concerns about the environment? What commitment, talents, and energy can you give to an environmental effort?

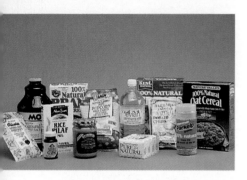

The term natural appears on many products. It is important to know that this term does not mean a product is safe or better than others.

United States agency sets up and enforces standards to help protect the environment from pollution. The EPA also does research on the effects of pollution.

Current Environmental Issues

Every person who lives on Earth has some responsibility for what happens to it. We vary greatly in our knowledge, skill, interests, and needs concerning the environment. So it is not likely that every person can learn all there is to know about each environmental issue that faces humankind. Perhaps there is an issue that is of great interest to you, or that is a particular problem in your area. Here are some major environmental issues that might be of interest to you:

- Futuristic thinking. Nations of the world need to consider the long-range effects of short-range decisions, such as unrestricted use of nuclear power. Many environmentalists are investigating alternate sources of energy for the future.

- Population growth. Throughout the world and in certain areas of the United States where there is rapid population growth, there is low quality of life and much human suffering. Rapid population growth also leads to rapid deterioration of the land and to a severe drain on resources, such as water and minerals.

- Development and environment. Most people realize that development brings jobs and helps the income of the local population. However, development also brings problems that can negatively affect land, resources, air, and water.

- Food and agriculture. Problems of hunger, poor food distribution, destruction of usable cropland, poor irrigation methods, and extensive use of chemicals are part of this area of concern.

- Biological diversity. There is concern throughout the world that the habitats of many species of plants and animals will be destroyed as population, mineral extraction, and development increases.

- Tropical forests. About half of all tropical forests are gone, and along with them, many species of plants and animals. Forest loss causes many problems for people, including soil erosion, flooding, shortages of fuelwood and timber, loss of food from tropical plants, and displacement of whole groups of people.

- Ocean and coastal resources. Overfishing is a major problem in the oceans of the world. Some species of whales are near extinction. Pollution from large municipal areas, oil spills, and waste dumping have all created major problems for aquatic life.

- Fresh water. Many people do not have access to clean water. Unsafe water causes millions of deaths. Surface and groundwater are being polluted by municipal, industrial, and chemical wastes. Increasing population creates more demand for water.

- Nonfuel minerals. More people and increased consumption from development results in a greater need for minerals such as copper, zinc, lead, and mercury. At the current rate, some of these minerals will be gone within 50 years. Mining of these minerals can also cause great environmental damage.

CONFLICT RESOLUTION

Catching a fish in a local river last June has impacted Tosh's life. The fish he caught was a carp with a huge tumor on its head. Tosh caught the carp downstream from an oil refinery and the city's sewage treatment plant. Tosh wants to convince the public that the river must be cleaned up. So he's gone fishing in the river just about every day. So far, more than half the fish Tosh has caught have had deformities, such as eroded fins, misshapen skeletons, tumors, and lesions. Tosh's kept a careful record of every catch and put the most gruesome examples in his parents' freezer.

How should Tosh use his evidence to convince local residents to act against the polluters?

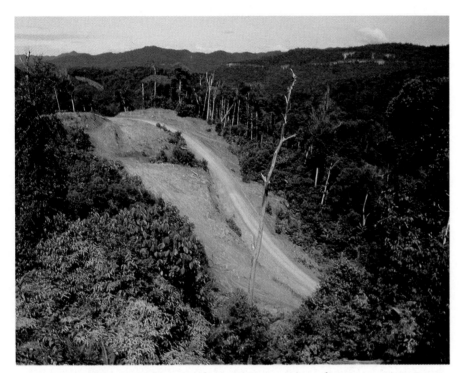

Many tropical forests are being deforested. Saving these forests is an environmental concern. Forest loss causes many problems.

- Energy. Industrial development and transportation are highly dependent upon fossil fuels. Use and need are increasing rapidly. War and pollution are just two of the problems associated with this issue.

- Air, atmosphere, and climate. Increased use of fossil fuels, chlorofluorocarbons, and other chemicals is severely damaging the ozone layer, and there is danger of seriously warming the earth's climate and changing the way of life for many people.

- Hazardous substances. Products such as plastics, pesticides, and radioactive wastes, while contributing to development, have created significant health problems for large groups of people.

- Solid waste management. The problems of insufficient space to dispose of all our waste and how that waste affects the air and water are major problems in the United States today. These problems will get worse as population increases.

KEEPING FIT

Cleaning Up After Large Events

Litter picked up after large events such as concerts and fairs is rarely recycled even though up to 60 percent of the debris is recyclable. According to the James River Corporation, after the International Special Olympics in Minneapolis, 2 million Styrofoam cups were picked up for recycling, as were 50,000 bottles and cans, 800,000 napkins, and 10,000 pounds of food.

The next time your school is planning a large event, make arrangements to make it an environmentally sound event. Precycle when planning for what will be sold. Recycle after the event, providing labeled bins for different kinds of trash, and cleaning up litter left behind.

Solid waste management is a major problem in the United States as communities try to determine what they should do with it.

Becoming Involved

Here are some practical suggestions for becoming involved in protecting the environment:

■ Become an informed consumer by evaluating advertising, labels, contents, and packaging as it relates to the environment. Give feedback to companies on positive ways they can affect the environment.

■ Get more information about environmental issues that are of concern to you.

■ Contact organizations that conserve resources, and educate people on environmental issues that are of interest to you. Ask for information and ideas for conservation.

■ Review how your own habits and life-style affect the environment.

■ Write letters to elected officials letting them know your environmental concerns.

■ Write letters to newspapers, and seek opportunities to have your opinions and concerns about the environment voiced on radio or public television.

K E E P I N G   F I T

Toxins in Art Supplies

According to the U.S. Public Interest Research Group, many art products do not contain warning labels mandated by the 1988 Labeling of Hazardous Art Materials Act. Yet the products have been known to cause serious health problems.

Before using any of the following products, you should look for safer, nontoxic alternatives, or provide proper ventilation while using them. These include

■ rubber cement

■ permanent markers
■ water-based spray paints
■ products with turpentine or toluene
■ products with spray adhesive
■ aerosol cleaners
■ antiquing solutions

Be aware of companies in your community that may be polluting the environment.

■ Join an environmental organization. Most of these organizations can provide you with resources for understanding current issues. Being part of such a group can often provide you with suggestions on ways you can promote environmental health. Planned activities will help you put your concerns into practice. There are many examples of action and change coming from the work of small local groups made up of individual citizens working on issues.

■ Take action against local polluters. The environmental problems in your community directly affect your health and your way of life. Targeting local polluters is a very effective way of protecting your health and that of your family and neighbors. Unfortunately, this is not an easy task. Local and national laws may not be adequately enforced. Some companies continue to pollute for years before the government can make them stop. Even then, the fines are often small compared with the cost of modernizing the facilities or cleaning up toxic wastes. Joining with others to let elected officials become aware of the problem is a start.

LESSON 2 REVIEW

Reviewing Facts and Vocabulary

1. Why can the term *biodegradable* be misleading to consumers?
2. Describe two current environmental concerns.

Thinking Critically

3. **Evaluation.** Explain whether or not you think individuals can make a difference in environmental problems. Support your opinion with examples.

4. **Analysis.** Compare the terms *natural* and *organic*.

Applying Health Knowledge

5. Begin a recycling project at your school. Make posters and pamphlets describing what can be recycled and where you can take recyclable materials.
6. Write a letter to your local newspaper stating your concerns and suggestions about an environmental problem in your community.

Self-Inventory

Are You Involved in Protecting the Environment?

HOW DO YOU RATE?

Number a sheet of paper from 1 through 20. Read each item below, and respond by writing *yes* if the statement is true most or all of the time or *no* if the statement is not true most or all of the time. Then proceed to the next section.

1. Do you consider waste when you buy things?
2. Do you store newspapers for recycling?
3. Do you litter?
4. Do you shut off lights in a room when you or someone else has left and does not plan to return?
5. Do you participate in any type of recycling program?
6. Do you accept unnecessary packaging in fast-food restaurants?
7. Do you use the toilet as a waste basket for paper, gum, and other waste?
8. Do you take a clean glass each time you get a drink at home?
9. Do you put on more clothing rather than turn up the heat when it is cold in the house?
10. Do you recycle aluminum cans?
11. Do you make others aware when they are littering?
12. Do you do anything specifically to conserve water in your home?
13. Do you shower longer than 5 minutes at a time?
14. Do you reuse paper that has been used only on one side?

15. Do you pick up litter even though you did not drop it?
16. Will you wear hand-me-down clothing?
17. Do you give used clothing and other items to friends or charitable organizations?
18. Do you let water run while shaving or brushing your teeth?
19. Do you clean the lint filter in your dryer after using it?
20. Do you buy recycled paper when you have a choice?

HOW DID YOU SCORE?

Give yourself 1 point for every *yes* answer to items 1, 2, 4, 5, 9, 10, 11, 12, 14, 15, 16, 17, 19, and 20.

Give yourself 1 point for every *no* answer to items 3, 6, 7, 8, 13, and 18. Then proceed to the next section.

18 to 20
Outstanding. Your concern for the environment is an example for others.

14 to 17
Very Good. You are doing much to protect the environment.

10 to 13
Good. You are on the right track. With some awareness and effort, you can improve.

5 to 9
Fair. While you are doing some things to help protect our environment, there is much more you can do.

0 to 4
Poor. Try to remember that we all have a shared responsibility for protecting Earth.

WHAT ARE YOUR GOALS?

If you received an *outstanding*, *very good*, or *good* score, complete the statements in Part A. If your score was rated *fair* or *poor*, complete Parts A and B.

Part A

1. I plan to learn more about protecting the environment by ____.
2. My timetable for accomplishing this is ____.
3. I plan to share my information with others by ____.

Part B

4. The attitude or behavior toward protecting the environment I would most like to change is ____.
5. The steps involved in making this change are ____.
6. My timetable for accomplishing this is ____.
7. The people or groups I will ask for support and assistance are ____.
8. My rewards for making this change will be ____.

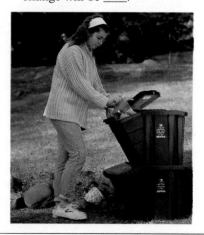

Building Decision-Making Skills

As part of a science fair program, Doug has discovered that his old school building has serious asbestos levels. He has proposed some solutions to the administration but has received little support. Doug isn't sure what he should do, but he has considered the following:

A. Organize a student protest.

B. Release his results to the news media.

C. Report his results to the health department.

D. Go to someone higher in the school administration.

E. Forget it, to avoid bad publicity for his school.

WHAT DO YOU THINK?

1. **Situation.** Why does a decision need to be made?

2. **Choices.** What other choices does Doug have?

3. **Consequences.** What are the advantages and disadvantages of each strategy?

4. **Consequences.** How might Doug's status in the school be affected by each strategy?

5. **Consequences.** How might Doug's relationship with his teacher or school principal be affected?

6. **Consequences.** How might Doug's parents be affected?

7. **Consequences.** How might Doug's health triangle be affected by this decision?

8. **Decision.** What do you think Doug should do? Explain your answer.

9. **Evaluation.** What do you do when you find yourself disagreeing with those in authority? What has been the outcome? What makes such a decision very difficult? What advice would you give Doug?

As part of a community service project by the school's service club, Brooke and some friends cleaned up a weedy area near the elementary school playground. While doing this they discovered a number of used hypodermic needles. Brooke's friends are looking to her for guidance in how to handle this situation. Brooke isn't sure, but she's considering the following:

A. Contact the health department immediately.

B. Contact the news media so attention can be drawn to this serious incident.

C. Let the administration handle it, though they want to keep everything quiet.

D. Keep quiet to avoid bad publicity for the school and town.

WHAT DO YOU THINK?

10. **Choices.** What other choices does Brooke have?

11. **Consequences.** What are the advantages and disadvantages of contacting the health department right away? What are the advantages and disadvantages of contacting the health department later?

12. **Consequences.** What are the advantages and disadvantages of contacting the news media?

13. **Consequences.** What are the advantages and disadvantages of letting the school administration handle the situation?

14. **Consequences.** What are the advantages and disadvantages of keeping quiet about this?

15. **Consequences.** What other people could be affected by this situation? Explain your answer.

16. **Decision.** What do you think Brooke should do?

17. **Evaluation.** How would you handle a situation in which keeping quiet about a problem could result in harm to others?

REVIEW

Using Health Terms

On a separate sheet of paper, write the term that best matches each definition given below.

LESSON 1

1. The process of reducing waste before it occurs by making environmentally sound decisions at the store.
2. Gases that harm the ozone layer.
3. An abundant metal that is expensive and polluting to produce.
4. Concern about saving or protecting the environment and its natural resources.
5. Treating or changing waste so it can be reused.

LESSON 2

6. Product not harmful or poisonous to humans.
7. Product that is derived from living organisms without the use of chemicals.
8. An item that can eventually be broken down by microorganisms.
9. Agency that enforces standards to help protect the environment from pollution.

Building Academic Skills

LESSON 1

10. **Writing.** Write a proposal to your principal on some aspect of conservation that can be utilized in your school, such as recycling paper or cans or turning lights off in rooms not in use.

LESSON 2

11. **Math.** Determine the number of gallons of gasoline burned by hypothetical families traveling 5, 15, 30, and 60 miles per day to work, school, and stores. Compute fuel consumption based upon 20 miles per gallon and compare with computations based upon 36 miles per gallon. How might these families reduce the amount of gasoline they consume? What factors will determine how much gasoline is needed by a particular family?

Recalling the Facts

LESSON 1

12. What does recycling involve?
13. Name two materials that are 100 percent recyclable.
14. What might old and worn tires be used for?
15. What is the distribution of energy use in an average household?
16. Which of the following situations demonstrates precycling and which shows recycling? Explain.
    a. Buying food products in bulk.
    b. Taking your own container to buy apple cider.
    c. Using the same piece of aluminum foil more than once.
    d. Using old envelopes for notes.
    e. Using cloth diapers.
    f. Collecting beverage cans and selling them.
    g. Using a cloth bag to carry home groceries and other items from the store.
17. What about modern life has enabled people to take the environment for granted?
18. What are significant benefits of conserving energy?
19. List three energy-saving actions an individual could practice at home, and tell how each helps protect the environment.

LESSON 2

20. Name three technological advances that were quick answers to problems and were immediately beneficial to humans but later caused environmental problems.
21. What are some issues that have become major problems for aquatic life?
22. What problems does forest loss cause people?
23. What is the Environmental Protection Agency and what does it do?
24. Identify three ways that conservation contributes to your life.
25. How can the term *biodegradable* be misleading?

REVIEW

Thinking Critically

LESSON 1

26. Evaluation. Some places of business offer incentives for recycling, such as selling a product for less money if you bring your own container. Why do you think incentives are necessary to get people to recycle? What incentives do you need to motivate you to recycle?

27. Analysis. Each person in the United States uses about 80 gallons of water a day with about 50 gallons wasted. How can you conserve water that you use?

LESSON 2

28. Synthesis. Summarize reasons that environmental laws are necessary.

29. Analysis. What could be misleading about labels that read "made from natural materials"?

30. Evaluation. Investigative reporting often brings public attention to environmental problems or companies that might be contributing to these problems. What value, if any, do you feel these stories have for the general public?

31. Evaluation. Of the current environmental concerns defined in this chapter, which do you feel you could make a commitment to? Support your answer.

Making the Connection

LESSON 2

32. Language Arts. Write to one of your community officials or state legislators to find out his or her position regarding local environmental issues. Discover what his or her proposals are for environmental health for the future. Share the response you receive with your class.

33. Social Studies. Research an environmental catastrophe of your choice. Report what happened and what we learned from the situation.

Applying Health Knowledge

LESSON 1

34. Identify the item in each pair that would be better for the environment. Explain.
  a. paper towels or cloth towels
  b. paper plates or Styrofoam plates
  c. popcorn or Styrofoam for packing material
  d. aluminum can or plastic bottle

35. Tell how the following items can be reused:
  a. plastic grocery bags
  b. plastic milk jugs
  c. paper grocery bags
  d. used envelopes

LESSON 2

36. What hazardous chemicals are used in your home? What disposal options for these substances are available in your community?

Beyond the Classroom

LESSON 1

37. Parental Involvement. Along with your parents, evaluate your home and life-style and determine several changes or behaviors you are willing to practice to help the environment. Use the suggestions in this chapter or some found in any other good sources about the environment.

LESSON 2

38. Further Study. Research any of the following or other environmental organizations of which you have interest: Greenpeace, World Wildlife Fund, Water Pollution Control Federation, Sierra Club, or the Cousteau Society. Find out what contributions the group is making toward saving the environment.

39. Further Study. Find and share examples of advertisements that reflect current societal concerns regarding the environment.

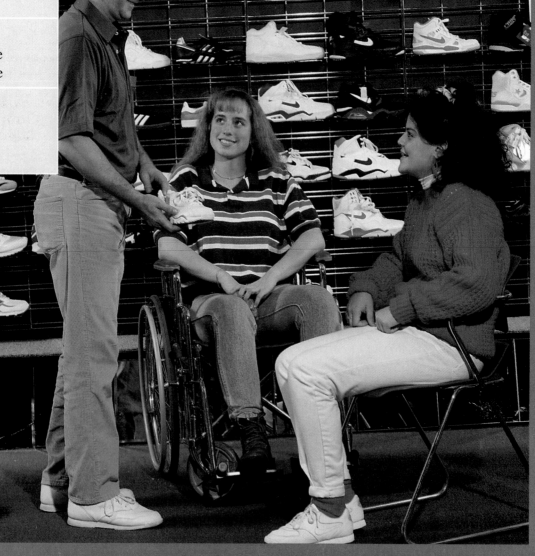

WHAT IS CONSUMER HEALTH?

A s you work to promote or take care of your health, you probably purchase many products and services. A **consumer** is anyone who uses a product or a service. Obviously, you have all been consumers for many years. When you consider the products that you buy that in some way affect your health, you also realize you are a *health* consumer.

Consumer health is concerned with helping you select products and services wisely, and with letting you know where to go or what to do if you have been treated unfairly or need help.

Benefits of Being a Wise Health Consumer

There are three major benefits to being a wise health consumer:

- Being a wise health consumer saves money and time, and increases your satisfaction. You are able to make the best purchases for the least amount of money and time. It may take preparation time to collect information and to compare products or services, but it usually pays off in the long run.
- Being a wise health consumer protects your health. A wise consumer is not swayed into buying health products that are worthless or that may be harmful. A wise consumer knows when to seek medical help and does so without delay. Recognition and treatment of early symptoms is an important consumer skill.
- Being a wise health consumer builds your self-confidence as you speak up for your rights. If you have been sold a defective product or service, you protect yourself, as well as others, from future deception when you take action. Much of the progress that has been made in protecting consumers has resulted from people's willingness to speak up when they were treated unfairly. Such basic assertiveness skills can be helpful to you in all facets of your daily life.

Your Rights as a Consumer

As a consumer you have rights. In 1962 President John Kennedy introduced the Consumer Bill of Rights. It includes the following:

- The right to safety. Consumers are protected from dangerous products.
- The right to be informed. Consumers are protected from misleading advertising. They can ask for all of the facts they need to make good choices.
- The right to choose. Consumers have the right to make their own choices.
- The right to be heard. Consumers can speak out when they are not satisfied. They have a voice in making consumer laws.

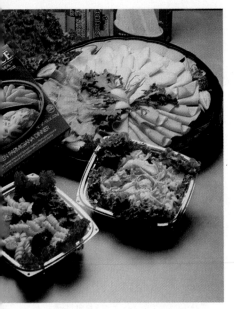

Generally, the more preparation that has been done for you, the higher the cost. Are there times when it pays to buy convenience foods?

During the 1970s President Richard Nixon added another right: the right to redress. This right means that consumers who have had a wrong done to them have the right to get that wrong corrected. There are many city, state, and federal agencies that help the consumer in these matters. President Gerald Ford also added a right—the right to consumer education.

What Factors Influence Your Purchasing Decisions?

Think of a health product you bought recently. What factors influenced your decision to buy that particular product? Did your friend have it? Was it on sale? Did you see it advertised?

Five main factors influence your choices as a consumer: price, convenience, family and friends, quality, and advertising. Be aware of these factors. You will be better able to make wise consumer health choices.

Price

Several factors influence price. Brand-name products cost more. They are usually well-advertised, and the cost of that advertising is passed on to the consumer. The size of the product also affects the price. Unit pricing tells how much different sizes of the same product cost per unit. The **unit price** is determined by dividing the price of the item by its weight, volume, or count—depending on how it is packaged. Many stores have unit pricing information on the shelves to help the consumer.

Another factor that affects price is where the product is sold. Products in convenience stores and specialty shops usually cost more than those in grocery stores or general department stores.

Convenience

Convenience, the labor-saving feature of a product, has a big impact on what we buy. In general, we pay more for convenience. Buying frozen macaroni and cheese may be more convenient than buying the ingredients and making it. When we are often in a hurry or want to save time, convenience becomes a significant factor in our purchases. Sometimes it is worthwhile to pay more, but making a habit of buying convenience products becomes expensive and can put a sizable dent in your budget.

Family and Friends

Your family influences your purchasing decisions. You may or may not buy an item because of comments family members may make. You also may choose to buy a certain brand of product if your family has used it a long time. Friends also influence your purchases. You probably have bought an item because your friend had one. You may have bought a certain type of shirt or jeans because everyone else had them, or you wanted to identify with a certain group.

Quality

Have you ever bought a product only to have it not work or fall apart? Decisions about the quality of a product can be difficult. Just because something costs more does not mean it is of better quality. Examining the ingredients or the parts of a product and the guarantees that accompany the product will help you assess its quality.

Advertising

Advertising is the way by which a manufacturer gains your attention for its product. You may not be aware of how much advertising you are exposed to in a day. Think of the signs, the T-shirts, or the bumper stickers you have seen today that advertise something.

Advertising works in subtle ways, often on the subconscious level. It takes a very sharp consumer not to be influenced by advertising. Catchy jingles, tunes, and rhymes have a way of staying with us. That recognition factor is just what the advertiser wants.

What other forms of advertising can you name? Which form do you think is most effective?

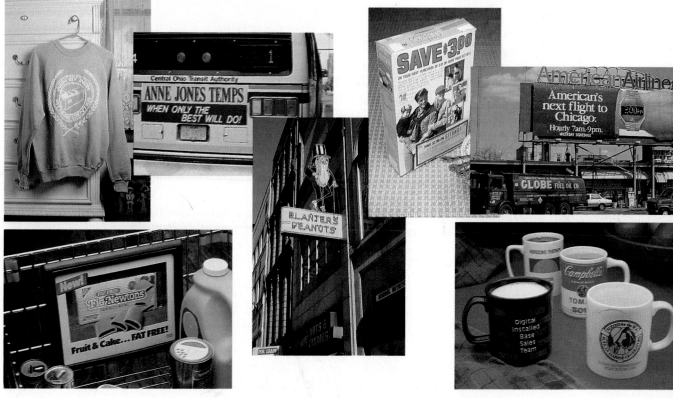

Margaret Lofner knows firsthand what it's like to be a health-care professional and not be able to get health insurance. Born and raised in England but living in Texas since 1972, she has worked as a nurse in both the British and American health-care systems. Mrs. Lofner left her job of 14 years when her medical insurance was canceled and no one would insure her. "My former job was in a family practice clinic. "I have a pre-existing condition called a Protein S. Deficiency, a deficiency in an anti-coagulant factor. This causes my blood to clot much faster than other people's blood, which can cause clots in the deep veins. It can be fatal. My condition was discovered when I was 18, but it hasn't stopped me. I lead a very full, active life. I've never missed a day of work. But insurance companies don't look at your health history or attendance record. They just look at your diagnosis.

"Then, in February, I had to have surgery for endometrial carcinoma, cancer of the endometrium, the lining of the uterus. The outcome was very favorable. The cancer hadn't spread. I didn't need radiation or chemotherapy. The surgery was very risky because of the blood clotting, but I sailed through it.

"Soon after that, our

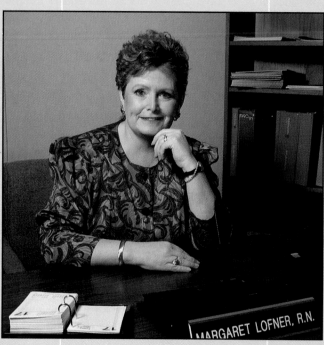

MARGARET LOFNER, R.N.

employers, who are physicians, called a meeting. They told us that the cost of the practice's health insurance premiums had skyrocketed, they were canceling the policies. I was told I couldn't get any coverage for three to five years—not just for cancer problems, either, but for anything at all. So I wrote to a consumer publication and called the American Cancer Society and was told there were a lot of other people just like me. Very soon I realized that if I was going to have health insurance, I'd need to be part of a large group where my high-risk premiums would be offset by lots of medium-risk or low-risk ones. It was a tough decision to make, but I knew I'd have to change jobs to get insurance. Leaving my job was an emotional decision just like the one I'd made in 1972 to come here from England and leave my family behind."

Mrs. Lofner concludes, "Good health insurance coverage should be foremost among the factors you consider in making a decision about which job to take."

1. Mrs. Lofner investigated options, then made the necessary changes to ensure that she could get health insurance. When you face obstacles, do you gather information, investigate options, and make necessary changes in the interest of your health? If so, how? If not, for what reasons?

2. What steps can you take to become an advocate for your own health care? What might the benefits to your self-esteem be? To your health?

Manufacturers spend billions of dollars to advertise their products. They use many different techniques to sell health products. Advertisements usually play on our emotions and our needs. They may promise popularity, sex appeal, or pain relief. Are you influenced by certain messages more than others? Do some ads turn you off? Look at some common techniques that are used in advertising.

Testimonials. Testimonials often use famous people to tell you how they use and like the product. A **testimonial** is a person's enthusiastic recommendation of a product. Because you like or identify with that person, you may be influenced to buy the product. The law says that the person who gives the testimonial must have actually used the product. This does not mean, however, that he or she really believes in the product or has purchased the product to use it. Companies pay famous people large sums of money for promoting their products.

Buy One, Get One Free. This is a common approach used in advertising. It makes consumers feel like they are getting something for nothing. Look closely at the advertisements. Often the price of one item has been raised, so you might pay more than you normally would. Remember, rarely, if ever, will you get something for nothing.

Emotional Pleas. Many ads play on people's emotional needs. Here are some examples:
- "Be the first on your block to have a . . . ."
- "Be happy, be smart, buy . . . ."
- "When you want only the best for you and your family . . . ."

All of these pleas encourage you to buy something for an emotional reason. Do not be tricked into spending more or buying something you normally would not buy.

LESSON 1 REVIEW

Reviewing Facts and Vocabulary

1. List two benefits of being a wise consumer.
2. What five factors influence one's choice of products or services?
3. What is a testimonial?

Thinking Critically

4. **Synthesis.** Could there be an honest purchasing system in our country if consumers had no rights? Explain your answer.
5. **Evaluation.** What criteria would you use to critique an ad for a particular product?

Applying Health Knowledge

6. Make a list of five common advertising slogans or jingles. Next to each one, write a consumer awareness warning. Your warning might point out something for the consumer to look for beyond what is being promoted in the ad.
7. Form a survey team to observe television commercials on different channels between 6:00 P.M. and 10:00 P.M. Answer the following questions, and then report your findings:
   a. How many commercials were for health products?
   b. How many were for beauty products?
   c. How many products used youth and beauty as part of the sales pitch?
   d. How many had pretty nature scenes?
   e. How many used music?
   f. Was the volume on the television louder during the commercials?

FRAUD IN THE MARKETPLACE

It is illegal to make false claims, promising that a medicine, a food, or a cosmetic will do something that it really cannot do. You have probably heard the terms **quack** and **quackery** used to describe a dishonest promoter of medicinal products and the useless products or treatments. Quackery plays on human emotions, weakness, and fear to get money from people who want fast cures or relief from pain. The most prevalent areas of quackery are those in which there is no cure or instant relief.

How Quackery Works

The promoter deals with magic, miracles, and fast painless cures. Amazingly, even intelligent people can become victims of these false claims. Many times it is because the people want to believe what they hear or because they are hoping for something that does not exist.

Take, for example, the person who is 20 pounds overweight and does not like to exercise. Exercise is hard work, especially for overweight people. Now "Slim-Ex," a new candy, claims that this person will lose weight without exercise and while continuing to eat whatever he or she likes. An overweight person may purchase the product, wanting to believe that there is an easy way to lose weight without exercising.

Popular Types of Product Fraud

Here are types of products that are most susceptible to quackery:

- Beauty aids. These play on people's fear of growing old or fat and promise youth, beauty, and sex appeal forever. Included are cures for baldness; products that promise quick, painless weight loss; and products for the prevention of wrinkles.
- Diet aids. Their appeal is to our need to be trim and energetic. They include vitamin and diet supplements.
- Food. Food fads represent one of the most lucrative areas of quackery. Relying on special foods, diets, or diet supplements is not only a waste of money—it also is not healthy.
- Fraudulent devices. This group of products includes devices that are promoted as being capable of curing ailments. For example, excess body weight is said to be melted away by wearing special clothing. Sometimes the devices are legitimate but are promoted improperly. Such cases involve, for example, getting eyeglasses, contacts, or dentures through the mail without seeing a doctor or dentist.

Medical Quackery

Quackery offers hope. Therefore, the most susceptible people are those suffering from diseases or conditions without known cures.

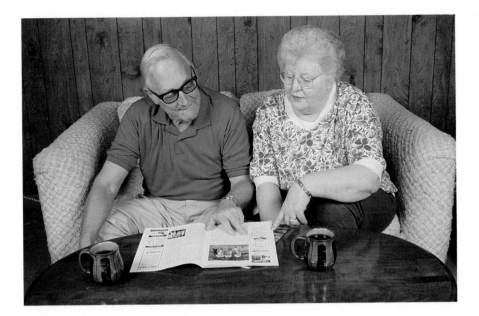

Even if a product claiming a fast cure will not do any harm; the danger is that the individual may postpone seeking medical attention.

The problem with quack products is not so much the harm that may be done. Medical authorities point to quackery as being dangerous because the patient delays seeking sound medical advice and treatment until it may be too late.

Quack cures are offered most often for diseases or conditions for which treatment is apt to be lengthy and unpleasant, with uncertain results. Three areas susceptible to quackery are cancer, arthritis, and weight problems.

Cancer

In contrast to the standard treatment for cancer, which may involve surgery, radiation, and chemotherapy—all of which may be painful and disfiguring—the quack remedy is usually simple and painless. It may be a pill, an injection, a trip to the mountains, or a special diet. The quack remedy offers hope. Often, because hope is vital to a patient's survival, there may be apparent remission of the disease. This effect makes people more likely to believe in the product and continue to use it.

Have you ever heard of a **placebo?** It is a substance that has no medical value, but which is given for its psychological effect. The placebo effect comes about when people think that they are taking medicine and

DID YOU KNOW?

- It is estimated that each year one in four Americans will use some kind of medical treatment that is considered quackery, or not medically sound.
- The American Medical Association estimates that 25 billion dollars a year is spent in the United States on quack medicines.

K E E P I N G   F I T

Be Alert to Health and Medical Frauds

Here are some ways that you can be alert to any signs of fraudulent practices or products. If you can answer yes to any of these questions, you should be wary.

- Is the product advertised as a scientific breakthrough without

any particular reference to a medical school, study, or journal? If one is mentioned, have you ever heard of it?

- Does the product claim to be effective for a large variety of ailments?

- Do the promised benefits seem too good to be true?
- Does a "health consultant" sell the product door-to-door?

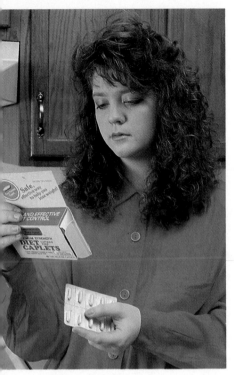

Weight control gimmicks attract a lot of attention.

therefore the symptoms are relieved. This effect illustrates the power of the mind over the body and the positive effect our beliefs can have on health. However, it also makes us quite susceptible to quackery.

Arthritis

The pain and suffering of arthritis, a condition that afflicts about 40 million Americans, makes sufferers of this disease a likely target for the quack's false promises. Medical science has no cure for arthritis, and even its control is complicated and not always effective. Some of the quack remedies are harmless enough, but they are still a waste of money. Wearing a copper bracelet, for example, is said to ease the discomfort of arthritis. It does no harm, but it cannot do what is claimed. However, other remedies that quacks offer are highly dangerous. The Arthritis Foundation estimates that arthritis victims spend millions of dollars a year on quack remedies.

Weight Problems

Unlike most quack remedies, many of the weight-loss plans that quacks offer may, if one faithfully follows them, actually work, resulting in a real loss of weight. The secret is not in the trick diet or the magic medicine the advertising features, but in the fact that most reduction plans involve a cutback in the amount of food consumed.

Weight control is perhaps the most lucrative area for unnecessary products and devices. There is only one way to lose weight—you must use up more calories than you consume. Buying products that claim to make weight loss effortless wastes your money and leads to more disappointment, making it even harder to deal successfully with the problem. Yet people spend billions of dollars annually on over-the-counter products that claim to aid in weight reduction.

LESSON 2 REVIEW

Reviewing Facts and Vocabulary

1. Name three types of product fraud, and describe what makes people susceptible to them.
2. What is the greatest danger to ill people who seek quack cures?
3. Why are cancer, arthritis, and weight loss the most susceptible areas of quackery?
4. What is a placebo?

Thinking Critically

5. **Evaluation.** What criteria would you use to select a shampoo or body lotion?

6. **Synthesis.** Imagine that advertising did not exist. Suggest some ways that our lives would be changed.

Applying Health Knowledge

7. Five classmates have been given $20 each to purchase health products. You are asked to give them some suggestions about the use of their money. What wise consumer practices would you share with them?
8. In a store you observe two people shopping for an item. What are some ways that you can tell if either one is a wise consumer?

HANDLING CONSUMER PROBLEMS

Each of us is a consumer. We depend upon others to provide us with products and services to protect our health. Many fine companies and businesses do their jobs well in providing us with what we want and need. Most businesses depend on satisfied customers to stay in business. Honest firms will make an effort to resolve problems, but you, as a consumer, must bring these problems to the attention of the company or store.

BEING AN ASSERTIVE CONSUMER

Being a wise consumer can protect your health and save you money, and it also can be fun and challenging. Think of a time when a salesperson was being pushy or pressuring you. How did you feel—uncomfortable, nervous, imposed upon? Next time, assert yourself. Challenge the person with consumer-oriented questions. If you are not interested or want to be left alone, simply state that. Compare what you stand to lose with your potential gains for being an assertive consumer.

Steps to Follow

Even the most careful shoppers find themselves buying products or securing services that do not work right or serve them well. Sometimes merchants and manufacturers are less than enthusiastic about resolving difficulties. This is why it is necessary for you, as a consumer, to know what to do and where to go for help. Here are some tips to follow:

1. Identify the problem and what you feel would be a fair way to solve it.
2. Have some documentation available to back up your complaint, for example, a sales receipt, a canceled check, or a warranty.
3. Go back to the person who sold you the item or performed the service. State the problem and how you would like to have it solved.
4. If this person is not helpful, ask to see the store manager or supervisor. Repeat your story. Most problems are resolved at this level.
5. If you are not satisfied with the response at this level, do not give up. If the company operates nationally or the product is a national brand, write a letter to the president or the director of consumer affairs of the company. Your letter should include these points:
   a. name and title of the person you're writing
   b. name of product and serial number or model number, or type of service
   c. date and location of purchase or service
   d. statement of the problem
   e. request for action within a reasonable time
   f. your address and phone number

LESSON 3 FOCUS

TERMS TO USE
- Better Business Bureau (BBB)
- Small-claims court
- Advocate
- Recall
- Food and Drug Administration (FDA)
- Federal Trade Commission (FTC)

CONCEPTS TO LEARN
- There are a variety of agencies that help protect the consumer.
- Consumer complaints need to be handled in an appropriate manner.

ATTITUDES AND BEHAVIORS TO EVALUATE
- Self-Inventory, page 648.
- Building Decision-Making Skills, page 649.

A well-written letter will usually bring positive results.

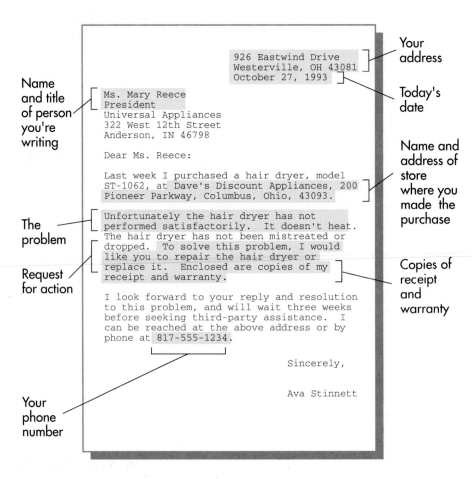

Your address
926 Eastwind Drive
Westerville, OH 43081
October 27, 1993
Today's date

Name and title of person you're writing
Ms. Mary Reece
President
Universal Appliances
322 West 12th Street
Anderson, IN 46798

Dear Ms. Reece:

Last week I purchased a hair dryer, model ST-1062, at Dave's Discount Appliances, 200 Pioneer Parkway, Columbus, Ohio, 43093.

Name and address of store where you made the purchase

The problem
Unfortunately the hair dryer has not performed satisfactorily. It doesn't heat. The hair dryer has not been mistreated or dropped. To solve this problem, I would like you to repair the hair dryer or replace it. Enclosed are copies of my receipt and warranty.

Request for action

Copies of receipt and warranty

I look forward to your reply and resolution to this problem, and will wait three weeks before seeking third-party assistance. I can be reached at the above address or by phone at 817-555-1234.

Sincerely,

Ava Stinnett

Your phone number

One of the first steps in solving a consumer complaint is to take the product back to the store and tell the clerk what the problem is and how you want it resolved.

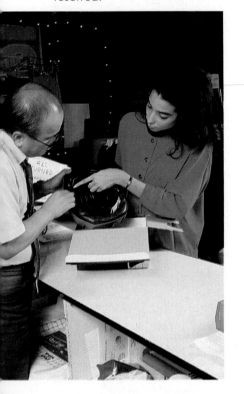

Getting Help

If you are not satisfied with the company's response, even after writing to the president, you may wish to contact one of several agencies outside the company for help. These sources vary greatly in services offered, approach taken, and type of complaint that will be handled. By becoming familiar with the existence and work of these agencies, you can improve your skill as a consumer.

The Better Business Bureau

The **Better Business Bureau (BBB)** is a nonprofit organization sponsored by private businesses. It offers a variety of services. These services include providing general information on products and services, reliability reports, background information on local businesses and organizations, and records of companies' complaint-handling performances.

The BBB attempts to settle consumer complaints against local business firms. It accepts written complaints and will contact a local firm on your behalf. The BBB considers a complaint settled when one of the following courses of action has taken place:

- The customer receives satisfaction.
- The customer receives a reasonable adjustment.
- The company provides proof that the customer's complaint is unreasonable or not backed by facts.

BBBs also handle false advertising cases. To find a BBB, check your local phone book, local consumer office, or local library. Most of them are located in major cities.

Media Programs

If you live in or near a large city, you may be aware of one of the more than 100 newspapers and 50 radio and TV stations that offer action or hot line services for consumers who need help. These programs often get successful results because of the powerful influence of the media. Unfavorable publicity may be one of the best encouragers to get a merchant or business to take action to resolve a consumer complaint.

"Call for Action" is one of the larger media help lines. Staffed by 800 volunteers, it helps about 250,000 people each year. The volunteers relay complaints to the proper individuals, business people, or public agencies, and then check back with you—usually in about two weeks. If you have been satisfied, the incident is closed. If not, then "Call for Action" will intervene in your behalf. It generally turns public attention on a case to get results.

Small-Claims Court

You might imagine that seeking satisfaction in small-claims court is an expensive and drawn-out procedure. It is not. If you have a complaint that you are not able to resolve, then consider going to the small-claims court. This is a very important alternative for consumers. Court procedures are simple, inexpensive, quick, and informal. There are court fees involved, but you often get most or all of them back if you win your case. Generally, you do not need a lawyer. In fact, in some states, lawyers are not permitted in small-claims courts.

Small-claims courts deal with claims that range from $100 to $3,000, with an average of around $500. Locate the small-claims court in your area in your local phone book. When you reach the court on the phone, ask the clerk how to use the court. Sit in on a court session before taking a case to small-claims court, so that you become familiar with the operation.

Occupational and Professional Licensing Boards

If you have a problem with professional or occupational services, such as with a physician, a dentist, or a physical therapist, you may be able to get some help from a state licensing or regulatory board. There are an estimated 1,500 state boards that license or register more than 550 health-related occupations. The practice of licensing was first started to protect the public in matters of health and safety and to guard the public from incompetency and fraud.

To be licensed, a professional must have a certain level of education and experience and must pass a qualifications test. State boards set licensing examinations; issue, deny, or revoke licenses; take disciplinary action; and handle consumer complaints.

If you contact a state board for help, it will usually bring your complaint to the attention of the person whom you filed against, known as

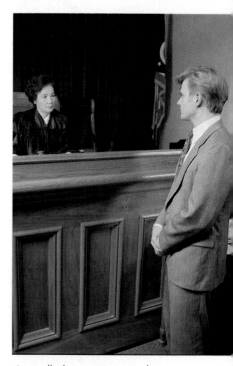

A small-claims court can be used for a quick, effective means of settling a minor claim.

If you have been unsuccessful in resolving a consumer problem where you originally did business, the next step is to contact the company's headquarters or the manufacturer of the product.

Often you can find the name and address of the manufacturer on the product's label. If not, check your local library for the *Thomas Register,* which lists the manufacturers of thousands of products or *Standard and Poor's Register of Corporations, Directors, and Executives,* which lists the addresses of over 50,000 American business firms.

the licensee. The board will seek a satisfactory solution to your problem. If necessary, the board can conduct an investigation. Some state boards even have consumer education materials to help you in selecting a health professional.

You can find out about a state licensing board by contacting your local consumer office. Check your phone book under state government offices or under professional listings. You can also ask professionals about the board that is responsible for their licensing. In fact, you should ask to see the person's license or registration before you use his o · her services.

State, County, and City Consumer Affairs Offices

If you are not satisfied with a company's or person's response to your complaint about a product or service, a good place for an inquiry or a complaint is the local consumer affairs office. Local consumer offices can be particularly helpful because a person can contact them easily by phone or in person, and they are usually familiar with local businesses and regulations. Keep all receipts and other papers to show or to use when talking to the local agency.

If there is no consumer office where you live, contact a state consumer office. These consumer offices are set up differently from state to state. Many state and local consumer offices have a large selection of educational materials and information available. Your phone book should give you a listing under city, county, or state government.

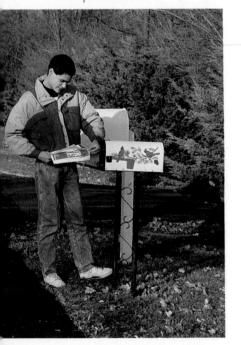

The postal service handles fraud or misleading promotions involving the use of the mail. If you have a complaint, contact your local postmaster.

Private Consumer Groups

In addition to the many governmental and business organizations that can be of assistance to the consumer, private consumer groups exist in all 50 states. In almost all cases, these are made up of individual consumer members who join together to support consumer interests. They are called advocates. An **advocate** is someone who speaks out for a position.

The private consumer groups are usually started and staffed by volunteers, although some have paid staff members. Some of the private consumer groups help individual consumers with complaints. Others are dedicated to serving the broad needs of special populations, such as the elderly, women, minorities, and low-income people. They represent consumers by using their collective energy to focus on critical consumer issues in the marketplace.

For more information about consumer groups in your area, you can contact your local or state government consumer affairs office. If you cannot locate a group in your area, you can try one of these organizations:

- The National Office of the Consumer Federation of America, 1424 16th Street, N.W., Washington, DC 20036
- National Consumers League, 815 15th St., N.W., Washington, DC 20005
- Ralph Nader's Public Citizen, P.O. Box 19404, Washington, DC 20036

Help through Government Services

The federal government has established a number of specialized agencies that deal with health-related products and services. Taxes support these agencies. You have a right as a citizen to make use of their services, and these agencies have a responsibility to help you.

The important skills of being an effective consumer are knowing where to get help and what services are provided. Such information will save you money, protect your safety and health, and often keep merchants honest in their dealings with consumers.

Product Safety. The Consumer Product Safety Commission (CPSC) protects consumers against the manufacture and sale of hazardous appliances, toys, games, and so forth. It has the power to ban hazardous products and also to order a recall when a product is thought to be dangerous to the public. A **recall** occurs when a product that is already on the market has been considered unsafe for use and the CPSC has instructed the manufacturer to take the product off the shelves.

It is the CPSC that requires oral prescription medicines and aspirin to be packaged in child-resistant containers. These containers are designed so that children will have difficulty opening them.

For more information about this agency, contact the Director, Office of Communications, Consumer Product Safety Commission, Bethesda, Maryland 20207.

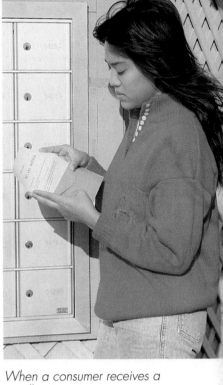

When a consumer receives a recall notice, it means a product that was bought has a defect. Ignoring a recall can put you at risk.

Consumer Information. The Consumer Information Center (CIC) distributes consumer information that the federal government publishes. It also works with other related agencies to develop and distribute new consumer information materials. The CIC publishes a listing of over 200 federal consumer publications, many of which are directly related to health. For a free copy of the Catalog of Consumer Information, send a postcard to Consumer Information Center, Pueblo, Colorado 81009.

Food, Cosmetics, and Medicines. The **Food and Drug Administration (FDA)** ensures that all food and food additives, other than meat and poultry or those containing meat and poultry, are safe, pure, wholesome, and honestly and correctly labeled. If you find unsanitary, contaminated, or mislabeled foods, contact the FDA and it will review the complaint, which may lead to an investigation.

The FDA also ensures that cosmetics are safe and pure. The FDA requires that cosmetics be truthfully labeled and that the ingredients be listed on each package. If you have an unusual physical reaction to a cosmetic, report it to the FDA.

In addition, the FDA ensures that medicines are properly labeled and safe and effective for their intended uses. The FDA determines whether a medicine should be a prescription medicine, one that is obtainable only with a doctor's order, or whether a medicine may be sold over-the-counter, so that it is available by individual choice. The FDA regulates the advertising of prescription medicines, while the Federal Trade Commission (FTC) regulates the advertising of over-the-counter medicines in all their forms.

For more information, contact the Director, Consumer Communications, Food and Drug Administration, 5600 Fishers Lane, Rockville, Maryland 20857.

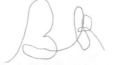

- When you are in the hospital, hospital staff will keep records about your condition, diagnosis, and treatment.
- Your chart may contain your medical history, lab test results, dietary restrictions, medications and other treatments, scheduled tests or therapies, and more.
- Though the chart technically belongs to the hospital, you have a right to know what is on it.

CONFLICT RESOLUTION

Travis is a bike-racing enthusiast. To help keep in shape over the winter, he saved his money for months to buy an exercise bike. Now, Travis has received the bike from the mail order company, and he's very disappointed. The bike doesn't seem worth the money he paid for it. Travis called the company to ask about sending it back and getting a refund. The sales rep he spoke with told him the bike was a nonreturnable sale item. Travis thinks he's being ripped off.

What can Travis do to get his money back?

HEALTH UPDATE

LOOKING AT THE ISSUES

Health Insurance

There are about 35 million people in the United States who have no health insurance—including 9 million children. As insurance companies become stricter about who they are willing to insure, more and more Americans are finding themselves unable to get insurance. Wanting to protect themselves from huge costs, insurance companies now often refuse to insure people with catastrophic illnesses like AIDS or cancer or even some people with chronic health problems such as diabetes or hypertension.

The issues of whether or not everyone should be insured and, if so, how this insurance should be financed remain in the forefront of health-care debates.

Analyzing Different Viewpoints

ONE VIEW. Some legislators propose making a requirement that employers have to provide health insurance for workers. In Hawaii, where a law was adopted requiring employers to insure all employees, the state's uninsured rate fell to 2 percent. Under the law, employees pay at least half the cost of health insurance for full-time workers. Hawaiians now have the greatest longevity in the United States and among the lowest health-care costs.

A SECOND VIEW. Other people in government propose a health-care plan covering every American that would be financed by a 5 percent payroll tax—80 percent on employers and 20 percent on employees.

A THIRD VIEW. Others call for a national health insurance program. They want a universal health-care plan for everyone who cannot afford their own insurance. They suggest moving Medicaid benefits into the universal health-care program. They call for coverage of basic benefits, including hospital and physician services. One such plan would call for everyone to pay based on income. They point to the Canadian system, which since 1971, has mandated that the government pay for all medically necessary doctor and hospital costs. It also allows the provinces and territories to run their own programs and set fees and hospital budgets.

A FOURTH VIEW. Others opposed to plans like the Canadian plan say that health-care insurance should remain in the private sector. They point out that in Canada, because of government restrictions, there are long waiting lists for elective surgery and equipment is often outdated.

Exploring Your Views

1. Do you think every United States citizen should have health insurance? Why or why not?
2. Who should pay for this insurance?
3. Are there certain kinds of procedures or tests you think health insurance companies should not pay for? If so, what are they? Why do you feel this way? Who should decide who should and should not get necessary care?

Meat and Poultry. The Food Safety and Inspection Service (FSIS) of the Department of Agriculture ensures that meat, poultry, and the products made from them are safe, wholesome, and labeled properly. This branch ensures that meat-packing plants are clean and that any potential hazards are kept at safe levels. If you have suffered from suspected food poisoning from meat or poultry, contact a doctor of the local public health office who will contact the Meatborne Hazard Control Center, Agriculture Research Center, Beltsville, Maryland 20705.

This same agency also provides information on its activities and publishes a variety of educational materials on such subjects as food safety and purchasing. For copies of any of these materials, contact the Information Division, Food Safety and Inspection Service, Department of Agriculture, Washington, DC 20250.

Advertising. As you have studied, advertising is designed to influence you and your decision about a product or service. Sometimes this advertising is honest, and sometimes it is not. The **Federal Trade Commission (FTC)** prevents the unfair, false, or deceptive advertising of consumer products and services. This includes television, radio, and print ads.

For more information about false advertising of consumer products and services, contact the Office of the Secretary, Federal Trade Commission, Washington, DC 20580.

Transportation. The Bureau of Consumer Protection of the Federal Aviation Administration (FAA) handles complaints against airlines. If you have been misled about discount fares or types of service, this is the agency with which to register a complaint. Usually you can get your problem taken care of by contacting the customer service representative of the airline. If this does not work, write to the airline's consumer affairs department. If this fails, then the Bureau of Consumer Protection is a good choice. Its address is Bureau of Consumer Protection, Federal Aviation Administraton, Washington, DC 20428.

> ## DID YOU KNOW?
>
> - In the past, women have often not been included in essential health research studies. Now The National Institutes of Health's Office of Research on Women's Health has been created, and up to 500 million dollars will be spent to study major health problems that afflict American women, including osteoporosis and breast cancer.

LESSON 3 REVIEW

Reviewing Facts and Vocabulary

1. Define the terms *advocate* and *recall*. Use each in a sentence.
2. What are the monetary limits of a case that could be taken to small-claims court?
3. How might an advocate group help the consumer?

Thinking Critically

4. **Analysis.** Compare five government agencies that protect consumers.

Applying Health Knowledge

5. Make up a situation in a store or restaurant in which a person is not treated well. Compose a letter of complaint to the appropriate place.
6. Identify three organizations that would be helpful to you as a consumer if you bought a package of pills that guaranteed weight loss, and the pills did not work.

Self-Inventory

Are You a Wise Consumer?

HOW DO YOU RATE?

Number a sheet of paper from 1 through 21. Answer *yes* or *no* to each of the items below. Total the number of *yes* responses. Then proceed to the next section.

1. I buy products I want only when I can afford them.
2. Before I buy food products, I compare ingredients.
3. Before I choose grooming products to buy, I compare ingredients.
4. Before I buy a product, I compare packaging.
5. I make an effort to avoid products sold with excess packaging.
6. I make an effort to purchase products packaged in recyclable containers.
7. I compare prices of different brands in the same store before I buy.
8. I compare prices of the same item in different stores.
9. I shop at stores that offer the best prices.
10. I read the local papers to find out where the best buys can be found.
11. I compare warranties before purchasing.
12. I read labels before I buy.
13. I am aware of factors such as advertising and peer pressure that might influence my purchase.
14. I return products if I am not satisfied with them or if they are defective.
15. I buy what I want or need without the influence of gimmicks.
16. I understand the purpose of advertising and how it is designed to make me want a product or feel that I need a product.
17. I check the material, product, or device before I buy it to be sure that the item is in good working order or is in its original packaging.
18. I read advertisements closely so that I am clear about what they are saying and not saying.
19. I avoid emotional or impulsive buying.
20. I am not intimidated by a high-powered, pushy salesperson.
21. I do not let myself be talked into things because they are on sale.

HOW DID YOU SCORE?

Give yourself 1 point for each *yes* response and 0 points for each *no* response. Total your points, and read the next column to see how you scored. Then proceed to the next section.

17 to 21
Excellent. You are an alert consumer and are probably getting the most for your money.

12 to 16
Good. You are on the right track.

Below 12
Needs Improvement. By changing a few of your behaviors you could get more for your money.

WHAT ARE YOUR GOALS?

Identify an area in which your score is low. Then complete the statements below.

1. The behavior I would most like to change or improve is ____.
2. The steps involved in making this change are ____.
3. My timetable for accomplishing this is ____.
4. People I will ask for support and assistance are ____.
5. The benefits I will receive are ____.
6. My reward at the end of each week will be ____.

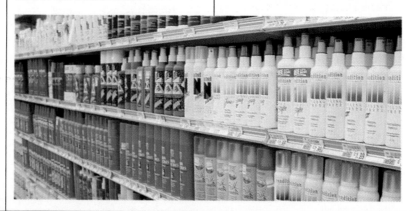

Building Decision-Making Skills

I n March Janet placed an order with ABC, Inc. Two months later, she still had neither heard nor received anything. She tried to contact the sales rep who helped her, but he was at lunch and never returned her phone call. Two weeks later she phoned customer relations to complain about the poor services and request a refund. Finally her order arrived, but it was incomplete. A refund check was enclosed to cover the missing items—but it was $50 more than it should have been. What should Janet do?

WHAT DO YOU THINK?

1. **Choices.** What choices does Janet have?

2. **Consequences.** What are the advantages of each choice?

3. **Consequences.** What are the disadvantages of each choice?

4. **Consequences.** How might Janet's self-esteem be affected by this decision?

5. **Decision.** What do you think Janet should do?

6. **Decision.** Do you think Janet's decision would be different if no one knew about this problem?

7. **Evaluation.** Have you ever had bad service or bought something that was broken or didn't work properly? What did you do? Was your action effective? What could you have done that would have been more effective?

T odd and his friend Joe are in a store looking at stereos. The salesperson asks if they need any help. They both say that they are just looking. The salesperson asks if they know the difference between the two models they're looking at. They shake their heads to indicate that they do not. The salesperson swings into a full-blown presentation complete with a "special deal" where they can charge a stereo and the charge won't appear for 60 days. Todd's mother has a charge account at this store. What should he do?

WHAT DO YOU THINK?

8. **Choices.** What are Todd's choices?

9. **Consequences.** Which of those choices is totally inappropriate? Why?

10. **Consequences.** What are the advantages and disadvantages of each choice

that is not identified as inappropriate?

11. **Consequences.** Who is likely to be affected by this decision?

12. **Decision.** What do you think Todd should do? Why?

13. **Decision.** What would you do if you were Todd?

14. **Evaluation.** Have you ever been in a situation where you were really tempted to buy something you didn't have money for? How did you handle the situation? Would you handle it differently now? Explain your answer.

J oyce and Meg were having lunch at a restaurant. They were seated in the nonsmoking section. Halfway through their meal a customer at the next table started smoking. The smoke was coming right across the girls' table. What should they do?

WHAT DO YOU THINK?

15. **Choices.** What are their choices?

16. **Consequences.** What are the advantages and disadvantages of each choice?

17. **Decision.** What do you think they should do? Why?

Using Health Terms

On a separate sheet of paper, write the term that best matches each definition given below.

LESSON 1

1. One's enthusiastic recommendation of a product.
2. Anyone who uses a product or a service.
3. The ability to state one's needs or wants in a positive, nonthreatening way.
4. The cost of a product per weight, volume, or content.

LESSON 2

5. Substance with no medical value but given for psychological effect.
6. One who dishonestly promotes medical products or treatments.

LESSON 3

7. Items such as sales receipts or canceled checks, which provide proof of a purchase or transaction.
8. A court that handles claims from $100 to $3,000.
9. A nonprofit organization that attempts to settle claims against local businesses.
10. The instruction to remove defective or harmful merchandise from store shelves.
11. A government agency that ensures the safety of foods and food additives other than meat and poultry.

Building Academic Skills

LESSON 3

12. **Reading.** A vital part of being a wise health consumer is deciding who to believe. Ralph Nader is a high-profile consumer advocate. Some people hold Nader in high esteem, others do not. Read an article about or by Ralph Nader. Decide if he is someone you would choose to regard highly. Support your opinion with statements from the information you have gathered.

Recalling the Facts

LESSON 1

13. What affects the price of a product?
14. What rights were given in President John Kennedy's Consumer Bill of Rights? How was it later amended and by whom?
15. What is one drawback of buying products for their convenience?
16. What are three common techniques used in advertising?
17. What does the right to be informed protect consumers from?
18. How might a consumer determine the quality of a product?

LESSON 2

19. What does quackery offer that consumers find difficult to resist?
20. What are some healthy ways to lose weight?

LESSON 3

21. What should a person do if a salesperson is pressuring him or her?
22. What is the Better Business Bureau and what services does it provide?
23. What federal agency ensures that meat and poultry and products made from them are safe?
24. What criteria must be satisfied before the Better Business Bureau considers a complaint settled?
25. How is unfavorable publicity helpful in getting a customer complaint resolved?
26. What are some advantages of going to small-claims court?
27. What federal agency protects consumers against the manufacture and sale of hazardous appliances and toys?
28. Where could you write to obtain more information about false advertising of consumer products?
29. How does the Food and Drug Administration protect the health of consumers?
30. Where should one go first when one is dissatisfied with a product or service?

REVIEW

Thinking Critically

LESSON 1

31. Evaluation. Which right under the Consumer Bill of Rights do you consider the most important? Explain your choice.

32. Synthesis. For two minutes, list all the advertising slogans and/or jingles you can think of. What conclusions can you draw from your list about the nature of advertising?

LESSON 2

33. Evaluation. Can education eliminate quackery? Support your answer.

34. Analysis. What emotions might a person experience if he or she spent money on a quack weight-loss remedy and lost weight but gained all of the weight back in a few months? Explain.

LESSON 3

35. Synthesis. BBBs are sponsored by private businesses. What advantages and disadvantages might there be to this sponsorship?

36. Evaluation. How would you distinguish between an effective complaint and an ineffective complaint?

37. Synthesis. Imagine that you have been cheated out of a large sum of money. Write a letter to a fictitious TV consumer reporter describing what happened. Predict how the problem might be solved "on the air."

Making the Connection

LESSON 1

38. Home Economics. Choose a health-care product and compare the price of that product in several different stores (convenience, specialty, supermarket). Summarize your findings in writing.

39. Math. Assume that all forms of promotion, including advertising, add 27 percent to the cost of the average grocery item. If a nationally advertised brand of paper towel sells for $1.03 a roll, how much should a generic brand sell for?

Applying Health Knowledge

LESSON 1

40. Which of the following is the best way to collect consumer information? Support your answer.
   a. Drive from store to store.
   b. Call various stores, requesting information.
   c. Write to various manufacturers.

41. Think of three purchases you have made recently. Which factors most influenced your decision? Do you feel these were good or bad?

42. Makers of name-brand products pay large sums of money to have their products used in movies. Do you feel this is fair advertising? Should it be permitted?

43. Write two ads about a product or service of your choice. In one, make misleading, faulty claims that attempt to entice the consumer. Write another that is honest and direct.

LESSON 2

44. An old expression is "Laughter is the best medicine." Some people claim to have actually been cured of diseases by watching movies that made them laugh. What do you think of this?

45. If a person became addicted to a placebo, would this be a physiological or psychological addiction? Explain.

46. It is the salesperson's job to ask if a customer needs help. What are some effective ways to decline? Explain.

Beyond the Classroom

LESSON 3

47. Community Involvement. See if your school or local libraries have a current copy of the Consumers Resource Handbook. If they do not, write to Consumer Information Center, Pueblo, Colorado 81009, requesting a copy of this free book or politely ask the librarians to do so.

HEALTH SERVICES AND HEALTH CARE

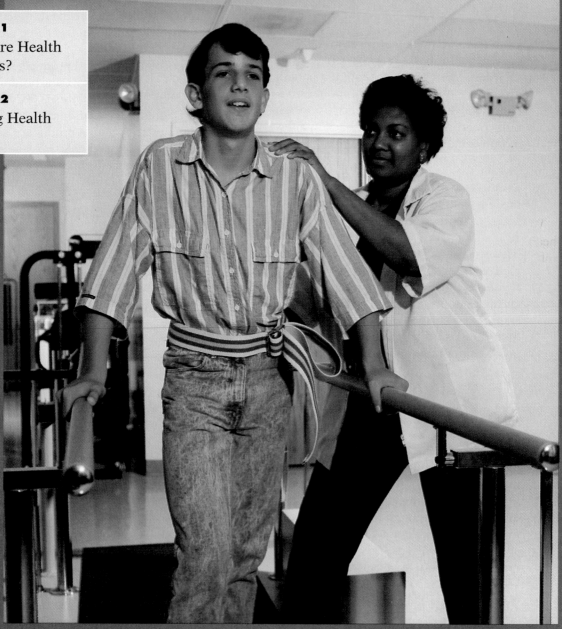

WHAT ARE HEALTH SERVICES?

A focus of health education is to provide health information in such a way that it influences people to take positive action about their health. Health services are another aspect of an overall health program. Health services involve prevention of disease, the maintenance and promotion of health, and the treatment and cure of disease.

The Range of Health Care

The American public spends about $756 billion per year on health care. About 7 million people are employed in some aspect of health-care delivery. The occupations and services range from very large hospitals to mobile vans, from air pollution controls in large cities to tuberculosis checks in small towns.

When a person is vaccinated against a disease that can spread, he or she is involved in preventive health services. People who are engaged in fitness programs are part of a health promotion program, while people who are being treated for cancer or obesity are in treatment or therapeutic types of programs. Health services can also be maintenance-oriented. Health maintenance includes the different types of assessments and examinations that are conducted periodically to make sure that individuals are free from disease.

Whatever the type of health service, it is a major part of the total health picture in the United States. Health service is more commonly referred to as **health-care delivery.**

Many different types of health resources exist in the United States. Health resources are places that people can go for various types of treatment. Think of some health resources in your community. Dentists' and doctors' offices, drugstores, nursing and retirement homes, hospitals, health maintenance organizations, poison-control centers, psychiatric outpatient clinics, public health clinics, mental health centers, suicide-prevention centers, and neighborhood health centers are all examples.

Types of Health Facilities

A **health facility** is a place a person goes to for health care. There are two basic types: facilities for inpatient care and facilities for outpatient care. The differences between inpatients and outpatients are as follows:

- **Inpatients** are people who require prolonged health care and are admitted to a facility and occupy a bed in it. Such people may need nursing service, extensive use of laboratory and X-ray services, or supervised rehabilitation.
- **Outpatients** receive various medical, dental, or other health services in a facility and return home the same day.

LESSON 1 FOCUS

TERMS TO USE
- Health-care delivery
- Health facility
- Inpatients
- Outpatients
- Medicare
- Medicaid

CONCEPTS TO LEARN
- Health care includes many different types of health services.
- Health facilities include hospitals and various kinds of nursing homes.
- Health insurance may be provided by government or private programs.

ATTITUDES AND BEHAVIORS TO EVALUATE
- Self-Inventory, page 666.
- Building Decision-Making Skills, page 667.

FINDING HELP

An RMH, a Ronald McDonald House, is a temporary housing facility for parents and families of children being treated for serious medical problems. Families staying at the house contribute a small donation, except in cases of financial hardship. Community donations help support each house.

The first Ronald McDonald House opened its doors in 1974 in Philadelphia through the joint efforts of the Philadelphia Eagles and McDonald's® Restaurants. It was named the Ronald McDonald House partly because of McDonald's fund-raising support and because of the McDonald's clown, Ronald.

There are over 125 Ronald McDonald Houses in the U.S. For more information, contact McDonald's Corporation, McDonald's Plaza, Oak Brook, IL 60521

Hospitals

The hospital is perhaps the most familiar type of health facility in a community. Hospitals are used for both inpatient and outpatient care and are often centers for education and medical research. Hospitals are often classified according to the length of time patients must stay, the kinds of services provided, and the type of ownership.

■ **Length of stay.** Hospitals can be long- or short-term care facilities. A long-term hospital is one in which patients stay more than 30 days. Having a spinal cord injury would involve a long-term hospital stay. A short-term hospital is one in which most patients stay less that 30 days. Having an appendectomy would involve a short-term stay.

■ **Kinds of services provided.** General hospitals provide health care for most types of illnesses and injuries. Care given at a special hospital is for certain kinds of health needs. A children's hospital is an example of a special hospital. Treating tuberculosis could occur in a hospital that specializes in this disease. Special hospitals also may provide other types of services, such as at a research hospital, where facilities are available for medical research.

■ **Type of ownership.** A nonprofit voluntary hospital may be owned by a church or other charitable group. A community hospital is owned by a community. Neither of these types of hospitals try to make a profit. These hospitals charge fees but also depend on donations to help cover costs of operation.

A private, or proprietary, hospital is operated like a business. This kind of hospital is expected to make a profit for the owners.

A government hospital is owned by federal, state, county, or local government. The staffs at these hospitals provide care for members of the armed forces and their dependents, veterans, and Native Americans. Many state hospitals care for patients who have tuberculosis or are mentally ill. Some county and local hospitals serve people who are economically disadvantaged and live near the hospital.

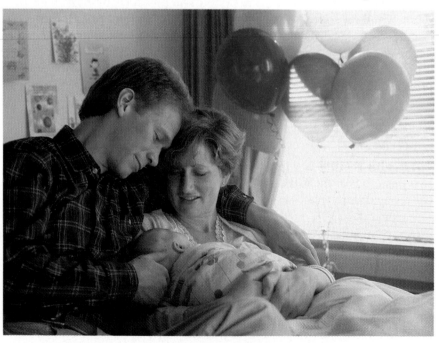

General hospitals provide health care for newborns and new mothers.

Other Health-Care Facilities

Other types of long-term health-care facilities are available. The following are the most common.

Nursing homes. Nursing homes are facilities in which care is provided for medical and nonmedical needs. Though most residents are 65 years of age or older, these facilities are used for people of all ages. A person with a serious, long-term illness or recovering from surgery may live at a nursing home. Some nursing homes are private and are run to make a profit. Others are nonprofit and may be owned by a church or other group.

There are basically three types of nursing home care. With personal residential care, the following is provided: assisted living in a sheltered environment, meals, and routine medical care and supervision, including use of medicines. A nursing home with intermediate care provides basic nursing care. Residents receive medical examinations more routinely. Programs for physical and speech therapy also may be provided. Social activities are planned for residents. At a skilled nursing facility, most of the residents have serious medical illnesses or disabilities. Consequently, medical care is needed more frequently. Twenty-four-hour nursing care is provided.

Health Insurance

Health insurance is a plan to pay for part or most costs of medical expenses and care associated with illness or disability. These costs can include medical tests, surgery, hospitalization, physician care, and medicines. Disability income insurance provides income for a period of time if a person is unable to continue working because of an illness or disability.

A person who is insured pays a premium, or fee, for insurance. This fee for the policy is paid either out-of-pocket, or through payroll deduction as part of a group plan with his or her place of employment. Health insurance plans vary widely, but there are two basic kinds of health insurance available—government programs and private programs.

Government Health Insurance

Medicare is a health insurance program that is available to people who are 65 years of age and older and to people who receive social security disability benefits. Taxes help cover the two parts of Medicare—hospital and medical insurance. Medicare covers costs of hospital or nursing home care. Additional Medicare insurance can be bought to help pay physicians and other costs. The patient is responsible for any uncovered balance.

Some people who receive Medicare also are eligible for Medicaid. **Medicaid** is an assistance program of medical aid for people of all ages who are unable to financially afford medical care. This includes people with low incomes who have dependent children, people with high medical costs in relation to their income, or people who are disabled.

Medicaid benefits vary from state to state in the United States. Types of cases that may be paid for by Medicaid include crack babies, AIDS patients, and nursing home patients. Medicaid is paid for through federal and state taxes and covers both physician and hospital fees.

Worker's compensation is insurance to cover costs of injury or illness that is job-related. Compensation may be made to cover lost wages or to a family in case of death. Employers pay the cost of worker's compensation insurance.

Private Health Insurance

There are two basic kinds of private health insurance programs—individual and group. A person may choose an individual program if he or she does not qualify for a group program or has health needs that cannot be met in a group plan or if a group program is not available. In individual health insurance programs, the individual pays the premium himself or herself.

In group plans, employers offer an insurance plan as part of a job benefit. Group plans also may include the insured person's spouse and children. The employer usually pays a portion of the premium. The premiums for group plans are usually lower than for individual plans because more people are covered in the plan, and the charge per person can be less for administrative costs. To keep costs as low as possible, most insurance policies have a deductible that must be met and paid for each year by the insured before the insurance company will begin to pay the balance of medical charges. Usually, the higher the deductible, the lower the premium of the health insurance.

KEEPING FIT

Adolescent Health Centers

Traditionally teens have been left out of the health-care system. Usually until age 12, patients visited a pediatrician. After that, they would visit either a family doctor or a specialist to deal with specific problems. There is a critical need for teaching teens lifelong health strategies. Adolescent clinics are a new option that helps meet this need. At best, adolescent health centers help teens get health care in an atmosphere that treats them as individuals with dignity and a capacity for self-cure. Across the country adolescent health centers come in many varieties, ranging from experimental drop-in centers to programs that are an offshoot of established children's hospitals.

Overcoming The Odds

Dr. Francisco Murphy-Rivera is a resident in family practice. He was graduated from the Universidad Central del Caribe, Cayey, Puerto Rico in 1991. He loves to spend the little free time he has with his wife and five-month-old twin daughters, Laura and Lourdes.

"All my life, I wanted to be a doctor," he begins. "I always told my mother I was going to be a doctor. All my games as a child had to do with this."

He continues, "Coming here was not easy. In Puerto Rico, there are good family practice residencies. My wife already had a good job. We had our own house, our families. When we decided to come to the U.S., we came alone by ourselves. We didn't know anyone. Then, twenty days after my residency started, my babies were born. But we have a very positive attitude. Having this positive attitude makes us remember that things could be worse. We have all the necessities."

Dr. Murphy-Rivera is committed to the idea of family practice. "Family practice is a specialty concerned with the continuous care of the patient from womb to tomb," he explains. "Family practice is concerned with how the patient is doing physically,

emotionally, and psychologically. It also means treating a patient as part of a total family system."

But being a family doctor is not always easy. Dr. Murphy-Rivera talks about the odds

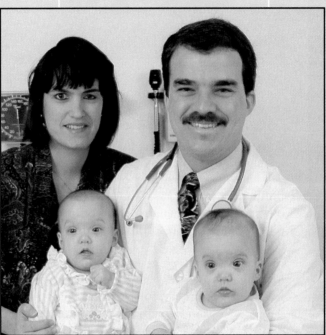

that many family practitioners today have to face. "There are too few family physicians in the U.S.," he says. "In some states there are a lot, but there is poor distribution. Some doctors don't want the 24-hour-a-day commitment. Others have amazing loans to repay for their medical educations and choose to go into specialties that pay more for this and other reasons."

With his busy schedule, Dr. Murphy-Rivera often gets only 5 or 6 hours of sleep each night. And he spends many

hours, sometimes even days, away from his family. He says, "It can be 48 to 56 hours before I see them again. But when I arrive home, I try to be with them as much as possible."

Dr. Murphy-Rivera concludes, "So many people care only about knowledge. But knowledge alone isn't enough. There are basic abilities that I think are very important for a doctor to have. They are to establish a good doctor-patient rapport, to communicate effectively, and to be a good listener. I also think that people have to think that in a way they are the real doctors. There's no reason for me to take care of you if you don't take care of yourself. People have to be more involved with their own health care. We are not here just to heal conditions," he says. "We are here to prevent people from getting sick."

1. What are the personal odds that Dr. Murphy-Rivera has overcome?
2. What three basic abilities does he think every doctor should have?
3. How would you sum up Dr. Murphy-Rivera's philosophy of medicine? Is his approach to medicine and his patients one that appeals to you?

Fighting Tuberculosis

Annie Dodge Wauneka, a Navajo, grew up on a reservation where tuberculosis, TB, was a major cause of death. Annie was elected to the Tribal Council and appointed chairperson of the health committee. She wrote a Navajo-English medical dictionary, and convinced Navajo healers to work with nonNavajo doctors. Through her efforts, many Navajo began to get X rays and treatment. In 1963 she was awarded the Freedom Award by President Kennedy for her war against TB. She also received the name of "Warrior Who Scouts The Enemy" from the Navajo people.

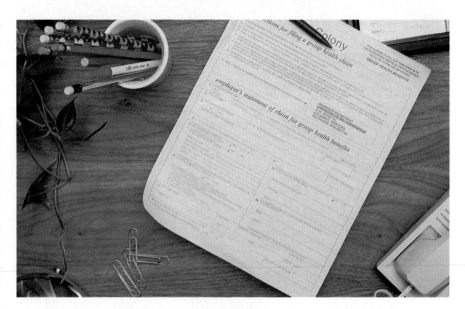

Health insurance claim forms can be confusing to fill out.

Insurance policies can be difficult to read and understand. Many consumers are not sure exactly what their insurance covers. It may come as a surprise to many consumers to discover that the insurance policy covers only a small portion of the medical bill. Some plans provide only minimal coverage. Hospital coverage is likely to be for a limited number of days. Other plans are quite comprehensive and may include coverage of dental bills, prescription drugs, and various kinds of psychiatric counseling.

The important point to remember for you as a consumer is to treat health insurance like any other purchase. Use your consumer skills. Read everything carefully before signing any agreement. Ask questions if you do not understand. Compare several different companies' prices and coverage.

LESSON 1 REVIEW

Reviewing Facts and Vocabulary

1. What is the primary concern of health services?
2. Explain what health insurance is and what may be covered.
3. What are the two parts of Medicare?

Thinking Critically

4. **Analysis.** Compare and contrast the three different types of hospitals.
5. **Evaluation.** Read current articles concerning health-care delivery in the United States. Summarize in a short report what you think is good about the system and what are some of the problems.

Applying Health Knowledge

6. Interview several adults about their reasons for selecting the health insurance they have. Find out what their policy deductible is. Find out what their insurance provides for them.
7. Find out what Medicaid benefits are available in your state. Discover the criteria used in order to grant Medicaid benefits.

LESSON 2

SEEKING HEALTH CARE

Today we have many facilities and medical specialists to care for our needs and to help us live longer. Presently, we have three major stages of health care and hundreds of different specialists in the health-care field.

Stages of Health Care

Following are the three stages of health care:

- Primary care. If you get sick and call a doctor, most likely you call a general practitioner, a doctor who is in family practice. This kind of care, which the patient seeks on his or her own, is called primary care. It most often takes place in a doctor's office or a clinic.
- Secondary care. If a primary-care doctor refers a patient to a specialist, this is secondary care. Secondary care may involve a stay in a hospital for more extensive testing than could be received in a clinic or a doctor's office.
- Tertiary care. When a patient's condition requires specialized equipment or treatment, this is tertiary care. This type of care takes place at hospitals equipped with special technology. Examples of tertiary care include kidney dialysis treatment, heart or brain surgery, and cancer or burn treatment.

Forms of Medical Practice

Traditionally, the doctor has been the central figure in the delivery of health care in the United States. Most doctors are in **private practice;** that is, they are self-employed, functioning in individual practices, operating out of their own offices, and not sharing personnel, facilities, or income with any other doctor.

The Specialist

Doctors work generally in five major clinical areas: internal medicine, obstetrics and gynecology, pediatrics, psychiatry, and surgery. These primary-care areas are further broken down into secondary or specialty areas. For example, under internal medicine, there is a specialist who diagnoses and treats almost every organ or system of the body. Some of the most common specialists are as follows:

- Allergist. Diagnoses and treats patients for asthma, hay fever, hives, and other allergies.
- Anesthesiologist. Administers anesthetics (drugs that cause insensitivity to pain) during surgery; checks the patient's condition before, during, and after surgery.

LESSON 2 FOCUS

TERMS TO USE
- Private practice
- Group practice
- Health maintenance organization (HMO)
- Hospice

CONCEPTS TO LEARN
- There are three stages of health care: primary, secondary, and tertiary.
- To choose a health care professional, you need to understand the various forms of medical practice.
- Many changes are occurring in the delivery of health care.

ATTITUDES AND BEHAVIORS TO EVALUATE
- Self-Inventory, page 666.
- Building Decision-Making Skills, page 667.

DID YOU KNOW?

- Like some fast-food restaurants, an emergency room at Doctors Hospital in Detroit, Michigan, promises that if you aren't seen within 20 minutes, your treatment will be free.
- Many schools have a school nurse. But some high schools now also have health centers. Students can use these by applying and with written parental permission. The centers are staffed by social workers, nurse practitioners, part-time physicians, dieticians, and mental health professionals.
- According to the Association of Independent Colleges and Schools, four of the five fastest-growing occupations in the '90s involve health care. These are medical assistant, physical therapist, physical therapy assistant, and home health aide.

- Cardiologist. Diagnoses and treats heart diseases.
- Dermatologist. Diagnoses and treats all forms of skin problems.
- Endocrinologist. Diagnoses and treats problems related to the endocrine glands.
- Gastroenterologist. Treats gastrointestinal (stomach and intestinal) disorders.
- Gynecologist. Diagnoses and treats problems related to female reproductive organs.
- Neurologist. Diagnoses and treats problems of the central and peripheral nervous systems.
- Obstetrician. Specializes in all aspects of childbirth—care of the mother before, during, and after delivery.
- Ophthalmologist. Diagnoses and corrects eye problems.
- Orthopedic surgeon. Performs surgery on bones and joints.
- Otolaryngologist. Treats ear, nose, and throat disorders.
- Otologist. Treats ear problems.
- Pathologist. Carries out laboratory tests of body tissues and fluids; studies the causes of death.
- Pediatrician. Specializes in the medical care of children.
- Plastic surgeon. Treats skin and soft tissue deformities; performs surgery to improve external features.
- Psychiatrist. Treats mental and emotional disorders.
- Radiologist. Examines and treats patients by using X rays and radium therapy.
- Thoracic surgeon. Performs surgery on the chest and the lungs.
- Vascular surgeon. Performs surgery on the heart and the blood vessels.
- Urologist. Treats disorders of the urinary tract (kidneys, ureters, urethra); also treats problems of the male reproductive organs.

Group Practice

While group practice has existed for many years, it has become more popular in recent years because of the rising costs involved in setting up

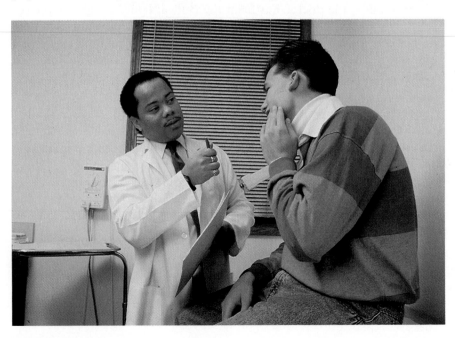

A dermatologist may be able to alleviate the problems associated with teenage acne.

660　CHAPTER 33 HEALTH SERVICES AND HEALTH CARE

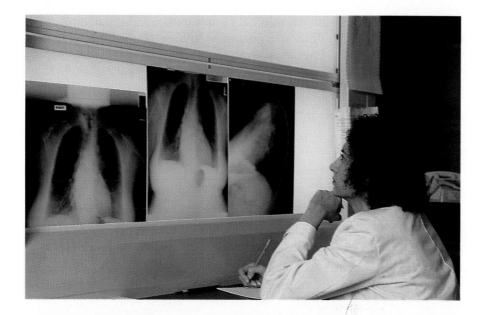

CHOOSING A HEALTH-CARE PROFESSIONAL

As you begin to take a more active and responsible role in promoting your personal health and wellness, it is important that you choose a health-care professional who will work with you in your efforts. The best time to select a health-care professional is before you need one. Following are some guidelines for selecting a health-care professional:

- Ask a number of people for recommendations.
- Use the yellow pages of the phone directory, in which doctors are categorized by their specialties.
- Call your local medical society. Most medical societies will provide three names, chosen in rotation from the society's membership roster.
- Ask your local librarian or consumer protection agency if a directory of doctors has been compiled for your community. It will provide detailed information about doctors.
- When you have compiled a list of several possible health-care providers, prepare a list of questions you would like answered, and call the office of each person to get the information you need to make your decision.

and maintaining a medical practice. The rapid advances in medicine and the demand for specialization also make this option more attractive today than in former years.

Group practice is an arrangement in which two or more doctors join together to provide medical care. They diagnose through consultation and treat through the joint use of equipment, support staff, and funds for the maintenance and development of the practice.

Health Maintenance Organizations

When you go to doctors who are in private practice or in a group practice, you pay for their services each time you use them. Another option is now available to consumers—a **health maintenance organization (HMO).** HMOs stress preventive medicine in an attempt to reduce the high cost of medical care. Preventive medicine involves the consumer taking personal responsibility for his or her own health.

Consumers pay regular fees and then are entitled to receive medical care for little or no additional cost. Consumers choose doctors who belong to the HMO. This may limit a person's choice of a doctor. However, within the HMO, a wide range of doctors and specialists is provided.

Members of HMOs are guaranteed treatment when they need it. HMOs save money by emphasizing preventive medicine and treatment for patients who do not need to be hospitalized—thus using expensive hospital care less often.

Trends in the Delivery of Health Care

In the last few years, other types of health-care outlets have developed. These outlets are designed to meet the needs of people who are not covered by other health-care supports. The people who receive service in these centers often make too much money to qualify for government medical benefits, but they do not make enough money to purchase their own private health insurance. Chief among these outlets are the following:

■ Adolescent health centers. Most of these centers are located in large cities. They are designed specifically to deal with problems relating to adolescence. These clinics address adolescents' physical, mental, and social health. The practitioners, for the most part, specialize in adolescent medicine.

■ Holistic health centers. These centers look at health in terms of the total person and put together a wellness plan for what an individual can do to improve personal health.

■ Neighborhood health centers. These centers are designed to meet local needs, particularly those of ethnic and social groups who have difficulty gaining access to existing health-care programs.

■ Alternative maternal-care birthing centers. Over 60 of these facilities exist throughout the United States. They are designed primarily to offer a homelike atmosphere, substantial savings on delivery costs, and opportunities to involve the entire family in the delivery of a baby.

■ Hospice care. Care for the terminally ill is becoming part of the mainstream of the health-care delivery system. The **hospice** provides a way of caring for the dying, not just a place where the dying are cared for. It unites the best techniques that have been devised for pain and symptom management with the provision of loving care.

K E E P I N G   F I T

Questions to Ask About Your Doctor

■ Does he or she make you feel valued?
■ Does he or she listen to you carefully?
■ Do you feel comfortable with him or her?
■ Does he or she seem to give you adequate time and attention?
■ Does he or she give thorough exams?
■ Does he or she ask you for information relating to your health problem?
■ Does he or she respond to and even encourage your questions and comments?
■ Does he or she encourage you to take an active part in your own health care?
■ Does he or she encourage you to exercise preventive medicine?

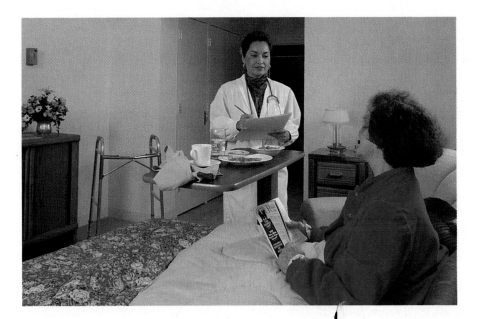

The following list describes characteristics of almost all hospice care outlets:

- They are open 24 hours a day.
- They provide a variety of services by health-care professionals.
- Hospice patients and their families are a central part of the care team.
- Volunteers are an integral part of the program.
- Emphasis is on optimal control of pain and other symptoms.
- A qualified doctor medically directs the programs.
- Programs provide inpatient and home care as needed.

ARE YOU IN CHARGE OF YOUR OWN HEALTH?

Throughout this book our discussions have centered on your taking an active role in preventing disease and in maintaining and promoting your own health. Each time you deal with a health concern, however, you need to know whose help, if any, you need. The list below will help you evaluate a given situation—but the key to successfully evaluating a health problem is being an informed consumer.

- Call an ambulance or rescue squad only if a situation is life-threatening or if the patient needs hospital care but cannot reach the hospital by car. Many communities as well as privately owned ambulance services charge for ambulance runs.
- Call your doctor's office when you need advice on whether to go to the hospital emergency room or when a condition for which you are being treated takes a bad turn. If you cannot reach your doctor, call a local emergency number and try to have an ambulance take you to the hospital with which your doctor is associated.
- Many large private clinics and HMOs staff their off-hour phones with nurses specially trained to give self-care information and to record questions and symptoms so that the doctor is well-informed when he or she returns your call.
- Call your doctor's office during regular hours when you need to ask if a problem requires an office visit or if you can get instructions for home treatment. You may be able to get assistance from a nurse practitioner, an office nurse, or a doctor's assistant.

Know how to respond to a health problem. Call emergency help if a situation is life-threatening.

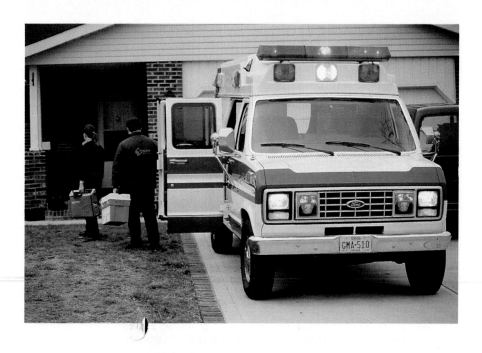

CONFLICT RESOLUTION

Last month, 16-year-old Raul spent the weekend home alone when his parents took a trip. While they were away, Raul developed severe stomach cramps, vomiting, and diarrhea. He wanted to call someone to stay with him or even take him to the hospital, but he was afraid his parents wouldn't allow him to stay home alone again. He also thought about how foolish he'd feel going to the emergency room just to find out he had a stomach virus. He wished he knew the difference between flu and food poisoning.

Where could Raul have called for information and to see if he needed medical attention?

HEALTH UPDATE

LOOKING AT TECHNOLOGY

What's Coming in Health Care?

There are many kinds of technology currently being considered, researched, or tested that may make great differences in Americans' health in the future. Among the new technologies are the following:

- "Computerized patients" may be used within the next ten years as part of medical students' training. Computer-generated hypothetical, or made-up, patients will be presented to students, including complete medical histories and current symptoms. Using voice commands, the medical student will be able to order tests, get results, diagnose, and propose treatments. When the process is over, the computer will evaluate the student's performance and the outcome for the "patient."

- Artificial organs will be developed using a combination of living cells and synthetic materials. This will decrease the need for organ donors and save the lives of the many people who need transplanted human organs but cannot get them.

- Antibodies that prevent clogged arteries may undo the need for much surgery that now removes arterial blockages. A new study using rats shows that the use of an antibody that neutralizes the buildup of such blockages may keep their arteries clear.

- Artificial blood is now being tested in clinical trials but does not yet have FDA approval. This "blood" will be especially useful for those people who refuse transfusions of human blood for religious reasons or because of fear of blood-transmitted infections.

The Consumer and Health Care

The demand for health care far exceeds available services. As a consumer, what can you do to relieve some of this demand on the health-care system? The most important thing you can do is take greater responsibility in protecting and promoting your own health. You can take greater responsibility in preventing disease by examining your life-style. Many health problems are related to life-style factors, such as food choices and amount of exercise a person gets.

By supporting health education programs in your school and community, you can help people learn about their bodies and their health. Health education programs also teach people the skills to make good choices. This provides the basis for individual responsibility in the protection and promotion of health. Health education programs also provide new and current information on preventive health care.

Knowing is not enough; people must act on the information they have to reduce health risks. Consider these questions:

- What good does it do to know that seat belts save lives if people sit on their belts?
- What good does it do to know that cervical cancer can be detected through Pap smears if women fail to have such tests performed on a regular basis?
- What good does it do to be aware of the mounting evidence that smoking is a direct cause of cancer and heart disease if people continue to smoke?

The health-care delivery system cannot be expected to care for your health if you are not willing to invest in your own health care. You must see the relationship between yourself and the health-care system as a partnership, with both committed and motivated to care for and be responsible for your health.

LESSON 2 REVIEW

Reviewing Facts and Vocabulary

1. Name the differences between primary, secondary, and tertiary care.
2. What are the major clinical specialties?
3. What is meant by *HMO?* Describe the service.

Thinking Critically

4. **Synthesis.** Develop a set of criteria for selecting a doctor or a dentist. Compare your list with your classmates' lists.
5. **Analysis.** Consider the differences between a specialist and a general practitioner. Highlight the advantages and disadvantages of each type of doctor.

Applying Health Knowledge

6. Make a list of the health services and health facilities in your community. Using the public health department as a resource, try to determine whether the facilities are adequate. What are the most pressing health-care needs in your area?
7. During the 1800s scientists made many important discoveries in the field of medicine. Choose a scientific discovery from this time, and discuss its impact on your health today.

Self-Inventory

Are You an Advocate for Your Own Health?

HOW DO YOU RATE?

Number a sheet of paper from 1 through 20. Read each item below and respond with a *yes* or *no*. Total the number of *yes* responses. Then proceed to the next section.

1. I eat a healthy diet.
2. I get enough sleep and rest.
3. I get regular exercise.
4. I use stress-management techniques.
5. I share my feelings with others.
6. I wear a seat belt and exercise other kinds of safety consciousness.
7. I do not use alcohol or other drugs.
8. I read the instructions carefully before taking any medicine.
9. I practice regular and proper health care.
10. I avoid situations that put my health at risk.
11. I get regular medical checkups.
12. I have been immunized against the common communicable diseases.
13. If I feel myself getting sick, I take some immediate action.
14. I have a medical doctor or other source of medical care that I can call for help or advice.
15. I am honest and thorough in communicating with my doctor(s).
16. I consider myself to be an active partner along with my doctor(s) in my medical care.
17. I am not afraid to tell my doctor(s) what I think is wrong or that I disagree with him or her.
18. I have a good relationship with my doctor(s).
19. I make certain I understand what my doctor is saying and what kind of treatment plan I am to follow.
20. If my family had no family doctor, or I could not get in touch with the doctor, I would be able to contact an appropriate substitute.

HOW DID YOU SCORE?

Give yourself 1 point for each *yes* response. Find your total and read below to see how you scored. Then proceed to the next section.

18 to 20
Excellent. You are taking very good care of your health.

15 to 17
Good. You are taking good care of your health.

12 to 14
Fair. You are taking only fair care of your health.

Below 12
Look out! You are not taking an active role in your own health care.

WHAT ARE YOUR GOALS?

If you scored 15 or higher, complete the statements in Part A. If you scored 14 or below, complete the statements in Part B. Regardless of your score, complete Part C.

Part A

1. One way in which I can become more active in my own health care is ____.
2. The steps I will take to become more active include ____.
3. My time frame for taking these steps will be ____.
4. My reward for taking these steps will be ____.

Part B

5. The reason I do not get medical care is ____.
6. The steps that I will take to try to get adequate medical care include ____.
7. The people, organizations, or other resources I will use to try to get this medical care include ____.
8. My time frame for accomplishing this goal is ____.
9. My reward for taking these actions on behalf of my own health will be ____.

Part C

10. One area in which I want to improve my communication or relationship with my doctor(s) is ____.
11. The steps I will take to make this improvement are ____.
12. My time frame for taking these steps is ____.
13. My health rewards for doing so will be ____.

Building Decision-Making Skills

J eff made an appointment with his family doctor because he has had a cold and sore throat for several days. The doctor examined him, took a throat culture, and gave Jeff two prescriptions. Jeff doesn't know what the medicines are expected to do or if they are available as generic brands. What should Jeff do before he leaves the doctor's office?

WHAT DO YOU THINK?

1. **Situation.** Why does Jeff need to make a decision?
2. **Situation.** How much time does Jeff have to decide?
3. **Choices.** What choices does Jeff have?

4. **Consequences.** How might Jeff's health triangle be affected by his decision?
5. **Consequences.** What are the advantages and disadvantages of each choice?
6. **Decision.** What do you think Jeff should do? Explain your answer.

7. **Evaluation.** Have you ever been in a situation in which you did not want to show your ignorance by asking questions? What decision did you make? Would you make the same decision again? Why or why not?

A few years ago, Melissa's father was in a car accident and now wears an artificial leg, which is getting very worn. He needs a new one. The cost of a new artificial leg is very high. Her father is now old enough to receive Medicare, but payments from Medicare do not cover the full cost. Melissa's family has no supplemental insurance or savings to make up the cost difference. What might Melissa do to help?

WHAT DO YOU THINK?

8. **Situation.** Why does a decision need to be made?
9. **Choices.** What choices does Melissa have?

10. **Consequences.** What are the advantages of each choice?
11. **Consequences.** What are the disadvantages of each choice?

12. **Consequences** How might Melissa's future be affected with each choice?
13. **Decision.** What do you think Melissa should do?

J uan's grandmother is in a nursing home. Juan thinks one of the LPNs who is assigned to his grandmother treats her poorly. She does not give the same care to his grandmother as Juan sees her give other patients. Because of his concern, Juan is trying to spend more time with his grandmother to make up for the nurse's lack of care. He was really angry, though, when he came to see his grandmother one afternoon last week. She was feeling very weak. Juan discovered that the nurse had not given his grandmother her lunch until very late. Juan's grandmother is diabetic and needs to eat regular meals. What should Juan do?

WHAT DO YOU THINK?

14. **Situation.** Why does a decision need to be made?
15. **Choices.** What choices are there to consider?

16. **Consequences.** What are the advantages and disadvantages of each choice?
17. **Decision.** What do you think Juan should do?

18. **Evaluation.** Have you ever had to confront a person in authority? If so, describe the situation and the outcome. What did you learn from that situation?

REVIEW

Using Health Terms

On a separate sheet of paper, write the term that best matches each definition given below.

LESSON 1

1. A place a person goes to receive health care.
2. People who receive prolonged health care and who are admitted to a health-care facility and occupy a bed there.
3. A type of nursing home that houses residents with serious medical illnesses.
4. Assistance program of medical aid for people who are unable to afford medical care.
5. Government health insurance for people 65 and older and for people who receive social security disability benefits.

LESSON 2

6. Health care that patients seek on their own.
7. The medical practice of a doctor who is self-employed.
8. A doctor who treats heart diseases.
9. A doctor who treats skin problems.
10. A situation in which two or more doctors work together to provide medical care.
11. A place that promotes a special way of caring for people who are dying.

Building Academic Skills

LESSON 1

12. **Writing.** Rewrite the following sentence using appropriate spelling, capitalization, and punctuation.

    One of the leding cauzes of Bankrupcty in the united states is the cost, of medical kare.

LESSON 2

13. **Reading.** In which of the following sentences does *committed* mean devoted?
    a. Claire is committed to improving her health triangle.
    b. Two witnesses said that a man wearing a ski mask committed the crime.

Recalling the Facts

LESSON 1

14. Label each of the following patients *outpatient* or *inpatient*.
    a. Dr. Ibani performs arthroscopy on Leonard Seaton at 10:00 A.M. on Thursday. Len and his wife go out to dinner that evening.
    b. Juanita spends two hours in her dentist's office on Monday having her wisdom teeth removed.
    c. Mrs. Jackson's labor pains begin at 8:00 P.M. on Saturday. Mr. Jackson drives her to the hospital. The baby is born at 7:00 A.M. on Sunday. Mr. and Mrs. Jackson bring their new baby home on Tuesday.
15. Who receives care from the staffs at government hospitals?
16. Explain the difference between long- and short-term care hospitals.
17. Explain how a nonprofit voluntary hospital is operated.

LESSON 2

18. What does an anesthesiologist do?
19. What kind of specialist should a pregnant female see?
20. Mrs. Marcello requires cataract surgery. What kind of specialist is likely to perform the surgery?
21. Should a person with a bladder infection consult a urologist or a radiologist?
22. What are two ways in which health maintenance organizations try to keep down the costs of health care?
23. Number the following steps that describe actions you might take for an injury or illness. Number the least serious action 1 and the most serious 5.
    a. Go to the nearest emergency room.
    b. Take care of the problem yourself.
    c. Call a physician during office hours.
    d. Go to a 24-hour clinic or a nonhospital emergency facility.
    e. Call an ambulance.

REVIEW

Thinking Critically

24. Analysis. How are general hospitals different from special hospitals? How are they the same?

25. Evaluation. What is the importance of health insurance?

26. Analysis. Label each of the following types of health care *primary*, *secondary*, or *tertiary*.

a. Sam has had what he believes is a bad cold. He calls his doctor, who tells him to take two aspirin and call him in the morning.

b. In the morning, Sam feels no better. His doctor makes an appointment for him with an allergist. The allergist cannot find any substance to which Sam is allergic.

c. Sam visits a psychiatrist. She decides his problems are not psychological.

d. Sam makes an appointment with an otolaryngologist. Dr. Hillman finds that Sam has a tumor, which may be cancerous.

e. Sam undergoes surgery to remove the tumor at a special cancer hospital in another state.

27. Analysis. What are the advantages and disadvantages of an HMO?

Making the Connection

28. Social Studies. Health care in the United States is among the best in the world, but it is also the most expensive. In countries where health care is free or more reasonably priced, patients may not choose their own doctors and may have to wait for care. Some specialized care may not be available to everyone. Is it better to have good care at high cost for some or minimal care for everyone at low cost? Explain your answer.

Applying Health Knowledge

29. Label each activity below as *health promotion*, *prevention*, *maintenance*, or *treatment*.

a. eating properly every day

b. not smoking

c. getting a flu shot

d. walking two miles three times a week

e. taking an antibiotic for an infection

f. having your teeth and gums examined by a dentist twice a year

g. dieting to reduce being overweight

30. Your grandfather is basically healthy, but he is no longer strong enough for the physical labor of housekeeping and yard work. He does not take any medications. What kind of nursing home facility might best fit your grandfather's needs? Why did you choose the facility you did?

31. Explain how prevention, maintenance, and treatment are related in a person's total health picture.

32. How would you interpret the following statement in relation to taking responsibility for your own health?

The doctor cannot do what the patient will not do.

Beyond the Classroom

33. Further Study. Interview someone who works in a health-care field. The person could be your family doctor, a nurse, or the pharmacist where you get your prescriptions filled. Find out what the person likes and dislikes about his or her work and what the requirements are for the particular job. Report to your class.

34. Community Involvement. Join the volunteer program at a health-service facility in your community.

CHAPTER

34 YOUR SAFETY AND WELL-BEING

LESSON 1
Safety at Home

LESSON 2
Safety Away from Home

LESSON 3
Safety on Wheels

LESSON 4
Personal Safety

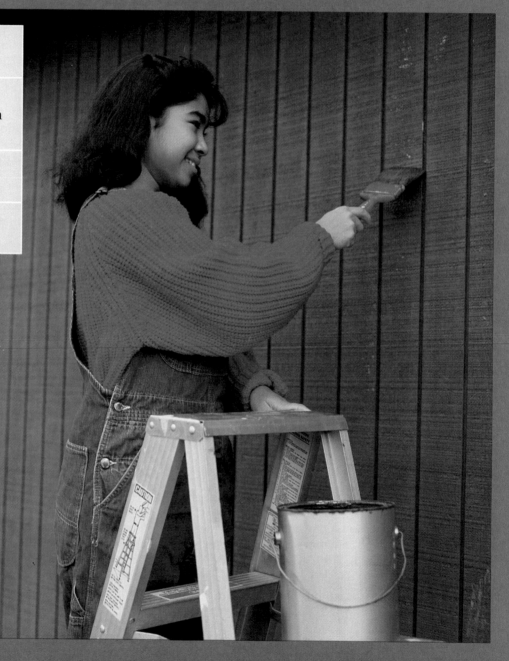

SAFETY AT HOME

Home should be the one place where you can feel safe and secure. Yet every year thousands of people are injured as a result of home accidents. These cause more disabling injuries than any other type of accident. Many are the result of hazards, such as objects carelessly placed or in poor condition.

Falls

Falls happen to people of all ages. They are the leading cause of accidental death and injury among the elderly. Small children, exploring on their own, are also at risk of injury. Although falls are not usually serious, in some instances they can be deadly.

Stairs are the most dangerous area in the home and the site of about one million injuries yearly in the United States. All stairways, indoors and out, should be well-lighted, in good repair, and equipped with sturdy handrails. Steps should have nonskid strips or well-fitting carpet.

Tripping hazards are a common cause of easily prevented falls. A loose rug is always a danger; if a room is not carpeted, area and throw rugs should be firmly fastened to the floor.

Bathtubs and showers also can be a source of falls. The use of safety rails and nonskid mats can help prevent these types of accidents.

People of all ages should avoid the temptation to use chairs, boxes, or other makeshift ladders to reach items on high shelves. Instead, a sturdy stepladder should be used.

Fire

What needs to be present in order for a fire to take place? That may seem like a simple question, but a very important set of elements must be present for a fire to start. By understanding that these three elements—fuel, heat, and air—must be present to make a fire burn, you have the basis of fire prevention.

Fuel for a fire can be carelessly stored rags, wood, coal, oil, gasoline, or paper. However, there still will not be a fire unless there is some heat to make the fuel burn. A heat source could be a match, an electrical wire, or a cigarette. Still there can be no fire unless air is present. The oxygen in the air feeds and fans the flames. If you remove any one of these elements, there can be no fire.

Fire Safety Devices

Because household fires kill thousands of people each year, it is essential that each home is equipped with two life-saving devices: a smoke detector and a fire extinguisher.

LESSON 1 FOCUS

TERMS TO USE
- Smoke detector
- Fire extinguisher

CONCEPTS TO LEARN
- A smoke alarm and fire extinguisher should be placed on every level of the home.
- Most fire deaths result from smoke inhalation rather than burns.

ATTITUDES AND BEHAVIORS TO EVALUATE
- Self-Inventory, page 688.
- Building Decision-Making Skills, page 689.

Smoke detectors save lives.

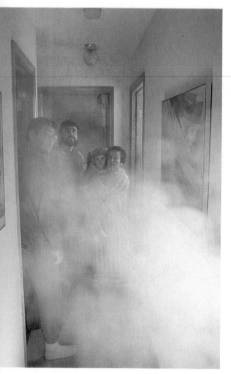

FIRE SAFETY PRECAUTIONS

The majority of home fires can be prevented if the following fire safety tips are observed.

Space Heaters
- Every gas or fuel-burning space heater must be properly vented, unless the unit is specifically designed to be unvented. In that case, make certain a window or door is opened slightly in the room in which the unit is operating.
- All space heaters should have tip-over shutoff switches and protective grilles around heating elements.
- Use only heavy-duty extension cords that match the electrical requirements of electric space heaters.

Matches and Lighters
- Keep matches and lighters where children cannot find them.
- Fill lighters in a well-ventilated area, away from flames. Try to avoid spills; if a spill occurs, wipe it up immediately.

Flammable Liquids
- Store gasoline outside the house and well away from ignition sources.
- Store gasoline only in containers designed specifically for this purpose.
- Never use gasoline for cleaning machine parts, clothing, or any other item.
- Use only fluids labeled as charcoal starters to light outdoor grills. Never throw any flammable liquid on a burning or smoldering fire.
- Use caution and observe good safety rules with other flammable liquids, such as nail polish remover, kerosene, rubbing alcohol, and paint thinner.

Upholstered Furniture
- Keep upholstered furniture away from stoves, ranges, space heaters, and fireplaces.
- Caution cigarette smokers against smoking when sitting on upholstered furniture, especially if the smoker is drowsy. A burning cigarette can be especially hazardous if the smoker is drinking alcohol or has been taking medication.

Clothing
- Do not wear loose-fitting long sleeves or full skirts around flames or a stove.
- Thin, lightweight fabrics ignite quicker than heavy, tightly woven fabrics like denim.
- By law, children's sleepwear (up to size 14) must be flame-resistant.

Smoke Detectors. The greatest danger from home fires occurs during the night when families are asleep. A **smoke detector** is an alarm used to awaken people and alert them in the event of smoke or flames. This device, mounted on a ceiling, sounds loudly if smoke passes into it. Smoke detectors are now recommended to be installed in new homes. They are economical to buy and easy to install. It is recommended that smoke detectors be placed on every level of the home, especially near sleeping areas. A smoke detector should be tested after it is installed and again at monthly intervals.

Fire Extinguishers. Each home should have a **fire extinguisher** on each floor. This is a portable device that puts out small fires by ejecting fire-extinguishing chemicals. If you are confident that you can control a fire quickly with an extinguisher, use it promptly and properly. Stand away from the flames, aim at the source of the fire, not at the flames, and move the spray from side to side. If there is any doubt at all, forget the extinguisher, get out of the house, and call the fire department.

When selecting a fire extinguisher for the home, be certain that you and your family understand the manufacturer's specifications and directions. Check the dial on the equipment periodically to be certain that it still has sufficient pressure to be useful in an emergency.

Fire Safety Actions

Most deaths caused by fire result from smoke inhalation rather than burns. Inhaling toxic fumes is not what kills, but rather the lack of oxygen. The chemical by-products of combustion combine quickly with oxygen, preventing smoke-inhalation victims from getting oxygen from the air. Since smoke rises, stay low to the floor to escape. If you cannot escape your room, place towels and clothing in door cracks and vents.

Planning Escape from Fire. Most fatal home fires occur during the night. At this time, it is easy to become disoriented when smoke or fire is first detected. The best protection against injury or death from home fires is to establish escape plans and periodically conduct practice drills.

You and your family should draw a floor plan, including doors, hallways, and windows, of each story of your home. Use arrows to point to two ways of escape, if possible, from each room. Alternate escape routes are necessary in case one route is blocked. For example, if an upstairs door is blocked by fire, a ladder or a readily available rope coil is essential for escape through windows.

All escape plans should include the following steps:

- Turn on the bedroom lights.
- Use a predetermined signal to alert everyone to the fire. Smoke detectors, which should be in every household, will do this job. You also can use whistles, which could be kept in every nightstand.
- Before opening a closed door during a fire, test for warmth. If the door is warm, do not open it. Escape through a window instead.
- Always stay close to the floor in a smoke-filled room. Smoke rises, so there is more oxygen near the floor and visibility is better.
- After escaping, meet outside at a safe prearranged place. Do not go back into the house.
- Call the fire department from a neighbor's house.
- If a person is trapped inside a burning building, rescue is safer and usually faster if left to the fire department.

Although most fire departments cannot conduct routine inspections of individual homes, they can provide a variety of fire safety information if requested.

If you are caught near or in a fire, acting quickly and remaining calm could save your life and that of others. Remember the following:

- If a fire starts in a frying pan, put a lid on the fire.
- If a fire starts in the oven, turn off the oven, and smother the fire with baking soda. Never put water on a grease fire, because it will make the grease and the fire spread.

DID YOU KNOW?

- According to the U.S. Consumer Product Safety Commission, in one recent year, more than 180,000 children and adults had toy-related injuries.
- In 1990 alone, more than 12,000 Americans were injured by fireworks. Injuries included severe burns, blindness, and damage to the nerves of the face.
- Stair-related injuries sent as many as one million Americans to the hospital in 1990.
- Serious burns from hot food and hot water result in 37,000 injuries among U.S. children each year.
- Each year, about 27,000 house fires in the U.S. are caused by children playing with matches or fire.

■ If your clothes catch on fire, remember: stop, drop, and roll. Roll on the ground or roll up in a rug or blanket to smother the flames. If you remain upright or run, the flames will spread.

Electrical Shock

Shocks from electrical appliances can kill. Every year electrical shock kills more than 1,000 people. In addition, electrical shock starts almost 62,000 fires.

If you become part of the circuit that an electric current travels, you will be shocked. You become part of the circuit when you touch an exposed wire while you are grounded because the current can then pass through you to the ground.

Here are some precautions to take when using home electrical appliances and power tools:

■ Any time anything seems to be wrong with an appliance or power tool, unplug it immediately.
■ Never touch pipes or metal with an electrical appliance or tool that is turned on.
■ Inspect cords occasionally for signs of cracked insulation. Have frayed cords replaced. Cords should not be placed under a carpet or rug because they can be damaged when walked on.
■ To avoid electrical shock, disconnect appliances by pulling on the plug, not on the cord.
■ Never use an electrical appliance or power tool if your body, clothing, or the floor is wet. This includes hair dryers, radios, and electric musical instruments.
■ Call an electrician rather than try to make electrical repairs yourself.

Poisons

Everyday products, not just those marked with a skull and crossbones, can be poisonous. Most of these products are typically found in the kitchen, bathroom, utility area, basement, and garage. In families with children, household products and medicines should be kept in locked cabinets, or out of the reach of children. Never rebottle or repackage products, such as storing cleaning solutions in soft drink bottles.

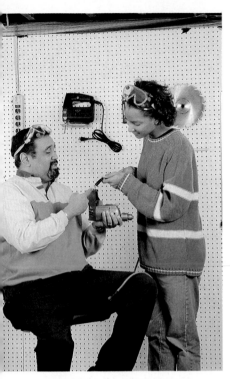
Unplug any appliance that does not seem to be working properly.

K E E P I N G   F I T

What to Do If There's a Fire

■ Crawl under the smoke.
■ Close doors between you and the smoke.
■ Don't open any door without feeling to see if it is hot. If it is, don't open the door.

■ Don't try to fight a large fire.
■ Don't stop to save anything except people.
■ Never go back into a burning building.

■ Call the fire department from outside your house unless the fire is very localized and small.
■ If you should catch on fire, stop, drop, and roll.

Five Elements of Accidents

In studying accidents over the years, one important point has become clear: accidents do not just happen. In fact, most accidents follow a specific pattern.

Five elements are present in almost all accidents. They are the situation, the unsafe habit or risk, the unsafe act, the accident, and possible injuries—and they combine to form an accident chain.

- **The situation.** You and your friend Mary are listening to CDs in your room. You had just bought a new one by your favorite artist and you wanted to share it with her.
- **The unsafe habit.** As is your routine when you come home from school, you put your textbooks on the eighth step of the open stairway leading to the second floor. This step is shoulder height for you and is right beside your path to the kitchen.
- **The unsafe act.** When you came home from school today, as usual, you threw your textbooks on the stairway. After grabbing an apple from the kitchen, you hurried to your room to pick up your clothes before Mary came over.
- **The accident.** Mary enjoyed listening to your new CD and looking at your CD collection. Time passed quickly, and suddenly Mary realized if she did not hurry, she would be late getting home. She said good-bye and grabbed her jacket. As she ran down the stairs, she failed to see your books. Falling head first to the bottom of the stairs, she landed on her shoulder.
- **The injuries.** Mary broke her collarbone, and you felt terrible about her injury.

In the five elements that make up an accident, consider the first three as links in an accident chain and the last two as the result. If you break any one of the links,—or change the element—you will prevent the accident in all likelihood.

The safety-conscious person is always alert to the risk of a given situation. The safety-conscious person breaks the accident chain by changing the situation, changing unsafe habits or avoiding unnecessary risks, and acting in a safe manner.

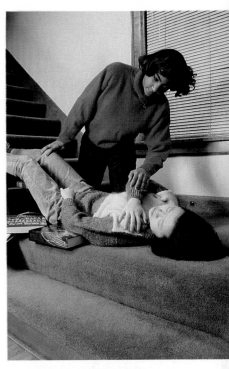

Breaking the accident chain can prevent accidents from happening.

LESSON 1 REVIEW

Reviewing Facts and Vocabulary

1. Give some examples of hazards that cause falls in the home.
2. Explain the purpose of a smoke detector and a fire extinguisher.

Thinking Critically

3. **Analysis.** One safety expert has said, "Safety begins at home." What assumptions did the writer make?

4. **Synthesis.** Summarize the necessary conditions for any fire.

Applying Health Knowledge

5. Design a fire escape plan for your home. Include two escape routes from each room.

SAFETY AWAY FROM HOME

Safety and accidents can touch every aspect of daily living. Although many accidents occur at home, the workplace also can pose a threat to your safety. Additionally, if you participate in recreational activities, you will want to be aware of the possible hazards. Whether at home or away, you should always follow basic safety rules.

At Work

If you have a part-time job, you know the importance of safety at work. Whether you work in a fast-food restaurant, in a local grocery store, or around heavy equipment, it is essential that you are provided with a safe environment in which to work.

The United States **Occupational Safety and Health Administration (OSHA)** is an agency that promotes safe and healthy conditions at work. This organization develops and enforces health regulations and job safety. It also is involved in keeping employers and employees aware of industrial hazards. OSHA deals with fire prevention, protective clothing, and acceptable levels of exposure to asbestos and lead. OSHA workers inspect work sites to ensure compliance with their standards.

Employers can reduce your risk of injury at work by eliminating health hazards that are causing or may cause serious physical harm or death. It is the employer's responsibility to train you and make you aware of hazards and to inform you of any new safety rules.

You can promote a safe work environment by arriving at work well-rested and alert, learning the proper use of all equipment, and following established safety rules.

Outdoors

Sports and recreation can be fun. However, if people do not follow basic safety behaviors, sports and recreation can end in accidents, injury, and even death. Prevention requires planning ahead and taking necessary precautions.

Here are five important points to remember:

- Know your abilities and skills as well as your limits, and stay within them. Many accidents happen when people become overly confident, try to show off in front of others, or get talked into trying something they are not able to do well.

- Use the proper equipment and know how to use it in the way it was intended.

- Take the time to warm up and stretch before you exercise or participate in a strenuous activity.

- Cool down properly after you exercise or participate in a strenuous activity.

- Learn the safety rules specific to your activity before getting started.

In and On the Water

Each year in the United States about 7,000 people die from drowning, and more than 1 million have close calls. Small children wander off and fall into unattended pools and ponds; boats overturn; swimmers panic when struck by a cramp, when caught in a current, or when they have swum out farther than they should.

Most of these drownings and near-drownings are avoidable. If people understand the risks of being around water and follow some basic rules of safety, the number of drownings would be greatly reduced.

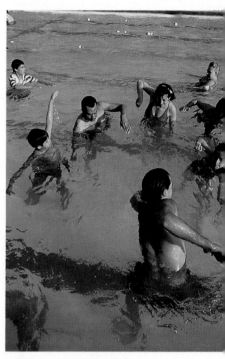

Learning to swim increases your confidence in the water.

WATER SAFETY PRECAUTIONS

Swimming

Learn to swim well. Being able to swim gives a person confidence in the water and reduces the chance of panic during an accident or emergency. Swimming lessons are usually available in your community, at school, or at municipal pools. While swimming, heed the following precautions:

- Follow the posted swimming rules.
- Always swim with someone, preferably someone who knows lifesaving techniques.
- Avoid pushing and shoving. Never participate in horseplay or give fake cries for help.
- If you get a muscle cramp, do not panic. Relax, float, and press and squeeze the muscle until it relaxes.
- Swim only when a lifeguard is on duty.
- If you are pulled offshore by rapid currents or undertows, swim at a 45° angle toward shore until you are freed by the current.

Diving

Sporting accidents are second to car accidents as the cause of spinal injuries that result in paralysis. Water sports—diving in particular—pose the most serious threat. Stay safe following these guidelines.

- Always check the water depth before diving.
- Never dive into unfamiliar water or into shallow breaking waves.
- Be sure the area is clear of swimmers and floating objects before diving.
- Always dive straight ahead and not off the side of the diving board.
- Never go down a water slide headfirst.

Boating

Follow these safety rules when out in a boat:

- Learn how to handle a boat or canoe correctly.
- Use only boats that are in good condition.
- Observe the load limit of the boat.
- Always wear a life jacket when boating.

K E E P I N G   F I T

Safety in the Workplace

When working at a part- or full-time job, keep these safety guidelines in mind:

- Do not use any machine you have not been fully trained to operate.

- Do not work without required protective equipment, such as goggles, earplugs, or gloves.
- Do not work at a pace that is too fast to maintain safety standards.

- Do not work without breaks.
- Do not work for long stretches at a time.
- Remember, you have a right to expect safe work conditions and protection from injury.

Overcoming The Odds

Jyh-Hann ("John") Chang is in his twenties. He knows firsthand about the importance of safety. A few years ago, he had a body-surfing accident that changed his life.

When he was 19, John decided to go body surfing in dangerous conditions. "It was just a day or two after a hurricane," John says. "I knew that the waves would be a lot rougher. I remember wading in the water and thinking I'd just wait for a large wave to come in. When I chose one, it was the one that ended up breaking my neck. The next thing I knew, I was drowning. A passerby thought I was a log, and he was going to clear this log from the wave, but then he realized it was a body—my body. I was very fortunate that he was there. I'm very fortunate that I'm alive."

John continues. "The next thing I knew, I was being flown to a shock trauma unit. I was completely paralyzed from the neck down. That night the doctor told me I probably wouldn't walk again. It really didn't hit me until I went home. Everything around me reminded me of what I couldn't do anymore."

But John learned to cope, and he excelled. "I got myself back into college," he says.

"The college initially didn't want me back. They'd never had a person in a wheelchair there before. But my parents begged. My first goal was to do well academically. I did.

"After my sophomore year,"

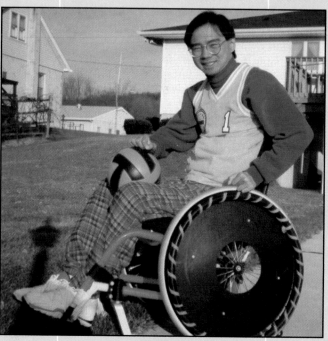

John says, "I knew I needed to improve my social life. I gradually got involved in committees and clubs. In my junior year, I became vice president of the student body, and senior year, I became president of the student council and senior class president. I felt good about myself because I realized people were finally looking at me, at my qualities, not just at my wheelchair. I'd felt for the longest time that I had to be happy all the time. But it was when I acted like a real person—with good

times and bad times, with both depression and humor—that people started responding to me.

"I was commencement speaker at graduation," John goes on. "I spoke in front of seven thousand people. Then I began speaking at schools, camps, and universities about being disabled. Before my accident, my dream was to be a doctor, but no medical school will take me because I can't fulfill some of the physical requirements. I'm now working on a PhD in clinical psychology. I'm going to specialize in neuropsychology and help the physically challenged."

Despite obstacles, John hasn't stopped enjoying new challenges. "This year, I began to go back into sports," he says. "I do some sculling on the river and I've gone airplane gliding as well. It took me six years to find that I could enjoy the things I used to enjoy. So I guess I should never set a limit on how much I can grow."

1. What obstacles has John faced since his accident? What are some of the personal lessons he has learned along the way?
2. How might more attention to safety have prevented his accident?

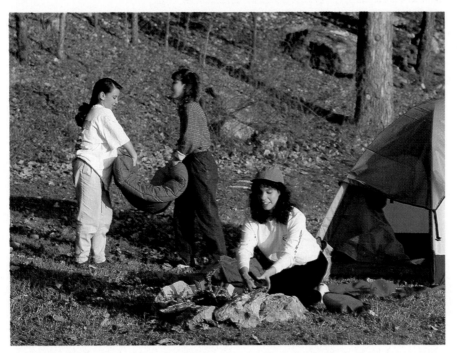
Camping is more fun when you follow safety precautions.

CONFLICT RESOLUTION

Ed was really happy when his uncle said he could borrow his tent to go camping with friends. Now out in the woods, his friend Larry has built a huge fire for them to cook their evening meal. Ed is concerned that wind will carry the fire to the trees. Larry says the fire will eventually die out overnight.

How should Ed handle this situation?

Camping

Unsafe behavior in and around campsites can lead to serious accidents. When camping, follow these guidelines:

- Stay in specified campsites.
- Never camp alone.
- Always let someone know where you are going and when you will return.
- Be knowledgeable about poisonous plants, insects, and snakes in the area.
- Carry plenty of fresh water.
- Never cook in a tent.
- Smother all fires with dirt and water.

LESSON 2 REVIEW

Reviewing Facts and Vocabulary

1. Describe the purpose of OSHA.
2. List basic rules of safety near water.

Thinking Critically

3. **Synthesis.** Develop a plan that would help reduce the number of drownings in your community.

4. **Analysis.** Compare safe and unsafe behavior when diving.

Applying Health Knowledge

5. Many communities offer swimming programs. Design a poster that advertises a swimming program in your area. Include information that would encourage someone to learn how to swim.

SAFETY ON WHEELS

TERM TO USE
- Human collision

CONCEPTS TO LEARN
- Most automobile accidents and deaths among young people do not involve a second vehicle.
- Many cyclists mistakenly ride on the wrong side of the road against traffic.

ATTITUDES AND BEHAVIORS TO EVALUATE
- Self-Inventory, page 688.
- Building Decision-Making Skills, page 689.

It is frightening to realize that automobile accidents are the leading cause of death for people between the ages of 15 and 24 in the United States.

Auto Safety

Most automobile accidents and deaths among young people do not involve a second vehicle. Instead, they result from the young person's overturning the vehicle, running the vehicle off the road, or colliding with fixed objects, such as trees, light poles, and concrete walls. Such accidents often involve high rates of speed.

Taking a driver's education course can help you develop better driving skills and habits. Such a course can help you learn to anticipate problems before they occur.

Drive within the Speed Limit

Speed kills. This is a plain and simple fact, yet one that people often ignore. By driving within the legal limit, you lower your risk of accidents and reduce your risk of injury to yourself and others. You also save gasoline and wear and tear on your car and tires.

Use Seat Belts

There are two kinds of collisions within a single accident. The first is the car collision, in which the car hits something, buckles and bends, and then comes to a stop. The second collision is the **human collision,** which happens when a person hits some part of the car or is thrown from the vehicle. It is the human collision that causes injury.

To help understand just how severe the human collision can be, imagine a person's head striking a post at 30 miles (48 km) per hour. In a 30-mile-per-hour (48-km-per-hour) crash of a vehicle, an occupant strikes the interior of the car with a force of several thousand pounds, resulting in serious injury or death. Because the car's interior has very little give, the human body must absorb most of the force of the impact.

Infants or children are even more likely than adults to become like flying missiles during a crash. This is true whether they are in the front or rear seats. If adults hold children on their laps, the children become cushions that protect the adults from colliding with the dashboard or windshield. In this case, the children receive the brunt of the crash, often suffering severe or fatal head injuries. Thus, families need to use car restraints or car seats for children.

Many people wear seat belts only on long trips or when weather conditions seem particularly dangerous. Serious accidents, however, occur at all speeds, on all kinds of trips, and under all kinds of conditions.

However, the chances are greater of being in an accident close to home. The accident rate is low on expressways where much high-speed, long-distance travel takes place.

For every 100 young people killed in a motor vehicle accident in the United States last year, 80 would still be alive if they had been wearing a seat belt. When you use a seat belt, you are practicing accident and injury prevention. If your friends do not buckle up, ask them to do so. Though air bags are now installed in many cars, it is still important to use seat belts. Most states have laws requiring their use.

Do Not Drink and Drive

Over one-half of all automobile fatalities involve drivers who had been drinking. If people followed the law and did not drink while driving, millions of accidents and deaths could be prevented.

People who drink and drive risk not only their own health but also that of anyone else who may be on the road. Judgment and physical skills are impaired. Driving is risky when sober—the risk increases when one is or has been drinking.

Motorcycle Safety

Motorcyclists are seventeen times more likely to be killed in an accident than are people traveling in a car. There are several reasons for this.

- A two-wheeled vehicle slides more easily than one with four wheels.
- A motorcycle is more difficult to see than a car.
- Motorcycles accelerate faster than cars.
- Motorcycles weigh less than cars.
- Motorcyclists are virtually unprotected.

Regardless of whose fault an accident is, the cyclist loses. Besides following safety rules on the road, cyclists can increase their protection by wearing safety helmets and proper clothing. Cyclists need to be especially careful in wet weather because of poor tire traction on wet surfaces.

Bicycle Safety

Bicycling is a lot of fun, and it can provide good exercise for the whole family. Bicycles also are an excellent means of transportation.

KEEPING FIT

Helmets: Using Your Head

Three out of every four bike deaths and 70 percent of the bike-related hospitalizations involve head injuries. Therefore, one of the most important things you can do when riding on a bicycle or motorcycle is to wear a good helmet. It is estimated that bicycle helmets alone could cut head injuries by 85 percent.

When looking for a helmet, look for one with a seal of either the Snell Foundation or American National Standards Institute. Don't use helmets intended for other sports. Also be sure to replace any helmet that has been damaged.

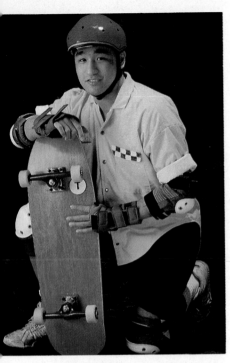

Wear protective equipment when skateboarding.

However, bicycles are involved in many injury accidents.

Four out of five collisions between bicycles and cars are caused by cyclists who disregard traffic rules. The most frequent mistake that cyclists make is riding on the wrong side of the road, against—rather than with—the flow of traffic.

Follow these guidelines for safe cycling:

- Ride on the right, keeping close to the side of the road. When riding with others, ride in a straight, single-file line.
- Always yield the right-of-way; you will not win against a car or truck.
- Watch for parked cars pulling into traffic and for car doors that swing open suddenly in your path.
- Obey the same rules as drivers, such as signaling before you turn and stopping for red lights and stop signs.
- Except when signaling, keep both hands on the handlebars at all times.

Three-fourths of all fatal bicycle accidents are due to head injuries. Wearing a hardshell helmet is a very important safety measure. Also, make sure your bike has a bright headlight and a red rear light and reflector for night riding. Wear reflective, or at least light-colored, clothing when riding at dawn, dusk, after dark, or in the rain. Be especially careful in wet weather. Bike tires have poor traction on wet surfaces.

Skating and Safety

Obey these safety rules when roller skating, skateboarding, or using in-line skates.

- Wear protective equipment—wrist guards, elbow and knee pads, hardshell helmet, and light gloves.
- If you fall, try to curl up into a ball and roll, staying loose. Tensing up will increase your chances of injury.
- Watch for and slow down around pedestrians.
- Keep your speed under control.

LESSON 3 REVIEW

Reviewing Facts and Vocabulary

1. What is a human collision?
2. List ways to prevent auto accidents.

Thinking Critically

3. **Evaluation.** Write a one-page paper that expresses your view on wearing a helmet when riding a motorcycle.
4. **Analysis.** The chances of being in an automobile accident are greater close to home. What support can you give to this statement?

Applying Health Knowledge

5. Collect several newspaper articles about accidents. Try to identify each of the links of the accident chain and ways the chain might have been broken.
6. A congressional representative has proposed that all cars have a device added to them so that no one can drive above the speed limit. Write a one-page response to this proposed legislation, based on what you have learned about accident prevention in this chapter.

LESSON 4

PERSONAL SAFETY

There are more cases of rape, thefts, shootings, murders, and gang violence than ever before. Because this violence is more widespread and more random than in the past, your chances of becoming a victim are very real.

Many causes for the increase in crime have been identified. For example, it is estimated that drugs and alcohol use are involved in two out of every three violent crimes. However, whatever the causes, we must all be concerned about not becoming victims.

Who are Victims?

Anyone can be a victim of a violent crime. No one is immune. That is the reason it is important to be prepared and know what to do not only to prevent but also to survive personal crimes. This is particularly necessary for teens because teens who are involved with or have friends who are involved with gangs, guns, alcohol, and/or drugs are more likely to be victims than other teens. However, everyone is at risk.

Consider these facts:

- According to the FBI, half of all rapes reported involve females under the age of 21.

- It is estimated that one out of three Americans will be the victim of a sexual attack or attempted attack sometime in his or her lifetime. Although this usually happens to females, males also are victims.

- Victims often know their attackers and may even be in ongoing relationships with them.

Preventing Becoming a Victim

It is wiser to give up jewelry, shoes, or a bike than to be shot. Other basic strategies are just common sense, such as always staying alert and aware of your surroundings.

Some Inner Tools of Self-Defense

When people talk about self-defense, they often mean learning physical strategies for stopping attacks. They imagine quick kicks and tricky tripping. However, mental or emotional strategies are also important. You may already have the following valuable self-defense tools within you.

- **Self-Esteem.** This includes the confidence you have in yourself. People with high self-esteem feel secure without being arrogant. They are not likely to be bullied or chosen as easy targets, particularly by people who know them.

TERMS TO USE
- Sexual assault
- Rape
- Date rape
- Acquaintance rape

CONCEPTS TO LEARN
- You have self-defense tools within you.
- Rape is an act of violence.

ATTITUDES AND BEHAVIORS TO EVALUATE
- Self-Inventory, page 688.
- Building Decision-Making Skills, page 689.

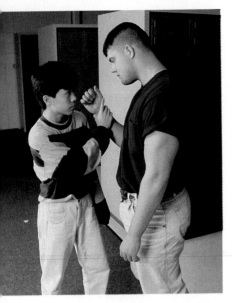

Use your self-defense skills. Let your assertiveness and body language show your self-protective attitude.

- **Assertiveness.** Assertiveness is bold and confident behavior. Assertive people speak with definite conviction, leaving no doubt as to their feelings or intentions. Verbal assertiveness may prevent a physical attack. Phrases such as "Leave me alone" or "I'm not going with you" may throw an attacker off guard. Many attackers want easy victims they can overpower quickly.
- **Body language.** Actions often speak louder than words. Your body language can project your thoughts in a forceful way. Making direct eye contact, using a strong voice, keeping your body erect and chin held high, and using a deliberate stride can send the message that you are in charge of your safety.
- **Intuition.** Many people who have been raped report sensing that something was wrong just before the attack. Learn to trust your intuition. If you sense danger, get away.
- **A self-protective attitude.** Realize that you are worthy and have a right to be treated with respect and to be safe. Don't be afraid of insulting someone by walking away or by being overly cautious. Better to be safe than to be a victim.

Preventing Violence in Teen Relationships

Sometimes it is difficult for teens to tell if their relationships are safe. Although teens often play rough and tease one another, behavior can sometimes change and become harmful. No matter how close you are to someone, if his or her behavior changes or threatens your safety, you have a responsibility to speak up. Demand changed behavior, or get away. If anyone slaps, pushes, or threatens you, take it seriously. Verbal threats, put-downs, and yelling often are followed by physical abuse. Abusive behavior can be confusing because it is not always constant. It may be followed by apologies or statements of intention to do better. However, the cycle usually continues, and abusive behavior happens again.

How can you prevent being in a violent relationship? Don't allow another person to control you in any way. Don't allow anyone to isolate you from your friends or to physically assault you. Confront the person. Let him or her know that the behavior is unacceptable and even illegal. Talk to your parents, or a trusted friend. End the relationship, even if you like the person. Encourage the abuser to get help.

KEEPING FIT

How to Avoid Being a Victim

- Don't walk alone at night.
- Avoid wooded areas or dark alleys.
- At night, have your car keys ready when you are going to your car.
- Check the back seats to make sure no one is inside your car.
- After getting in the car, lock it.
- Park in well-lighted areas.
- Take down license plate numbers and descriptions of suspicious cars in your neighborhood and report them to the police.
- When walking at night, walk under lights and by the curb. Avoid doorways.
- Don't put your wallet or purse in an easy-to-grab place.
- Lock your car when you park it.

WHAT IS SEXUAL HARASSMENT

The term *sexual harassment* means different things to different people. It may take many forms, such as telling obscene jokes or stories, deliberate touching, pressure for dates, unwanted letters or calls, or rape.

Sexual harassment is a widespread problem. Its occurence is often controversial and open to debate because people hold different views of what it really is. Sexual harassment has become a major problem in the workplace and many companies now hold education and awareness programs for their employees. Sexual harassment is a form of abuse and should not be tolerated.

Preventing Sexual Assault and Rape

Sexual assault is attempted or actual physical attack with violent, sexual intent. **Rape** is sexual intercourse by force or threat. Rape is an act of violence and it is illegal. Frequently rapes occur when people are drunk or on drugs.

Victims of rape often know their attacker. When rape occurs between two people who are dating, it is called **date rape. Acquaintance rape** is rape by someone who is known casually by the victim or someone thought to be a friend.

There are preventive measures you can take.

- Have sexual limits and communicate them clearly.
- Do not drink or use drugs or date anyone who does.
- Do not go out alone or ride in a car with a person you do not know well.
- Do not put other's feelings ahead of your own safety.
- Take classes in karate or other forms of self-defense.
- Never open your door to anyone you do not know or trust.
- Use locks on doors and windows.
- Do not let strangers use your phone.
- Do not get into an elevator alone with a stranger.

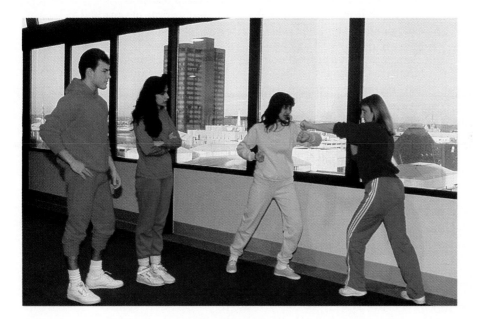

Learn all you can to protect yourself.

Culturally Speaking

Personal Space
Our idea of how much "personal space" we need is culturally influenced. Many Americans like to be about an arm's length from someone when they talk informally. People from some Middle Eastern cultures are comfortable standing inches apart. Test yourself: 1. Ask someone to walk toward you and tell them to stop when they are a comfortable distance away. 2. What factors make this distance change? Does the age or sex of the other person have an effect? Does it matter if the person is a friend?

- According to the U.S. Bureau of Prisoners, in 1991, there were over 65,000 prisoners in U.S. federal prisons. In 1995, that number is expected to be over 99,000.
- Since 1983, the number of murders committed by juveniles has increased threefold, the number of rapes by juveniles has doubled, and the number of robberies has increased five times.
- In 1989, Heath Wilkins and Kevin Stanford, then 16 and 17, were sentenced as adults and received the death penalty for the murder they committed. The Supreme Court upheld this death sentence in *Stanford* vs. *Kentucky*.
- According to the F.B.I. Uniform Crime Reports, in this country there is a murder committed every 25 minutes, a rape every 6 minutes, a robbery every minute, a car theft every 22 seconds, and a burglary every 10 seconds.
- The age group of 14 to 24 is responsible for the majority of violent crimes in our society.

- Do not hitchhike or pick up hitchhikers.
- Do not park your car, walk, or jog in remote areas.
- If you are being followed, hurry to a place where there are other people, such as to a store.
- Get to know your neighbors. Look out for each other.
- If your car is rammed from behind or breaks down, stay in your car with doors locked and flasher lights on.
- Keep a "Call Police" sign in your car and place it in the rear window in an emergency situation.

Escaping and Surviving an Attack

If you are attacked, try to run for help. If you cannot run, decide on another course of action. Scream, yell "fire," and/or physically disable or stun the person in some way. Watch for a moment when the attacker may be caught off guard so you can escape. Use your wits. Try different approaches. Don't assume you can't get away. You have a greater chance of escaping than you might think. If all else fails you may have to submit in order to survive.

HEALTH UPDATE

LOOKING AT TECHNOLOGY

DNA Banks: Genetic Information on File

DNA, or deoxyribonucleic acid, is a complex molecule found in all cells, mainly in their nuclei. It is the substance that makes up genes, the material that carries hereditary information that determines what characteristics a person will develop.

In the past, convicting criminals was often based on fingerprints, witness testimony, obvious physical evidence, and/or admissions of guilt, but often there was no absolute proof that a suspect committed a certain crime. With advancements in DNA testing, however, some criminals are now being located and convicted on the basis of a kind of genetic testing called DNA profiling. DNA profiling tests can be run on small amounts of blood or other body fluids such as semen. If the DNA from these samples matches body fluids left at the scene of the crime or on the victim, it is highly probable that the profiled suspect committed the crime.

Increasingly, DNA profiling information is being used in courtroom testimony. Now some states are taking steps to create extensive DNA computerized files known as DNA banks. Such information could be scanned and retrieved quickly when trying to identify suspects.

Many crime experts and law enforcement officials believe that DNA banks will take the guesswork out of much investigative work, get criminals identified and off the streets more quickly, and make the whole trial process more scientific. Others, however, believe that DNA profiling is a violation of the right to privacy as well as a violation of the Fourth Amendment to the United States Constitution, which states that citizens are protected against unreasonable searches.

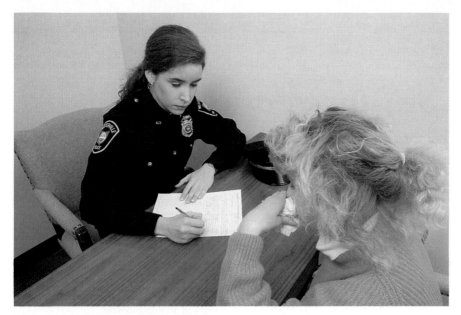
Always seek help in case of attack.

What to Do After a Rape

If you or someone you know is raped, get help from your family or a friend after an attack and get it quickly. Do not take a shower or bath or discard any physical evidence. Get medical help right away. You may be hurt or infected and not know it. Have medical tests for pregnancy, STDs, and HIV infection. The male involved should also be tested for STDs and HIV. Report the rape to the police even if it is a date or acquaintance rape. You may want to request that someone of your sex take your report.

Call a rape crisis center and get counseling or join a support group. You will need help to recover from the emotional shock of being raped. Be patient. It takes time to recover from the trauma of an attack. Remember that you did not cause the rape and have no reason to be ashamed.

LESSON 4 REVIEW

Reviewing Facts and Vocabulary

1. What are three characteristics that are self-defense tools and may add to your chances of not becoming a victim?
2. What does it mean to be assertive?

Thinking Critically

3. **Evaluation.** Why do you think most incidences of rape are not reported?

4. **Synthesis.** Develop a plan that will help you reduce the chances of being physically assaulted or raped.

Applying Health Knowledge

5. Read an article about a rape situation. Identify three general concepts about rape that you learned from your reading.
6. Create a public service announcement about preventing date rape and acquaintance rape.

Self-Inventory

Staying Safe

HOW DO YOU RATE?

Number a sheet of paper from 1 through 22. Read each item below, and respond by writing *MT* if the statement describes you *all or most of the time*, *ST* if the statement describes you *some of the time*, and *N* if the statement *seldom or never* applies to you. Total the number of each type of response. Then proceed to the next section.

1. I avoid acting in an unsafe manner.
2. I avoid showing off.
3. I share personal safety concerns with trusted adults.
4. I am self-confident and sure of my self-worth.
5. I am assertive, especially when around aggressive individuals.
6. I use body language to send a message that I am in charge of my personal safety.
7. When I drive a vehicle or a motorcycle, I avoid tailgating. If I do not drive but ride a bicycle, I follow safety guidelines.
8. I follow posted speed limits when driving or cycling.
9. I use seat belts.
10. I do not drink and drive.
11. I avoid riding with drivers who speed or who drink and drive.
12. I allow myself sufficient time to get places without having to speed or be distracted.
13. I stay within my abilities and limits when taking part in sports and recreational activities.
14. I take the time to warm up before and cool down after physical activities.
15. I follow safety rules specific to my favorite activities.
16. I avoid touching plumbing or metal and an electrical appliance or tool at the same time.
17. I disconnect appliances by pulling on the plug, not on the cord.
18. I do not use an electrical appliance if my body, clothing, or the floor is wet.
19. I keep poisons out of the reach of children.
20. I do not rebottle or repackage products, which might cause harm to someone else.
21. I do not open the door of my home to anyone I do not know or trust.
22. When going out with someone I do not know well, I make sure we go with other friends of mine.

HOW DID YOU SCORE?

Give yourself 2 points for each statement that describes you *all or most of the time*, 1 point for each statement that describes you *some of the time*, and 0 points for each *seldom or never* response. Find your total and read below to see how you scored. Then proceed to the next section.

35 to 44
Excellent. Your safety-conscious attitude and behavior deserve high praise. Keep it up.

25 to 34
Good. You are doing a good job of practicing safe behavior, and it appears that you generally have a safe attitude.

15 to 24
Fair. You need to make safety attitudes and behavior more a part of your daily life.

Below 15
Poor. You are a serious threat to your own health and safety and that of others.

WHAT ARE YOUR GOALS?

If you received an *excellent* or *good* score, complete the statements in Part A. If your score was rated *fair* or *poor*, complete Parts A and B.

Part A

1. I plan to learn more about safety behavior in the following ways: ____.
2. My timetable for accomplishing this is ____.
3. I plan to share my information with others by ____.

Part B

4. The unsafe or risky behavior I would like to change most is ____.
5. The steps involved in making this change are ____.
6. My timetable for making this change is ____.
7. The people or groups I will ask for support and assistance are ____.
8. My rewards for making this change will be ____.

Building Decision-Making Skills

Amy has just started driving to school and has discovered that some of the students engage in driving games. These games include a driver trying to squeeze his or her car into the line of traffic as others try to squeeze the driver out. Quick starts, stops, and cuts are the rule, along with loud music, and passengers hanging out the window or the sun roof while yelling at people in other cars. Some drive faster than the posted limit, some tailgate, and some try to pass when they shouldn't. What should Amy do?

A. Tell her friends that she is not going to take part and insist that passengers in her car use seat belts.

B. Find a reason to be late leaving after school every day to miss the crowd and this game.

C. Learn the game so that she gets a reputation for risk-taking and others know she is not afraid.

WHAT DO YOU THINK?

1. **Situation.** Why does a decision need to be made?
2. **Choices.** What other solutions or choices could Amy try?
3. **Consequences.** How will people react to the direct approach? Will they respect her? Will they make fun of her?
4. **Consequences.** Is this an issue that the students should resolve on their own or do adults need to be involved? How will people react if they find out Amy brought adults into it?
5. **Consequences.** What are Amy's legal liabilities? What will happen if she gets a ticket or wrecks her car? What if someone gets badly hurt? How will this affect her driving privileges, her life-style, or her financial situation?
6. **Consequences.** How will Amy feel about herself in each situation? How will others feel about her, including her friends, other drivers, her parents, school officials, and so on?
7. **Consequences.** How would Amy's health triangle be affected by this decision?
8. **Decision.** What action do you think Amy should take and just how should she do it?

Lynn is walking home from school when a stranger drives up and asks if she is Lynn Andrews, daughter of Marcy Andrews. When she says yes, the man says her mother has been involved in a serious auto accident and has asked him to bring Lynn to the hospital. What should Lynn do?

A. Say no and get to a phone and call home, then call the hospital.

B. Go with him, since the man knew both Lynn's and her mother's name.

C. Call the police and report the license number and description of the car and the man.

WHAT DO YOU THINK?

9. **Situation.** What are the dangers here?
10. **Choices.** What other choices does Lynn have?
11. **Consequences.** What are the consequences of each choice?
12. **Decision.** Which choice do you think is best for Lynn?
13. **Decision.** What should Lynn do if the man becomes more insistent?
14. **Evaluation.** How do you think you would handle a similar situation?

REVIEW

Using Health Terms

On a separate sheet of paper, write the term that best matches each definition given below.

LESSON 1

1. A device that sounds an alarm if smoke passes into it.
2. A portable device that can be used to extinguish small fires by ejecting fire-extinguishing chemicals.

LESSON 2

3. An agency that promotes safe conditions in the workplace.

LESSON 3

4. When a person hits some part of the car or is thrown from the vehicle.
5. Devices installed in automobiles to protect people during collisions.

LESSON 4

6. An act of violence involving sexual intercourse by force or threat.

Building Academic Skills

LESSON 2

7. **Writing.** Write two paragraphs describing camping trips. In one paragraph, describe a safe camping trip. In the other paragraph, describe an unsafe camping trip.

LESSON 3

8. **Math.** According to statistics, if 585 young people have been killed in motor vehicle accidents, how many would have been alive if they had worn a seat belt?
9. **Writing.** Write a newspaper article convincing bicycle riders to wear helmets.

LESSON 4

10. **Math.** By September 15, 1991, 100 murders had been committed in Columbus, Ohio, during the year. If this rate continued for the remainder of the year, how many people would have been murdered in this city during 1991?

Recalling the Facts

LESSON 1

11. What can be done to reduce the number of falls that occur on stairways?
12. What safety phrase should you remember if your clothing catches fire? What does this phrase mean?
13. What is a good way to prevent smoke inhalation during a fire?
14. How should poisonous products in the home be stored to minimize their dangers?

LESSON 2

15. How can employers minimize the risk of work-related accidents?
16. How can employees minimize the risk of work-related accidents?
17. Why should everyone learn to swim?
18. What are the two major causes of spinal injuries that result in paralysis?

LESSON 3

19. What is the leading cause of death among people between the ages of 15 and 24?
20. List three advantages of driving within the speed limit.
21. List five guidelines for riding a bicycle safely.
22. How can bike riders minimize the risk of injury in case of an accident?
23. What five pieces of protective equipment should people wear when roller skating or skateboarding?
24. What should you do if you fall while using in-line skates?
25. What are the benefits of taking a course in driver's education?

LESSON 4

26. What fraction of violent crimes involve drugs and alcohol?
27. Name four self-defense tools you can use to help protect yourself from others.
28. Give examples of body language that can help protect someone from harm.
29. What measures can you take to help prevent rape?
30. What strategies can you use if you are attacked?

REVIEW

Thinking Critically

LESSON 1

31. Evaluation. Some argue that falls among the elderly would be eliminated if the elderly were put in nursing homes. Do you agree with this strategy? Explain your reasoning.

32. Synthesis. Name three flammable liquids that might be used in or around a home. Tell what precautions should be taken in using each.

33. Synthesis. What would you include in a home fire escape plan? Explain your answer.

34. Analysis. What parts of the accident chain are the easiest to break?

LESSON 2

35. Synthesis. Plan a project to illustrate the importance of bicycle safety in elementary school.

36. Evaluation. How would you measure the worth of seat belts as a safety measure?

LESSON 3

37. Evaluation. Some states have laws requiring a person to use a seat belt while driving or riding in a car and to wear a helmet while operating a motorcycle. What is your opinion of such laws and why?

38. Analysis. What are the health advantages and disadvantages of riding a bicycle?

LESSON 4

39. Evaluation. If someone is raped, that person should seek help. List, in order, the five most important things you think this person should do after an attack. Why did you rate each one as you did?

Making the Connection

LESSON 1

40. Math. Survey several classes in school to find out how many homes have smoke detectors. Compute the percentage of homes that have smoke detectors.

Applying Health Knowledge

LESSON 2

41. Mario wants to participate in the gymnastics program at Jefferson High. His parents must sign a paper giving him permission to do so. Before they sign the paper, they are required to watch a film showing the possible dangers of injury in all the sports programs offered at Jefferson. After viewing the film, they are reluctant to sign the paper. What arguments can Mario use to convince them his participation in gymnastics will be safe?

Beyond the Classroom

LESSON 1

42. Community Involvement. Find the telephone numbers for the fire department, the police department, and the poison control center in your community. Post these and other emergency numbers in your home by the phone. Interview a person from each of these agencies to find out what action they take when they receive a call.

LESSON 2

43. Parental Involvement. Talk to your parents about safety precautions that are necessary on their jobs. Ask them what they are required to do regarding safety in their work.

LESSON 3

44. Further Study. Several years ago the speed limit on interstate highways was 70 miles per hour. Then the federal government passed a law changing this limit to 55 miles per hour. Recently, states have been permitted to increase this limit to 65 miles per hour in certain areas. Do some research to find out what effect the reduction from 70 to 55 miles per hour had on highway accidents and injuries. Based on your research, what do you think will be the effect of increasing the speed limit from 55 to 65 miles per hour?

CHAPTER

35

FIRST AID

LESSON 1

Administering
First Aid

LESSON 2

First Aid for
Poisoning

LESSON 3

First Aid for
Other Injuries

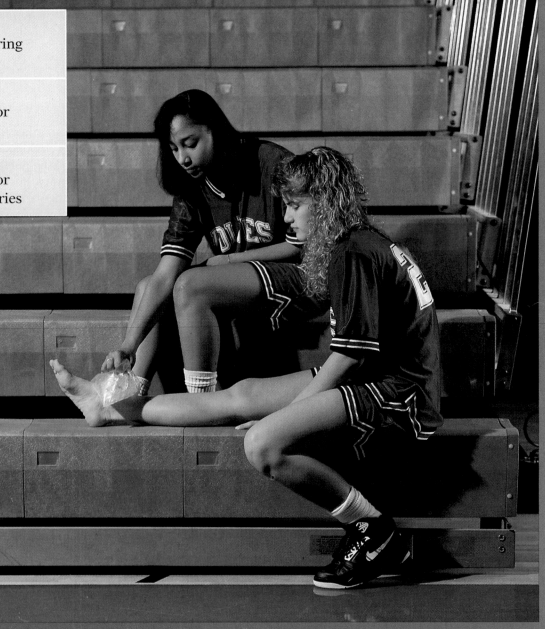

ADMINISTERING FIRST AID

Imagine you happened upon the scene of a traffic accident in which people had been hurt. Suppose you were on a bus and someone fainted. Would you know what to do in either of these emergency situations? **First aid,** or emergency care, is the immediate, temporary care given to a person who has become sick or who has been injured. First aid continues until a proper medical authority arrives at the scene of the emergency. Such authorities include persons on an emergency vehicle, a nurse, a physician, police officers, or firefighters.

Administering first aid is a serious job. It can mean the difference between life and death or between temporary and permanent disability. Because first aid can make life-changing differences, it is important to know—and know well—what you are doing when you give first aid.

Priorities in an Emergency

The first five minutes of an emergency situation are the most critical. During this crucial time it is important to remain calm and keep these six priorities in mind:

1. Check the immediate surroundings for possible dangers. Move the victim only if his or her life is threatened. Some life-threatening conditions include water deep enough for drowning to occur, a car that might catch on fire, or a room filled with smoke or poisonous fumes.
2. Check to see if the victim is conscious. If not, call for an ambulance at once.
3. Check breathing. Be sure the victim has an open airway. If he or she does not have an open airway, attempt to clear the airway; then administer rescue breathing if necessary. You will learn about this technique in Chapter 36.
4. Control severe bleeding. If blood is bright red and spurting, an artery has been damaged. You can control the bleeding by applying direct pressure to the wound. This lifesaving measure will be covered in depth later in this lesson.
5. Check the victim for poisoning. A **poison** is any substance—solid, liquid, or gas—that causes injury, illness, or death when introduced into the body. Treatment for poisoning is in the next lesson.
6. Send for medical help. Emergency Medical Services (EMS) can be summoned in many areas by dialing either 911 or 0. Learn the number for EMS in your area.

After the Priorities

Once you have taken steps to ensure the victim's safety and have administered life support procedures, you should attend to the following secondary measures:

LESSON 1 FOCUS

TERMS TO USE
- First aid
- Poison
- Pressure-point technique
- Shock

CONCEPTS TO LEARN
- Actions taken during the first five minutes of an emergency can save a person's life.
- The most important considerations in treating open wounds are stopping the bleeding, treating the victim for shock, and seeking medical care.

ATTITUDES AND BEHAVIORS TO EVALUATE
- Self-Inventory, page 710.
- Building Decision-Making Skills, page 711.

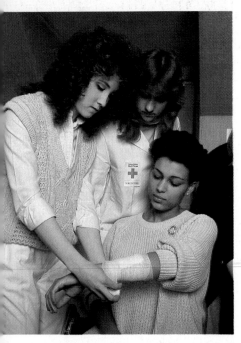

Knowing how to administer first aid is a valuable skill for anyone.

- Learn as much as you can about what happened, and devise a plan of action. Give the victim a reason for each thing you do. This reassurance will provide much needed encouragement.
- See to the victim's continued safety and comfort. Keep the victim still and in the position most suited to his or her injury or condition. Add privacy if you can, sheltering the victim from disturbance and unnecessary handling.
- Make sure the victim maintains normal body temperature. Provide blankets or a coat for warmth; provide shade for cooling protection from a hot sun.
- Loosen tight or binding clothing, taking care not to jar the victim's neck or spine.

As you work, remember to reassure the victim. Part of your job is to keep him or her calm. Above all else, know your own limits and abilities. Do not try to do more than you have been trained to do.

READ MY WRIST

Another important procedure when treating an accident victim is to look for a piece of emergency medical identification on or near the victim. He or she may have a bracelet, necklace, or card carried in a wallet or purse advising of a medical condition that demands special attention.

People with diabetes or heart conditions and those subject to seizures or severe allergic reactions are among those who wear or carry emergency medical identification. The tag or card gives vital information to those who might be called upon to give the wearer first aid.

Treating Open Wounds

Open wounds are usually a result of external physical forces. Auto accidents, falls, and mishandled tools or other sharp objects are the most common causes of open wounds.

Types of Open Wounds

There are four basic types of open wounds:

- **Scrape.** (abrasion) This type of wound damages outer layers of skin. Abrasions are accompanied by little or no bleeding but may become infected. Abrasions are caused by scraping or rubbing.
- **Cut.** (incision or laceration) A cut can have jagged or smooth edges. Cuts are caused by sharp objects, such as knives or broken glass. A cut also can result when a hard blow from a blunt object opens the skin. Cuts result in bleeding. Deep cuts can damage nerves, large blood vessels, and other soft tissues. Heavy bleeding may result.
- **Puncture.** When a pin, splinter, or other pointed object pierces the skin, the resulting wound is a puncture. While external bleeding is usually limited, puncture wounds carry the potential for internal bleeding and damage to internal organs as well as an increased possibility of infection. The risk of infection increases when the object remains in the skin.

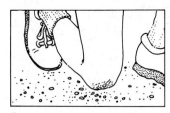

- **Avulsion.** This is a wound that results when tissue is separated partly or completely from the victim's body. Avulsions often occur in auto accidents and from animal bites. Since severed body parts can sometimes be reattached surgically, they should be sent along with the victim to the hospital.

Scrape

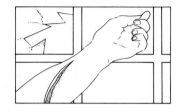

First Aid for Open Wounds

There are four steps in applying first aid to open wounds. They include: stopping the bleeding, protecting the wound from infection, treating the victim for shock, and seeking medical care.

Cut

Stopping the Bleeding. Applying direct pressure to the wound is the best method for stopping bleeding, because this method prevents blood loss without interfering with circulation. Direct pressure involves applying force directly to the top of the wound. To protect yourself from communicable diseases, wear disposable latex gloves, and wash your hands as soon as possible after giving care.

To apply direct pressure, follow these steps:

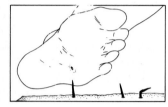

1. Place a thick, clean cloth over the wound.
2. Place the palm of your hand over the cloth and press firmly. If blood soaks through, place added layers of cloth over the first. Never remove the original cloth; doing so might disturb blood clots that have formed.
3. Continue applying pressure to the wound until the bleeding stops.

Puncture

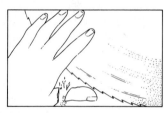

Avulsion

WHEN THE PRESSURE IS ON

Sometimes the direct-pressure method is not enough to stop the bleeding. In such cases, the **pressure-point technique** can be a lifesaver. For this technique, apply pressure to the main artery supplying blood to the affected limb. The main arteries supplying the limbs are the brachial artery, which brings blood to the arms, and the femoral artery, which brings blood to the legs.

To apply pressure at a pressure point, use your fingers or the heel of your hand. Press the artery toward the bone. Remember to keep applying direct pressure while you use the pressure-point technique.

K E E P I N G   F I T

How to Stop a Nosebleed

The most effective procedure to stop a nosebleed is to pinch both nostrils shut with a thumb and index finger. The victim should sit down and lean slightly forward or stand up. Leaning backward or tipping the head back will cause the blood to run down the throat, causing nausea or choking. Pinching provides direct pressure to the wound, which is a broken surface capillary.

Sometimes people who have chronic nosebleeds have the problem area inside the nose cauterized. If a nosebleed is severe and cannot be stopped, medical help should be sought.

Overcoming The Odds

Todd Drake is 22. He is a senior at Texas A&M majoring in accounting. He loves to play baseball, basketball, golf, and racquetball. In fact, you might say he just plain loves life—especially since he almost lost his.

Todd tells about the accident that changed and almost claimed his life. "I was 11 years old when I got electrocuted. I was goofing around with a long aluminum pole when it touched a low-hanging wire. That's when 14,400 volts of electricity went through me and blew me about ten feet back onto the ground on my back."

The shock caused Todd to stop breathing. "My neighbor's uncle rushed out and gave me CPR. That saved my life. I remember nothing except being put in the ambulance and seeing my mom.

"The doctors assessed that I needed to go to Parkland Hospital Burn Unit in Dallas, Texas. I remember only that I was in the emergency room and had an incredible thirst and that they gave me a pain killer. Before I was through, I had 15 reconstructive surgeries and was in the hospital from April till July."

Todd's injuries were very severe. "They amputated my right arm below the elbow and all my toes except one. They took ligaments and tendons

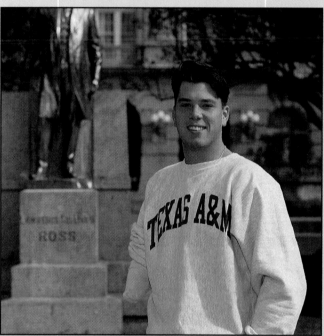

out of my right leg and my bicep muscle out of my left arm because they had been destroyed. My left hand had no movement because the nerves were burned. I had third-degree burns over 40 percent of my body. At one time, they didn't know if I was going to make it. Slowly, due to the surgeries, all the great care, and family love, I got better. I had incredible support from my family, my community, my church, and my friends—and that helped me a lot."

Despite the severity of his injuries, Todd wasn't about to be stopped. "In the hospital," he says, "all I could think of was getting out so I could play sports again." Playing baseball remains Todd's passion, and neither rejection by others nor having just one hand have stopped him. "In high school, when I tried out for the baseball team, I got cut twice. But I was determined, and I made it my senior year. Today, when I play baseball, I do it all: I bat, play outfield, and catch."

Todd knows he is fortunate to be alive, and he is grateful that someone nearby knew CPR. "I've got a second chance on life. I'm trying to make the best of my education and do something for the world. I fully intend to go on to law school or graduate school, so I can be the most well-rounded person I can be."

Todd also advises teens to listen to warnings from adults about health and safety. "Listen to your parents and your teachers," he concludes, "because they are telling you what's good for you and safe for you."

1. How might you feel if someone you know was in a life-threatening situation, and you didn't know what to do? If you do not know basic first aid, what steps can you take to learn it as soon as possible?
2. What attitude has helped Todd through his ordeal? How might you apply this attitude to your life?

Unless the injury involves a fracture, or broken bone, the bleeding body part should be elevated above the level of the victim's heart. The force of gravity helps slow the flow of blood.

Protecting the Wound. Normally, a clean cloth over an open wound will help protect it from infection. If a cloth is not available, a coat or any other clean covering will do.

Treating for Shock. **Shock** is the failure of the cardiovascular system to keep adequate blood circulating to the vital organs of the body. Shock can result from severe bleeding, heart attack, electrocution, poisoning, burns, or sudden changes of temperature.

You can recognize shock by these signs or symptoms: confused behavior, very fast or very slow pulse rate or breathing, trembling and weakness in the arms and legs, skin that is pale or clammy, pale or bluish lips and fingernails, and enlarged pupils.

When treating for shock, do the following:

- Keep the victim lying down.
- Make sure the victim maintains normal body temperature.
- Get medical help as soon as possible.

Unless you suspect a head injury, place the shock victim on his or her back with the feet elevated about 8 to 12 inches (20 to 30 cm) above the head. Elevating the feet in this manner helps return blood to the heart. A shock victim with a possible head injury should not be moved. Since emergency surgery may be required, shock victims should never be given food or drink.

Seeking Medical Care. See to it that the wounded victim gets immediate medical attention. Send someone for help, or if you are alone, shout for help. Leave the victim only after you have performed first aid and feel that you have lessened the risk of further injury or death.

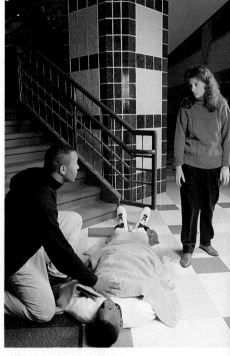

Shock victims should be kept quiet and warm, with their feet elevated. Seek medical help immediately.

LESSON 1 REVIEW

Reviewing Facts and Vocabulary

1. Define *first aid, poison,* and *shock.*
2. List the six tasks that should be completed when one first encounters an emergency situation.
3. Name the four types of open wounds.

Thinking Critically

4. **Evaluation.** Tell some of the things you would include if you were assembling a first-aid kit. Explain your choices.

Applying Health Knowledge

5. Imagine you were asked to give a talk on first aid to a group of third graders. What points would you stress in your talk?
6. While cycling fast, your friend takes a bad spill. You rush to help and find that her skin is clammy and blood is spurting from her head. Describe the first aid you would administer.

FIRST AID FOR POISONING

LESSON 2 FOCUS

TERM TO USE

- Poison control center

CONCEPTS TO LEARN

- Poisons are hazardous to your health and can be life-threatening.
- Victims of poisoning need immediate treatment.

ATTITUDES AND BEHAVIORS TO EVALUATE

- Self-Inventory, page 710.
- Building Decision-Making Skills, page 711.

What do medicines, snakebites, auto exhaust, household cleaners, and many plants have in common? All are potentially poisonous to the human body. Do you remember from the last lesson what a poison is? A poison is any substance that causes injury, illness, or death when introduced into the body.

The American Red Cross estimates that between 1 and 2 million poisonings occur every year. Some poisons are swallowed or inhaled while others enter the body through insect or animal bites. Even touching certain substances, such as poison ivy, can cause poisoning. Most poisonings involve children under the age of 6.

Swallowing a Poison

Today most household cleaners, medications, and other potentially dangerous products come in containers with safety tops that are hard for children to remove. Yet in spite of these precautions, many poisonings still occur.

While the signs of oral poisoning are not as obvious as those in many other emergency situations, telltale symptoms do exist. These symptoms include sharp abdominal cramps, extreme drowsiness followed by a loss of consciousness, vomiting, chemical odor on the breath or chemical burns on the lips, and the presence of an open container of a potentially poisonous substance.

First Aid for Swallowing a Poison

When you suspect someone has swallowed a poison, do the following:

- Call the nearest **poison control center.** It is part of a nationwide network that has been set up in and around large cities. People can contact these centers 24 hours a day. The number of the poison control center nearest you should be posted in a highly visible place in your home.
- Be prepared to give information about the victim and the poison to the person on the phone. This information should include the age and weight of the victim, the name of the suspected poison, and the amount of poison swallowed, if known. The staff person at the control center will then offer assistance with the situation and tell you where to go for further help. Specific treatments for each type of poison are available.
- Treat the victim for shock. Use the same procedure you read about in the section on treating wounds in Lesson 1. It may also be necessary to help the victim maintain respiration and circulation through rescue breathing or CPR. You will learn about these techniques in the next chapter.

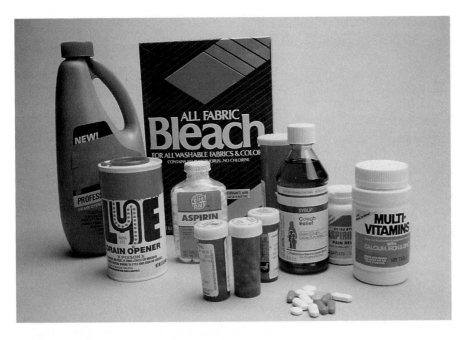

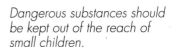

Dangerous substances should be kept out of the reach of small children.

A DO AND A DON'T

If you suspect someone has swallowed a poison, do look for and save the container of the suspected poison. You will need to give information about the poison to your telephone contact at the poison control center. Don't induce vomiting in the victim unless the poison control center advises you to do so. Some poisons, such as strong acids (bleach, toilet bowl cleaner) or strong alkalis (liquid drain cleaner), can do as much damage coming up as going down.

Poisoning by Snakebite

People who think of snakebites as hazards of life exclusively in rural areas are only partly right. Suburban environments and city parks can also be home to poisonous snakes.

Of the hundreds of varieties of snakes, only four poisonous types are found in the United States. These are the rattlesnake, the copperhead, the water moccasin (also called the cottonmouth), and the coral snake. More than half of all poisonous snakebites occur in Texas, North Carolina, Florida, Georgia, Louisiana, and Arkansas.

Culturally Speaking

Sandbox Trees

Sandbox trees, found in parts of Latin America, have poisonous bark with short spines. Their leaves also are poisonous. The sap of these trees is acidic and can burn skin and cause blindness. Exploding seed capsules from the tops of the trees have injured humans and animals. Nevertheless, sandbox trees are useful to humans. They are cut for wood, although people must wear masks and heavy gloves to protect themselves from the sap. The sap also is used to stun fish in streams so that they can be gathered for food. The poison does not affect the people who eat the fish.

KEEPING FIT

To Prevent Accidental Poisoning of Children

- Keep all medicines out of their reach.
- Install childproof locks on cabinets and closets that contain anything that could poison a child.
- Buy medicines with child-proof caps.
- Do not give children empty medicine bottles to use to play doctor. Next time they play, they might mistakenly use full ones.
- Don't remove labels from medications. You may need to identify what a child has accidentally swallowed.
- Crawl around your house at the child's level. See what potentially hazardous substances children may see.

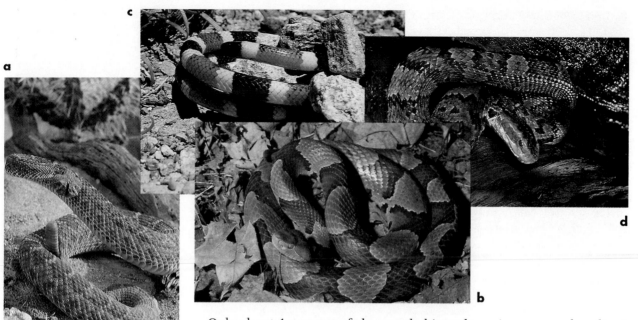

Know which snakes are poisonous: a. rattlesnake, b. copperhead, c. coral snake, d. water moccasin.

Only about 1 percent of the people bitten by poisonous snakes die. A large number of deformities and amputations do result from poisonous snakebites, so they should be treated immediately.

SNAKE SAVVY

A first line of defense against a poisonous snakebite is to know your enemy. A handy rule of thumb is summed up in the following rhyme: "Red and yellow mean a poisonous fellow; red and black, poison lack." In other words, if a snake's coloring includes consecutive bands of red and yellow, the snake is poisonous; a snake with consecutive red and black bands, on the other hand, will be nonpoisonous.

Once a victim has been bitten, a bite usually can be identified as one from a poisonous snake by the shape of the puncture wounds. A poisonous bite will also be accompanied by extreme pain and swelling, followed soon after by any or all of these symptoms: shortness of breath, nausea, dimness of vision, convulsions, a tingling sensation, or unconsciousness.

First Aid for Snakebite

If you are unsure about whether a snakebite came from a poisonous snake or not, treat the bite as though it were from a poisonous snake. You can administer first aid by following these steps:

1. Keep the victim calm. Your most important task is to get the victim to the hospital. Until you can complete this task, keep the victim as quiet as possible, preferably in a reclining position. The more the victim moves, the greater the risk that the venom will be circulated throughout the body.
2. Keep the bitten area at or below the level of the heart. If the bitten area is on a limb, keep the affected part immobile.
3. Call, or have someone call, EMS. Dialing 911 or 0 in many localities puts you in touch with EMS. Take careful note of any instructions you are given.

4. Delay the absorption of venom. Because snakes are coldblooded animals, their venom does the most damage in a cold environment. For this reason, avoid putting anything cold on the bite or giving the victim alcohol or sedatives. Aspirin, which can adversely affect blood coagulation, should also be avoided.

5. Maintain breathing, and prevent aggravation of the wound. If you are the victim of a snakebite and are alone, walk slowly and rest periodically. This will help keep blood circulation to a minimum.

Poisoning by Touching

Poisons that come into contact with the skin fall into two categories: those found on plants and those found in certain chemicals. The effects of touching these poisons are likewise twofold. In some cases the damage is limited to the area of the skin that touches the poison, whereas in others the whole body is affected.

First Aid for Touching a Poisonous Plant

The most common poisonous plants have the word *poison* in their names. These are poison ivy, poison oak, and poison sumac. A first defense against poisoning by any of these plants is to learn what they look like.

Interestingly, some people exhibit no reaction to poisonous plants. Those who do react develop a severe skin rash at the point of contact, followed later by various symptoms, which may include blistering, swelling, burning, and itching. In extreme cases, a fever occurs.

First aid for plant poisoning consists of three key steps:

1. Remove any clothing that may be contaminated.
2. Pour large quantities of water over the affected areas.
3. Wash the affected areas thoroughly with soap and water.

Calamine lotion can be used to relieve itching if a rash develops. If inflammation or pain is severe, seek medical attention.

First Aid for Touching a Poisonous Chemical

Pesticides, solvents, household cleaning agents, and highly abrasive cleaners are among the chemicals that can cause poisoning. A protec-

KEEPING FIT

Poison-Proofing Your Home

To poison-proof your home:
■ Check to see that any chemicals, cleaners, or other poisons are clearly marked and completely out of a child's reach.

■ Properly dispose of any old, unused poisonous substances.
■ Use the phone book and write the phone number of

the nearest poison-control center on a card. Place it next to the phone on the family's emergency number list.

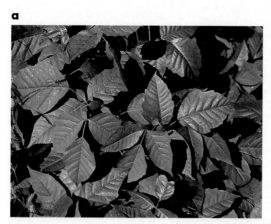

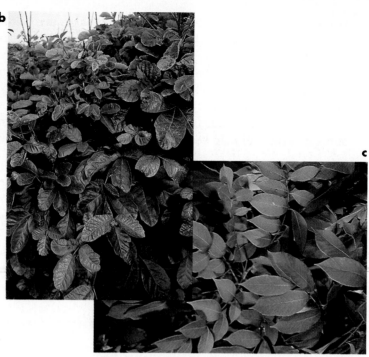

Learn to recognize these poisonous plants: a. poison ivy, b. poison oak, c. poison sumac.

tion against such poisoning is to make sure safety caps on these products are securely in place when the products are not being used. They should also be stored out of the reach of small children.

Poisoning through direct contact with a chemical is usually characterized by a burning of the skin, which appears similar to a sunburn. Treatment, which should begin as soon after the contact as possible, parallels first aid for plant poisoning:

1. Remove any clothing that has come into contact with the chemical.
2. Remove as much of the chemical from the surface of the skin as you can by continuously flooding the area with water for 15 minutes.
3. Contact the nearest poison control center for information on how to treat the resulting burn. A toll-free number for the poison control center in your state may be listed in your local telephone directory. Otherwise, call the emergency room of your local hospital.

LESSON 2 REVIEW

Reviewing Facts and Vocabulary

1. Define *poison* and give three examples.
2. Name four ways poisoning occurs.

Thinking Critically

3. **Analysis.** In what ways are first aid for swallowing a poison and touching a poison similar? How are they different?
4. **Evaluation.** Which first-aid techniques would be especially important for a camper or a hiker to know? Explain your choices.

Applying Health Knowledge

5. Use an encyclopedia to learn more about other forms of poisoning, such as lead or mercury. In an oral report to your class, explain how to identify and avoid these types of poisons.

First Aid for Other Injuries

In addition to such life-threatening emergencies as severe bleeding and poisoning, life has its share of minor mishaps. You are baby-sitting and the child you are watching gets a nosebleed. You and your friend are going out the door when your friend slips and sprains an ankle. You are mowing the lawn when a piece of debris flies into your eye. You have been exercising in the heat and begin to get painful heat cramps.

As with major emergencies, knowing proper first aid in these and other common emergencies can help prevent further injury or complication.

Nosebleeds

Nosebleeds can happen when the nose is struck. Although people whose noses bleed often should see their health-care professional, infrequent, minor nosebleeds are not a cause for alarm.

To treat a nosebleed, do the following:

1. Keep the person quiet. Walking, talking, and blowing the nose may cause an increase in bleeding.
2. Place the person in a sitting position and have him or her lean forward. You do not want to tilt the head back, because doing so may cause the person to choke as the blood runs down the throat.
3. Apply direct pressure by pressing on the bleeding nostril.
4. Apply a cold towel to the person's nose and face.

If these measures fail to stop the bleeding, the person should seek medical help.

Animal Bites

A dog may be a person's best friend—but not when the dog bites. Dogs and other animals can transmit diseases to humans by biting them.

Any animal bite, and especially one in which the animal's teeth have pierced the skin, should be washed with soap and warm water, then covered with a clean dressing or bandage.

In addition to treating the wound, it is important to observe the victim for signs of illness. Many animals carry **rabies**—a viral disease of the nervous system that eventually causes madness and death. Dogs, squirrels, and rats are common carriers of this disease.

If you know the whereabouts of the animal that inflicted the wound, have the proper authorities capture that animal. Do not try to capture the animal yourself. Once the animal has been captured, call the local health center to learn where the animal has been taken for examination. Then call to find out if treatment for tetanus or rabies is needed.

LESSON 3 FOCUS

TERMS TO USE

- Rabies
- Sprain
- Frostbite
- Gangrene (GANG•green)
- Hurricane
- Tornado
- Earthquakes
- Blizzard

CONCEPTS TO LEARN

- Each type of injury has its own set of general and specific first-aid procedures.
- Natural disasters and severe weather activity are threats to health, safety, life, and property.
- Disaster preparedness can greatly reduce the potential negative effects of natural disasters and severe weather.

ATTITUDES AND BEHAVIORS TO EVALUATE

- Self-Inventory, page 710.
- Building Decision-Making Skills, page 711.

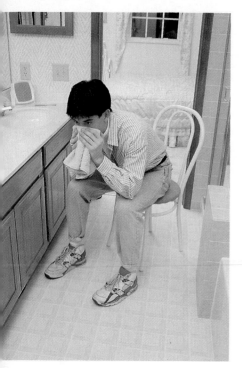

Infrequent nosebleeds are not a cause for alarm, but should be treated properly.

Bee Stings

In most cases bee stings are minor emergencies and are easily treated. For people who are allergic to bee stings, however, stings can be serious and sometimes even fatal. To treat bee stings, do the following:

1. Using a piece of cardboard or other flat, sharp-edged object, scrape against the stinger until you pull out the venom sac. Do not use tweezers because they may rupture the venom sac, forcing painful venom into the skin.
2. Wash the area thoroughly with soap and water.

Once the stinger is out, watch for allergic reactions. An allergic person will usually carry a kit with adrenaline to open the airways.

Fractures

When a body part, such as a leg or an arm, is under stress and you hear a popping sound, it is usually a good indication that a bone has been fractured. Always treat such an injury as if the bone were broken.

In applying first aid to fractures, your main objective is to keep the bone end from moving. Never attempt to set the bone. Follow these guidelines for first aid for a fracture:

1. Keep the body part in the position it is in, and immobilize it with a splint. You can fashion a splint from everyday materials, such as rolled newspapers and heavy cardboard.
2. Seek medical care immediately.

Sprains

A **sprain** is a condition caused by a stretching or tearing of the soft tissue bands, or ligaments, that hold bones together at a joint. Wrists, knees, and ankles are among the areas most frequently sprained. To treat a sprain, follow these steps:

1. Immobilize the injured area. If the sprain is in the leg, make sure the victim stays off his or her feet.
2. Elevate the injured part to help reduce swelling.
3. Apply cold packs. This will also help keep swelling down. Never apply heat, which makes swelling worse.
4. Seek medical attention.

Burns

Critical burns need immediate care. Critical burns include those that involve breathing difficulties, burns covering more than one body part, and burns to the head, neck, hands, and feet. They also include chemical burns. There are three descriptions for burns:

- Superficial (first-degree) burns, like most sunburns, involve the top layer of skin. Healing takes five to six days.

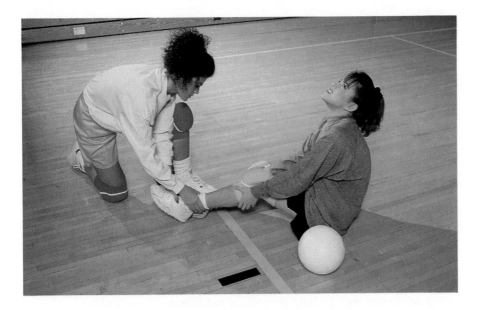

Is it a fracture or a sprain? How can you tell? What should you do for each?

- Partial-thickness (second-degree) burns involve the top layers of skin. The skin will have blisters and appear blotchy. Healing takes three to four weeks.
- Full-thickness (third-degree) burns destroy all layers of skin as well as nerves, muscles, fat, and bones. The burn looks black or brown.

First Aid for Burns

First aid for all burns includes the following:

1. Stop the burning by removing the victim from the source of the burn.
2. Cool the burn by soaking the burned area in cool water or using wet towels.
3. Cover the burn with dry, sterile dressings. This action helps prevent infection and reduces pain.

Protect a person with severe burns from drafts. Unless the victim is having trouble breathing, lay the person down. If possible, the burned area should be raised above the level of the heart.

Chemical burns should be flushed with large quantities of cool running water. Take off any clothing that has the chemical on it.

Fainting

Fainting is a temporary loss of consciousness brought on by a reduced supply of blood to the brain. People who faint usually recover within a few minutes. First aid for fainting includes the following steps:

1. Do not prop up the person. Leave him or her lying down on the back. If possible, elevate the legs 8 to 12 inches.
2. Loosen any tight or binding clothing.
3. Maintain an open airway. (Refer to Chapter 36.)
4. Sponge the person's face with water. Do not splash water over the face, because this may cause the person to choke.
5. If the person fails to revive promptly, seek medical help.

DID YOU KNOW?

- If a tick is attached to your skin, you can remove it by pulling slowly and firmly with tweezers.
- Some sea life, including some jellyfish and the Portuguese man-of-war, discharge venom on contact even after they are dead.
- One way to stop the pain from a jellyfish sting is to rub meat tenderizer, vinegar, salt, or sand on the area.

Objects in the Eye

If a foreign object comes into contact with the surface of your eye, resist the impulse to rub the eye. Doing so may scratch the cornea. Instead, gently flush the eye with water, starting at the edge nearest the nose and working outward. If this measure fails to dislodge the object, cover both eyes and seek medical attention.

Heat Cramps

When a person is exposed to high temperatures over a prolonged period, the body loses essential water and salt. The resulting condition is known as heat cramps. Heat cramps are characterized by muscle cramps, heavy sweating, headache, and dizziness.

Here are some procedures to follow when heat cramps strike:

1. Move the victim, or help the victim move, out of the heat.
2. Using your hands, apply firm pressure to the cramped muscle. Gently massage the muscle to relieve the spasm.
3. Give the victim sips of a commercial sports drink, which will replace salt and water. The victim should consume about 4 ounces (118 ml) every 15 minutes. Be careful that the victim does not take in too much of the liquid at any one time. Excessive amounts of salt may induce vomiting. Do not give the victim salt tablets.

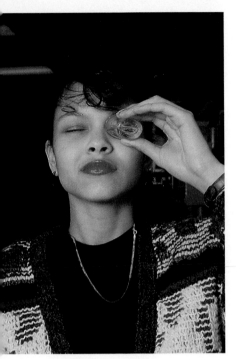

To remove a foreign object from the eye, gently flush with water.

Frostbite

Have you ever noticed on bitter winter days that your fingers and toes are the first parts of your body to get cold? In extremely cold conditions, the body tries to conserve heat for its more vital internal organs. As a result, less blood is sent to the extremities.

If the temperature in body cells gets low enough, **frostbite** may occur. Frostbite is a condition in which ice crystals form in the spaces between the cells. This ice expands and kills tissue, and in the process, causes the skin to lose color and become insensitive to any feeling. Frostbite is common among those who spend long periods of time outdoors in temperatures at or below freezing. Several factors play a role in frostbite: the temperature, the length of time the person is exposed to the cold, the wind velocity, the humidity level, the amount of protective clothing worn, and the dampness of the clothing.

K E E P I N G   F I T

Weather Problems

For years, blizzards have been common in the North, and tornadoes and hurricanes have been common along the coastline of the South. Weather patterns are changing now, and many areas of the country are vulnerable to new weather-related disasters. An earthquake in the Adirondack mountains of New York state destroyed a portion of a road and several cars. Hurricanes have whirled inland, carrying devastation to the central part of the country. Snowstorms have caused loss of life and property in Georgia. These changes point out the need to understand the required emergency behavior for many types of danger.

First Aid for Frostbite

Frostbitten skin is yellowish or gray in color and feels clammy or doughy. A frostbite victim will usually experience numbness in the frostbitten body part. Treat frostbite by doing the following:

1. Never rub the affected area. Rewarm the frozen body part by soaking it in water that is about 100° to 105°F (37.8° to 40.6°C).
2. Bandage the injured part, placing sheets of gauze between the warmed fingers and toes.
3. Seek professional medical attention as soon as possible.

If a frostbitten body part goes untreated, **gangrene** may set in. Gangrene is the death of tissue in a part of the body. Gangrene often requires amputation of the affected part.

COLD WEATHER ADVISORY

When you plan to spend prolonged periods outdoors during cold weather, it is vital that you dress properly. Wearing several layers of clothing will help retain body heat. Footgear and headgear are also important.

Be mindful, too, of the windchill. Any windchill of −25°F (−31.7°C) or colder presents a danger, with −72°F (−57.8°C) presenting a critical danger. Here are some temperature equivalents at different wind speeds. All are based on a thermometer reading of −10°F (−23.3°C).

When the wind blows at . . .	the windchill makes it feel like . . .
5 mph (8 km/h)	−15°F (−26.1°C)
10 mph (16 km/h)	−33°F (−36.1°C)
15 mph (23 km/h)	−45°F (−42.8°C)
20 mph (32 km/h)	−53°F (−47.3°C)

More Weather-Related Emergencies

Weather poses a threat not just to individuals but to entire communities. Hurricanes, tornadoes, and other natural disasters can cause widespread injury and death as well as property damage and loss.

Most communities have emergency sirens to warn of potentially dangerous situations. Some environmental conditions, however, occur without warning. Does your community have an emergency warning system? Do you know what to do in such an emergency?

Hurricanes and Tornadoes

A **hurricane** is a powerful rainstorm, characterized by driving winds. Hurricanes occur near coastal areas of the United States, mainly on the eastern and southern seaboards.

A **tornado** is a powerful, twisting windstorm that generally occurs in the central part of the United States. Tornadoes occasionally are associated with hurricanes. In recent times, tornadoes have been known to strike sporadically in all areas of the country. Knowing what to do in case of a hurricane or a tornado could save your life.

When severe weather conditions exist, the National Weather Service issues advisories called watches and warnings. A hurricane watch or a tornado watch means that atmospheric conditions exist so that these events could develop. A warning means one has been sighted. Warnings are often accompanied by instructions. Do exactly as you are told without delay.

In general, preparation for a hurricane includes securing your property and then either going to a shelter or evacuating the area as the National Weather Service instructs. The farther inland you go, the safer you will be. Hurricanes have been known to build up enough momentum to carry their destructive winds inland for hundreds of miles.

A storm cellar or basement is the safest place to go for protection from a tornado. If neither option is available, a hallway or bathtub away from windows will suffice. If you are caught outside, get into a ditch and lie face down. Cover yourself, if possible, with a mattress, blanket, rug, or bulky winter clothing to protect yourself from flying objects.

Earthquakes

Heavy ground tremors from **earthquakes** occur often in some parts of the United States. California averages almost 5,000 weak but notice-

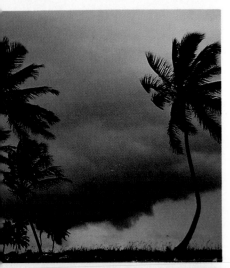
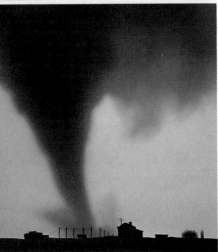

Hurricanes (top) and tornadoes (bottom) are dangerous weather storms.

able quakes per year. Knowing what to do during and after an earth-quake is important to your safety.

Most casualties during an earthquake are not a direct result of the ground movement but result from falling objects or collapsing structures. If you are inside a building and begin to feel a tremor, follow these safety procedures:

1. Stay in the building.
2. Select a safety spot within a few steps of where you are standing, and go to it. Safety spots are areas that provide some measure of safety from falling matter. Try to find a heavy desk or table with enough space for you to fit underneath. Crawl under it and then hold on to this shelter to keep it from moving away from you.
3. If no such piece of furniture is handy, choose a corner of the room away from bookcases, tall shelves, sliding doors, chimneys, or anything else that may collapse.
4. If you live in an area prone to tremors, safeguard your home by bolting bookcases and other tall or heavy furniture to the wall. If you are outdoors when an earthquake hits, stay away from buildings, trees, and power lines.

Blizzards

A **blizzard** is a snowstorm with winds of 35 miles per hour (56 km per hour) or greater. Visibility is less than 500 feet (152 m), so it is easy for a person to get lost. The safest place to be during a blizzard is indoors. If you are caught outside, try to keep your mouth and nose covered, and keep moving so that you do not freeze. Try to follow a road or a fence to the closest safe place.

If you must go outside in a blizzard, wear protective clothing. All of the following will help protect you from freezing temperatures and frostbite: thermal, woolen undergarments; outer garments that will repel wind and moisture; head, face, and ear coverings; extra socks; warm boots; and wool-lined mittens.

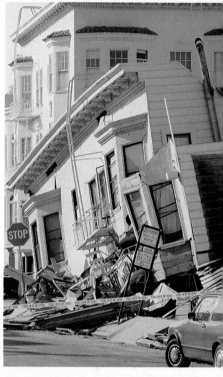

Most earthquake injuries are caused by falling objects and collapsing buildings .

LESSON 3 REVIEW

Reviewing Facts and Vocabulary

1. Define *frostbite, gangrene, hurricane watch,* and *earthquake.*
2. What should you *not* do in treating a fracture? In treating a heat cramp?
3. Describe the three types of burns and the first aid for each.

Thinking Critically

4. **Evaluation.** Tell which of the first-aid measures you read about in this lesson you feel are most important to know. Give reasons.

5. **Analysis.** Compare and contrast hurricanes, tornadoes, and earthquakes.

Applying Health Knowledge

6. Research the kinds of natural disasters common to your area of the United States. Speak with someone at your local chapter of the American Red Cross about what action should be taken in disasters of this type. Summarize your findings, and share them with the class. If there is no chapter in your community, find out who is responsible for handling disasters or emergencies.

Self-Inventory

Emergency Behaviors and Attitudes

HOW DO YOU RATE?

A measure of the health of any community is the ability of its members to aid themselves and others in an emergency. Do you contribute to your personal health and to the health of your community? Number a sheet of paper from 1 through 15. Read each item below, and respond by writing *yes* or *no*. Total the number of *yes* and *no* responses. Then proceed to the next section.

1. I make a point of knowing the names of all my family's health-care professionals.
2. I keep a list of emergency phone numbers near a telephone in my home.
3. I know how to reach the police, the fire department, and emergency medical help from a public telephone.
4. I keep a fully stocked first-aid kit in my home.
5. I believe that first aid is everyone's responsibility.
6. I use only those first-aid skills for which I have had training.
7. I know how to treat different kinds of wounds.
8. I am aware of the five priorities related to an emergency situation.
9. I know what steps to take to stop heavy bleeding.
10. I have the ability to help someone who has swallowed a poison.
11. I can administer first aid for different types of bites and stings.
12. I know how to help a victim of nosebleed, fainting, heat cramps, and frostbite.
13. I am able to tell the difference between minor and serious burns and can treat each kind.
14. I know first aid for sprains and fractures.
15. I know what action to take in the event of hurricanes, tornadoes, and other natural disasters.

HOW DID YOU SCORE?

Give yourself 1 point for every *yes* answer and 0 points for every *no* answer. Find your total, and read below to see how you scored. Then proceed to the next section.

12 to 15
Excellent. You have the makings of a lifesaver in emergency situations.

8 to 11
Good. Many of your skills and attitudes are healthy; others need work.

4 to 7
Fair. You need to develop more emergency skills. By developing your first-aid skills, you could save a life.

Below 4
Poor. By your responses, you would be of little help in most emergency situations.

WHAT ARE YOUR GOALS?

Identify an area in which your score was low, and use the goal-setting process below to pave the way for a change.

1. The skill or attitude I would like to change is ____.
2. If this skill or attitude were changed, I would look, feel, or act differently in the following ways: ____.
3. The steps involved in making this change are ____.
4. My timetable for making this change is ____.
5. People I will ask for help or assistance are ____.
6. The benefits I will receive as a result of making this change are ____.

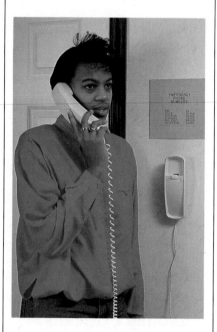

Building Decision-Making Skills

Sandy and some of her friends are playing volleyball on the beach after school. Sandy receives a volley from her brother Leo, and she successfully spikes the volleyball over the net. Unfortunately, on her way down from her jump, Sandy's left foot hits a rock that is hidden in the sand. A severe pain shoots through her ankle, and she screams in pain. She lies on the ground, clutching her ankle. Her brother runs to her. He can see that Sandy is in extreme pain. What should Leo do?

A. Tell Sandy to "shake it off" and get up and continue the game.

B. Ask Sandy if she heard a crack or a popping sound when she fell so that he can determine whether she has broken her ankle or only sprained it. Then administer the appropriate first-aid measures.

C. Tell Sandy to lie still while someone goes for help.

WHAT DO YOU THINK?

1. **Situation.** Why does a decision need to be made?
2. **Choices.** What other choices does Leo have?
3. **Consequences.** How might Leo's decision affect Sandy's health triangle?
4. **Consequences.** How might Leo's decision affect his own health triangle?
5. **Consequences.** What are the advantages of each choice?
6. **Consequences.** What are the disadvantages of each choice?
7. **Decision.** What decision do you think is best for Sandy?
8. **Evaluation.** Have you ever found yourself in a situation where a friend was injured and you had to decide what to do? What did you do? What would you do differently if you found yourself in a similar situation?

Carlos is baby-sitting his twin cousins, Pedro and Pilar. He has put them to bed upstairs and is watching a video in the living room. Suddenly, he hears a crash. He races upstairs to find the twins in the bathroom with an open and half-empty bottle of pills on the floor. What should Carlos do?

A. Send the twins back to bed, and put the remaining pills back in the medicine chest.

B. Read the label on the bottle of pills to find out whether the pills could be harmful to children.

C. Call a poison control center, and describe the pills the twins may have taken.

WHAT DO YOU THINK?

9. **Situation.** Why does a decision need to be made?
10. **Situation.** Who will be affected by Carlos's decision?
11. **Situation.** Where can Carlos find the phone number for the poison control center?
12. **Choices.** What other choices does Carlos have?
13. **Consequences.** How might Carlos's decision affect the twins' health?
14. **Consequences.** What are the advantages of each choice?
15. **Consequences.** What are the disadvantages of each choice?
16. **Consequences.** What risks are involved in this situation?
17. **Consequences.** How will the twins' parents probably react to Carlos's decision?
18. **Decision.** What do you think Carlos should do?
19. **Evaluation.** Have you ever been in a situation similar to Carlos's? How did you handle it? What would you do differently if you encountered a similar situation in the future?

REVIEW

Using Health Terms

On a separate sheet of paper, write the term that best matches each definition given below.

LESSON 1

1. A jagged, irregular tear with heavy bleeding.
2. Type of wound in which the skin is pierced.
3. A broken bone.
4. A condition that occurs when vital organs are deprived of blood.

LESSON 2

5. Part of a nationwide network that provides information on treatment in cases of poisoning.
6. Snakes with bands of red and yellow.
7. Snakes with bands of red and black.
8. An over-the-counter medication that can be applied to relieve itching caused by exposure to poisonous plants.

LESSON 3

9. A viral disease of the nervous system that leads to madness and death.
10. A condition caused by a sudden stretching of soft tissues around a joint.
11. The temporary loss of consciousness due to a lack of blood to the brain.
12. Loss of essential water and salt from the body when it is exposed to high temperatures over a prolonged period of time.
13. A twisting windstorm.
14. A snowstorm during which visibility is less than 500 feet and wind speeds reach 35 miles per hour.

Building Academic Skills

LESSON 1

15. **Writing.** Emergency Medical Technician is a career that you or someone in your school may wish to pursue. Interview an Emergency Medical Technician in your community. Summarize your interview in an article for your school or local newspaper.

Recalling the Facts

LESSON 1

16. In your own words, describe four secondary measures one should attend to in an emergency situation.
17. Explain the function of emergency medical identification and who is likely to wear it.
18. Tell the four steps in treating an open wound.
19. What are possible situations in which shock might be an outcome? What are the symptoms of shock?

LESSON 2

20. What is the proper first aid for poisoning by swallowing?
21. What information should you give when you call a poison control center?
22. When treating a victim of poisoning by swallowing, why should one not induce vomiting unless directed to do so by someone at the poison control center?
23. Given the following symptoms, what would you conclude happened to the victim: puncture wounds, extreme pain and swelling, shortness of breath, nausea, dimness of vision, convulsions, a tingling sensation, and unconsciousness?
24. What is a characteristic of chemical poisoning by touch?

LESSON 3

25. If one suspects someone has suffered a fracture, should the victim be told to move the injured part to see if it works? Why or why not?
26. Which of the following should you *not* do in treating a burn victim?
    a. Submerge the burned area in cool water.
    b. Apply butter or oil to the burned area.
    c. Apply a clean, dry dressing.
    d. Pop any blisters that form and remove the burned skin.
27. What is the first-aid procedure for fainting?
28. What factors can play a role in frostbite? Which of these factors is within a person's control?

REVIEW

Thinking Critically

LESSON 1

29. **Synthesis.** Develop a series of principles that every good first aider should follow in an emergency.

30. **Analysis.** Methods of first aid sometimes change as new information becomes available. What implications does this have for anyone who has ever studied first aid?

LESSON 2

31. **Synthesis.** Why do you think over half of poisonous snakebites occur in Texas, North Carolina, Florida, Georgia, Louisiana, and Arkansas?

32. **Analysis.** How would treatment for poison ivy and treatment for battery acid on the skin differ?

LESSON 3

33. **Evaluation.** In some areas, emergency medical technicians decide whether to transport emergency victims to a hospital for further treatment. In other areas, anyone who calls for emergency help is transported to a hospital. Which procedure do you feel is better? Support your answer.

Making the Connection

LESSON 1

34. **Dramatics.** Work with several other students to prepare a skit dramatizing an accident involving an open wound and its treatment.

LESSON 3

35. **Art.** Make a poster illustrating the procedures to be followed in one of the following: hurricane, tornado, or earthquake.

36. **Speech.** Do some research to learn more about the American Red Cross. Prepare a speech describing its history and its involvement in weather-related disasters in your area if possible. Find out how the ARC recruits its workers and what you could do to become an ARC volunteer.

Applying Health Knowledge

LESSON 1

37. Discuss why it would be unwise to put one's own safety at risk when helping a victim.

38. Tell what type of wound would most likely result from each situation below.
    a. A dog bite.
    b. Wrestling on a carpet.
    c. Getting your hand too close to moving lawnmower blades.
    d. Being slashed with a knife.

LESSON 2

39. What is a highly visible place in your home where the phone number for the poison control center could be posted?

LESSON 3

40. Why do you suppose a cold towel applied to a person's nose or face is part of the first aid for a nosebleed?

41. For a sprain, first aid includes applying a cold pack. What is a cold pack? How can you make one? Should you put ice directly on a sprain? Explain.

Beyond the Classroom

LESSON 1

42. **Parental Involvement.** Share with your parents information you have learned in this chapter. Then, together, make your home more first-aid ready. Find and post the phone numbers for the nearest poison control center and other emergency numbers. Assemble or update a first-aid kit.

LESSON 3

43. **Community Involvement.** You have learned first aid for many different kinds of wounds in this chapter. Make a separate poster for each kind of first aid discussed in the chapter. Post each one where it is most appropriate. For example, a poster on how to treat chemical burns may be best suited for the chemistry lab.

CHAPTER 36

HANDLING EMERGENCIES

LESSON 1
Acting in an
Emergency

LESSON 2
Cardiopulmonary
Resuscitation

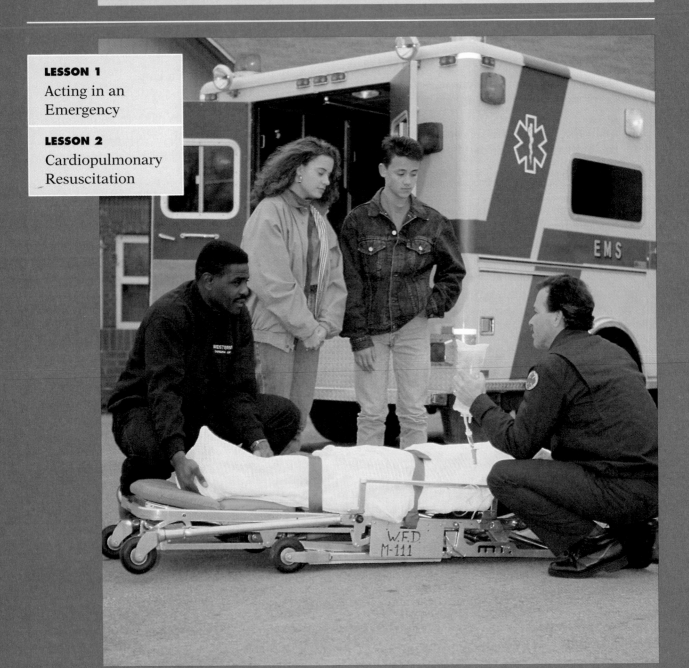

ACTING IN AN EMERGENCY

Consider these life-threatening situations: A family is seated at dinner when someone at the table begins to choke. A group of people are standing on a busy city street corner when suddenly a middle-aged man among them clutches his chest and slumps to the ground. Scenes like these happen in the United States thousands of times each year, and thousands of times the victim dies—needlessly.

The most common cause of sudden death is heart attack. Drowning, electrical shock, drug overdose, stroke, smoke inhalation, and suffocation can also stop a person's breathing and circulation and result in sudden death. A knowledge of first aid in these cases is, literally, a matter of life and death.

First Aid for Choking

More than 3,000 Americans choke to death annually. Many of the deaths reported involve children under 4 years of age. Choking is the sixth leading cause of death in the overall population. It is a leading cause of accidental death in the home for children under 1 year of age.

These statistics are sobering. What is perhaps even more sobering is that a great many of these deaths could have been prevented.

In order for a choking victim to survive, immediate recognition and treatment are a must. A gasping for breath or a weak coughing noise, accompanied by an inability to talk, are indications that a person is choking. The victim may become pale, turn blue, or even lose consciousness. You can learn to recognize these signs and give aid.

The universal distress signal for choking is clutching the neck between the thumb and index finger. Learning this signal can help you save a choking victim. It can also help another person save you.

LESSON 1 FOCUS

TERMS TO USE
- Abdominal thrusts
- Rescue breathing
- Carotid pulse

CONCEPTS TO LEARN
- The abdominal thrust should be administered only to conscious victims; it can also be self-administered.
- Maintaining an open airway and supplying a victim with oxygen are the main objectives for rescue breathing.

ATTITUDES AND BEHAVIORS TO EVALUATE
- Self Inventory, page 726.
- Building Decision-Making Skills, page 727.

NO CHOKE

You can reduce your chances of becoming a choking victim by observing some simple safety tips:

- Take small bites of food when you eat.
- Eat slowly, chewing each mouthful of food thoroughly.
- Do not talk or laugh with food in your mouth.
- Do not go to sleep with chewing gum or food in your mouth.

Choking in Children and Adults

Hard as it may be to believe, many choking deaths result from mistaken identity. That is, people witnessing someone choking fail to administer first aid for choking because they wrongly believe that the victim is

Abdominal thrusts force out the substance blocking the airway.

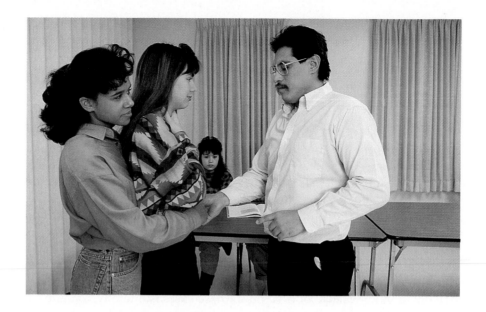

suffering a heart attack. This is why fatal choking accidents in restaurants have been called "café coronaries."

If you suspect a child or adult is choking, ask the person, "Are you choking?" If the victim cannot breathe, cough, or speak, begin first aid immediately by administering **abdominal thrusts.** Also called the Heimlich maneuver, after the chest surgeon who developed the technique, these quick, upward thrusts force the diaphragm upward and force out the substance blocking the airway.

When administering abdominal thrusts to conscious victims, this is what to do:

1. Wrap your arms around the victim's waist, with the thumb side of your wrist against the victim's abdomen. Place your hand halfway between the lower tip of the victim's breastbone, or sternum, and the navel.
2. Grasp your fist with your other hand, and press into the abdomen with quick, upward thrusts until the blockage is dislodged. Abdominal thrusts on a conscious adult should be repeated until the object is coughed up or the person becomes unconscious.

Note that the abdominal thrust technique can be self-administered. If no other person is present, a choking victim can perform abdominal thrusts on himself or herself by leaning over the back of a chair or over the edge of a table.

Choking in Infants

Very young children often place buttons and other small objects in their mouths. Because of this, families with infants, children up to 1 year of age, should take a course in first aid for choking. Your local Emergency Medical Services (EMS) or local chapter of the American Heart Association or American Red Cross provides training in the use of effective techniques for infants who are choking. Use the following techniques only on conscious, choking infants:

1. Turn the infant to a downward angle over your arm.
2. Using the heel of your other hand, give four quick blows to the baby's back between the shoulder blades.

Learning the signal for choking can save another person's life and maybe your own.

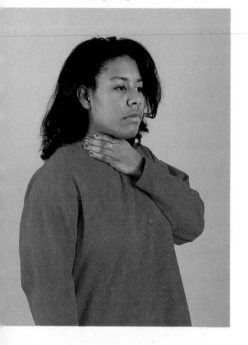

3. Turn the infant over, supporting its head, neck, and back between the shoulders. Press two fingers into the middle of the baby's sternum. This action is known as a chest thrust. Repeat the action four times.
4. Alternate administering back blows and chest thrusts until the object is dislodged.

Respiratory Failure

In some emergencies, such as choking, drowning, and electrical shock, a victim's breathing stops or becomes blocked. You can recognize breathing failure by a number of signs, including an absence of breathing movements, dilated pupils, and a bluish color to the lips, tongue, or fingernails.

When respiratory failure occurs, it is essential to give the victim oxygen immediately. Lack of oxygen to the brain can cause permanent brain damage within minutes after breathing stops. The most practical method in such an emergency is mouth-to-mouth or mouth-to-nose respiration. This technique, known variously as **rescue breathing,** artificial respiration, or resuscitation, has two main objectives:

Rescue Breathing for Adults

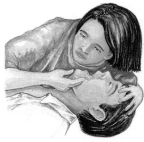 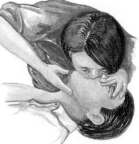 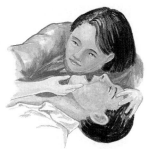

1. If the victim is unconscious, tilt the victim's head back while lifting the chin upward. Look, listen, and feel for signs of breathing.

2. If the victim is not breathing, close the victim's nostrils shut. Place your mouth over the person's mouth, forming a seal. Give two full breaths.

3. Look, listen, and feel again. Feel the carotid pulse. If there is a pulse but no breathing, give one breath every five seconds.

Rescue Breathing for Infants and Children

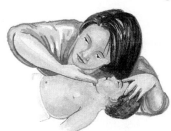 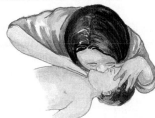

1. Position the head to clear the airway.

2. Cover and form a seal with your mouth over the victim's mouth and nose. Give one breath every three seconds for an infant. Give one breath every four seconds for a child.

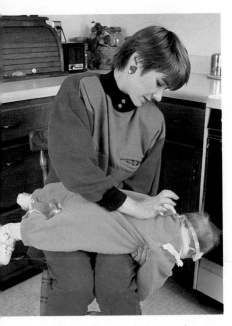

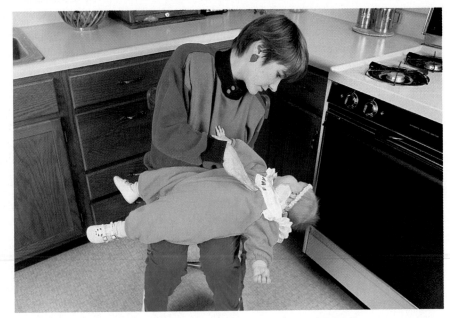

If an infant is choking, alternate back blows and chest thrusts.

■ to maintain an open airway
■ to supply the victim with oxygen necessary for his or her survival

Additional measures are called for when a person is not breathing and has no pulse. You will learn about these measures in the next lesson.

Rescue Breathing for Adults

Rescue breathing for adults is different in some respects from rescue breathing for small children. The steps a person should follow when administering rescue breathing to adults are as follows:

1. Check to see whether the victim is conscious. Tap the person's shoulder and ask, "Are you all right?" If there is no response, direct someone to call EMS for help.
2. Place one hand on the bony part of the victim's chin and one on the forehead, and tilt the victim's head back while lifting the chin upward. This action moves the jaw and tongue forward, opening the airway.
3. Place your ear and cheek close to the victim's mouth and nose. Look, listen, and feel. Look at the chest to see whether it is rising and falling. Listen for air being exhaled from the lungs. Feel for exhaled air on your cheek.

K E E P I N G   F I T

How to Report an Emergency

If you have to report an emergency, keep these guidelines in mind:
■ Give the emergency dispatcher the complete address and phone number where help is needed.
■ Try to speak clearly and loudly.

■ Try to stay as calm as possible.
■ If the victim is unconscious or not breathing, tell the dispatcher. Many dispatchers are trained to tell people over the phone what to do until help can get there.

■ If there are two or more of you who are uninjured, send one person to turn on the outside lights and another to the entrance or street to direct the ambulance to you.

Overcoming The Odds

Tracey Maichle is 29. She has many hobbies and feels good about herself, partly because of her passion for her work. Tracey is a city firefighter.

Yet Tracey didn't always have as much confidence in herself, "Even though I had a terrific childhood," she begins, "I had a lot of problems as a child knowing that I was adopted. But when I was 18, I found my biological mother, then my biological father, and that helped me a great deal. It helped me find out and accept who I am."

Tracey had an early experience with fire that has stuck with her into adulthood. "My adoptive parents had a trailer down at the beach," she says. "One night, when I was about 13, my mother had put my little cousin down to sleep. I'd gone to bed. My mother had draped a towel over a light to make it dimmer for my cousin. I smelled smoke. At that point, there was no one else in the trailer but my cousin and me. I ran in and got my cousin, who was near the fire, and took him outside. It made me feel good, even though I was young. I'd always been taught the basics by my parents, like if you smell smoke, get out, get help, and stay calm. The basics worked."

Tracey's interest in rescuing

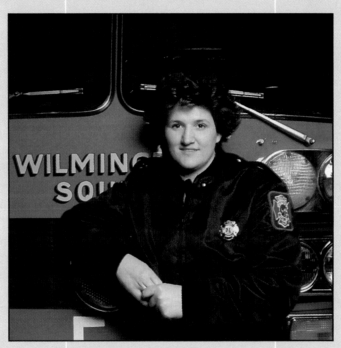

people in trouble continued. "I dated a volunteer firefighter for a number of years. I got tired of waiting in the car or waiting at the fire house. I began to want to help victims that were in car accidents or people whose houses were on fire." So Tracey went through fire school, got a certificate, then went through advanced training.

Tracey loves to talk about her experiences. "We had a 14- or 15-year-old male who had drowned. He had been under water for about 20 minutes. I did CPR until the paramedics got there and could use electric shock on him. They brought him back and took him to the hospital."

Having her own children has given Tracey new perspec-

tive on the importance of safety and safety training. She says, "My 14-year-old son went to get certified by the Red Cross for infant CPR because I have another son who is 18 months. Now the 14-year-old is really turned on to safety."

Tracey offers this advice. "If you are faced with an emergency, know who to call for help. In many areas that's 911. Try not to panic. Try to keep your wits about you. Most important, try to get training beforehand."

Tracey now feels very competent. "I have a lot of confidence in myself knowing that, when I come across an emergency, I can exhaust every possibility of trying to help that person, whether it be to save a life, get someone proper care, or save someone's property."

1. How do you react in emergencies? Do you think the way you react helps or hurts the situation? If you do not think you react in a calm or effective way, what steps can you take to change your reactions?
2. Do you feel trained to handle basic medical emergencies until professional help arrives? Do you know who to call to get help?

4. If the victim is not breathing, pinch the victim's nostrils shut with your index finger and thumb. Place your mouth over the victim's mouth, forming a seal. Give the person two breaths with only enough air to make the chest rise (1 to 1½ seconds each). Check pulse and breathing together for 5 to 10 seconds.

5. Keeping the victim's head tilted, look, listen, and feel again. Determine whether the victim's heart is beating by feeling for the **carotid pulse.** This pulse is the heartbeat found on each side of the neck. You can locate the carotid pulse by placing your index and middle fingers on the Adam's apple and sliding them into the groove at the side of the neck. Do not use your thumb to feel for the pulse. You may feel your own pulse if you do.

6. If there is a pulse but still no breathing, begin giving the victim one breath every five seconds.

Periodically check the chest to see whether it is rising or falling. If it is moving, you know that air is getting into the lungs. Continue artificial respiration until the victim has started breathing again or medical help takes over.

Rescue Breathing for Infants and Children

Rescue breathing for infants and children parallels rescue breathing for adults, with these exceptions:

- When positioning the victim's head to clear the airway, do not tilt the head back as far as you would for an adult.
- For infants, cover and form a seal with your mouth over both the victim's mouth and nose rather than over the victim's mouth alone.
- Breathe in only enough air to make the chest gently rise. Breathe air into the infant's nose and mouth at the rate of one breath every three seconds. For a child, give one breath about every four seconds.

LESSON 1 REVIEW

Reviewing Facts and Vocabulary

1. Give another name for each of these terms: *abdominal thrust* and *artificial respiration.* Then use each term in an original sentence.
2. What are some signs of choking? Of respiratory failure?
3. What are the main objectives of rescue breathing?

Thinking Critically

4. **Evaluation.** Name two factors that might explain why two-thirds of all choking deaths involve small children.

5. **Analysis.** Compare first aid for choking in infants with first aid for choking in children and adults.

Applying Health Knowledge

6. Interview someone trained in emergency medical care. Write a report describing how he or she helps someone who is not breathing. In your report include equipment that is used to help perform rescue breathing.

CARDIOPULMONARY RESUSCITATION

Among the most serious life-threatening situations a person can encounter is failure of the cardiovascular system. Cardiovascular failure, as this condition is called, can be brought on by breathing failure, a drug overdose, a blockage in a blood vessel, electrical shock, or poisoning. Attempting to rescue a victim of cardiovascular failure is one of the most critical and weighty responsibilities a person can face.

Cardiopulmonary resuscitation (CPR), the lifesaving technique administered to victims of cardiovascular failure, requires no special tools, instruments, or equipment. It involves breathing for the victim and forcing the heart to pump blood through the body by applying pressure on the victim's sternum.

CPR for Adults

CPR consists of three steps. A good way of remembering these steps and the order in which they occur is to think of them as the ABCs of CPR: *A* stands for *airway, B* stands for *breathing*, and *C* stands for *circulation*.

Airway—Step A

When you witness a person collapsing or come upon a person who has collapsed, your first task is to determine if the victim is conscious. Tap the victim's shoulder and ask loudly, "Are you all right?" If the victim does not respond, and before beginning CPR, dial 911 for help or contact your local EMS. If someone is nearby, direct them to call.

If the victim is not lying flat on his or her back, you need to roll the victim to this position. Take care to roll the body as an entire unit. For example, do not turn the upper body first, followed by the lower body. Once the victim is flat on his or her back, open the airway by tilting the person's head back, and at the same time, lifting up on the chin.

Breathing—Step B

Check for breathing by looking, listening, and feeling.

- *Look* for the rise and fall of the chest.
- *Listen* for the sound of air being exhaled from the lungs.
- *Feel* for exhaled air on your cheek.

If the victim shows no sign of breathing, you must get air into his or her lungs at once by administering the steps outlined on pages 718 and 720 for rescue breathing.

| **LESSON 2 FOCUS** |

TERMS TO USE

- Cardiopulmonary resuscitation (CPR) (CARD•ee•oh•PULL•muh•ner•ee ree•sus•uh•TAH•shun)
- Xiphoid (ZY•foyd) process

CONCEPTS TO LEARN

- CPR involves breathing for the victim while forcing the heart to pump blood to the body by applying pressure on the victim's sternum.
- Adjustments are made when administering CPR to infants and children.

ATTITUDES AND BEHAVIORS TO EVALUATE

- Self-Inventory, page 726.
- Building Decision-Making Skills, page 727.

Circulation—Step C

The third and most critical step in CPR is to move blood through the body to supply oxygen to the cells. The heart is located beneath the sternum. Compressions on the sternum force blood out of the heart and into the blood vessels. Remember that a person should be properly trained and certified before administering this procedure to anyone.

First, check the victim's carotid pulse for five to ten seconds. This is a very important step because chest compressions can harm the victim if his or her heart is beating. If you find no pulse, begin artificial circulation.

Finding the correct position to give effective compressions is essential. The pressure must be directly on the sternum to avoid injury to the ribs and above the xiphoid process so internal organs will not be damaged. The **xiphoid process** is located at the lower end of the sternum where the lower ribs meet the sternum. Refer to the illustrations and captions on this page.

After finding the correct position for hand placement, you should also position your body properly to administer compressions. Your shoulders should be directly over your hands and your elbows locked. When you push down, the weight of your body will compress the victim's chest. Push straight down. Each compression should push the sternum down $1\frac{1}{2}$ to 2 inches (3.8 to 5.1 cm). Give compressions at a rate of 80 compressions per minute.

CPR is a combination of rescue breathing and chest compressions. You would alternate 2 full breaths and 15 chest compressions until the victim has recovered or until help arrives.

As you kneel facing the victim's chest, use your hand nearest the victim's feet. Find the xiphoid process, which is the lower end of the sternum that projects downward. Place two fingers at this point on the sternum.

Place the heel of your other hand on the victim's sternum just above your two fingers already positioned on the sternum.

Interlock the fingers of your two hands so that only the heel of the bottom hand is resting on the victim's sternum.

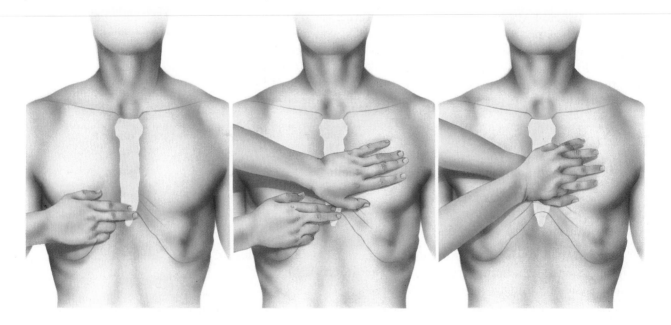

LOOKING AT TECHNOLOGY

Computerized Cardiac Defibrillators

A computerized cardiac defibrillator is a device used to evaluate and sometimes revive patients suffering from cardiac arrest by restoring their heart rhythms. Now available in many ambulances, these defibrillators help paramedics and emergency medical technicians avoid the need for guesswork in trying to determine what kind of immediate emergency care should be given.

When a person in the ambulance is not breathing and does not have a heartbeat, action has to be taken immediately. The paramedic or emergency medical technician attaches electrodes to the patient's body. The computer unit analyzes the patient's medical situation and determines whether an electric shock to jolt the heart is needed. If the computer decides that the patient does need such a shock, the paramedic or emergency medical technician pushes a button and the machine itself delivers the shock. If that isn't strong enough, the attendant pushes the button again. Another shock is administered. If after three tries the heart hasn't restarted, the attendant stops and does CPR, or cardiopulmonary resuscitation, until the patient gets to the hospital. Then doctors and other health-care workers take over.

The computerized cardiac defibrillator is one big step in emergency medicine. It means that many decisions once left up to paramedics or other emergency medical technicians, are now decided by the computer and based on careful, accurate scientific information. Ambulance attendants have a predetermined protocol to follow in dealing with cardiac patients that instructs them in exactly what steps to follow when using the computerized device and in what order. Despite the services provided by the computer, however, their training and input is still critical in helping cardiac arrest victims to get correct and lifesaving treatment.

KEEPING FIT

CPR in the Age of Hepatitis and AIDS

Many people who can perform CPR may be afraid to do so for fear of contracting hepatitis, HIV, or other communicable diseases.

A pocket mask makes performing CPR much safer. This device can be placed over the mouth or nose and mouth area. Some lay people carry these with them in the event an emergency may arise. Professional rescuers and others who feel they are likely to stop at the scene of an accident also use them.

The American Red Cross encourages the public to use something as a barrier between someone's blood and other body fluids and themselves when performing emergency lifesaving techniques.

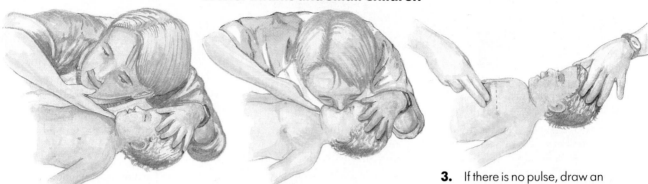

CPR for Infants and Small Children

1. Tip the infant's head back a little in order to open the airway.

2. Cover your mouth over the baby's mouth and nose and give puffs of air.

3. If there is no pulse, draw an imaginary line between infant's nipples. Place two or three fingers on sternum, one finger's width below the middle of the imaginary line. Compress downward ½ to 1 inch at a rate of 100 compressions per minute for an infant and 80 to 100 for a young child.

CPR for Infants and Children

Because of differences in size, some adjustments need to be made when administering CPR to infants and children up to age 8.

Airway

Tip the child's head back only a little. Tilting the head back too far will close the airway.

Breathing

Cover your mouth over the child's nose and mouth rather than pinching the nose shut. For infants give small puffs of air.

Circulation

In infants, check the pulse at the inner arm just above the elbow. For a child, check the carotid pulse. If no pulse is detected, administer chest compressions as follows:

- Infants. Draw an imaginary line between the victim's nipples. Place two or three of your fingers on the sternum, one finger's width below the imaginary line. Compress ½ to 1 inch (1.3 to 2.5 cm) at a rate of 100 compressions per minute.
- Children. Place your middle and index fingers on the xiphoid process, and place the heel of your hand next to your index finger. With one hand, compress the sternum about 1 to 1½ inches (2.5 to 3.8 cm) at a rate of 80 to 100 compressions per minute.

For both infants and children, administer a breath after every five chest compressions.

DID YOU KNOW?

- Access to your medical information might save your life in an emergency—especially if you are unconscious. One solution is Medic Alert, a worldwide nonprofit ID service that includes a bracelet or neckchain engraved with Medic Alert's 24-hour hot line and the person's critical medical facts. In an emergency, medical personnel can read the engraved information and call for medical details.

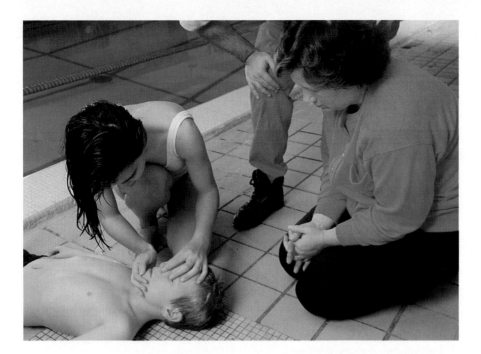

First-aid training may help you save a life.

PROTECTING THE GOOD SAMARITAN

Even when first aid has been administered properly, complications sometimes arise. To protect rescuers from being sued in the event of such complications, Good Samaritan laws have been established in most states throughout the United States. According to these laws, no person who administers emergency care in good faith is liable for civil damages unless such acts are willfully or deliberately negligent.

This protection means that if you know first aid and are a layperson—that is, someone other than a medical professional who receives pay for services rendered—and you act in good faith, you cannot be held responsible for complications that might occur.

LESSON 2 REVIEW

Reviewing Facts and Vocabulary

1. Tell what *CPR* stands for. Then define the term and use it in an original sentence that also contains the term *xiphoid process*.
2. Who can administer CPR?
3. What are the ABCs of CPR?

Thinking Critically

4. **Analysis.** Compare the CPR given to an adult with that given to an infant or small child.
5. **Synthesis.** You are in the supermarket when a clerk suddenly slumps to the floor. Assuming you have been trained in CPR, what do you do first?

Applying Health Knowledge

6. Learn what you can about CPR and rescue breathing courses taught in your community. Prepare a directory of such courses, including the name of the organization, kind of instruction offered, and when and where classes are held.

CARDIOPULMONARY RESUSCITATION **725**

Self-Inventory

Are You a Lifesaver?

HOW DO YOU RATE?

There are many things you can do to save your own life and the lives of others. Number a sheet of paper from 1 through 12. Read each item below, and respond by writing *yes* or *no*. Total the number of *yes* and *no* responses. Then proceed to the next section.

1. I take small bites of food when eating.
2. I eat slowly, chewing each bite of food thoroughly before swallowing.
3. I try not to talk or laugh when I have food in my mouth.
4. I avoid taking sips of water or other beverages while there is food in my mouth.
5. I never eat or drink while in a reclining position.
6. I never go to sleep with chewing gum in my mouth.
7. I do not chew gum while playing sports.
8. I swim only in places where there is a trained lifeguard on duty.
9. I know what action needs to be taken to aid victims of choking, and I can perform that action.
10. I am trained in rescue breathing for adults and children.
11. I hold certification in CPR and know the procedure well.
12. I periodically review rescue breathing and CPR techniques.

HOW DID YOU SCORE?

Give yourself 1 point for every *yes* answer and 0 points for every *no* answer. Find your total, and read below to see how you scored. Then proceed to the next section.

10 to 12
Excellent. Your health choices show that you try to avoid risky situations and are prepared when emergencies arise.

7 to 9
Good. Your health choices are good, but you could be more cautious.

4 to 6
Fair. You are prone to health risks that could have serious consequences for yourself and others.

Below 4
Watch it! You are unprepared for life-threatening emergencies.

WHAT ARE YOUR GOALS?

Identify an area in which your score was low, and use the goal-setting process to pave the way for a change.

1. The behavior I would like to change is ____.
2. If this behavior were changed, I would look, feel, or act differently in the following ways: ____.
3. The steps involved in making this change are ____.
4. My timetable for making this change is ____.
5. People I will ask for help or assistance are ____.
6. The benefits I will receive as a result of making this change are ____.

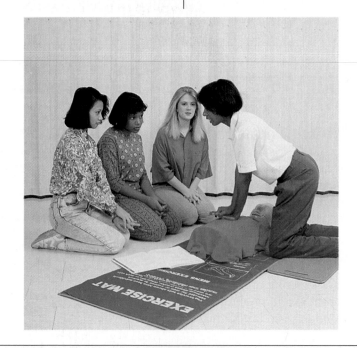

Building Decision-Making Skills

Dan likes to play football. On Saturdays he and some friends from his neighborhood often meet in the park to play. Last week they met as usual, divided into teams, and were having a great time. Dan was really pumped. He loved being a receiver and had scored one touchdown that afternoon. He was hoping for another. On the next play, his team had possession of the ball. Gina was quarterback. Her pass was long, but Dan stretched and caught it in his fingertips. He went down holding the ball, but he did not get back up. His friends ran to where he lay. Dan was not breathing. Gina ran for help. What should his friends do?

A. Try to keep Dan warm and comfortable.
B. Raise his head with a pile of jackets.
C. Run for Dan's parents.
D. Check Dan's breathing and pulse. Begin rescue breathing if necessary.

WHAT DO YOU THINK?

1. **Situation.** Why does a decision need to be made? How much time is there to decide?
2. **Choices.** What other choices do Dan's friends have?
3. **Consequences.** What are the advantages of each choice?
4. **Consequences.** What are the disadvantages of each choice?
5. **Consequences.** What risks are involved in this decision?
6. **Decision.** What is the best solution for Dan? Explain your answer.
7. **Evaluation.** How would you handle a similar situation? What steps need to be taken in order to be prepared to help someone? What would be your concerns about helping someone?

Greta's brother Dave was driving her and a carload of her friends home from a concert. Suddenly, a car passed Dave at a high speed. Unfortunately the driver's speed did not allow time to maneuver a right curve in the road, and an accident occurred. Dave pulled over and ran to the wrecked car. A family was trapped inside. Two of the people in the car were unresponsive. What should Greta and her friends do?

A. Stay quietly in Dave's car and wait for Dave to tell them what to do.
B. Follow Dave to see what they can do to help.
C. Leave Dave and take the car to find a phone to call for emergency help.
D. Try to flag down a passing motorist to send for help.

WHAT DO YOU THINK?

8. **Situation.** What decisions need to be made? What are the dangers involved?
9. **Consequences.** What are the advantages and disadvantages of each choice listed above?
10. **Choices.** What other possibilities exist for Greta and her friends?
11. **Consequences.** What are the probable consequences of each of these choices?
12. **Choices.** What choices will Dave have to make? Who will be affected by his choices?
13. **Consequences.** How will others feel about Dave in each of his choices?
14. **Decision.** What is the best choice for Greta and her friends to make?
15. **Evaluation.** How would you respond if you were Dave or Greta in this situation? What factors should you consider?
16. **Evaluation.** Have you ever been in a similar situation? If so, how did you handle it? What did you learn from it?

REVIEW

Using Health Terms

On a separate sheet of paper, write the term that best matches each definition given below.

LESSON 1

1. Organization that provides training in the use of effective techniques for choking.
2. Signs of breathing failure.
3. Choking accidents in restaurants have been called this.
4. Rate of rescue breathing for a child under 8 years old.
5. Muscle located right below the lungs.
6. A quick upward movement used on an adult choking victim.
7. Major artery located in a person's neck.
8. The act or process of reviving.

LESSON 2

9. Breastbone.
10. Condition in which the heart and/or cardio-vascular system do not function properly.
11. The posterior part of the sternum.

Building Academic Skills

LESSON 2

12. **Writing.** Imagine that you have become a spokesperson for the American Red Cross. Write a speech to be given to area high schools, persuading your peers of every-one's need to know procedures for choking, artificial respiration, and CPR. Make sure your speech is clear and concise and sup-ports your ideas.
13. **Math.** For cardiopulmonary resuscitation on an adult, one should administer 80 com-pressions per minute. Estimate and then calculate how many this would be per sec-ond. Now record the time it takes to do 2 full breaths. Allowing for the breaths, estimate and then calculate how many compressions one would need to do if one had to perform CPR for 19 minutes; for 52 minutes.

Recalling the Facts

LESSON 1

14. When respiratory failure occurs, why is it important that the victim receive oxygen quickly?
15. Explain how one should feel for a victim's pulse.
16. When performing the Heimlich maneuver, why is it important not to give up after one or two tries?
17. What is the significance of look, listen, and feel when administering rescue breathing?
18. If one is alone and choking, what is the best thing to do?
19. What are the steps for aiding an adult choking victim?
20. What is the procedure for aiding a choking infant?
21. Outline the steps to follow in giving artificial respiration to adults.
22. In your own words, tell four ways a person might avoid becoming a choking victim.
23. What is the proper technique for perform-ing an abdominal thrust?
24. What are the two main objectives for res-cue breathing?

LESSON 2

25. What are some situations that can bring on cardiovascular failure?
26. When should cardiopulmonary resuscita-tion be administered?
27. What is the purpose of cardiopulmonary resuscitation?
28. How does administering cardiopulmonary resuscitation to young children differ from that for infants?
29. Briefly explain the steps in administering cardiopulmonary resuscitation to an adult.
30. Outline the steps for administering artificial circulation to an adult.
31. Why must one be careful not to press on the xiphoid process?
32. What are the measurements for compres-sion when performing cardiopulmonary resuscitation on an infant, child, and adult?

Thinking Critically

LESSON 1

33. Analysis. What is the importance of knowing any universal distress symbol, such as the one for choking?

34. Analysis. Why do you suppose abdominal thrusts cannot be performed on an infant?

LESSON 2

35. Evaluation. What are some reasons one might be hesitant to become involved in an emergency situation?

36. Evaluation. Of all the reasons given for why people choose not to get involved in emergency situations, which do you feel are valid? Explain your answer.

37. Analysis. When administering CPR, two people can be better than one. What do you think is the reason for this?

38. Evaluation. It is part of some religious beliefs that any kind of medical intervention should not be conducted. Imagine that a physician in an emergency room administered first aid to a person whose faith forbids it, and that victim sues the rescuer. The rescuer is protected by the Good Samaritan laws. In your opinion, is it a good law? Explain your answer.

Making the Connection

LESSON 1

39. Science. Draw the respiratory system showing how the abdominal thrust forces the diaphragm upward and dislodges a foreign object.

40. Language Arts. Research the universality of body language. Make a notebook of eight words and their interpretation in body language. Learn these words and share them with the class.

41. Home Economics. Make a list of items that need to be kept away from small children to prevent choking. Make a poster to display this information. Share your poster with your class.

Applying Health Knowledge

LESSON 1

42. Make a list of at least five items that may cause choking in small children.

43. A person should not use his or her thumb to take a pulse. Find out why.

44. When one is administering artificial respiration to an infant, why is it important not to breathe full breaths into the baby?

LESSON 2

45. Now that you have studied artificial respiration and cardiopulmonary resuscitation, identify three places where emergency situations that require these techniques might take place. Check to see whether the people at these locations are trained and certified to administer these procedures.

46. When administering CPR to an adult, it is important to kneel over the victim so that the rescuer's shoulders are directly over the victim's chest. Why is this necessary?

47. List reasons you can think of that no one should give CPR without proper training and certification.

Beyond the Classroom

LESSON 2

48. Parental Involvement. Describe to your parents the importance of learning cardiopulmonary resuscitation. Take a basic first aid course or a CPR class with your parents.

49. Community Involvement. Check to see who is the closest person to your home, school, and/or workplace who knows CPR. Ask the person if you could call on her or him for assistance if the need arises. Get the person's phone number and keep it in a place close to the phone.

50. Further Study. Research and write a short report on the beginnings of the American Red Cross or the American Heart Association. Find out what role the organization plays today in your community.

Glossary

A

Abdominal thrusts. Quick, upward thrusts that force the diaphragm upward and force out the substance blocking the airway; Heimlich maneuver.

Absorption. The passage of digested food from the digestive tract into the circulatory system.

Abstinence. Choosing not to be sexually active; choosing not to use alcohol or other drugs.

Acquaintance rape. Rape by someone known casually by the victim or someone thought to be a friend.

Acquired immune deficiency syndrome (AIDS). A fatal communicable disease caused by HIV, with no known effective treatment or cure.

Active immunity. Immunity developed by one's body to protect one from disease.

Addiction. A physiological or psychological dependence on a substance or activity.

Additive interaction. An interaction that occurs when medicines work together in a positive way.

Adolescence. The stage between childhood and adulthood.

Adoption. The act of taking a child into one's family and legally assuming responsibility for that child, agreeing to raise him or her to adulthood.

Adrenal glands. Glands responsible for secreting hormones that help maintain the body's sodium and water balance, affect metabolism, and cope with stressors.

Adrenaline. A hormone secreted by the adrenal glands to prepare the body to respond to a stressor; the emergency hormone.

Advertising. The way by which a manufacturer gains one's attention for its product.

Advocate. Someone who speaks out for a position or product.

Aerobic exercise. Vigorous activity that uses continuous oxygen; activity that increases the lung's capacity to hold air.

Aesthetic. Artistic; responding to or appreciating that which one perceives as beautiful.

Age norm. Things a person is expected to be doing at a particular chronological age.

Aggravated assault. Unlawful attack often with a weapon, and having the intent to hurt or kill.

Aggressive. Being overly forceful, pushy, or hostile.

AIDS dementia complex. A progressive disorder that destroys the brain tissue of a person with AIDS.

Al-Anon. A worldwide self-help organization for family members and friends of alcoholics.

Alateen. An offshoot of Al-Anon specifically for teens and preteens between the ages of 12 and 20, whose parents or other family members or friends have drinking problems.

Alcoholics. People with alcoholism; people addicted to alcohol.

Alcoholics Anonymous (AA). A worldwide organization or support group that has played a major role in helping people to get and stay alcohol- and drug-free.

Alcohol-impaired driving. Driving under the influence of alcohol.

Alcoholism. Addiction to alcohol; a physical and psychological dependence on alcohol.

Allergens. Substances to which the body's immune system overreacts.

Alveoli. A cluster of thin-walled air sacs found at the end of each bronchiole.

Alzheimer's disease. A progressive, degenerative disorder that causes general mental deterioration.

Amino acids. Chemical substances that make up proteins.

Amphetamines. Stimulants that speed up the heart and breathing and cause anxiety, sleeplessness, and loss of appetite.

Anabolic steroids. Synthetic derivatives of testosterone.

Anaerobic exercise. Intense physical activity in which the body's supply of oxygen to produce energy does not meet the demand; activity that improves muscular strength, muscular endurance, and flexibility.

Analgesics. Medicines that relieve pain without loss of consciousness.

Angina pectoris. A condition in which one experiences pain and tightness or pressure in the chest as a result of the heart's not getting enough oxygen.

Anorexia nervosa. A psychological disorder that involves the irrational fear of becoming obese and results in severe weight loss from self-induced starvation.

Antagonistic interaction. An interaction that occurs when the effect of a medicine is canceled or reduced when taken with other medicine.

Antibiotics. Medicines that kill or reduce harmful bacteria in the body.

Antibodies. Proteins that destroy or neutralize pathogens in your body.

Antidiuretic hormone. One of two hormones secreted by the posterior lobe of the pituitary gland.

Antisocial personality disorder. A condition characterized by a person's constant conflict with society.

Antivenins. Blood fluids that contain antibodies and act more quickly than vaccines.

Anxiety disorders. Disorders in which real or imagined fears prevent a person from enjoying life.

Appendicitis. The inflammation of the appendix.

Appendicular skeleton. The bones of the shoulders, arms, hands, hips, legs, and feet.

Aqueous humor. In the eyeball, watery fluid that fills the cavity between the cornea and the lens.

Arteries. The largest of the blood vessels and those that carry blood away from the heart.

Arteriosclerosis. A condition in which the walls of arteries become thick and lose their elasticity.

Arthritis. Inflammation of a joint; conditions that cause aching, pain, and swelling in joints and connective tissue throughout the body.

Artificial respiration. See *rescue breathing*.

Assertive. Standing up for one's own rights in a firm, but positive, way.

Atherosclerosis. A condition in which the artery wall thickens due to fatty deposits that restrict blood flow.

Athlete's foot. An infection of the skin between the toes caused by the ringworm fungus.

Autonomy. The confidence that one can control one's own body, impulses, and environment.

Axial skeleton. The bones of the skull, sternum, ribs, and vertebrae.

Axon. The part of the neuron that carries impulses away from the cell body.

B

Balloon angioplasty. A procedure that involves threading a balloon-tipped catheter through the body to the site of a blockage, inflating the balloon, and opening a path for the blood to flow through; officially known as percutaneous transluminal coronary angioplasty.

Basal metabolism. The absolute minimum amount of energy required to maintain the life processes in one's body.

Battery. The use of physical force to control someone through the use of power.

B cells. Lymphocytes that are produced and that mature in bone marrow; stimulated by T helper cells to make antibodies.

Benign. Noncancerous.

Better Business Bureau (BBB). A nonprofit organization sponsored by private businesses.

Bile. A bitter fluid produced in the liver that is important to the breakdown of fats.

Binaural hearing. The ability to determine the direction a sound comes from by being able to hear it with both ears.

Biodegradable. Able to be broken down by microorganisms.

Biofeedback. Biological feedback about one's body; the process of becoming aware of physical events in one's body that one is normally not aware of, with the intent of gaining voluntary control of such events.

Biological age. One's age as determined by how well different parts of one's body are functioning.

Biopsy. A procedure in which a small amount of tissue is removed and examined for the presence of abnormal or cancerous cells.

Biosphere. The thin layer of soil, water, and air near the earth's surface.

Birth defects. Genetic conditions and many other types of diseases and disorders that are caused by a variety of other factors.

Bladder. A muscular organ that stores urine.

Blastocyst. A cluster of cells that has a hollow space in the center; the stage following the zygote stage.

Blended family. A type of nuclear family in which one or both parents have been married before and in which each may have a child or children from a previous marriage.

Blizzard. A snowstorm with winds of 35 miles per hour (56 km per hour) or greater.

Blood alcohol concentration (BAC). The amount of alcohol in a person's blood expressed by a percentage.

Blood pressure. The force of blood against the

walls of blood vessels as blood flows through the cardiovascular system.

Body composition. The percent of fat, lean muscle, bone, connective tissue, water, and so forth in the body.

Body system. A group of organs that work together to perform a common function.

Brain death. The loss of function of the entire brain, including the brain stem.

Brain stem. The division of the brain that connects the spinal cord to the brain.

Bronchi. Bronchial tubes that lead into the lungs.

Bronchioles. Divisions of the bronchial tubes within the lungs.

Bruise. An injury to tissue under the skin.

Bulimia. An eating disorder in which the victim follows a very restrictive diet, then binges in response to hunger, followed by self-induced vomiting, purging through laxative abuse, or following severely restrictive diets.

C

Calorie. A unit to measure the energy in food and the energy one's body burns.

Cancer. Abnormal, uncontrolled cell growth.

Capillaries. The smallest blood vessels.

Carbohydrate loading. Storing extra glycogen in the muscles before strenuous exercise.

Carbohydrates. Sugars, starches, and fiber that are the body's preferred source of energy.

Carbon monoxide. A colorless, odorless, poisonous gas that can be found in cigarette smoke and automobile exhaust fumes.

Carcinogenic. Cancer-causing or poisonous.

Carcinogens. Cancer-causing agents.

Carcinomas. Cancers that develop in epithelial tissue—tissue that forms the skin and linings of body organs.

Cardiac arrest. A condition in which the heart stops completely.

Cardiac muscle. Striated tissue that forms the walls of the heart.

Cardiopulmonary resuscitation (CPR). The lifesaving technique that involves breathing for the victim of cardiovascular failure and forcing his or her heart to pump blood by applying pressure on the victim's sternum.

Cardiorespiratory endurance. The ability of the heart, lungs, and blood vessels to send fuel and oxygen to the body's tissues during long periods of vigorous activity.

Cardiovascular diseases. Diseases of the heart and blood vessels.

Carjacking. The hijacking or stealing of a car by force with a weapon.

Carotid pulse. The heartbeat that can be felt on each side of the neck.

Cartilage. A strong, flexible material that allows for smooth movement in joints, supports the nose and ears, connects the ribs to the sternum, and acts as a cushion between adjoining vertebrae.

Catheter. A thin, flexible plastic tube that can be guided through blood vessels to certain body organs.

Cell. The basic unit of structure of all living things.

Cell body. The part of a neuron that has a nucleus and is the center for receiving and sending nerve impulses.

Cerebellum. The part of the brain that functions as a center for the coordination of skeletal muscle movement.

Cerebral palsy. A group of nonprogressive neurological disorders that are the result of damage to the developing brain either before or during birth.

Cerebrum. The largest, most complex part of the brain, consisting of the right and left hemispheres, that controls muscular activity and receives sensory input.

Cervix. The round, muscular neck, or bottom part, of the uterus.

Chancre. A reddish sore at the place where a pathogen enters the body.

Chemotherapy. The use of anticancer medications in the treatment of cancer.

Child abuse. Physical harm, including sexual abuse, and/or emotional harm to children.

Chlamydia. A sexually transmitted disease that attacks the reproductive organs.

Chlorofluorocarbons (CFCs). Compounds of chlorine, fluorine, and carbon believed to be a major factor in ozone reduction.

Cholesterol. Fatlike substance.

Choroid. The middle layer of the eyeball wall, containing the iris, the suspensory ligaments, and the ciliary muscles.

Chromosomes. Tiny structures within the nuclei of cells, which carry genetic information.

Chronic bronchitis. A condition in which the bronchi are irritated.

Chronic fatigue syndrome (CFS). A type of fatigue that is long-term and for which the cause is unknown.

Chronological age. One's age as determined by the number of birthdays one has had.

Chyme. A substance formed when food and gastric juices mix together.

Circumcision. A procedure in which the foreskin is surgically removed.

Cirrhosis. Scarring; a condition of the liver in which scarring reduces blood flow in the liver.

Clinical death. The cessation of a person's body functions.

Clinical depression. A condition in which feelings of sadness and hopelessness last for more than a few weeks and interfere with one's daily activities and interests.

Clinical psychologist. A psychologist who diagnoses and treats emotional and behavioral disorders.

Cliques. Exclusive friendship groups that usually share common interests and backgrounds.

Cluttered-nest syndrome. A phenomenon in which grown children return home to live with their parents.

Codependency. Being overly concerned with other people's behavior and problems and feeling driven to fix and control those problems.

Communicable diseases. Diseases caused by the direct or indirect spread of pathogens from one person to another.

Communication. A process through which messages are sent and received; openness among family members, including displays of tenderness, warmth, and humor.

Compromise. A way of solving a problem in which each person gives up something in order to find a solution that satisfies everyone.

Compulsion. An urgent, repeated behavior.

Congenital. Existing at or dating from birth.

Congenital syphilis. A condition in which a pregnant female who had syphilis transferred the infection to her unborn child.

Conjunctiva. A protective mucous membrane attached to the inner surface of the eyelids that continues over the outer surface of the eyeball.

Consequence. The result of an action.

Conservation. Preserving the environment.

Consumer. Anyone who uses a product or service.

Consumer health. The process of helping one select health products and services wisely, and letting one know where to go or what to do if one has been treated unfairly or needs help.

Cooling down. Gradually decreasing activity after exercise in order to allow one's pulse rate to slow down.

Cornea. A colorless, transparent part of the sclera in the front part of the eye.

Coronary angiography. Procedure used to help evaluate the extent of coronary artery disease.

Coronary bypass surgery. A procedure to create detours around obstructed or narrowed coronary arteries so that blood can reach the heart.

Crisis. An extreme change in a person's life.

Cross-contamination. Spreading bacteria from one food to another.

D

Daily Food Guide. A publication that offers an easy way to choose a varied, balanced, and moderate diet.

Date rape. Rape that occurs between two people who are dating.

Deafness. The loss of the ability to hear.

Decision. The act of making a choice or coming to a solution.

Defense mechanisms. Strategies used to deal with stressful situations.

Deforestation. The destruction of forests.

Dendrites. The part of the neuron that receives and carries impulses toward the cell body.

Dentin. Material that surrounds the pulp.

Depressants. Sedatives; drugs that tend to slow down the central nervous system.

Dermis. The inner, thicker layer of skin.

Desertification. The conversion of grasslands, rain-fed cropland, or irrigated cropland to desertlike conditions.

Designer drugs. Drugs made with synthetic substances by street chemists.

Detoxification. The process of removing drugs from one's body.

Developmental task. Something that needs to occur during a particular stage for a human being to continue his or her growth toward becoming a healthy, mature adult.

Diabetes. A chronic disease that affects the way body cells convert food into energy.

Diaphragm. A muscle that separates the chest and abdominal cavity.

Diet. Everything a person eats and drinks.

Digestion. The physical and chemical breakdown of foods into smaller pieces.

Digestive enzymes. Proteins that speed up the breakdown of food.

Discrimination. A form of prejudice in which people are singled out and treated negatively as a result of one factor, such as age, sex, race, ethnicity, or some physical trait.

Distress. Negative stress.

Divorce. The legal dissolution, or ending, of the marriage contract.

Dormant. Inactive.

Down syndrome. A condition, characterized by mild to serious mental retardation, that is the result of a chromosomal abnormality.

Drug. Dangerous and often illegal substance, including alcohol and tobacco.

Drug dependence. Drug addiction.

E

Earthquakes. Heavy ground tremors.

Electrocardiogram (EKG or ECG). A test that produces a graph of the electric activity of the heart.

Elimination. The expulsion of undigested food or body wastes.

ELISA. Enzyme-linked immunosorbent assay; a test to detect the presence of HIV infection.

Embolus. A blood clot that moves from the point where it was formed.

Embryo. A cluster of cells, or blastocyst, that has implanted itself in the uterus.

Emotions. Feelings that influence everything one does.

Empty-calorie foods. Foods that have little or no nutritional value.

Empty-nest syndrome. The phenomenon of children entering adulthood and leaving home.

Enabling. Trying to protect the person having trouble with alcohol or drugs from facing the consequences of his or her drug-related problems.

Enamel. The hardest material in the body; material that covers the crown of the tooth.

Encephalitis. An inflammation of the brain caused by a virus and sometimes by a bacteria.

Endocrine glands. Ductless glands that secrete hormones into the bloodstream.

Endocrine system. The body system consisting of ductless glands and the hormones they produce.

Enriched. A product that has had nutrients lost in processing added back.

Environment. All of one's surroundings, including family, location, and experiences.

Epidermis. The outer, thinner layer of skin.

Epilepsy. A disorder of the nervous system characterized by a sudden burst of nerve impulses in the brain that results in a seizure.

Esophagus. A muscular tube that extends from the pharynx to the stomach and is situated behind the trachea and heart.

Estrogen. A female hormone first released during puberty.

Estuaries. Ecosystems where seawater mixes with fresh water.

Eustress. Positive stress.

Exploited. Used for someone else's benefit.

Extended family. A family with one or more relatives in addition to the nuclear or single-parent family.

Extensors. Muscles that straighten a limb.

External auditory canal. A passageway about 1 inch long that leads to the eardrum and protects the ear by keeping out foreign substances.

External respiration. The exchange of oxygen and carbon dioxide between the blood and the air in the lungs.

F

Fallopian tubes. A pair of tubes through which a mature ovum travels.

Family. A group of people related by blood, marriage, or adoption.

Fatigue. A tired feeling that lowers one's level of activity.

Fatty liver. A condition in which fats have built up in the liver, preventing normal functions of liver cells.

Federal Trade Commission (FTC). A federal agency that prevents the unfair, false, or deceptive advertising of consumer products and services.

Feedback. Messages from others that tell how others feel about a person or idea.

Fertilization. The union of an egg cell and a sperm cell that can occur only if sperm cells are present when the ovum is in the Fallopian tube; conception.

Fetal alcohol syndrome (FAS). A condition in which a fetus has been adversely affected by its mother's heavy alcohol use during pregnancy.

Fetus. An embryo from the eighth week after conception to birth.

Fibrillation. A rhythmic disturbance that occurs when the muscle fibers of the heart contract in an uncoordinated manner.

Fire extinguisher. A portable device that puts out small fires by ejecting fire-extinguishing chemicals.

First aid. Emergency care; the immediate, temporary care given to a person who has become sick or who has been injured.

Fitness. Readiness. Fit people are better equipped than nonfit people to handle day-to-day situations.

Flexibility. The ability to move a body part through a full range of motions.

Flexors. Muscles that bend a limb.

Fluoroscope. A machine that provides a live picture, often used by doctors to look directly at the heart shadow.

Follicle. A small pocket that holds the hair root in the dermis.

Food additives. Substances added to food intentionally to produce a desired effect.

Food allergy. A condition in which the body's immune system overreacts to allergens in some foods.

Food and Drug Administration (FDA). A federal agency that ensures all food and food additives, other than meat and poultry, are safe, pure, wholesome, and honestly and correctly labeled.

Foodborne illness. A condition caused by eating food contaminated with bacteria; food poisoning.

Fortification. The process of adding nutrients not naturally present.

Fraternal twins. Two embryos with different genetic makeup.

Friendship. A significant relationship between two people, based on caring, consideration, and trust.

Frostbite. A condition in which ice crystals form in the spaces between the cells.

Functional disorder. A mental disorder that occurs as a result of psychological causes in which no brain damage is involved.

G

Gallbladder. An organ that stores bile.

Gallstones. Small crystals formed from bile that can block the bile duct between the gallbladder and the duodenum.

Gangrene. The death of tissue in a part of the body.

Gastric juices. Liquids that contain hydrochloric acid, digestive enzymes, and mucus and that start the digestion of proteins.

Gastritis. A disorder in which the mucous membrane that lines the stomach becomes inflamed.

Genes. Small sections of chromosomes that control hereditary characteristics.

Genetic condition. Disease or disorder, illness, or other condition of malfunction with which one is born.

Gerontologist. People who study the process of aging.

Glucose. A sugar formed in the body during digestion.

Glycogen. The form in which carbohydrates are stored in the body.

Goal. An aim that requires planning and work to attain; definite plan one has in one's life.

Gonorrhea. A sexually transmitted disease caused by bacteria that live in warm, moist areas of the body.

Group practice. A situation in which two or more physicians unite to provide medical care.

H

Halitosis. Bad breath.

Hallucinogens. Psychedelics; drugs that alter mood, thought, and the senses.

Hashish. Dark brown resin collected from the tops of the cannabis plant.

Health. The state of total physical, mental, and social well-being.

Health care delivery. Health service.

Health education. The providing of health information so as to influence people to change attitudes so that they take positive action about their health.

Health facility. A place a person goes for health care.

Health maintenance organization (HMO). A health plan in which one pays regular fees and then receives medical care for little or no additional cost.

Health resources. Places that people can go for various types of treatment.

Health services. The aspect of an overall health program concerned with the prevention of disease, the maintenance and promotion of health, and the treatment and cure of disease.

Heart attack. A common way to refer to a number of disorders that involve the heart and blood vessels, but in general occurs because the heart muscle cells are not getting the oxygen and nutrients they need.

Hemodialysis. A technique in which a person is connected to an artificial kidney machine.

Hemoglobin. The oxygen-carrying substance in red blood cells.

Hepatitis. A serious inflammation of the liver that is most often caused by viral infection.

Heredity. The passing of characteristics from parents to offspring.

Hernias. Weak areas in the muscle supporting various organs; ruptures.

Herpes simplex type 2 virus. An STD in which a virus causes blisterlike sores, called genital herpes, in the genital area.

Hiatal hernia. A condition in which the upper part of the stomach pushes through the diaphragm.

Hierarchy of needs. A ranked list of things human beings must have to survive and thrive.

High blood pressure. Hypertension.

Histamine. A substance released when a cold-causing virus invades one's respiratory system.

Holistic. Whole; considering physical, mental, and social influences on the whole person and his or her health.

Homicide. The willful killing of one human being by another.

Hormones. Body chemical produced by ductless glands that regulate the activity of different body cells; the cause of physical and emotional changes.

Hospice. A place that promotes a special way of caring for the dying.

Host. The plant or animal on which a parasite feeds.

Human collision. In an accident, the act of a person hitting some part of the car or being thrown from the vehicle.

Human immunodeficiency virus (HIV). The virus that attacks the body's immune system and leads to AIDS.

Hurricane. A powerful rainstorm characterized by driving winds.

Hurricane watch. A National Weather Service advisory that means atmospheric conditions exist so that a hurricane could develop.

Hypertension. High blood pressure.

Hypochondria. A somatoform disorder in which one experiences a preoccupation with the body and fear of presumed diseases.

I

Identical twins. Two embryos with the same genetic makeup.

Implantation. The process by which cells attach to the lining of the uterus.

Indigestion. A condition in which one's body does not properly break down foods.

Inhalants. Substances with fumes that are sniffed and inhaled to give a hallucinogenic high.

Inpatients. People who require prolonged health care and are admitted to a facility and occupy a bed in it.

Insulin. A hormone produced in the pancreas that aids the body in converting glucose into energy to be used by the cells.

Integumentary system. The system that includes the skin, hair, nails, and sweat glands.

Internal respiration. The exchange of gases between the blood and the body cells.

Interneurons. Nerve cells within the brain and spinal cord that relay impulses from sensory neurons to motor neurons.

Intervention. The act of interrupting the addiction continuum before the alcoholic or addict hits bottom.

Involuntary. Not within a person's conscious control.

K

Kidneys. Organs that filter blood to remove harmful substances from the substances one's body can use.

L

Labyrinth. The inner ear; consists of the vestibule, semicircular canals, and cochlea.

Lacrimal gland. A gland located above the eye that is responsible for producing tears.

Lactose intolerance. A condition in which the body is unable to digest milk sugar.

Larynx. The voice box.

Leukoplakia. Thickened, white, leathery-appearing spots on the inside of a smokeless tobacco user's mouth.

Life expectancy. The average number of years a group of people is expected to live.

Life-style factors. Repeated behaviors related to the way a person lives, which affect one's level of health.

Ligaments. Strong bands or cords of tissue that connect bones to bones at a joint.

Lipids. Fatty substances that do not dissolve in water.

Look-alike drugs. Drugs made from legal substances to look like illegal drugs.

Lymph. A clear, yellow fluid that flows through lymphatic vessels.

Lymph nodes. Masses of tissues that filter lymph.

Lymphocytes. A type of white blood cell that multiplies in lymph nodes and lymph tissue to destroy invading pathogens.

Lymphomas. Cancers that develop in blood-forming tissues and the lymphatic system.

M

Mainstream smoke. Smoke that a smoker blows off.

Malignant. Cancerous.

Manic-depressive disorder. A condition in which a person's moods shift dramatically from one emotional extreme to another for no apparent reason.

Manipulation. An indirect, and often sneaky or dishonest, means of trying to control another's attitudes or behaviors.

Marijuana. A hemp plant that is smoked, eaten, or drunk for intoxicating effects.

Marital adjustment. How well people within a marriage adjust and adapt to the marriage and to each other.

Marriage. The joining of a man and a woman according to custom or law.

Mastication. The process of chewing.

Medicaid. An assistance program of medical aid for people of all ages who are unable to financially afford medical care.

Medicare. A health insurance program available to people who are 65 years of age and older and to people who receive social security disability benefits.

Medicine. A substance that, when taken into or applied to the body, helps prevent or cure some disease, injury, or medical problem.

Medicine misuse. Using medicine in a way that is not intended.

Megadoses. Very large amounts of nutrient supplements.

Melanoma. Skin cancer.

Meningitis. An inflammation of the meninges.

Menstrual cycle. The time from the beginning of one menstrual period to the onset of the next.

Menstruation. The process of shedding the lining of the uterus.

Mental disorders. Mental and emotional problems.

Mental health. The process of accepting and liking oneself and adapting to and coping with the emotions, challenges, and changes that are part of life.

Mental illness. Medical disease or disorder that affects one's mind and prevents a person from enjoying life.

Metabolism. The sum total of all chemical reactions within a cell.

Metastasis. The process of cancer cells spreading.

Mobile. Likely to move from place to place.

Motor neurons. Nerve cells that carry impulses from interneurons within the brain and spinal cord to muscles and glands.

Multiple sclerosis. A progressive disorder in which the myelin sheath that surrounds nerve fibers is destroyed.

Multiplier effect. The act of taking drugs or medicines with alcohol.

Muscular endurance. The ability of muscles to keep working over a period of time without causing fatigue.

Muscular strength. The ability to exert force against resistance.

Mycobacterium avium intracellulare (MAI). An opportunistic infection that is the leading cause of wasting syndrome, a gradual deterioration of all body functions; associated with AIDS.

N

Narcotics. Drugs made from the opium poppy flower and medicines used to relieve pain and induce sleep.

Nephrons. The functional units of the kidneys.

Neurologist. A doctor who specializes in organic disorders of the brain and nervous system.

Neurons. Nerve cells that are the functional and structural parts of the nervous system.

Neutrophils. One type of phagocyte that is most actively involved in the process of phagocytosis.

Nicotine. The addictive drug in cigarettes that raises blood pressure and increases heart rate.

Noncommunicable diseases. Diseases that are not caused by pathogens and not transmitted through contact.

Nongonococcal urethritis (NGU). A sexually transmitted disease caused by several different kinds of bacterialike organisms that infect the urethra in males and the cervix in females.

Nontoxic. Not harmful or poisonous to humans.

Nonverbal communication. The act of sending messages through facial expressions and body movements.

Nuclear family. Parents and one or more children sharing a household.

Nutrient-dense. High in nutrients relative to caloric content.

Nutrients. Substances in food that the body needs to function properly.

Nutrient supplements. Pills, powders, and liquids that contain nutrients.

Nutrition. The science of looking at how the body uses nutrients and at how and why people eat.

O

Obesity. Excess body fat.

Obsession. A very damaging emotional and social preoccupation.

Occupational Safety and Health Administration (OSHA). A federal agency that promotes safe and healthy conditions at work.

Open-dating. The practice of putting dates on food packages to indicate expiration, freshness, packing, or last sale date of product.

Organ. Two or more tissue types that perform a specific job.

Organic. Derived from living organisms without the use of chemicals.

Organic disorder. A mental disorder caused by a physical illness or an injury that affects the brain.

Ossicles. Three small bones that are linked together and located behind the eardrum that connect the eardrum with the inner ear.

Ossification. A process by which cartilage cells are replaced by bone cells and minerals.

Osteoarthritis. A condition in which the mechanical parts of a joint suffer from wear and tear.

Osteomyelitis. An inflammation of the soft inner surface of the bones.

Osteoporosis. A condition that results from a lack of calcium in the bone.

Otosclerosis. A hereditary disease that is a common cause of partial deafness.

Outpatients. People who receive medical, dental, or other health services in a facility and return home the same day.

Ovaries. Female sex glands that house the ova and produce female sex hormones.

Overweight. Weighing more than 10 percent over the standard weight for height.

Ovulation. The process in which the ovaries release one mature ovum each month.

Ovum. An egg cell.

Oxytocin. One of two hormones secreted by the posterior lobe of the pituitary gland.

P

Pancreas. A gland that serves the digestive and endocrine systems.

Papillae. Small projections that cover the tongue's surface.

Parasite. Microorganism that uses a living plant or animal as a food supply.

Parathyroid glands. The glands located on the lobes of the thyroid gland and that regulate the body's calcium and phosphorous balance.

Parkinson's disease. A progressive disorder that interferes with the transmission of nerve impulses from the motor areas of the brain.

Passive. Giving up, giving in, or backing down without standing up for one's own rights and needs.

Passive-aggressive personality disorder. A condition in which one is often uncooperative with others and displays anger indirectly.

Passive immunity. The temporary immunity an infant acquires from its mother.

Passive smoke. Cigarette, cigar, or pipe smoke inhaled by nonsmokers.

Pathogens. Tiny microorganisms that invade the body and attack its cells and tissues, causing many common diseases.

Peer pressure. The control and influence people of the same age or social group have over one another.

Peers. People one's own age.

Pelvic inflammatory disease (PID). A painful infection of the Fallopian tubes, ovaries, and/or the uterus as a result of untreated gonorrhea or chlamydia.

Penis. The male external reproductive organ composed of spongy tissue that contains many blood vessels.

Peptic ulcers. Ulcers that develop in the digestive system.

Percent body fat. The amount of fat in the body in relation to total body weight.

Percutaneous transluminal coronary angioplasty (PTCA). See *balloon angioplasty*.

Periodontal disease. An inflammation of the periodontal structures.

Periodontium. The area immediately around the teeth; the gums, periodontal ligament, and the jawbone.

Peripheral. Located away from the center.

Peristalsis. A series of involuntary muscle contractions that moves food through the esophagus and the entire digestive tract.

Personal identity. Factors that one believes make one unique ordifferent from everyone else.

Personality. A complex set of characteristics that makes each person unique and distinctive from everyone else.

Phagocytosis. The process in which certain white blood cells surround and eat up invading bacteria.

Pharmacist. A person concerned with the preparation, distribution, and sale of medicine.

Pharynx. The throat.

Phobia. An extreme fear that causes a person to limit normal functioning to avoid the fear.

Phonocardiograph. A test that involves placing a microphone on a person's chest to record heart sounds and signals, transferring them through photography to graph paper.

Photochemical smog. Pollution that occurs when vehicle exhausts, activated by sunlight, combine with other hydrocarbons in the atmosphere.

Physical fitness. The ability to carry out daily tasks easily and have enough reserve energy to respond to unexpected demands.

Physiological dependence. A chemical need of the body for a drug.

Phytoplankton. Microscopic organisms found in open, sunlit waters that are the basis of food webs in freshwater and marine life and are a factor in maintaining the composition of the atmosphere.

Pituitary gland. The gland that is situated at the base of the brain and that regulates other endocrine glands; the master gland.

Placebo. A substance that has no medicinal value, which is given for its psychological effect.

Placenta. A blood-rich tissue developed from an outer layer of cells from the embryo and tissue from the mother.

Planned pregnancy. A pregnancy in which a decision is made to get pregnant before the baby is conceived.

Plaque. Fatty deposits that can build up along the inner lining of the arteries; on teeth–a sticky, colorless film that acts on sugar to form acids that destroy tooth enamel and irritate gums.

Plasma. The liquid part of blood.

Platelets. The smallest parts of the blood; crucial to clotting of the blood.

Platonic relationship. A friendship in which there is affection but not romance.

Pneumocystis carinii pneumonia (PCP). An opportunistic infection associated with AIDS.

Poison. Any substance that causes injury, illness, or death when introduced into the body.

Poison control center. A center that one can call for information about what to do when someone has ingested a poison.

Poliomyelitis. A viral infection that affects motor neurons in the spinal cord and brain stem.

Post-traumatic stress disorder. A condition in which a person who has experienced a traumatic event feels severe and long-lasting aftereffects.

Precaution. A planned, preventive action taken before an event to increase the chances of a safe outcome.

Precycling. Reducing waste before it occurs by making environmentally sound decisions about purchases.

Prejudice. A negative feeling toward someone or something that is based on stereotypes, not experience.

Pressure-point technique. Method used to stop bleeding by applying pressure to the main artery supplying blood to the affected limb.

Prevention. The act of practicing healthy habits to keep oneself well and free from disease and other ailments.

Primary care. The care one seeks on one's own, usually administered by one's family doctor.

Private practice. The medical practice of a doctor who is self-employed.

Progesterone. A female hormone first released during puberty.

Proteins. A vital part of every body cell.

Psychiatrist. A medical doctor who deals with mental, emotional, and behavioral disorders.

Psychoactive drugs. Drugs that affect the central nervous system and alter normal functioning of the brain.

Psychological dependence. The belief that one needs a drug in order to feel good or function normally.

Psychosomatic. Involving both the body and the mind.

Puberty. The beginning of adolescence; the period of time when males and females become physically able to reproduce.

Pulmonary circulation. The flow of blood from the heart to the lungs and back to the heart.

Pulmonary emphysema. A condition in which the tiny air sacs in the lungs through which oxygen is absorbed into the body are destroyed.

Pulp. Very sensitive, living tissue inside the tooth.

Pulse recovery rate. The rate at which one's heart beats following activity.

Q

Quack. A dishonest promoter of useless medicinal products or treatments.

Quackery. The act of dishonestly promoting useless medicinal products.

Quality of life. The level of health and satisfaction that a person has in being alive.

R

Rabies. A viral infection of the brain and spinal cord transmitted to humans through the bite of an infected animal.

Random violence. Violence committed for no particular reason and/or against anyone who happens to be around at the time.

Rape. Sexual intercourse by force or threat.

Recall. The process of instructing a manufacturer to take its product that is already on the market, but considered to be unsafe, off the shelves.

Recommended Dietary Allowances (RDA). Guidelines for the amounts of 19 essential nutrients that most people need daily and for calories and estimated intake for seven other vitamins and minerals.

Recovery. The process of getting well again; the process of learning to live an alcohol- or drug-free life.

Recycling. Treating or changing waste so that it can be reused.

Reflex. A spontaneous response of the body to a stimulus.

Refusal skills. Techniques and strategies that help one say no effectively.

Relapses. For people in recovery, periodic returns to drinking and drug use.

Relationship. A bond or connection between people.

Rescue breathing. The process of providing oxygen for a victim who has stopped breathing.

Resident bacteria. Bacteria that live in one's mouth and intestines and on one's skin and help protect one from harmful bacteria.

Resting heart rate. One's heart rate while one is not active.

Retina. The layer of the eyeball wall that contains the nerve cells and the processes responsible for vision.

Rheumatoid arthritis. A destructive and disabling inflammation of the joints.

Risk. A behavior with an element of danger that may cause injury or harm.

Risk factor. A characteristic that has been shown to increase the chances of getting heart disease.

Role. A part that one plays, especially in a relationship.

S

Saliva. A secretion that starts the digestion of carbohydrates.

Saprophytes. Bacteria that digest nonliving food materials, such as milk and meat.

Sarcomas. Cancers that develop in connective and supportive tissues, such as bones, muscles, and tendons.

Saturated. In the case of fatty acids, having hydrogen linked to all the carbon atoms on the chain.

Schizophrenia. A severe mental disorder in which one exhibits abnormal emotional responses or no emotional responses.

Sclera. A white, tough membrane that helps the eye keep its spherical shape and helps protect the eye's delicate inner structure.

Scoliosis. A side-to-side curvature of the spine.

Scrotum. A sac outside the male's body that contains the testes and protects sperm by regulating the temperature of the testes.

Sebaceous glands. Glands that produce an oily secretion called sebum and that are connected to hair follicles.

Secondary care. The care one receives when one is referred by a primary-care doctor to a specialist.

Secondary sex characteristics. Body hair and the development of breasts in the female and muscles in the male.

Self-actualization. The continuing process of striving to develop one's capabilities to their fullest.

Self-esteem. The confidence and worth one feels about oneself; influences everything you do, think, feel, and are.

Semen. A mixture of fluids from the seminal vesicles, the prostrate gland, and Cowper's glands combined with sperm; seminal fluid.

Sensory deafness. Hearing loss caused by excessive noise over a long period of time.

Sensory neurons. Nerve cells located in the skin and other sensory organs that have specialized receptor ends.

Sexual assault. Attempted or actual physical attack with violent, sexual intent.

Sexually transmitted disease (STD). A communicable disease that is spread from person to person through sexual contact.

Shock. The failure of the cardiovascular system to keep adequate blood circulating to the vital organs of the body.

Sidestream smoke. Smoke that comes from burning tobacco.

Single-parent family. A family in which children live with one parent at a time.

Skeletal muscles. Voluntary muscles attached to bones that cause body movement.

Small-claims courts. Courts that deal with consumer complaint claims that range from $100 to $3,000.

Small intestine. An organ in which a major part of digestion and absorption occurs.

Smoke detector. An alarm used to awaken people and alert them in the event of smoke or flames.

Smooth muscles. Involuntary muscles located in such places as intestines and blood vessels.

Social age. One's age as determined by a person's life-style.

Sprain. An injury to soft tissues surrounding a joint.

Stereotype. An exaggerated and oversimplified belief about an entire group, such as an ethnic group, a religious group, or a certain sex.

Sterility. A condition in which a person is unable to reproduce.

Stigma. A mark of shame.

Stimulant. A drug that increases the action of the central nervous system, the heart, respiratory rates, and blood pressure, and causes the pupils to dilate and appetite to decrease.

Strain. A condition in which muscles have been overworked.

Stress. The body's and mind's reactions to everyday demands.

Stressor. A stimulus that produces a stress response.

Stroke. A condition in which the blood supply to a part of the brain is cut off, and as a result, the nerve cells in that part of the brain cannot function.

Sweat glands. Glands that secrete perspiration through ducts to pores on the surface.

Synapse. A narrow gap between the axon end on one neuron and the dendrite of another over which an impulse must cross.

Synergistic effect. The interaction of two or more medicines that results in a greater effect than when the medicines are taken independently.

Synthetic. Made from laboratory chemicals.

Syphilis. A sexually transmitted disease that attacks many parts of the body.

Systemic circulation. The flow of blood to all body tissues except the lungs.

T

Tar. A thick, sticky, dark fluid produced when tobacco burns.

Target heart rate. Seventy to 85 percent of one's maximum heart rate.

Tartar. A very hard substance that irritates the underlying bone as well as the surrounding gums of one's teeth; calculus.

T cells. Lymphocytes produced in the bone marrow that travel to the thymus gland where they mature, then fight specific pathogens.

Tendinitis. A condition when a tendon—the connective tissue of the muscles and bones—is stretched or torn.

Tendons. Bands of fiber that connect muscles to bones.

Tertiary care. The care one receives when one's condition requires specialized equipment or treatment.

Testes. Two small glands that produce sperm; testicles.

Testimonial. A person's enthusiastic recommendation of a product.

Testosterone. A male hormone that causes the testes to produce sperm and is responsible for physical changes during puberty.

Thanatology. The study of death and adjustments that need to be made in association with the death of a loved one.

Therapy. Treatment technique.

Thrombosis. The presence or formation of a blood clot that forms in a blood vessel and usually remains attached to its point of origin.

Thyroid gland. The largest gland in the endocrine system that regulates the metabolism of carbohydrates, fats, and proteins in body cells.

Time-management skills. The ability to effectively arrange one's time.

Tinnitus. A condition characterized by a ringing noise in one's ears.

Tissue. Cells with similar structure that do similar work.

Tolerance. A condition in which the body becomes used to the effects of a medicine or drug.

Tooth decay. A disease of the digestive tract that weakens the tooth and affects the way one can bite and chew food.

Toxins. Poisons produced by some bacteria.

Trachea. The windpipe.

Tranquilizers. Depressants that reduce muscular activity, coordination, and attention span.

Transition. Change.

Tumor. A mass of tissue caused by the uncontrolled division of abnormal cells.

Type I diabetes. Diabetes that usually occurs in people under 15 years of age and that requires daily injections of insulin to sustain life.

Type II diabetes. Diabetes that usually occurs in adults over 40 years of age and can often be controlled by diet and exercise.

U

Ulcer. An open sore on the skin or in the mucous membrane.

Umbilical cord. Cord that connects the embryo to the placenta and through which nutrients and oxygen from the mother are carried through blood vessels to the embryo, and waste products from the embryo are carried to the mother.

Undernutrition. Not consuming enough essential nutrients or calories for normal body functions.

Underweight. Being 10 percent or more below normal weight.

Unit price. The amount that a unit of a product costs.

Unit pricing. The practice of showing the cost per unit of different-sized packages of a product.

Unplanned pregnancy. A pregnancy in which a baby is conceived accidentally.

Uremia. A series of symptoms caused by the kidneys' inability to rid wastes from the body.

Ureters. Tubes that lead from the two kidneys to the bladder.

Urethra. A small tube that extends from the bladder to the outside of the body.

Urine. Liquid waste material that collects in the bladder until it is ready to be passed out of the body.

Uterus. A small, muscular, pear-shaped organ in a female body.

V

Vaccination. The process by which a vaccine is injected into the body.

Vaccine. A preparation containing weakened or dead pathogens of a particular disease given to prevent one from contracting that disease.

Vagina. A muscular, very elastic tube in the female that is a passageway from the uterus to the outside of the body; the birth canal.

Values. Principles that one considers important and that guide one's life.

Veins. The vessels that carry the blood back to the heart.

Verbal communication. Sending messages using words.

Violence. The use of physical force to injure or abuse another person or persons.

Viruses. Small, simple life-like forms.

Vitreous humor. A fluid found behind the lens that keeps the eyeball firm.

Voluntary. Within a person's conscious control.

W

Warming up. Engaging in activity that prepares the muscles for the work that is to come.

Weight cycling. The cycle of losing, regaining, losing, and regaining weight; seesaw or yo-yo dieting.

Wellness. An overall state of well-being; total health.

Western blot. A test that is very specific in identifying HIV antibodies.

Withdrawal. A physical reaction that occurs when a person stops taking a drug or medicine on which he or she is physiologically dependent.

X

Xiphoid process. The lower part of the sternum that projects downward.

Z

Zygote. A fertilized egg cell.

A

Abdominal thrusts/empujones abdominales: empujones rápidos hacia arriba que hacen subir el diafragma y hacen que salga la sustancia que esté bloqueando la tráquea; maniobra de Heimlich.

Absorption/absorción: paso del alimento digerido desde el sistema digestivo hasta el sistema circulatorio.

Abstinence/abstinencia: la opción de no tener relaciones sexuales; la opción de no usar alcohol ni otras drogas.

Acquaintance rape/violación por un conocido: violación por algún conocido de la víctima o por alguien a quién se considera como amigo.

Acquired inmune deficiency syndrome (AIDS)/Síndrome de inmunodeficiencia adquirida (SIDA): enfermedad letal contagiosa, causada por el VIH, para la cual aún no hay cura o tratamiento eficaz.

Active immunity/inmunidad activa: inmunidad que desarrolla el cuerpo para protegerse de las enfermedades.

Addiction/adicción: dependencia psicológica o fisiológica en una sustancia o actividad.

Additive interaction/ interacción aditiva: una reacción que ocurre cuando las medicinas obran juntas de modo positivo.

Adolescence/adolescencia: etapa entre la niñez y la vida de adulto.

Adoption/adopción: acoger en la familia a un(a) niño(a) y asumir su responsabilidad de forma legal, comprometiéndose a criarlo(a) hasta la edad de adulto.

Adrenal glands/glándulas suprarrenales: las glándulas responsables de secretar hormonas que ayudan a mantener el equilibrio entre el sodio y el agua del cuerpo; afectan el metabolismo y ayudan a hacer frente al estrés.

Adrenaline/adrenalina: hormona que secretan las glándulas adrenales para preparar al cuerpo a responder a algo que cause estrés; la hormona de la emergencia.

Advertising/publicidad: el modo por el cual un fabricante logra que nos fijemos en su producto.

Advocate/defensor: alguien que apoya o defiende una posición o un producto.

Aerobic exercise/ejercicio aeróbico: actividad vigorosa que consume oxígeno continuamente; actividad que aumenta la capacidad de los pulmones para contener oxígeno.

Aesthetic/estético: artístico; que responde o aprecia aquello que uno percibe como hermoso.

Age norm/edad cronológica típica: lo que se espera que una persona sea capaz de desarrollar a cierta edad cronológica.

Aggravated assault/agresión grave: ataque ilegal cometido, a menudo, con un arma y en el cual la intención del agresor es causar daño o matar a la víctima.

Aggressive/agresividad: conducirse con contundencia, insistencia u hostilidad.

AIDS dementia complex/complejo de demencia ocasionado por el SIDA: trastorno progresivo que destruye los tejidos del encéfalo de una persona con el SIDA.

Al-Anon/Al-Anon: organización mundial de ayuda para los familiares y amigos de los alcohólicos.

Alateen/Alateen: una rama de Al-Anon específicamente para los adolescentes y pre-adolescentes, entre las edades de 12 y 20 años, cuyos padres u otros familiares, o amigos tienen problemas con el alcohol.

Alcoholics/alcohólicos: las personas que padecen de alcoholismo; las personas adictas al alcohol.

Alcoholics Anonymous(AA)/Alcohólicos Anónimos (AA): una organización mundial o grupo de apoyo que ha jugado un gran papel en ayudar a la gente a dejar el alcohol y las drogas y no volverlos a usar.

Alcohol-impaired driving/conducir impedido por el alcohol: conducir bajo la influencia del alcohol.

Alcoholism/alcoholismo: adicción al alcohol; la dependencia física y psicológica del alcohol.

Allergens/alergenos: sustancias en las comidas contra las cuales reacciona el sistema inmune del cuerpo.

Alveoli/alvéolos: conjunto de sacos con paredes delgadas para el aire ubicados en la punta de cada bronquiolo.

Alzheimer's disease/trastorno de Alzheimer: un trastorno progresivo, degenerativo que causa deterioro mental por completo.

Amino acids/aminoácidos: sustancias químicas que componen las proteínas.

Amphetamines/anfetaminas: estimulantes que aceleran el corazón y la respiración y causan ansiedad, insomnio y la pérdida del apetito.

Anabolic steroids/esteroides anabólicos: derivados sintéticos de la testosterona.

Anaerobic exercise/ejercicio anaeróbico: actividad física intensa en la cual el abastecimiento de oxígeno del cuerpo para producir energía no cumple con la demanda; actividad que mejora la fuerza muscular, la resistencia muscular y la flexibilidad.

Analgesics/analgésicos: medicinas que alivian el dolor sin la pérdida del conocimiento.

Angina pectoris/angina de pecho: una condición en la cual uno experimenta un dolor y tirantez o presión en el pecho cuando el corazón no recibe suficiente oxígeno.

Anorexia nervosa/anorexia nerviosa: un trastorno psicológico que incluye el miedo irracional a estar gordo y que resulta en la pérdida excesiva de peso debido a la autoinanición.

Antagonistic interaction/interacción antagónica: una reacción que ocurre cuando los efectos de una medicina se cancelan o se reducen al tomarse con otra medicina.

Antibiotics/antibióticos: medicinas que matan o reducen las bacterias perjudiciales en el cuerpo.

Antibodies/anticuerpos: proteínas que destruyen o neutralizan los patógenos en el cuerpo.

Antidiuretic hormone/hormona antidiurética: una de dos hormonas que secreta el lóbulo posterior de la glándula pituitaria.

Antisocial personality disorder/trastorno de personalidad antisocial: una condición caracterizada por el constante conflicto de una persona con la sociedad.

Antivenins/antitoxina: fluidos sanguíneos que contienen anticuerpos y que actúan más rápidamente que las vacunas.

Anxiety disorders/trastornos de ansiedad: trastornos en el que las fobias, sean imaginadas o reales, impiden que la persona disfrute la vida.

Appendicitis/apendicitis: la inflamación de la apéndice.

Appendicular skeleton/esqueleto apendicular: los huesos de los hombros, los brazos, las manos, las caderas, las piernas y los pies.

Aqueous humor/humor acuoso: en el ojo, sustancia acuosa que llena la cavidad entre la córnea y el cristalino.

Arteries/arterias: los más grandes de los vasos sanguíneos que parten del corazón.

Arteriosclerosis/arteriosclerosis: una condición en la cual las paredes de las arterias se endurecen y pierden su elasticidad.

Arthritis/artritis: inflamación de una articulación; condición que causa molestia, dolor e hinchazón en las articulaciones y los tejidos conjuntivos del cuerpo.

Artificial respiration/respiración artificial: ver *respiración de rescate.*

Assertive/afirmativo: defender sus propios derechos de una forma firme, pero positiva.

Atherosclerosis/aterosclerosis: una condición en la cual la pared de la arteria se ensancha debido a depósitos de grasa que impiden la circulación de la sangre.

Athlete's foot/pie de atleta o tiña podal: una infección de la piel entre los dedos de los pies causada por el hongo de la tiña.

Autonomy/autonomía: la certidumbre de que uno puede controlar su propio cuerpo, sus impulsos y el ambiente.

Axial skeleton/esqueleto axil: los huesos del cráneo, del esternón, las costillas y las vértebras.

Axon/axón: la parte de una neurona que lleva los impulsos desde las células del cuerpo.

B

Balloon angioplasty/angioplastia con globo: un procedimiento que incluye ensartar un catéter con un globo en la punta, a través del cuerpo hasta donde está el bloqueo, y luego inflar el globo para abrir el camino para que la sangre fluya; conocido oficialmente como angioplastia coronaria transluminal y percutánea.

Basal metabolism/metabolismo basal: la cantidad mínima absoluta que se requiere para mantener los procesos vitales del cuerpo.

Battery/acometimiento: el uso de fuerza física para controlar a alguien.

B cells/células B: los linfocitos que se producen y maduran en la médula ósea; estimulados por las células T ayudantes para producir anticuerpos.

Benign/benigno: no canceroso.

Better Business Bureau (BBB)/Oficina de Mejoramiento de los Negocios: una organización sin fines de lucro patronizada por negocios privados.

Bile/bilis: un fluido amargo producido por el hígado cuya función es esencial para la descomposición de las grasas.

Binaural hearing/audición binaural: la habilidad para determinar la procedencia de un sonido al poderlo oír con ambos oídos.

Biodegradable/biodegradable: capaz de ser descompuesto por microorganismos.

Biofeedback/retroalimentación biológica: retroalimentación biológica acerca de tu propio cuerpo; el proceso de enterarse de los acontecimientos de tu propio cuerpo que, por lo general, desconoces con el fin de lograr control voluntario de ellos.

Biological age/edad biológica: la determinación de nuestra edad basándose en cuán bien funcionan las distintas partes del cuerpo.

Biopsy/biopsia: un procedimiento por el cual se extirpa un poco de tejido para analizarlo y ver si contiene células anormales o cancerosas.

Biosphere/biosfera: la fina capa de tierra, agua y aire cerca de la superficie de la tierra.

Birth defects/defectos de nacimiento: condiciones genéticas y muchos otros tipos de enfermedades y trastornos que son causados por una variedad de distintos factores.

Bladder/vejiga: un órgano muscular que contiene la orina.

Blastocyst/blástula: un conjunto de células que tienen una cavidad en el centro; la etapa que sigue a la del cigoto.

Blended family/familia mixta: un tipo de familia nuclear en la que uno o ambos padres han estado casados anteriormente y en la que cada uno tiene hijos del matrimonio anterior.

Blizzard/ventisca: una tormenta de nieve con vientos de 35 millas (56 km) o más por hora.

Blood alcohol concentration (BAC)/concentración de alcohol en la sangre (CAS): la cantidad de alcohol en la sangre de una persona según se expresa en porcentajes.

Blood pressure/presión sanguínea: la fuerza de la sangre contra las paredes de los vasos sanguíneos al fluir la sangre por el sistema cardiovascular.

Body composition/composición corporal: el porcentaje de grasa, músculo magro, hueso, tejido conjuntivo y agua en el cuerpo.

Body system/sistema corporal: un grupo de órganos que obran conjuntamente para lograr una función común.

Brain death/muerte encefálica: la pérdida de la función del encéfalo entero, incluyendo el bulbo raquídeo.

Brain stem/bulbo raquídeo: la división del encéfalo que conecta la espina dorsal al encéfalo.

Bronchi/bronquios: tubos bronquiales que conducen a los pulmones.

Bronchioles/bronquiolos: divisiones de los tubos bronquiales dentro de los pulmones.

Bruise/magulladura: una lesión al tejido subcutáneo.

Bulimia/bulimia: un trastorno de la alimentación en el cual la víctima sigue una dieta muy estricta, luego come en exceso como reacción al hambre, y procede a provocar el vómito, darse purgantes y a seguir dietas exageradamente rigurosas.

C

Calorie/caloría: una unidad para medir la energía en los alimentos y la energía que quema el cuerpo.

Cancer/cáncer: crecimiento anormal y descontrolado de las células.

Capillaries/capilares: los vasos sanguíneos más pequeños.

Carbohydrate loading/almacenamiento de carbohidratos: almacenar glicógeno extra en los músculos antes de hacer ejercicio extenuoso.

Carbohydrates/carbohidratos: azúcares, almidones y fibra que son la fuente de energía preferida del cuerpo.

Carbon monoxide/monóxido de carbono: un gas venenoso, incoloro e inodoro, que se encuentra en el humo de cigarrillo y en el humo de escape de los automóviles.

Carcinogenic/carcinogénico: que causa cáncer o envenena.

Carcinogens/carcinógenos: agentes que causan cáncer.

Carcinomas/carcinomas: cáncer que se desarrolla en el tejido epitelial—tejido que compone la piel y las membranas que cubren los órganos del cuerpo.

Cardiac arrest/paro cardíaco: una condición en la cual el corazón se para por completo.

Cardiac muscle/músculo cardíaco: tejido estriado que forma la pared del corazón.

Cardiopulmonary resuscitation (CPR)/resucitación cardiopulmonar (RCP): la técnica salvavidas que incluye respirar por la víctima de un fallo cardiovascular y, mediante la aplicación de presión sobre el esternón de la víctima, forzarle a que el corazón bombée sangre.

Cardiorespiratory endurance/resistencia cardiovascular: la habilidad del corazón, los pulmones y los vasos sanguíneos de enviar energía y oxígeno a los tejidos del cuerpo durante largos períodos de actividad vigorosa.

Cardiovascular diseases/enfermedades cardiovasculares: enfermedades del corazón y los vasos sanguíneos.

Carjacking/robo de un auto: hurtar un auto por la fuerza, utilizando un arma.

Carotid pulse/pulso de la carótida: el latido cardíaco que se puede sentir a cada lado del cuello.

Cartilage/cartílago: un material fuerte y flexible que permite el suave movimiento de las articulaciones, sostiene la nariz y las orejas, conecta las costillas al esternón y actúa como un cojín entre las vértebras contiguas.

Catheter/catéter: tubo de plástico, delgado y flexible, que se puede conducir a través de los vasos sanguíneos hasta ciertos órganos del cuerpo.

Cell/célula: la unidad básica de estructura de todo ser viviente.

Cell body/cuerpo celular: la parte de una neurona que tiene un núcleo y es el centro para recibir y enviar impulsos nerviosos.

Cerebellum/cerebelo: la parte del encéfalo que funciona como centro para la coordinación del movimiento esqueletomuscular.

Cerebral palsy/parálisis cerebral: un grupo de trastornos neurológicos no progresivos que son el resultado del daño sufrido por el encéfalo durante su desarrollo antes o en el momento del nacimiento.

Cerebrum/cerebro: la parte mayor y más compleja del encéfalo, que consiste de los hemisferios derecho e izquierdo, que controla la actividad muscular y recibe información sensorial.

Cervix/cérvix: el cuello redondo y muscular, la parte inferior, del útero.

Chancre/chancro: una llaga rojiza en el sitio donde los patógenos invaden el cuerpo.

Chemotherapy/quimioterapia: el uso de medicamentos anticancerosos en el tratamiento del cáncer.

Child abuse/abuso de los niños: daño físico, incluyendo el abuso sexual, y/o el daño emocional que se le haga a los niños.

Chlamydia/clamidia: una enfermedad transmitida sexualmente que ataca los órganos reproductores.

Chlorofluorocarbons(CFCs)/clorofluorcarbonos: compuestos de cloro, flúor y carbono, los que se piensa que son un factor principal en la reducción del ozono.

Cholesterol/colesterol: sustancia semejante a la grasa.

Choroid/coroides: la capa intermedia de la pared del ojo, la cual contiene el iris, los ligamentos suspensorios y los músculos ciliares.

Chromosomes/cromosomas: pequeñas estructuras dentro de los núcleos de las células, las cuales contienen información genética.

Chronic bronchitis/bronquitis crónica: una condición en la cual los bronquios están irritados.

Chronic fatigue syndrome (CFS)/síndrome de fatiga crónica: un tipo de fatiga que es de largo plazo y para la cual se desconoce la causa.

Chronological age/edad cronológica: la edad de una persona basada en la cantidad de años que haya cumplido.

Chyme/quimo: la sustancia que se forma cuando se mezclan los alimentos y los jugos gástricos.

Circumcision/circuncisión: el procedimiento por el cual se extirpa quirúrgicamente el prepucio de los varones.

Cirrhosis/cirrosis: cicatrización, una condición del hígado en la cual las cicatrices reducen el flujo de sangre en el hígado.

Clinical death/muerte clínica: el paro de las funciones del cuerpo de una persona.

Clinical depression/depresión clínica: una condición en la cual los sentimientos de tristeza y de desesperanza duran por más de unas semanas e interfieren con los intereses y actividades diarias de la persona.

Clinical psychologist/psicólogo clínico: persona que diagnostica y trata trastornos del ánimo y de conducta.

Cliques/grupos exclusivos o pandillas: grupos de amistades exclusivas que por lo general comparten intereses y orígenes.

Cluttered-nest syndrome/síndrome del nido revuelto: el fenómeno en el cual los hijos adultos regresan a vivir en el hogar de los padres.

Codependency/codependencia: preocuparse excesivamente de la conducta y problemas de otras personas; las ansias agudas de arreglar y controlar esos problemas.

Communicable diseases/enfermedades contagiosas: enfermedades causadas por la transmisión, directa o indirecta, de patógenos de una persona a otra.

Communication/comunicación: un proceso a través del cual se envían y se reciben mensajes; la franqueza entre los miembros de la familia, lo que incluye la demostración de ternura, afecto y simpatía. También significa ser capaz de expresar sentimientos negativos.

Compromise/concesión: un modo de resolver un

problema en el cual cada persona rinde algo de modo que se halle una solución que satisfaga a todos.

Compulsion/compulsión: una conducta urgente que se repite.

Congenital/congénito: que existe o que se inicia al nacer.

Congenital syphilis/sífilis congénita: una condición en la cual una mujer embarazada que tiene sífilis transmite la infección al feto.

Conjunctiva/conjuntiva: una membrana mucosa protectiva pegada a la superficie interior de los párpados que continúa sobre la superficie exterior del ojo.

Consequence/consecuencia: el resultado de una acción.

Conservation/preservación: la conservación del medio ambiente.

Consumer/consumidor: cualquier persona que usa un servicio o un producto.

Consumer health/salud del consumidor: el proceso de ayudar a uno a elegir con juicio los productos y servicios de salubridad; y el permitirle a uno saber dónde ir o qué hacer si a uno lo han tratado injustamente o si uno necesita ayuda.

Cooling down/enfriamiento: la reducción gradual de actividad tras hacer ejercicio de modo que se permita que el pulso disminuya.

Cornea/córnea: la parte incolora y trasparente de la esclera en la parte delantera del ojo.

Coronary angiography/angiografía coronaria: procedimiento que se usa para evaluar cuan extensa es la enfermedad de la arteria coronaria.

Coronary bypass surgery/cirugía del puente coronario: un procedimiento para crear una desviación alrededor de las arterias coronarias obstruidas, de modo que la sangre pueda llegar al corazón.

Crisis/crisis: un cambio extremo en la vida de una persona.

Cross-contamination/contaminación cruzada: la propagación de bacterias de un alimento a otro.

D

Daily Food Guide/Guía Diaria de Alimentos: una publicación que ofrece una forma fácil de escoger una dieta variada, balanceada y moderada.

Date rape/violación durante una cita: la violación que ocurre entre dos personas que están saliendo juntas.

Deafness/sordera: la pérdida de la habilidad de oír.

Decision/decisión: el acto de hacer una elección o llegar a una solución.

Defense mechanisms/mecanismos de defensa: estrategias que se usan para hacer frente a situaciones de mucho estrés.

Deforestation/tala: la destrucción de los bosques.

Dendrites/dendritas: la parte de una neurona que recibe y lleva impulsos hacia las células del cuerpo.

Dentin/dentina: el material que rodea la pulpa.

Depressants/depresivos: sedantes; drogas que tienden a retardar el sistema nervioso central.

Dermis/dermis: la capa más gruesa y profunda de la piel.

Desertification/desertificación: la conversión de prados o tierras de regadío, a condiciones desérticas.

Designer drugs/drogas diseñadas: drogas hechas con sustancias sintéticas por químicos clandestinos.

Detoxification/desintoxicación: el proceso de sacar las drogas del cuerpo.

Developmental task/tarea de desarrollo: algo que necesita ocurrir durante una etapa en particular para que un ser humano continúe su desarrollo, hasta convertirse en un adulto saludable y maduro.

Diabetes/diabetes: una enfermedad crónica que afecta la forma en que las células del cuerpo convierten los alimentos en energía.

Diaphragm/diafragma: un músculo que separa el pecho de la cavidad abdominal.

Diet/dieta: todo lo que una persona come y bebe.

Digestion/digestión: la descomposición física y química de los alimentos a pedazos más pequeños.

Digestive enzymes/enzimas digestivas: proteínas que aceleran la descomposición de los alimentos.

Discrimination/discriminación: una forma de prejuicio por el cual se elige a ciertas personas y se les trata mal como resultado de un factor, como la edad, el sexo, la raza, la etnia o algún rasgo físico.

Distress/estrés negativo: estrés que causa angustia.

Divorce/divorcio: la disolución legal o la terminación del contrato matrimonial.

Dormant/latente: inactivo.

Down syndrome/síndrome de Down: una condición caracterizada por un retraso mental de ligero a agudo que resulta de anormalidades de los cromosomas.

Drugs/drogas: sustancias peligrosas y a menudo ilegales, que incluyen el alcohol y el tabaco.

Drug dependence/dependencia de las drogas: la drogadicción.

E

Earthquake/terremoto: temblores de tierra severos.

Electrocardiogram(EKG)/electrocardiograma (ECG): una prueba que produce una gráfica de la actividad eléctrica del corazón.

Elimination/eliminación: la expulsión de alimentos no digeridos o desperdicios del cuerpo.

ELISA/ELISA: muestra inmuno-sorbente relacionada a la enzima; una prueba para detectar la presencia de la infección del VIH.

Embolus/émbolo: un coágulo de sangre que se mueve del lugar donde se formó.

Embryo/embrión: un conjunto de células o blástula que se ha implantado en el útero.

Emotions/emociones: sentimientos que influyen en todo lo que uno hace.

Empty-calorie foods/comidas sin valor nutritivo: comidas que tienen escaso valor nutritivo.

Empty-nest syndrome/síndrome del nido vacío: el fenómeno en el cual los hijos al hacerse adultos se van de la casa.

Enabling/responsabilizarse: tratar de proteger a la persona que tiene problemas con el alcohol o las drogas, de las consecuencias de su problema de adicción.

Enamel/esmalte: el material más duro del cuerpo; el material que cubre la corona de los dientes.

Encephalitis/encefalitis: una inflamación de encéfalo causada por un virus y a veces por una bacteria.

Endocrine glands/glándulas endocrinas: glándulas de secreción interna que secretan hormonas en el torrente sanguíneo.

Endocrine system/sistema endocrino: el sistema del cuerpo que consiste de glándulas de secreción interna y las hormonas que producen.

Enriched/enriquecido: un producto al cual se le agregan los nutrimentos que ha perdido durante el procesamiento.

Environment/ambiente: todo nuestro entorno, incluyendo la familia, la ubicación y las experiencias.

Epidermis/epidermis: la capa exterior de la piel la cual es la más delgada.

Epilepsy/epilepsia: un trastorno del sistema nervioso caracterizado por un arrebato de impulsos nerviosos en el encéfalo como resultado de un ataque.

Esophagus/esófago: un tubo muscular que se extiende desde la faringe hasta el estómago y el cual está situado detrás de la tráquea y el corazón.

Estrogen/estrógeno: una hormona femenina que se libera por primera vez durante la pubertad.

Estuaries/estuarios: ecosistemas donde el agua de mar se mezcla con el agua dulce.

Eustress/estrés positivo: estrés benéfico.

Exploited/explotado: usado para el beneficio de otro.

Extended family/parentela: una familia con más de un pariente además de la familia nuclear o la consistente de un solo padre.

Extensors/extensores: músculos que enderezan las extremidades.

External auditory canal/canal auditivo externo: una vía, de más o menos, una pulgada de largo que conduce al tímpano y la cual protege el oído al mantener fuera los cuerpos extraños.

External respiration/respiración externa: el intercambio de oxígeno y dióxido de carbono entre la sangre y el aire en los pulmones.

F

Fallopian tubes/trompas de Falopio: un par de tubos a través de los cuales viaja el huevo maduro.

Family/familia: un grupo de gente relacionada por sangre, matrimonio o adopción.

Fatigue/fatiga: una sensación de cansancio que le reduce a uno el nivel de actividad.

Fatty liver/hígado grasoso: una condición en la cual las grasas se han acumulado en el hígado, evitando el funcionamiento normal de las células del mismo.

Federal Trade Commission (FTC)/Comisión Federal de Comercio (CFC): una agencia federal que impide que se anuncien de forma injusta y fraudulenta los productos y servicios de consumo.

Feedback/retroalimentación: mensajes de otras personas que nos indican cómo se sienten acerca de una persona o una idea.

Fertilization/fecundación: la unión de una célula de huevo y una célula de esperma que solo puede ocurrir si las células de esperma están presentes cuando el óvulo está en la trompa de falopio; concepción.

Fetal alcohol syndrome(FAS)/síndrome de alcoholismo fetal: una condición en la cual un feto ha sido adversamente afectado debido a que su madre hizo uso excesivo del alcohol durante el embarazo.

Fetus/feto: un embrión a partir de las ocho semanas de concepción hasta el nacimiento.

Fibrillation/fibrilación: una perturbación rítmica que ocurre cuando las fibras musculares del corazón se contraen de una manera no coordinada.

Fire extinguisher/extinguidor de fuego: un aparato portátil que apaga pequeños fuegos al disparar sustancias químicas para ese fin.

First aid/primeros auxilios: cuidados de emergencia; los cuidados inmediatos y momentáneos que se le da a una persona que ha caído enferma o que se ha lesionado.

Fitness/estar en forma: soltura física. Las personas que están en buena forma física se encuentran en mejores condiciones de sobrellevar las situaciones cotidianas, que las personas que no están en buena forma.

Flexibility/flexibilidad: la habilidad de mover cualquier parte del cuerpo por todo un campo de movimiento.

Flexors/flexores: músculos que doblan una extremidad.

Fluoroscope/fluoroscopio: una máquina que provee un retrato en vivo, con frecuencia empleada por los médicos para ver directamente la sombra del corazón.

Follicle/folículo: una pequeña bolsa que sujeta la raíz del pelo a la dermis.

Food additives/aditivos: sustancias que se le agregan a los alimentos con el propósito de producir un efecto deseado.

Food allergy/alergia por alimento: una condición en la cual el sistema inmune del cuerpo reacciona a los alergenos en algunos alimentos.

Food and Drug Administration (FDA)/Administración de Alimentos y Drogas: una agencia federal que asegura que todas las comidas y los aditivos, a no ser las carnes y las aves, son fiables, puros, íntegros y que han sido etiquetados con precisión y honradez.

Foodborne illness/enfermedad transmitida por alimentos: una condición causada por ingerir comida contaminada por bacteria; envenenamiento por comida contaminada.

Fortification/fortificación: el proceso de agregar nutrimentos donde no suelen ocurrir por naturaleza.

Fraternal twins/mellizos fraternales: dos embriones con composición genética distinta.

Friendship/amistad: una relación significativa entre dos personas basada en el cariño, la consideración y la confianza.

Frostbite/congelación: una condición en la cual se forman cristales de hielo en los espacios entre las células.

Functional disorder/trastorno funcional: un trastorno mental que ocurre como resultado de causas sociológicas sin que exista lesión encefálica.

G

Gallbladder/vesícula biliar: el órgano que aloja la bilis.

Gallstones/cálculo biliar: pequeños cristales que se forman de la bilis y que pueden bloquear el conducto biliar entre la vesícula y el duodeno.

Gangrene/gangrena: la muerte del tejido en una parte del cuerpo.

Gastric juices/jugos gástricos: líquidos que contienen ácido clorhídrico, enzimas digestivas y mucosa y que comienzan la digestión de las proteínas.

Gastritis/gastritis: un trastorno en el cual la membrana mucosa que cubre el estómago se inflama.

Genes/genes: pequeñas secciones de cromosomas que controlan las características hereditarias.

Genetic condition/condición genética: una enfermedad, trastorno, quebranto o estado de mal funcionamiento con el que se nace.

Gerontologist/gerontólogo: persona que estudia el proceso de envejecimiento.

Glucose/glucosa: un azúcar formado en el cuerpo durante la digestión.

Glycogen/glucógeno: la forma en la cual los carbohidratos se almacenan en el cuerpo.

Goal/meta: algo que requiere planificación y trabajo para poder lograrlo; plan definitivo que uno tiene para su propia vida.

Gonorrhea/gonorrea: una enfermedad transmitida sexualmente causada por bacterias que viven en áreas calientes y húmedas del cuerpo.

Group practice/grupo de médicos: una situación en la cual dos o más doctores se unen para proveer cuidado médico.

H

Halitosis/halitosis: mal aliento.

Hallucinogens/alucinógenos: psicodélicos; drogas que alteran el humor, el pensamiento y los sentidos.

Hashish/hashís: resina marrón oscura que se recoge de la parte del cáñamo (cannabis).

Health/salud: estado de pleno bienestar físico, mental y social.

Health care delivery/rendimiento de cuidados de salud: servicio de salud.

Health education/educación de la salud: proveer información sobre la salud para lograr influir a la gente para que cambien su actitud y tomen pasos positivos respecto a su salud.

Health facility/ambulatorio: un lugar a donde va una persona para recibir atención médica.

Health maintenance organization (HMO)/organización para el mantenimiento de la salud: un plan de salud en el cual uno paga una cuota regularmente y luego recibe cuidados médicos por poco o ningún costo adicional.

Health resources/recursos de salud: lugares a los que la gente puede ir para obtener varios tipos de tratamiento.

Health services/servicios de salud: los aspectos de un programa general de la salud que incluye la prevención, tratamiento y cura de las enfermedades, y el mantenimiento y promoción de la salud.

Heart attack/ataque al corazón: nombre común para referirse a varios trastornos que tienen que ver con el corazón y los vasos sanguíneos, pero que generalmente ocurre porque las células del músculo cardíaco no están recibiendo el oxígeno y nutrimentos que necesitan.

Hemodialysis/hemodiálisis: una técnica en la cual a una persona la conectan a una máquina de riñón artificial.

Hemoglobin/hemoglobina: la sustancia que porta oxígeno en los glóbulos rojos.

Hepatitis/hepatitis: una inflamación grave del hígado que por lo general la causa una infección viral.

Heredity/herencia: el paso de características de los progenitores a los descendientes.

Hernias/hernias: áreas débiles en el músculo que sostiene a varios órganos; ruptura.

Herpes simplex type 2 virus/virus tipo 2 de herpes simplex: una ETS en la cual un virus causa llagas como especie de ampollas en el área genital, las cuales se denominan herpes genital.

Hiatal hernia/hernia hiatal: condición en la cual la parte superior del estómago se empuja sobre el diafragma.

Hierarchy of needs/jerarquía de necesidades: una lista que anota, por orden de importancia, las cosas que los seres humanos necesitan para sobrevivir y tener bienestar.

High blood pressure/tensión arterial alta: la hipertensión.

Histamine/histamina: una sustancia liberada cuando un virus que causa resfriado le invade a uno el sistema respiratorio.

Holistic/integral: que toma en consideración la influencia física, mental y social sobre la persona por completo y su salud.

Homicide/homicidio: el acto premeditado en que un ser humano mata a otro ser humano.

Hormones/hormonas: sustancias químicas que se producen en el cuerpo por las glándulas endocrinas las cuales regulan la actividad de distintas células del cuerpo; la causa de cambios físicos y emocionales.

Hospice/hospicio: un lugar que promueve un modo especial de cuidar a los moribundos.

Host/huésped: la planta o animal del cual se alimenta un parásito.

Human collision/choque humano: durante un accidente, el hecho de una persona darse contra cualquier parte del auto o ser arrojada del mismo.

Human immunodeficiency virus (HIV)/virus de inmunodeficiencia humana (VIH): el virus que ataca el sistema de inmunidad del cuerpo y conduce al SIDA.

Hurricane/huracán: una tormenta potente con lluvias caracterizada por ráfagas.

Hurricane watch/vigilancia de huracán: un pronóstico del Servicio Meteorológico Nacional que significa que existen las condiciones atmosféricas para que se desate un huracán.

Hypertension/hipertensión: tensión arterial alta.

Hypochondria/hipocondría: un trastorno somatoforme en que uno experimenta una preocupación con el cuerpo y un temor a supuestas enfermedades.

I

Identical twins/gemelos idénticos: dos embriones con la misma composición genética.

Implantation/implantación: el proceso por el cual las células se adhieren al forro del útero.

Indigestion/indigestión: una condición en la cual el cuerpo no descompone bien los alimentos.

Inhalants/inhalantes: sustancias con vapores que al olerlos e inhalarlos producen un estado de alucinación.

Inpatients/pacientes internos: pacientes que requieren cuidado médico prolongado y que se admiten en un hospital y ocupan una cama.

Insulin/insulina: una hormona producida por el páncreas que ayuda al cuerpo a convertir la glucosa en energía para que las células la usen.

Integumentary system/sistema integumentario: sistema que incluye la piel, el pelo, las uñas y las glándulas sudoríparas.

Internal respiration/respiración interna: el intercambio de gases entre la sangre y las células del cuerpo.

Interneurons/interneuronas: células nerviosas en el encéfalo y el bulbo raquídeo que transmiten impulsos desde las neuronas sensoriales a las neuronas motoras.

Intervention/intervención: el hecho de interrumpir la continua adicción antes que el alcohólico o el narcómano empeore.

Involuntary/involuntario: fuera del control consciente de la persona.

K

Kidney/riñón: órgano que filtra la sangre para quitarle las sustancias dañinas de aquellas que el cuerpo puede usar.

L

Labyrinth/laberinto: el oído interno; consiste del vestíbulo, los canales semicirculares y la cóclea.

Lacrimal gland/glándula lagrimal: una glándula situada encima del ojo cuya función es producir lágrimas.

Lactose intolerance/intolerancia láctica: una condición en la cual el cuerpo no puede digerir el azúcar de la leche.

Larynx/laringe: órgano productor de la voz.

Leukoplakia/leucoplasia: lesión caracterizada por manchas blanquecinas, ligeramente elevadas dentro de la boca de los que mascan tabaco.

Life expectancy/expectación de vida: el promedio de años que se espera que un grupo de personas viva.

Life-style factors/factores del estilo de vida: conductas repetidas relacionadas al modo de vivir de una persona que afectan el nivel de su salud.

Ligaments/ligamentos: bandas fuertes o cordones de tejidos que conectan los huesos en una articulación.

Lipids/lípidos: sustancias grasas que no se disuelven en agua.

Look-alike drugs/drogas parecidas: drogas hechas de sustancias legales con el propósito de parecerse a las ilegales.

Lymph/linfa: un líquido transparente y amarillo que fluye por los vasos linfáticos.

Lymph nodes/nódulos linfáticos: masas de tejidos que filtran las linfas.

Lymphocytes/linfocitos: tipo de glóbulos blancos que combaten los patógenos.

Lymphomas/linfomas: cánceres que se desarrollan en los tejidos que forman la sangre y el sistema linfático.

M

Mainstream smoke/humo directo: humo que el fumador exhala.

Malignant/maligno: canceroso.

Manic-depressive disorder/trastorno maníaco depresivo: una condición en la cual el humor de una persona cambia dramáticamente de un extremo emocional a otro sin ninguna razón aparente.

Manipulation/manipulación: un medio indirecto, y a veces solapado o bajo, de tratar de controlar la conducta o la actitud de otra persona.

Marijuana/mariguana: la planta del cáñamo (cannabis) que se fuma, se come, o se bebe por sus efectos de intoxicación.

Marital adjustment/ajuste matrimonial: lo bien que las personas dentro del matrimonio se ajustan y se adaptan al matrimonio y mutuamente.

Marriage/matrimonio: la unión de un hombre y una mujer de acuerdo con las tradiciones y la ley.

Mastication/masticación: el proceso de masticar.

Medicaid/Medicaid: programa de asistencia médica para personas de todas las edades que no pueden pagar por el cuidado médico.

Medicare/Medicare: programa de seguro de salud accesible a personas mayores de 65 años de edad y a personas que reciben beneficios para lisiados a través del seguro social.

Medicine/medicina: una sustancia que, cuando se ingiere o se aplica al cuerpo, ayuda a prevenir o a curar una enfermedad, lesión, o problema médico.

Medicine misuse/mal uso de medicinas: el uso de un medicamento contrario a su propósito.

Megadose/megadosis: grandes cantidades de suplementos nutricionales.

Melanoma/melanoma: cáncer de la piel.

Meningitis/meningitis: la inflamación de las meninges.

Menstrual cycle/ciclo menstrual: el tiempo desde el inicio del período menstrual al inicio del próximo período.

Menstruation/menstruación: el proceso de despojar el forro del útero.

Mental disorders/trastornos mentales: problemas mentales y emocionales.

Mental health/salud mental: el proceso de aceptarse y gustarse uno mismo y adaptarse y hacer frente a las emociones, los retos y los cambios que forman parte de la vida.

Mental illness/enfermedad mental: enfermedad o trastorno médico que afecta la mente e impide que la persona disfrute la vida.

Metabolism/metabolismo: la suma total de todas las reacciones químicas dentro de una célula.

Metastasis/metástasis: el proceso de propagación de las células cancerosas.

Mobile/móvil: capaz de moverse de un sitio a otro.

Motor neurons/neuronas motoras: células nerviosas que llevan impulsos desde las interneuronas dentro del encéfalo y la espina dorsal a los músculos y glándulas.

Multiple sclerosis/esclerosis múltiple: un trastorno progresivo en el cual la membrana de mielina que rodea las fibras nerviosas se va destruyendo.

Multiplier effect/efecto multiplicador: el hecho de tomar drogas o medicinas con alcohol.

Muscular endurance/resistencia muscular: la habilidad de los músculos para seguir trabajando a lo largo de un período de tiempo sin fatigarse.

Muscular strength/fortaleza muscular: la habilidad de ejercer fuerza contra la resistencia.

Mycobacterium avium intracellulare (MAI)/micobacteria avium intracelular: una enfermedad oportunista que es la causa principal del síndrome de debilitación, del deterioro gradual de todas la funciones del cuerpo y que está asociada con el SIDA.

N

Narcotics/narcóticos: drogas hechas de la flor de la amapola del opio y las medicinas que se emplean para aliviar el dolor e inducir el sueño.

Nephrons/nefrones: las unidades funcionales de los riñones.

Neurologist/neurólogo: un médico que se especializa en trastornos orgánicos del encéfalo y del sistema nervioso.

Neurons/neuronas: células nerviosas que forman la parte funcional y estructural del sistema nervioso.

Neutrophils/neutrófilos: un tipo de fagocito; los cuales están más activamente involucrados en el proceso de fagocitosis.

Nicotine/nicotina: la droga adictiva en los cigarrillos que hace subir la presión y aumenta la palpitación cardíaca.

Noncommunicable diseases/enfermedades no transmisibles: enfermedades no causadas por patógenos y que no se transmiten por contacto.

Nongonococcal urethritis (NGU)/uretritis no gonococa: una enfermedad transmitida sexualmente causada por varios tipos de organismos parecidos a las bacterias que infectan la uretra en los hombres y el cuello de la matriz en la mujer.

Nontoxic/no tóxico: no dañino o venenoso para los humanos.

Nonverbal communication/comunicación no verbal: el hecho de enviar mensajes por medio de expresiones faciales y movimientos corporales.

Nuclear family/familia nuclear: los padres y uno o más hijos que comparten el hogar.

Nutrient-dense/denso en nutrimentos: rico en nutrimento respecto al contenido calórico.

Nutrients/nutrimentos: sustancias en los alimentos que el cuerpo necesita para funcionar adecuadamente.

Nutrient supplements/suplementos nutritivos: píldoras, polvos y líquidos que contienen nutrimentos.

Nutrition/nutrición: la ciencia de ver cómo el cuerpo usa los nutrimentos y cómo y por qué la gente come.

O

Obesity/obesidad: exceso de grasa en el cuerpo.

Obsession/obsesión: una preocupación emocional y social muy perjudicial.

Occupational Safety and Health Administration (OSHA)/Departamento de Seguridad y Salud Ocupacional: una agencia federal que promueve condiciones seguras y saludables en el lugar de trabajo.

Open-dating/fechado abierto: la práctica de poner la fecha en los paquetes de alimentos para indicar la fecha de caducidad, la frescura, la fecha de envase o el último día para la venta del producto.

Organ/órgano: dos o más tipos de tejido que realizan una tarea específica.

Organic/orgánico: derivado de organismos vivientes sin el uso de sustancias químicas.

Organic disorder/trastorno orgánico: un trastorno mental causado por un quebranto físico o una lesión que afecta el encéfalo.

Ossicles/osículos: tres huesillos que se unen, situados detrás del tímpano y que lo conectan con el oído interno.

Ossification/osificación: el proceso por el cual las células cartílagas se reemplazan por células óseas minerales.

Osteoarthritis/osteoartritis: una condición en la cual las partes mecánicas de una articulación sufren deterioro cotidiano.

Osteomyelitis/osteomielitis: la inflamación de la superficie blanda del interior de los huesos.

Osteoporosis/osteoporosis: la condición que resulta de la falta de calcio en los huesos.

Otosclerosis/otosclerosis: una enfermedad hereditaria que es la causa común de la sordera parcial.

Outpatient/pacientes ambulatorios: gente que recibe servicios médicos, dentales o de otro tipo en un local médico y luego se van a su casa el mismo día.

Ovaries/ovarios: glándulas sexuales femeninas que contienen los óvulos y producen las hormonas sexuales femeninas.

Overweight/sobrepeso: pesar más del 10 por ciento sobre el estándar de peso para la estatura.

Ovulation/ovulación: el proceso por el cual los ovarios liberan un óvulo maduro todos los meses.

Ovum/óvulo: una célula de huevo.

Oxytocin/oxitocina: una de dos hormonas formadas por el lóbulo posterior de la glándula pituitaria.

P

Pancreas/páncreas: una glándula que sirve al sistema digestivo y al endocrino.

Papillae/papilas: pequeñas proyecciones que cubren la superficie de la lengua.

Parasite/parásito: microorganismo que se alimenta de una planta o animal vivo.

Parathyroid glands/glándulas paratiroides: las glándulas situadas en los lóbulos de la glándula tiroides que regulan el equilibro de calcio y fósforo en el cuerpo.

Parkinson's disease/enfermedad de Parkinson: un trastorno progresivo que interfiere con la transmisión de impulsos nerviosos desde las áreas motoras al encéfalo.

Passive/pasivo: darse por vencido, acceder o retroceder sin defender los derechos y necesidades.

Passive-aggressive personality disorder/trastorno de la personalidad pasivo-agresiva: una condición en la cual uno a menudo no coopera con los demás y demuestra la ira indirectamente.

Passive immunity/inmunidad pasiva: la inmunidad temporal que un bebé obtiene de su madre.

Passive smoke/humo indirecto: humo de cigarrillo, de cigarro o de pipa que inhala la persona que no fuma.

Pathogens/patógenos: microorganismos que invaden el cuerpo y atacan sus células y tejidos, causando muchas enfermedades comunes.

Peer pressure/presión paritaria: el control e influencia que la gente de la misma edad o grupo social se ejercen mutuamente.

Peers/compañeros o contemporáneos: personas de la misma edad.

Pelvic Inflammatory Disease (PID)/Enfermedad Pélvica Inflamatoria: una infección dolorosa de las trompas de falopio, los ovarios y/o del útero como resultado de la gonorrea o la clamidia sin tratamiento.

Penis/pene: el órgano externo del macho para la reproducción compuesto de tejido esponjoso que contiene muchos vasos sanguíneos.

Peptic ulcers/úlceras pépticas: úlceras que se forman en el sistema digestivo.

Percent body fat/por ciento de grasa corporal: la cantidad de grasa en el cuerpo con relación al peso total del cuerpo.

Percutaneous transluminal coronary angioplasty (PTCA)/angioplastia coronaria transluminal percutánea: ver *angioplastia con globo*.

Periodontal disease/enfermedad periodontal: una inflamación de las estructuras periodontales.

Periodontium/periodontio: el área que rodea los dientes; las encías, los ligamentos periodontios y la quijada.

Peripheral/periférico: alejado del centro.

Peristalsis/peristalsis: una serie de contracciones de los músculos involuntarios que mueve los alimentos a través del esófago y por todo el sistema digestivo.

Personal identity/identidad personal: factores que creemos que nos hacen singulares o distintos de todo el mundo.

Personality/personalidad: un conjunto complejo de características que hacen que cada persona sea única y distinta de los demás.

Phagocytosis/fagocitosis: el proceso en el cual ciertos glóbulos blancos rodean y se comen las bacterias invasoras.

Pharmacist/farmacéutico: una persona que tiene que ver con la preparación, distribución y venta de medicina.

Pharynx/faringe: la garganta.

Phobia/fobia: un temor extremo que hace que una persona limite sus funciones normales para evitar el miedo.

Phonocardiography/fonocardiografía: una prueba que incluye colocar un micrófono en el pecho de una persona para anotar los sonidos y señales del corazón, transmitiéndolos a través de fotografía a un papel de gráfica.

Photochemical smog/smog fotoquímico: la contaminación que ocurre cuando el escape de los autos, activados por el sol, se combinan con otros hidrocarbonos en la atmósfera.

Physical fitness/bienestar físico: la habilidad de desempeñar las tareas cotidianas con facilidad y tener energía suficiente para responder a demandas inesperadas.

Physiological dependence/dependencia fisiológica: la necesidad química que siente el cuerpo por una droga.

Phytoplankton/fitoplancton: organismos microscópicos que se hallan en aguas abiertas y soleadas y que son la base de las redes de alimento de la vida marina y de agua dulce y que son un factor en el mantenimiento de la composición de la atmósfera.

Pituitary gland/glándula pituitaria: la glándula situada en la base del encéfalo que regula las otras glándulas endocrinas; la glándula maestra.

Placebo/placebo: una sustancia que no tiene valor medicinal, la cual se administra por su efecto psicológico.

Placenta/placenta: tejido rico en sangre, que se desarrolla de la capa exterior de las células del embrión y de los tejidos de la madre.

Planned pregnancy/embarazo planificado: un embarazo en el cual antes de concebir, se toma la decisión de estar embarazada y de tener un bebé.

Plaque/placa: depósitos de grasa que se acumulan a lo largo del forro interior de las arterias; en los dientes—una película pegajosa e incolora que actúa sobre el azúcar para formar ácidos que destruyen el esmalte de los dientes e irrita las encías; sarro.

Plasma/plasma: la parte líquida de la sangre.

Platelets/plaquetas: las partes más pequeñas de la sangre; de suma importancia para la coagulación.

Platonic relationship/relación platónica: una amistad en la cual hay afecto pero no romance.

Pneumocystis carinii pneumonia (PCP)/pulmonía neumocística de carinii: una infección oportunista asociada con el SIDA.

Poison/veneno: cualquier sustancia que causa daño, quebranto o muerte cuando se introduce en el cuerpo.

Poison control center/centro de control de envenenamientos: un centro al cual se puede llamar para pedir información acerca de qué se debe hacer cuando alguien ha ingerido un veneno.

Poliomyelitis/poliomielitis: una infección viral que afecta las neuronas motoras en la espina dorsal y la corteza encefálica.

Post-traumatic stress disorder/trastorno de estrés postraumático: una condición en la cual la persona que ha experimentado un suceso traumático sufre los efectos posteriores durante un largo tiempo.

Precaution/precaución: una acción preventiva planificada que se toma antes de un acontecimiento para aumentar las posibilidades de que todo salga sin percances.

Precycling/preciclaje: la reducción de desperdicios previo a que ocurran al tomar decisiones beneficiosas para el medio ambiente respecto a compras.

Prejudice/prejuicio: un sentimiento negativo hacia alguien o algo basado en estereotipos y no en la experiencia.

Pressure-point technique/técnica del punto de presión: método empleado para parar una hemorragia al aplicar presión a la arteria principal que suple sangre a la extremidad afectada.

Prevention/prevención: el hecho de practicar hábitos saludables para mantenerse bien y libre de enfermedades y quebrantos.

Primary care/cuidado primario: cuidado que uno busca de su cuenta, generalmente administrado por el médico de cabecera.

Private practice/práctica privada: la práctica médica de un doctor que tiene su propia consulta.

Progesterone/progesterona: una hormona femenina que se libera inicialmente durante la pubertad.

Proteins/proteínas: una parte vital de todas las células del cuerpo.

Psychiatrist/psiquiatra: un doctor en medicina que trata los trastornos mentales, emocionales y de la conducta.

Psychoactive drugs/drogas psicoactivas: drogas que afectan el sistema nervioso central y alteran el funcionamiento del encéfalo.

Psychological dependence/dependencia psicológica: la creencia de que uno necesita una droga para sentirse bien y funcionar con normalidad.

Psychosomatic/psicosomático: que concierne tanto al cuerpo como a la mente.

Puberty/pubertad: el comienzo de la adolescencia; el período de tiempo cuando el varón y la hembra son capaces de reproducirse físicamente.

Pulmonary circulation/circulación pulmonaria: el flujo de sangre desde el corazón a los pulmones y de vuelta al corazón.

Pulmonary emphysema/enfisema pulmonar: una condición en la cual se destruyen los sacos de aire diminutos en los pulmones, por los cuales el oxígeno se absorbe en el cuerpo.

Pulp/pulpa: tejido viviente dentro del diente muy sensitivo.

Pulse recovery rate/razón a la cual el pulso se repone: la razón a la cual el corazón late tras alguna actividad.

Q

Quack/curandero: un promovedor deshonrado de productos y tratamientos médicos.

Quackery/curanderismo: el hecho deshonrado de promover productos médicos inútiles.

Quality of life/calidad de vida: el nivel de salud y satisfacción que una persona tiene al estar viva.

R

Rabies/rabia: una infección viral del encéfalo y la espina dorsal trasmitida a los humanos por la mordida de un animal infectado.

Random violence/violencia al azar: violencia cometida sin ninguna razón en particular y/o en contra de cualquiera que se encuentre en el lugar equivocado.

Rape/violación: coito por la fuerza o bajo amenaza.

Recall/devolver al fabricante: el proceso de instruir a un fabricante a que retire de la venta un producto que ya lanzó al mercado debido a que se le considera perjudicial.

Recommended Dietary Allowance (RDA)/Ración Dietética Recomendada: pautas para las cantidades de los 19 nutrimentos esenciales, para las calorías y la cantidad estimada de otras siete vitaminas y minerales que la mayoría de la gente necesita a diario para mantenerse saludables desde la infancia hasta la adultez.

Recovery/recuperación: el proceso de volver a estar bien; el proceso de aprender a vivir una vida libre de alcohol y drogas.

Recycling/reciclaje: tratar o cambiar los deshechos de modo que se puedan volver a usar.

Reflex/reflejo: la reacción espontánea del cuerpo a un estímulo.

Refusal skills/destrezas de rechazo: técnicas y estrategias que nos ayudan a decir que no eficazmente.

Relapses/recaídas: para las personas en recuperación, es la vuelta periódica al uso del alcohol o las drogas.

Relationship/relación: un vínculo o conexión entre las personas.

Rescue breathing/respiración de rescate: el proceso de proveerle oxígeno a una víctima que ha dejado de respirar.

Resident bacteria/bacteria residente: bacterias que viven en la boca, los intestinos y en la piel y que nos protegen de las bacterias dañinas.

Resting heart rate/frecuencia de los latidos del corazón en reposo: latidos del corazón cuando no está activo.

Retina/retina: la capa de la pared del ojo que contiene las células nerviosas y los procesos responsable de la visión.

Rheumatoid arthritis/artritis reumatoide: una inflamación destructiva de las articulaciones que incapacita.

Risk/riesgo: una conducta con un elemento de peligro que puede causar lesión o daño.

Risk factor/factor de riesgo: una característica que se ha demostrado que aumenta los chances de que ocurra un ataque al corazón.

Role/papel: la parte que uno desempeña, especialmente en una relación.

S

Saliva/saliva: una secreción que da comienzo a la digestión de carbohidratos.

Saprophytes/saprofitos: bacteria que digiere materiales comestibles no vivos, tales como la leche y la carne.

Sarcomas/sarcomas: cánceres que se desarrollan en los tejidos conjuntivos y en los de soporte, tales como los huesos, los músculos y los tendones.

Saturated/saturado: en el caso de ácidos grasos, que tiene hidrógeno enlazado a todos los átomos de carbono en la cadena.

Schizophrenia/esquizofrenia: trastorno mental severo en el cual uno exhibe reacciones emocionales anormales o no exhibe ninguna reacción emocional.

Sclera/esclera: una membrana blanca y fuerte que contribuye a mantener la forma esférica del ojo y protege su delicada estructura interna.

Scoliosis/escoliosis: una curvatura de lado a lado de la espina dorsal.

Scrotum/escroto: una bolsa en el exterior del

cuerpo del varón que contiene los testículos y protege los espermatozoides al regular la temperatura de los testículos.

Sebaceous glands/glándulas sebáceas: glándulas que producen una secreción oleaginosa llamada sebo y que están conectadas a los folículos del pelo.

Secondary care/cuidado secundario: el cuidado que uno recibe cuando la doctora de cuidado primario lo refiere a uno a un especialista.

Secondary sex characteristics/características sexuales secundarias: vello corporal y el desarrollo de senos en la hembra y de músculos en el varón.

Self-actualization/autorrealización: el proceso continuo de luchar por alcanzar el máximo de la capacidad propia.

Self-esteem/autoestima: la confianza y sentimiento de valer que uno tiene acerca de sí mismo; influye en todo lo que hacemos, pensamos, sentimos y somos.

Semen/semen: una mezcla de fluidos de las vesículas seminales, la glándula próstata, las glándulas de Cowper combinada con la esperma; fluido seminal.

Sensory deafness/sordera sensorial: la pérdida de la audición causada por el ruido excesivo a través de largo período de tiempo.

Sensory neurons/neuronas sensoriales: células nerviosas situadas en la piel y en otros órganos sensoriales que tienen puntas receptoras especializadas.

Sexual assault/agresión sexual: atentado de ataque sexual o acto en sí con intención de violencia sexual.

Sexually transmitted disease (STD)/enfermedad transmitida sexualmente: una enfermedad contagiosa que se propaga de una persona a otra a través del contacto sexual.

Shock/choque: el fallo del sistema cardiovascular para mantener suficiente sangre circulando a los órganos vitales del cuerpo.

Sidestream smoke/corriente de humo secundaria: el humo que proviene de quemar tabaco.

Single-parent family/familia con solo la madre o el padre: familia en la cual los hijos solo viven con uno de los padres a la vez.

Skeletal muscles/músculos del esqueleto: músculos voluntarios pegados a los huesos que causan los movimientos del cuerpo.

Small-claims courts/cortes de litigios pequeños: cortes que tratan las demandas sobre las quejas de los consumidores que van desde $100 hasta los $3,000.

Small intestine/intestino delgado: un órgano donde toma lugar la mayor parte de la digestión y la absorción.

Smoke detector/detector de humo: una alarma que se usa para despertar a la gente y alertarlos en el caso de incendio.

Smooth muscles/músculos lisos: músculos involuntarios situados en tales lugares como los intestinos y los vasos sanguíneos.

Social age/edad social: la edad de una persona según lo determina su estilo de vida.

Sprain/esguince: una lesión de los tejidos suaves que rodean una articulación.

Stereotype/estereotipo: una creencia exagerada y simplificada acerca de un grupo entero, como un grupo étnico, religioso, o cierto sexo.

Sterility/esterilidad: una condición en la cual una persona no puede reproducirse.

Stigma/estigma: una marca de vergüenza.

Stimulant/estimulante: una droga que aumenta la acción del sistema nervioso central, el corazón, la respiración y la presión arterial y que causa que las pupilas se dilaten y que disminuya el apetito.

Strain/tensión: una condición en la cual los músculos han trabajado demasiado.

Stress/estrés: la reacción física o mental del cuerpo hacia situaciones diarias.

Stressor/causante de estrés: un estímulo que produce una reacción de estrés.

Stroke/ataque de apoplejía: una condición en la cual la sangre que va al encéfalo se ve interceptada, y como resultado, las células nerviosas en esa parte del encéfalo no pueden funcionar.

Sweat glands/glándulas sudoríparas: glándulas que secretan sudor a través de conductos hasta los poros en la superficie de la piel.

Synapse/sinapsis: un espacio estrecho entre la punta del axón de una neurona y la dendrita de otra neurona a través de la cual tiene que cruzar un impulso.

Synergistic effect/efecto sinergístico: la reacción de dos o más medicinas que resulta en un efecto más fuerte que cuando se toman por separado.

Synthetic/sintético: hecho de sustancias químicas de laboratorio.

Syphilis/sífilis: una enfermedad transmitida sexualmente que ataca muchas partes del cuerpo.

Systemic circulation/circulación sistémica: el flujo de sangre a todos los tejidos del cuerpo con excepción de los pulmones.

T

Tar/alquitrán: un fluido grueso, pegajoso y oscuro que se produce al quemar tabaco.

Target heart rate/meta de frecuencia cardíaca: de 70 a 80 por ciento de la frecuencia cardíaca de una persona.

Tartar/sarro: una sustancia muy dura que irrita los huesos subyacentes tanto como las encías que rodean los dientes: cálculo.

T cells/células T: linfocitos producidos en la médula ósea que van a la glándula del timo donde maduran y luego combaten patógenos específicos.

Tendinitis/tendonitis: una condición en la cual el tejido conjuntivo de los músculos y los huesos o los tendones se estira o se desgarra.

Tendons/tendones: bandas de fibra que conectan los músculos a los huesos.

Tertiary care/cuidado terciario: el cuidado que se recibe cuando uno tiene una condición que requiere tratamiento o equipo especializado.

Testes/testículos: dos glándulas pequeñas que producen esperma.

Testimonial/testimonio: la recomendación entusiasta de una persona que endosa un producto.

Testosterone/testosterona: una hormona masculina que hace que los testículos produzcan esperma y la responsable de los cambios físicos durante la pubertad.

Thanatology/tanatología: el estudio de la muerte y los ajustes necesarios en conexión con la muerte de un ser querido.

Therapy/terapia: técnica de tratamiento.

Thrombosis/trombosis: presencia o formación de un coágulo de sangre que se forma en un vaso sanguíneo y que, por lo general, no se mueve del lugar de origen.

Thyroid gland/glándula tiroides: la glándula más grande del sistema endocrino la cual regula el metabolismo de carbohidratos, grasas y proteínas en las células del cuerpo.

Time-management skills/destrezas para el manejo del tiempo: la habilidad para aprovechar con eficacia el tiempo que uno tenga.

Tinnitus/tintineo: una condición caracterizada por un retintín en los oídos.

Tissue/tejido: células con las mismas estructuras y que hacen la misma función.

Tolerance/tolerancia: una condición en la cual el cuerpo se acostumbra a los efectos de una medicina o droga.

Tooth decay/caries dentales: una enfermedad de las vías digestivas que debilita los dientes y afecta el modo en que uno puede morder y masticar la comida.

Toxins/toxinas: venenos producidos por algunas bacterias.

Trachea/tráquea: conducto que transporta aire a los pulmones.

Tranquilizers/tranquilizantes: depresivos que reducen la actividad muscular, la coordinación y el lapso de atención.

Transition/transición: cambio.

Tumor/tumor: una masa de tejido causada por la división incontrolada de células anormales.

Type I diabetes/diabetes tipo I: diabetes que por lo general le ocurre a personas menores de 15 años de edad y que requiere inyecciones diarias de insulina para poder sobrevivir.

Type II diabetes/diabetes tipo II: diabetes que por lo general le ocurre a las personas de más de 40 años de edad y que se puede, con frecuencia, controlar con dieta y ejercicio.

U

Ulcer/úlcera: una llaga abierta en la piel o en la membrana mucosa.

Umbilical cord/cordón umbilical: cordón que conecta el embrión a la placenta y a través del cual los nutrimientos y el oxígeno fluyen desde la madre hasta el embrión, a través de los vasos sanguíneos; y los desechos del embrión son transportados hasta la madre.

Undernutrition/subnutrición: el no consumir los suficientes nutrimentos esenciales o calorías para el buen funcionamiento del cuerpo.

Underweight/bajo peso: estar 10 por ciento o más por debajo del peso normal.

Unit price/precio por unidad: la cantidad que una unidad de un producto cuesta.

Unit pricing/indicación del precio por unidad: la práctica de mostrar el precio por unidad de los distintos tamaños de envases de un producto.

Unplanned pregnancy/embarazo no planificado: un embarazo en el cual un bebé se concibe por accidente.

Uremia/uremia: una serie de síntomas causados por la inhabilidad de los riñones para deshacerse de los desperdicios del cuerpo.

Ureters/uréteres: tubos que conducen desde los dos riñones hacia la vejiga.

Urethra/uretra: un pequeño tubo que se extiende desde la vejiga al exterior del cuerpo.

Urine/orina: desecho líquido que se recoge en la vejiga hasta que está lista para salir del cuerpo.

Uterus/útero: órgano pequeño y muscular en forma de pera en el cuerpo de la hembra.

V

Vaccination/vacunación: el proceso por el cual se inyecta una vacuna en el cuerpo.

Vaccine/vacuna: una preparación que contiene patógenos debilitados o muertos de una enfermedad en particular y que se da para evitar que se contraiga esa enfermedad.

Vagina/vagina: tubo muscular y muy elástico en la hembra que sirve como conducto desde el útero hacia el exterior del cuerpo; el canal de nacimiento.

Values/valores: principios que uno considera importantes y que nos sirven de guía en la vida.

Veins/venas: los vasos que portan la sangre de regreso al corazón.

Verbal communication/comunicación verbal: el envío de mensajes por medio de la palabra.

Violence/violencia: el uso de la fuerza física para causar daño o abusar de otra persona o personas.

Virus/virus: una forma de vida muy pequeña y simple.

Vitreous humor/humor vítreo: un fluido que se encuentra detrás del cristalino del ojo que lo mantienen firme.

Voluntary/voluntario: dentro del control consciente de una persona.

W

Warming up/calentamiento: participar en actividad que prepara los músculos para el trabajo venidero.

Weight cycling/ciclo de peso: bajar, aumentar, volver a bajar y volver a aumentar de peso.

Wellness/bienestar: un estado de bienestar general; plena salud.

Western blot/prueba Western blot: una prueba que es muy específica para identificar los anticuerpos del VIH.

Withdrawal/síndrome de abstinencia: una reacción física que ocurre cuando una persona cesa de tomar una droga o medicamento del cual ha llegado a depender.

Xiphoid process/proceso xifoides: la parte baja del esternón que se proyecta hacia abajo.

Z

Zygote/cigoto: una célula de huevo fertilizada.

Halitosis, 282, 317
Hallucinogens, 481, 486-87
Handicapped, 14, 233, 235
Hangnails, 201
Hardening of the arteries, 259. *See also* Arteriosclerosis
Harvard Medical School, 578
Hashish, 481, 488
Havighurst, Robert, 161
Hazardous substances, 625
HDL, 446
Headaches, 70, 226, 229
 and biofeedback, 530
 and food, 228
Head lice, 201
Head of household, 86-87
Health
 centers, for adolescents, 656, 660
 clubs, 345
 continuum, 6
 definitions of, 3-5
 education, 4
 facilities, 653-55
 of family and society, 83, 89
 and fitness, 337
 foods, 416-17
 habits, 7
 insurance, 636, 646, 655-56
 and marriage, 124
 and parenting, 128-29
 physical, 5, 371
 and relationships, 101
 self-management of, 663
 and stress, 71
 teacher, 5
 triangle, 6
Health care resources, 653-56, 659-65
 for adolescents, 656
 for infants, 128
Health Maintenance Organizations (HMOs), 661-62
Health-risk appraisal, 5
Hearing impaired, 329, 330
Hearing loss, 148
 problems, 183
 See also Ears
Heart, 249-50
 and aging, 183
 strengthening, 357
Heart attack, 571-72
Heartburn, 282
Heart disease, 8, 255, 261, 378, 446
 congenital, 256
 and technology, 260
 See also Cardiovascular disease
Heart-lung machine, 576
Heart murmurs, 256
Heart rate, 355, 358
Heart valve surgery, 577
Heat, risks to health from, 362-63
Heat cramps, 706
Heating, and energy conservation, 616
Height, 150, 239, 241
Heimlich maneuver, 716
Help, and families, 93. *See also* Family counseling; Parents Anonymous
Help, when to seek, 28, 697
Hemodialysis, *See* Dialysis
Hemoglobin, 251, 259, 379
Hemophilia, 150, 261, 557
Hemophiliac, 562

Hemorrhoids, 286
Hepatitis, 286, 519, 531
 and CPR, 723
Heredity, 35, 144-50
 and alcoholism, 498
 and cancer, 585
 and disease, 497
 and hypertension, 569
 and obesity, 404
 See also Genetics
Heritage, 31
Hernia, 362
 abdominal, 282
 hiatal, 282
Herpes, 544-45
Heroin, 481, 486. *See also* Drugs
Hiccups, 228, 267
Hierarchy of needs, 32
Hinge joints, 206
Histamine, 432
HIV, Human immunodeficiency virus, 264, 555-63
 origin, 555-56
 and pregnancy, 141
 prevention, 559
 and rape, 687
 testing, 560-61, 562
 transmittal, 556-59
 See also AIDS
Hodgkin's disease, 264, 579
Holistic approach, 6
Holistic health centers, 662
Homeless, 29, 41, 77, 93
Homicide, 107
Hormones, 37, 159, 238-43, 302, 379
 and aging, 183
Hospice care, 662-63
 and death, 190
Hospital administrator, 663
Hospital records, 646
Hospitals, 654
Hospital stay, 584, 654
Host organisms, 517
Househusbands, 127. *See also* Parenting
Human collision, 680
Human immunodeficiency virus. *See* HIV
Humor, as attitude, 7. *See also* Laughter
Hunger, 281
Hurricanes, 707-708
Hydrochloric acid, 278, 285
Hygiene, personal, 301, 308
 and disease prevention, 528
Hyperopia, 324
Hypertension, 569-70. *See also* Blood pressure
Hyperventilation, 267
Hypochondria, 50
Hypodermis, 199
Hypothalamus, 66, 228, 281
Hypothermia, 707

I

Ice, 481, 483
Identification, 74
 emergency medical tag, 694, 724
I Have a Dream Foundation (IHAD), 12
Ileum, 278

Illness, and elderly, 180. *See also* Diseases
Illustrator, medical, 539
Immune deficiency, 264
Immune system, 524
 and aging, 183
Immunity, 527
Immunization, 425, 426, 527-31
Incision, 694, 695
Incontinence, 289
Incus, 326, 327
Independence, in adults, 175-76
 and aging, 186
Indigestion, 282
Industry, in childhood, 153
Infancy, 152
Infant care, 128
Infection. *See* Pathogens; Symptoms; names of individual diseases
Inferiority, in childhood, 153
Inflammatory response, 524
Ingredient listing, 394-96
Ingrown toenail, 201
Inhalants, 482, 489
Initiative, in childhood, 153
Injuries
 avoiding, 360-65
 head, 231
 prevention of, 237
 spinal cord, 231-32
 toy-related, 673
Inner ear, 327-28
Inpatient, 653
Insecticides, as inhalant, 482
Institute of Scrap Recycling, 618
Insulin, 238, 241, 243, 427, 586
Insurance, health, 636, 655-656, 658
Integumentary system, 197-203. *See also* Skin
Intelligence, in babies, 141
Interbrain, 228
International Special Olympics, 625
Interneurons, 221
Intervention, 500
Intestinal viruses, 416
Intestines, 278-79. *See also* Digestive system
Intoxication, 459, 460. *See also* Alcohol; Driving
Involuntary muscles, 212
Iodine, 240, 242, 383
Iris, 320, 321
Iron, 251, 258, 280, 379, 383, 385, 418
Islets of Langerhans, 241
Isokinetic, 346
Isometric exercise, 346
Isotonic exercise, 346

J

Jaundice, 286
Jejunum, 278-79
Jellyfish sting, 705
Jenner, Edward (Dr.), 528
Job, 30. *See also* Career
Jock itch, 200
Joints, 206
 and aging, 183
 and arthritis, 589-91
 injuries to, 207-08

Journal, 42
   and weight control, 407
Journal of the American Medical Association, 66
Journey from Darkness, 323

K

Kennedy, John (President), and consumer rights, 633
Kidney disease, and diabetes, 586
Kidneys, 288-91
   and aging, 183
   artificial, 284
   effects of alcohol on, 460
   stones, 290-91
Kids Against Pollution, 623
Killed-Virus Vaccine, 529
Knee-jerk reflex, 230
Knee surgery, 208
Kübler-Ross, Elisabeth, 188-90

L

Labeling
   definitions, 395-97
   food and, 393-97
Labeling of Hazardous Art Materials Act, 626
Labyrinth, 327
Laceration, 694, 695
Lacrimal glands, 319
Lactic acid, 517
Lactobacilli, 517
Lactose intolerance, 282, 285, 409
Laetrile, 585
Landfill, and recycling, 617-18
Land use, and environmental issues, 604-09
Lang, Eugene, 12
Langerhans, Paul, 241
Laparoscopy, 308
Large intestine, 279
Larynx, 265
Laser surgery, 317
Laughter, 67
Laws
   and drugs, 504
   and immunizations, 529
   and marriage, 119, 543
   and tobacco, 451-53
Lawsuits, and STDs, 541
Laxative abuse, 412
LDL, 446
Lead exposure, 676
Lead poisoning, 598
Lean, label definition, 395
Left-handedness, 228
Legumes, 380
Leigh's disease, 149
Lens, 321
Lenses, corrective, 322
Leukemia, 259-61, 584
Leukoplakia, 447
Leuteinizing hormone (LH), 240
Lewis, F. John (Dr.), 576
Lice, 519
   head, 201

pubic, 546
Licensed Practical Nurse (LPN), 672
Licensing Boards, 643-44
Life cycle, 137-50, 175-91
Life expectancy, 7-8, 182
   and AIDS, 560
Life-style, 7, 183
   and cancer, 286
   sedentary, 286, 337
Ligaments, 206
Lighting, and energy conservation, 616
Limitations, in physical activities, 364
Lipase, 281
Lipids, 377
Liquor, 459
Listening, 111-112. *See also* Communication
Lithotripsy, 291
Litter, 625
Little People of America, 147
Liver, 279-80
   conditions, 286
   effects of alcohol on, 459-60, 461-62
   transplant, 280
   and viruses, 519
Live-virus vaccine, 528
Lobes
   cerebral, 225
   of lung, 266
   of pituitary gland, 239-240
Lockjaw, 518
Longevity, and relationships, 101
Look-alike drugs, 490
Love
   loss of, and suicide, 168
   and marriage, 121
   and parenting, 131
Lumps, 580
   and cancer detection, 300, 306, 309
Lung cancer, 444, 445, 581, 583
Lungs, 266-67
   and high altitudes, 356
   strengthening, 357
Lyme disease, 529
Lymphatic system, 262-64, 526
   and cancer, 581
Lymphocytes, 262, 263, 526, 555
Lymphoma, 579
Lysergic acid diethylamide (LSD), 481, 487

M

Magnesium, 383
Magnetic resonance imaging (MRI), 358, 580
Mainstream smoke, 448
Malaria, 259, 521
Malignant tumor, 579
Malleus, 326, 327
Malocclusion, 317
Mammogram, 309
Manganese, 383
Manic-depressive disorder, 51
Manipulation, 105
Marijuana, 469, 481, 484, 488-89
Marine biologist, 600
Marital adjustment, 121
Markers, felt-tip, as inhalant, 482

Marriage, 119-24
   adolescent preparation for, 161
   blood test prior to, 543
   and health, 124
   in midlife, 179
Marrow, 204-206
Maslow, Abraham, 32-34, 101
Massage, 362
   foot, 213
Mastication, 275
Mastoid process, 327
Maternal care, 662
Maturity, and marriage, 122
MDMA, 489
Meals, 390-92. *See also* Food; Nutrition
Measles, 519
Measles, vaccine, 528
Meat, 386, 391
   and consumer safety, 647
   in diet, 386
Meatborne Hazard Control Center, 647
Mechanical mechanisms, 523
Medicaid, 656
Medic Alert, 724
Medical
   ethics, 190
   history, 646
   identification bracelet, 694
   illustrator, 539
   laboratory technician, 518
   therapy, and mental disorders, 56-59
Medical Group Management Association, 663
Medical quackery. *See* Quackery
Medicare, 656
Medicines, 425-35
   absorption of, 427-28
   and consumer safety, 645
   misuse, 430
   reaction to, 428-29
Medulla oblongata, 226, 228
Megadose, 419
Melanin, 198
Melanoma, 580-581
Memories, 14
Memory skills, in adolescence, 160
Meninges, cranial 225
Meningitis, 234
Menopause, and calcium deficiency, 418
Menstruation, 303-304
   and iron loss, 418
Mental disorders, 49-59
Mental health, 5, 27-43
   connection to physical, 42
   and exercise, 338, 341
   facilities, 655
   professionals, 55-59
Mental Health Association, 53
Mental illness, 49
Mentally ill, residence of, 59
Mental retardation, 140, 148, 498
Mentor, 185
Mercury poisoning, 601
Metabolism, 240
   and aging, 183
   basal, 340
   and calorie requirements, 403
   and exercise, 340
   and fat, 409
Metastasis, 579

Methadone, 481, 486
Methamphetamine, 483-84
Michael and Charles Barnett Center, 149
Micronutrients. *See* Vitamins
Midbrain, 187, 228
Middle age, mid-life. *See* Adulthood
Middle ear, 326-27
Middle East, 277
Minerals, 204, 209, 240, 280, 382-83
  and environmental issues, 624
Miscarriage, 141, 307
  and STDs, 543
Mites, 519, 546
Moles, 200, 580
Molybdenum, 383
Money, and adolescents, 165
Moniliasis, 546
Mononucleosis, 519, 526
Monosodium glutamate (MSG), 228
Mood, 53, 228
  as attitude, 7
  and food, 38
  See also Blues; Emotions
Morphine, 427, 481, 486
Mothers. *See* Parenting
Motorcycles, and accidents, 18
Motorcycle safety, 681
Motor neurons, 221
Mourning, 191
Mouth, 275, 315-18
Mucous membranes, 278, 523
Mucus
  in tears, 319
Multiple sclerosis (MS), 232, 233
Multiplier effect, 462
Mumps, 519
Murder, 107, 683
Muscle
  mass, 413, 415
  tension, and biofeedback, 530
  tissue, 211, 359
  tone, 210
  types, 211-12
Muscles
  and adolescent development, 159
  and aging, 183
  and exercise, 353-59
Muscular dystrophy, 150, 212, 214, 215
Muscular Dystrophy Association, 212
Muscular strength and endurance, 342-44
Muscular system, 210-15
  injuries to, 361-62
Myasthenia gravis, 213-15
Mycobacterium avium intracellulare
  (MAI), 562
Myelin, 223, 233
Myofibrils, 210
Myopia, 324
Myosin, 210
Myxedema, 242

N

Nails, 183, 198, 201-203
Naming a baby, 138
Narcolepsy, 483
Narcotics, 427, 481, 485-86. *See also*
  Drugs
Narcotics Anonymous (Nar-Anon), 503,
  511

Nasal cavity, 265
National Academy of Sciences, 602
National Adolescent Student Health
  Survey, 547
National Aeronautics and Space
  Administration (NASA), 337
National Association of Cardiovascular
  Pulmonary Technology, 260
National Association of Emergency
  Medical Technicians, 723
National Association of Social Workers,
  36
National Association of Student
  Councils, 21
National Association of Town Watch,
  687
National Cancer Act, 583
National Cancer Institute, 388, 583
National Captioning Institute, 328
National Center for Health Statistics,
  589
National Childcare Association, 127
National Clearinghouse for Alcohol and
  Drug Information, 74
National Consumers League, 644
National Council on Alcoholism and
  Drug Dependence, 74, 461
National Diabetes Data Group, 586
National Education Association, 5, 76,
  112
National Institute on Drug Abuse, 490
National Institutes of Health (NIH), 146,
  647
National Marrow Donor Program, 577
National Mental Health Association, 28,
  53, 128
National Multiple Sclerosis Society,
  233
National Office of the Consumer
  Federation of America, 644
National Recreation Association of
  Japan, 75
National Rehabilitation Hospital, 233
National Society to Prevent Blindness,
  325
National Weather Service, 707
Natural, label definition, 395
Natural catastrophes, 609
Natural products, 622, 624
Nausea, 282, 283
Nearsightedness, 324
Need, for drugs. *See* Addiction
Needles, 556
Needs, 32-34
Neighborhood health centers, 662
Nephritis, 290
Nephrons, 288
Nerve deafness, 330
Nerve impulse, 223-24
Nervous system, 221-37
  and exercise, 338
  problems and care, 231-37
Nest. *See* Empty-nest syndrome;
  Cluttered-nest syndrome
Neurologist, 56, 660
Neurons, 210, 221-24
Neurosyphilis, 542
Neutrophils, 524
Niacin, 380
Nicotine, 442, 449, 450
Night blindness, 321

Nixon, Richard (President), 583
  and consumer rights, 634
Nocturnal emission, 299
Noise, 329
Noncommunicable diseases, 569-91
Nongonococcal urethritis (NGU), 545-47
Nonsmokers' rights, 450, 453
Nonspecific resistance, 523
Nontoxic products, 622
Nosebleeds, 695, 703
Nuclear energy, 606-607
  and waste from, 607
Nuclear family, 83
Nursing homes, 655
Nutrient-dense foods, 407, 413
Nutrients, 376-84
  definition, 371
  food sources of, 380, 381, 383
  and mood, 38
  supplements, 418
  See also Vitamins
Nutrition, 371, 375
  and sports, 415
Nutrition Information Label, 393-94,
  395, 397
  on shelves, 397

O

Obesity, 389, 404-406, 578, 588. *See also*
  Overweight
Obsession, 506
Obsessive-compulsive disorder, 50
Obstetrician, 140, 660
Occupation. *See* Career
Occupational Safety and Health
  Administration (OSHA), 676
Occupational therapist, 504
Oceanic Society, 618
Oceans, and environmental issues, 624
Oil, in skin, 198-99
Oil
  recycling, 619
  spills, 602
Oils, 377-78. *See also* Fats
Old age. *See* Elderly; Aging
Ombudsman, 643
Open-dating label, definition, 396
Ophthalmologist, 660
Opium, 481, 485-86
Opportunistic infection, 561
Optic nerve, 321, 322
Optometric technician, 320
Oral hygiene. *See* Mouth; teeth
Organ of Corti, 328
Organic
  disorders, 49
  foods, 417
  products, 622
Organs, artificial, 664
Orthodontics, 317
Orthopedic surgeon, 660
Ossicles, 326
Ossification, 204
Osteoarthritis, 591
Osteoblasts, 204
Osteomyelitis, 207
Osteoporosis, 207, 418
Otolaryngologist, 660

Photo Credits

Cover, © David Madison 1992;
Back Cover, Steve Whalen-Viesti
  Associates

2, Terence Turner/FPG International;
4, 8, Rod Joslin;
9, Custom Medical Stock Photo;
11, file photo;
13, Mak-I Photo Design;
14, 15, Gabe Palmer/The Stock Market;
17, Mak-I Photo Design;
18, Aaron Haupt;
20, Mak-I Photo Design;
26, Matt Meadows;
29, Mak-I Photo Design;
30, Gabe Palmer/The Stock Market;
34, (t) Rod Joslin, (b) Doug Martin;
38, Mak-I Photo Design;
41, 42, Crown Studios;
45, Ed Wheeler/The Stock Market;
48, 50, Mak-I Photo Design;
51, file photo;
57, Dr. Warren Rhodes;
58, 61, Mak-I Photo Design;
64, Doug Martin;
66, Mak-I Photo Design;
68, Doug Martin;
71, Crown Studios;
72, Bob Mullenix;
73, Crown Studios;
75, Mak-I Photo Design;
78, Crown Studios;
82, Aaron Haupt;
84, 85, 88, Bob Mullenix;
90, Gail Meese/Meese Photo Research;
91, Bob Mullenix/Photographic
  Illustrators,Inc.;
92, Doug Martin;
94, Mak-I Photo Design;
95, First Image;
96, Gabe Palmer/The Stock Market;
100, Bob Mullenix;
103, Photographic Design Group;
104, Kenji Kerins;
109, Bob Mullenix;
110, Matt Meadows;
114, Bob Mullenix;
118, Doug Martin;
120, Sandy Roessler/The Stock Market;
121, 122, Mak-I Photo Design;
127, Aaron Haupt;
129, Rod Joslin;
130, Mak-I Photo Design;
132, 136, file photo;
139, © Vladimir Lange/The Image Bank;

141, Mak-I Photo Design;
142, Lennart Nilsson/The Incredible
  Machine/National Geographic
  Society;
147, Doug Martin;
149, Robin Laskey Chipman;
151, 152, 153, Gale Zucker;
154, 158, Doug Martin;
161, Mary Lou Uttermohlen;
162, Doug Martin;
163, Aaron Haupt
166, David Frazier;
168, Bryan Peterson/The Stock Market;
169, 171, Mak-I Photo Design;
174, Bob Mullenix;
176, Rod Joslin;
179, Matt Meadows;
181, Ronnie Kaufman/The Stock
  Market;
184, The Presidential Sports/Fitness
  Festivals;
185, Roy Morsch/The Stock Market;
186, Catherine Ursillo/Photo
  Researchers, Inc.;
189, (t) Matt Meadows, (b) Gale Zucker;
190, George Disario/The Stock Market;
191, Matt Meadows;
193, Rod Joslin;
196, Doug Martin;
199, David Stoecklein/The Stock
  Market;
200, Biophoto Associates/Science
  Source/Photo Researchers, Inc.;
201, Custom Medical Stock;
203, Bob Mullenix/Photographic
  Illustrators,Inc.;
206, Aaron Haupt;
212, First Image;
214, Darlene Sullivan/Canine Partners
  for Life;
216, Margaret Kois/The Stock Market;
220, Aaron Haupt;
227, Paul Facenda Photography;
230, 232, Bob Mullenix;
234, Will & Deni McIntyre/Photo
  Researchers, Inc.;
236, Gail Meese/Meese Photo Research;
237, Bob Mullenix;
243, Hattie Youne/Science Photo
  Library/Photo Researchers, Inc.;
244, Joe Sohm/The Stock Market;
248, Aaron Haupt;
251, Matt Meadows;
253, Mak-I Photo Design;

254, Matt Meadows;
258, Science Source/Photo Researchers,
  Inc.;
259, file photo;
268, Crown Studios;
270, Rod Joslin;
274, Bob Mullenix;
283, file photo;
284, Ted Bartoshesky;
287, Elaine Shay;
291, Werner H. Muller/Peter Arnold,
  Inc.;
296, Bob Mullenix;
299, John Walsh/Science Photo
  Library/Photo Researchers, Inc.;
301, Michael Keller/The Stock Market;
306, Matt Meadows;
307, Thibeault:Design,Inc.;309,
  American Cancer Society/Ken
  Frick;
310, Spandorfer & Jordan/Photo
  Researchers, Inc.;
314, Doug Martin, courtesy Dr. Clayton
  N. Hicks;
317, (t) Michael Philip Manheim/The
  Stock Market, (b) Van
  Bucher/Photo Researchers, Inc.;
323, Muncy & Muncy Inc.;
325, 329, Crown Studios;
330, Bob Mullenix;
331, Crown Studios;
332, Doug Martin;
336, Bob Mullenix;
337, Mak-I Photo Design;
339, 341, 344-345, Bob Mullenix;
347, Kenji Kerins;
349, Rod Joslin;
352, Bob Mullenix;
354, Doug Martin;
356, 359, Bob Mullenix;
361, (l) David Madison,(r) File photo;
362, Mak-I Photo Design;
363, Bob Mullenix;
364, First Image;
366, David Madison;
370, Bob Mullenix;
373, (tl-tr) Aaron Haupt, (bl) file photo,
  (br) Gabe Palmer/The Stock
  Market;
374, Doug Martin;
377, 379, Platinum Productions;
381, Mak-I Photo Design;
384, Bob Mullenix;
386, USDA;

388, Bob Mullenix;
389, 394-397 Platinum Productions;
402, Hickson & Associates;
404, Mak-I Photo Design;
405, Craig Hammell/The Stock Market;
407, Bob Mullenix;
408, Aaron Haupt;
412, Mak-I Photo Design;
413, Aaron Haupt;
414, Anthony Edgeworth/The Stock Market;
417, Henley & Savage/The Stock Market;
418, Elaine Shay;
419, 424, Bob Mullenix;
426, Matt Meadows;
427, Aaron Haupt;
429, 431, 433, Matt Meadows;
434, Elizabeth Zeschin;
435, Rod Joslin;
436, Mak-I Photo Design;
437, Rod Joslin;
440, Mak-I Photo Design;
443, (t) Martin Rotker/Phototake, (b) Camera M.D. Studios;
445, Doug Martin;
446, Mak-I Photo Design;
448, Bob Mullenix;449, Mak-I Photo Design;
450, (t) Jules T. Allen, (b) Bob Mullenix;
453, Bob Mullenix;
458, Hickson & Associates;
460, Matt Meadows;
463, 465, Kenji Kerins;
466, Doug Martin;
469, Mak-I Photo Design;
471, Gabe Palmer/The Stock Market;
472, Bob Mullenix;
473, Wes Thompson/The Stock Market;
478, Aaron Haupt;
480, Mak-I Photo Design;
484, Focus on Sports;
485, Doug Martin;
487, Biomedical Communications/Photo Researchers, Inc.;
489, Alon Reininger/Woodfin Camp & Associates, Inc.;
490, Jerry Wachter/Focus On Sports;
496, Aaron Haupt;
499-501, 503 Doug Martin;
505, Mak-I Photo Design;
507-508, 511, Doug Martin;
512, Mak-I Photo Design;
516, Doug Martin;
518, Bob Mullenix;
519, file photo;

520, Harry Smith;
521, Elaine Shay;
522, Aaron Haupt;
523, (t) Elaine Shay, (b) Alan Carey;
524, 528, Bob Mullenix;
529, file photo;
530, 532, Bob Mullenix;
536, Doug Martin;
538, James Westwater;
542, 543, Custom Medical Stock Photo;
545, Matt Meadows;
548, Doug Martin;
549, Mak-I Photo Design;
550, 554, 556, Matt Meadows;
557, Jennifer Nicols;
558, Sharon Remmer;
561, (l) AP/Wide World Photos, (r) Rick Rickman/Duomo Photography, Inc.;
564, Bob Mullenix;
568, Doug Martin;
570, Bob Mullenix;
572, Larry Mulvehill/Photo Researchers, Inc.;
575, Superstock;
577, Custom Medical Stock Photo;
580, American Cancer Society/Ken Frick;
582, Philippe Plally/Science Photo Library/Photo Researchers, Inc.;
583, William Roy/The Stock Market;
584, William's Photography;
587, 589, Custom Medical Stock Photo;
590, Hickson & Associates;
591, (l) Allen Lee Page/The Stock Market, (r) CNRI/Science Photo Library/Photo Researchers, Inc.;
592, Ken Frick;
596, Bob Winsett/Tom Stack & Associates;
598, Superstock;
602, Joe Sohm/Chromosohm 1990/The Stock Market;
605, Rafael Macia/Photo Researchers, Inc.;
607, Jerry Irwin/Photo Researchers, Inc.;
608, Jeffre J. Dean;
609, Ken Frick;
610, Bob Mullenix;
611, Joe Sohm/Chromosohm 1990/The Stock Market;
614, 617, Mak-I Photo Design;
620, Matt Meadows;
623, Kids Against Pollution;
624, Matt Meadows;
625, Nigel Dickinson/Tony Stone Worldwide;
626, 627, E. R. Degginger;

628, Jon Riley/Tony Stone Worldwide;
632, Doug Martin;
634, Elaine Shay;
635, (tl) Bob Mullenix, (tr) Harry Haralambou/Peter Arnold, Inc., (cl) Aaron Haupt, (cr, br, bc, bl) Bob Mullenix;
636, David J. James/Texas Inprint;
639, Mak-I Photo Design;
640, Aaron Haupt;
642, Mak-I Photo Design;
643, Bob Mullenix/Photographic Illustrators, Inc.;
644, 645, Elaine Shay;
648, Bob Mullenix;
652, Doug Martin;
654, Tom Stewart/The Stock Market;
655, Matt Meadows;
657, Jim Dallas Studio;
658, 660, Bob Mullenix;
661, Matt Meadows;
663, Jeff Bates;
664, Bob Mullenix;
670, Mak-I Photo Design;
672, Bob Mullenix;
674, Crown Studios;
675, Mak-I Photo Design;
677, Bob Daemmrich;
678, Juh-Hann Chang;
679, Bob Daemmrich;
682, Kenji Kerins;
684, Mak-I Photo Design;
685, Matt Meadows;
687, Rod Joslin;
692, Doug Martin;
694, Blair Seitz/Photo Researchers, Inc.;
696, Photo by Chandler Arden, Texas A & M Photo Services;
696, Tim Thorp;
697, Mak-I Photo Design;
699, Rod Joslin;
700, 702, E. R. Degginger;
704, 705, Rod Joslin;
706, Bob Mullenix;
708, E. R. Degginger;
709, David Weintraub/Photo Researchers, Inc.;
710, Aaron Haupt;
714, Bob Mullenix;
716, Matt Meadows;
718, Aaron Haupt;
719, First Image;
725, Rod Joslin;
726, Matt Meadows.